Handbook of Exercise in Diabetes

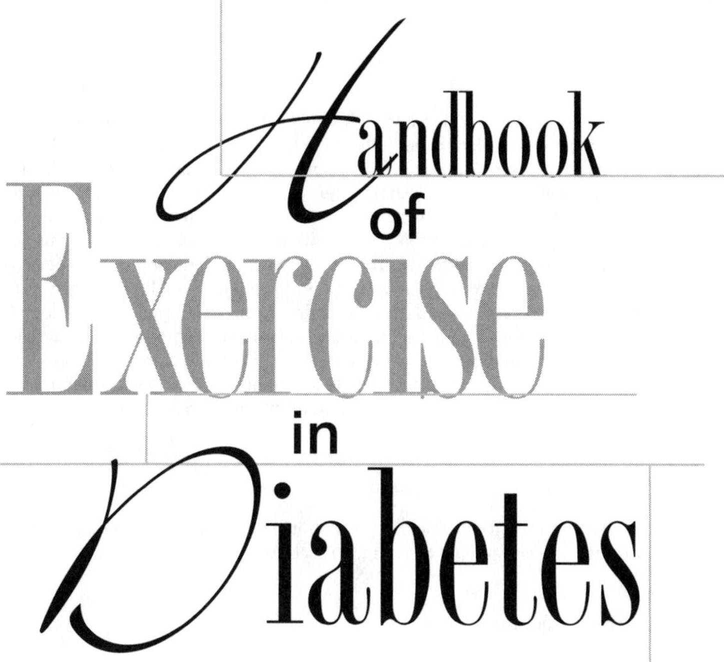

Handbook of Exercise in Diabetes

Editor-in-Chief
Neil Ruderman, MD, DPhil

Editors
John T. Devlin, MD
Stephen H. Schneider, MD

Contributing Editor
Andrea Kriska, PhD

American Diabetes Association®
Cure • Care • Commitment℠

Director, Book Publishing, John Fedor; *Associate Director, Professional Books,* Christine B. Welch; *Editor,* Joyce Raynor; *Project Manager/Editor,* Wendy M. Martin; *Production Manager,* Peggy M. Rote; *Composition,* Circle Graphics, Inc. ; *Text and Cover Design,* Bremmer & Goris; *Printer,* Transcontinental Printing.

Printed in Canada
1 3 5 7 9 10 8 6 4 2

♾ The paper in this publication meets the requirements of the ANSI Standard Z39.48-1992 (permanence of paper).

ADA titles may be purchased for business or promotional use or for special sales. For information, please write to Lee Romano Sequeira, Special Sales & Promotions, at the address below.

American Diabetes Association
1701 North Beauregard Street
Alexandria, Virginia 22311

Library of Congress Cataloging-in-Publication Data

Handbook of exercise in diabetes / Neil Ruderman, editor-in-chief ; John T. Devlin and Stephen H. Schneider, editors ; Andrea Kriska, contributing editor.—[2nd ed., rev. and expanded].

p. cm.

First ed. published under title: Health professional's guide to diabetes and exercise.
Includes bibliographical references and index.
ISBN 1-58040-019-1 (hc : alk. paper)

1. Diabetes—Exercise therapy—Handbooks, manuals, etc. I. Ruderman, Neil. II. Devlin, John T. III. Schneider, Stephen H. IV. Kriska, Andrea M. V. American Diabetes Association. VI. Health professional's guide to diabetes and exercise.

RC661.E94 H36 2001
616.4'620624—dc21

2001045789

Contents

Preface to the Second Edition

The initial edition of this book, *The Health Professional's Guide to Diabetes and Exercise*, was intended to provide a practical yet comprehensive guide to diabetes and exercise for health care professionals involved in patient care. A major hurdle in writing many of the chapters was the lack of existing literature. Thus, the many chapters dealing with exercise in people with diabetic complications and special patient groups in large part represented the distilled experience of each author. In essence, the authors (and editors) had the sometimes daunting task of creating a database and making "prudent recommendations" that ultimately would require scientific validation.

In the six years since the first edition was published, remarkable progress has been made. Key biochemical events that regulate muscle metabolism during exercise have been delineated, the approach to prescribing exercise has been significantly altered, and perhaps most important, published reports have provided strong support for the use of exercise in the treatment and prevention of type 2 diabetes and its complications. In August 2001, the preliminary results of the Diabetes Prevention Program (DPP) were nationally announced, signifying a major advancement in the area of type 2 diabetes prevention ("Diet and Exercise Dramatically Delay Type 2 Diabetes; Diabetes Medication Metformin Also Effective"; HHS News Announcement; US Dept of Health and Human Services, August 6, 2001). The DPP was a randomized clinical trial of diabetes prevention in 3,234 overweight individuals aged 25–85 years with impaired glucose tolerance, a condition that often precedes diabetes. Of the participants enrolled in the DPP, 45% were from minority groups that suffer disproportionately from type 2 diabetes, including African Americans, Hispanic Americans, Asian Americans and Pacific Islanders, and American Indians.

One of the treatment arms of this trial included diet and exercise. DPP volunteers were asked to reduce their weight by 7% through a low-fat diet and to exercise for 150 minutes per week with moderate activity similar to that of a brisk walk. This exercise goal is similar to the public health recommendations that call for an increase in moderate levels of physical activity such as walking for about 30 minutes on most days (*Physical Activity and Health: A Report of the Surgeon General*).

The exciting results of the DPP clearly demonstrated that diet and exercise can effectively delay diabetes in a diverse, multiethnic American population of overweight individuals at high risk for type 2 diabetes. The results both continued and extended those of the exercise studies reviewed elsewhere in this volume. The fact that the DPP demonstrated a substantial decrease in the development of diabetes in individuals with impaired glucose tolerance at baseline through moderate, feasible, levels of activity, diet and weight loss speaks to the importance of exercise in diabetes.

As a result of these and other findings, the second edition, *Handbook of Exercise in Diabetes*, has been significantly revised and expanded. A new section dealing with diabetes prevention has been added and contains several chapters that, among other things, provide in-depth analyses of three recent studies demonstrating the efficacy of lifestyle modification (exercise and diet) in preventing the progression of impaired glucose tolerance to overt diabetes (see chapters by Kriska and Horton, and Eriksson et al.). In addition, an emerging body of evidence suggesting that regular exercise diminishes mortality and cardiovascular disease in patients with diabetes is discussed (see chapters by Skerrett and Manson, Després et al., and Ruderman), as are the likely mechanisms responsible for these benefits (see chapters by Després et al. and Ruderman).

Another area given added attention is the treatment plan. Recommendations as to how to prescribe and maintain exercise have changed radically in the past six years, and the exercise programs now recommended are far more user-friendly and easier to prescribe. New chapters by Marrero, Kriska and Horton, Després, and Schneider and Shindler address this subject, as does the revised chapter on the exercise prescription by Gordon. Additional new chapters deal with exercise in women with gestational diabetes (Buchanan), children and adolescents (Riddell and Bar-Or), patients with disabilities (Stein), and patients using insulin pumps (Zinman). In addition, Goodyear and Horton describe the changes in cell signaling induced by exercise, and they discuss the enzyme AMP-activated protein kinase, which recent data suggest plays a key role in regulating glucose transport and lipid metabolism in exercising muscle and may contribute to many of the beneficial effects of exercise in diabetic patients.

As before, this book is intended to reflect the interests and opinions of the American Diabetes Association's Council on Exercise and the American College of Sports Medicine. The individual chapters were reviewed by the four senior editors and, in some instances, outside referees. We thank the following reviewers: Michael Berger, MD; Thomas Buchanan, MD; Robert Eberhardt, MD; Stephen Gabbe, MD; Robert Haimovici, MD; John Ivy, PhD; and Richard Nesto, MD. The editors are especially indebted to the many authors who also wrote chapters in the first edition. Without exception, they accepted the challenge of contributing to this volume, and whatever success it achieves is in no small measure due to their enthusiastic support as well as the high quality of their chapters. The editors also gratefully acknowledge the efforts of a number of individuals who have made this edition possible. At Boston University: Ruth Van Hatten, an indefatigable undergraduate student, who essentially functioned as an assistant editor and was the principal liaison between the editors, the ADA, and the authors from the planning stages of the book to near its completion; Sharon Mosher, who constantly supported Neil Ruderman and Ruth Van Hatten with her practical wisdom throughout this project; and Christina Giuliano, Angie Liu, and Deanna Chung, who provided secretarial and administrative support. At the ADA: Robert Anthony, Sherrye Landrum, and later, Christine Welch guided the book through its formative stages, and Wendy Martin both edited the final text and, together with Christine Welch, steered it through its path during the final stages before publication. Finally, we thank the many health care professionals, and patients, who made use of the first edition. Their positive response to it and their encouragement were in large part responsible for our decision to do it again. It is to them that this book is dedicated.

NEIL RUDERMAN, MD, DPhil
Editor-in-Chief

JOHN T. DEVLIN, MD, and STEPHEN H. SCHNEIDER, MD
Editors

Preface to the First Edition

The concept for this book was developed by the American Diabetes Association's Council on Exercise to fill an important niche in the diabetes and exercise literature; namely, the need for a comprehensive, yet practical, resource for health care professionals involved in the management of physical activity in patients with diabetes. We recognized early the dual loyalties of many of our members and readers in the diabetes/metabolism and sports medicine communities. Thus, this book was conceived as a joint effort with the American College of Sports Medicine, and the guidelines in it represent a consensus opinion written by the two organizations. It is our hope that this effort will lay the foundation for future cooperation between these organizations in the preparation of Position Statements, Technical Reviews, and other important publications.

Throughout the book, our aim has been to provide "hands-on" advice to health care providers in their daily clinical practices. The intended audience includes clinical and research scientists, physicians, nurses, dietitians, physical therapists, and exercise physiologists, among others. With these considerations in mind, we have included voices usually silent in diabetes and exercise manuals, namely, those of the diabetic athletes themselves. The section "Sports: Practical Advice and Experience" includes individual descriptions of therapeutic regimens used by successful, competitive athletes. Although this information may not be applicable to the general population of patients with diabetes, the insights gained from a difficult trial-and-error process, the "tricks of the trade," are a unique part of this volume.

In assembling the contents of this book, it became clear to us how far our knowledge of diabetes and exercise has advanced in the past several years and how much additional work is still needed. This seems to be especially true for such areas as the effects of exercise on the microvascular complications of diabetes, the incorporation of an exercise routine into intensive insulin treatment regimens (in increasing demand following publication of the Diabetes Control and Complications Trial results), and the effects of exercise in special patient populations, such as diabetic women. Although specific recommendations can now be made in these areas, it is equally clear that current, seemingly prudent, recommendations will need to be modified as ongoing scientific research sheds new light on these subjects.

Also included in this book are topics that are presently the focus of very active investigation. One of these is the role of exercise in the possible prevention of diabetes in high-risk groups. Ongoing large collaborative trials, such as the National Institutes of Health–sponsored multicenter Diabetes Prevention Trial-Type II, should provide valuable insights into the ability of physical exercise programs to reduce the incidence rate of diabetes. The results could have potentially far-reaching implications from a public health standpoint. Other chapters deal with topics that have received far too little attention, such as the psychological effects of exercise in patients with diabetes. Much of the previous research effort in the field of diabetes and exercise has been devoted to characterizing the metabolic benefits of increased levels of physical activity, especially in patients with type 2 diabetes. Now that the benefits have been identified, more research is needed to define techniques for motivating the desired lifestyle changes (i.e., exercise and diet) and increasing the likelihood of maintaining these healthier behaviors over the lifetime of the patient.

The editors intend this book to reflect the broad range of interests and opinions and the numerous disciplines represented by the ADA Council on Exercise and the American College of Sports Medicine. If this book serves as a catalyst for ongoing discussion and debate and stimulates new scientific endeavors by these groups, our efforts will have been well worth it.

The individual chapters were written over the past 2 years, reviewed by outside experts, and then revised by the authors and edited. The editors gratefully acknowledge these efforts and those of a number of other people who made this possible: at Boston University, Joan Judge and Maryse Roudier, who provided secretarial and administrative assistance, and Aimee Montoya and Linda Abraham, who assisted them in these tasks; at Maine Medical Center, Diane Devlin, who typed manuscripts, and Judy Barrington, who assisted with figures; at the American Diabetes Association, Christine Welch and Sherrye Landrum, who guided the book through its formative stages, Laurie Guffey, who helped with copyediting and rewriting, and Karen Ingle, who expertly edited the manuscript and shepherded it through publication. Our thanks also to Barbara Campaigne of the American College of Sports Medicine and Lois Lipsett of the American Diabetes Association, who made the interactions between the two organizations, with respect to this book and other exercise-related matters, both pleasant and productive; and to Dr. Bernie Zinman of the book's International Advisory Committee, whose services above the beyond the call of duty freed up the editors to complete the book.

NEIL RUDERMAN, MD, DPhil, and JOHN T. DEVLIN, MD
Editors

Introduction

1

Exercise Physiology and Diabetes: From Antiquity to the Age of the Exercise Sciences

MICHAEL C. RIDDELL, PhD,
NEIL RUDERMAN, MD, DPhil,
MICHAEL BERGER, MD, and
MLADEN VRANIC, MD, DSc, FRCP, FRSC

Knowledge of the body's physiological responses to exercise in individuals with diabetes has increased rapidly over the last several decades. However, even before this, the effects of physical activity on the health and well-being of patients with diabetes had been of major interest to physicians and scientists. Recommendations that physical activity should be considered as "therapeutic" for individuals with what was almost certainly diabetes had been proposed in ancient times and throughout the 19th and 20th centuries, and many reports of its potential utility had appeared. In 1979, the American Diabetes Association published the proceedings of the First International Conference on Exercise and Diabetes (held by the Kroc Foundation in Santa Ynez Valley, CA, in March 1978). This early conference was instrumental in stimulating a vast number of subsequent studies, including epidemiologic and clinical trials and molecular biological and genetic investigations, many of which are cited in the subsequent chapters in this book. The aim of this introductory chapter is to highlight some of the key discoveries made before the Kroc Symposium.

The history of exercise and diabetes has been divided into four somewhat overlapping periods for the purposes of this review: *1*) an *ancient period* including early physicians and philosophers such as Sushruta, Celsus, and Aretaeus; *2*) an *early therapeutic period* including physicians and diabetologists like Stockvis, Külz, and Allen, which essentially spans the time between 1800 and when insulin was initially used to treat diabetes; *3*) a *late therapeutic period* including diabetologists such as Banting, Joslin, and Lawrence, which extends to the present time during which insulin and oral antidiabetic agents are in use; and finally *4*) an *exercise sciences period* in which experimental studies of the physiological responses to acute exercise and physical training in individuals with type 1 and type 2 diabetes were carried out by physiologists and physicians such as Issekutz, Björntorp, and Wahren.

Ancient Period (600 B.C. to 1800 A.D.)

As early as 600 B.C., the Indian physician Sushruta recommended that physical activity, along with dietary modifications, be considered as therapy for his overweight patients with "overabundant urine" (polyuria). He also noted that there was no cure for those patients who were lean and had polyuria (presumably those with type 1 diabetes). Approximately 600 years later, the Roman physician and philosopher Celsus (30 B.C. to 50 A.D.) prescribed exercise for patients with polyuria and weakness. In the 2nd century A.D., the great Greek physician Aretaeus of Cappadokia noted that exercise may benefit these individuals with "sweet urine." Aretaeus is also known to have coined the term "diabetes," which he described as "an awkward affection melting down the flesh and limbs into the urine." Little else was reported about exercise and diabetes during the ancient period until 1798, when the English physician John Rollo published his famous study on an account of two cases of diabetes.[1] Rollo, considered an authority on diabetes at that time, recommended only mild physical activity and a diet consisting exclusively of meat to correct excessive urine production and the "peculiar odor" of the patient's breath. In addition, possibly because of his experience with more severe cases of diabetes, he clearly recommended bed rest or confinement rather than physical exertion, at least until the condition improved. As discussed later in this book (see Chapter 20), this recommendation still holds for poorly controlled patients with type 1 diabetes.

Early Therapeutic Period (1801 A.D. to 1920 A.D.)

In the 19th century, leading diabetologists such as Stockvis[2] commented on the importance of exercise for individuals with diabetes, although little evidence existed that physical activity could improve metabolic control. In an article published in 1865, the French physician Bouchardat (1806–1886) stressed the importance of moderate undernourishment and exercise in the treatment of "grape" sugar in the urine (glycosuria).[3] Incorrectly, however, he agreed with Rollo's theory that diabetes was a digestive disease that caused too much sugar in the patient's blood and urine. Bouchardat made the observation that glycosuria disappeared in some of his patients during the siege of Paris as a result of the lack of food. He also observed that exercise had some therapeutic value for some patients by increasing carbohydrate intake tolerance. Another well-known French physician, Trousseau (1801–1867), reported that exercise can cause a decrease in glycosuria in those individuals with diabetes.[4] The observational talents of Bouchardat, Trousseau, and others were impressive considering that the knowledge of metabolism in diabetes was in its infancy and there were no analytical procedures to determine glycemic control. The esteemed physician and scientist R.E. Külz (1845–1895) found in some patients a decline and in others an increase of glucosuria during exercise.[5] Based on his in-depth examinations of hundreds of patients with diabetes, he concluded that exercise is beneficial in strong patients with mild diabetes and has no effect in severe cases. Interestingly, this was noted by Külz without having any knowledge that the glucosuric response depends on the individual's initial metabolic control. von Noorden (1858–1944), a clinician from Vienna who was interested in metabolism, further developed Külz's notion in 1907 by reporting that glucosuria, under the influence of exercise, is reduced in mild cases of diabetes but increases in severe cases of the disease.[6] von Noorden also found that ketonuria was influenced by exercise and that "muscular exercise" could induce coma in those with the most marked glucosuria.[7] He also believed that the liver as well as the thyroid play an important role in the disease, which could be altered by oatmeal ingestion. Just before the discovery of insulin, the well-known American physician F.M. Allen, in a landmark publication based on his own clinical research, clearly demonstrated that exercise could be therapeutic for individuals with mild to moderate diabetes.[8]

His approval of physical exercise for patients was the first recommendation of this type that was widely accepted by diabetologists in the therapeutic age.

Late Therapeutic Period (1921 A.D. to present)

After the discovery of insulin by F. Banting and C. Best with J.B. Collip in J.J.R. MacLeod's laboratory at the University of Toronto, several key observations were made on the interaction of insulin and exercise in type 1 diabetes. For example, Hetzel and Long,[9] Lawrence,[10] and Bürger and Kramer[11] all reported that exercise caused blood glucose concentrations to fall rapidly after insulin administration. Arguably, the most dramatic of these observations was that of the British diabetologist R.D. Lawrence in 1926.[10] Having diabetes himself, Lawrence observed that exercise not only enhanced the lowering of his blood glucose levels by insulin, but also could induce severe hypoglycemia. He concluded that exercise enhanced the effect of subcutaneously injected insulin, a phenomenon that is still of major concern for today's patients with type 1 diabetes. Two years later, Bürger and Kramer[11] illustrated that a 1-h bout of strong exercise was associated with an increase in glucose concentration in untreated individuals with diabetes and a decrease in glucose levels when the individuals were insulin treated. According to these authors, the exaggerated effects of insulin during exercise are caused by increased capillary blood flow and insulin delivery to the working muscles. At that time, there was no realization that the effects of exercise might be independent of insulin and that exercise alone can increase glucose uptake in muscle.

It was these early reports of the blood glucose–lowering effect of exercise, together with his own clinical experience, that led the famous American physician E.P. Joslin to emphasize the importance of exercise in the management of diabetes.[12] His idea was that together with diet and insulin, exercise was necessary for victory over the disease. This notion was best illustrated in Joslin's patient award, called the "Victory Medal" (Fig. 1.1), which was created for individuals celebrating the "extension of life and good health with insulin" after 25 years of diabetes. The three wild horses that pull the diabetic chariot signify that an individual must master control via insulin, exercise, and diet to achieve successful management of diabetes.

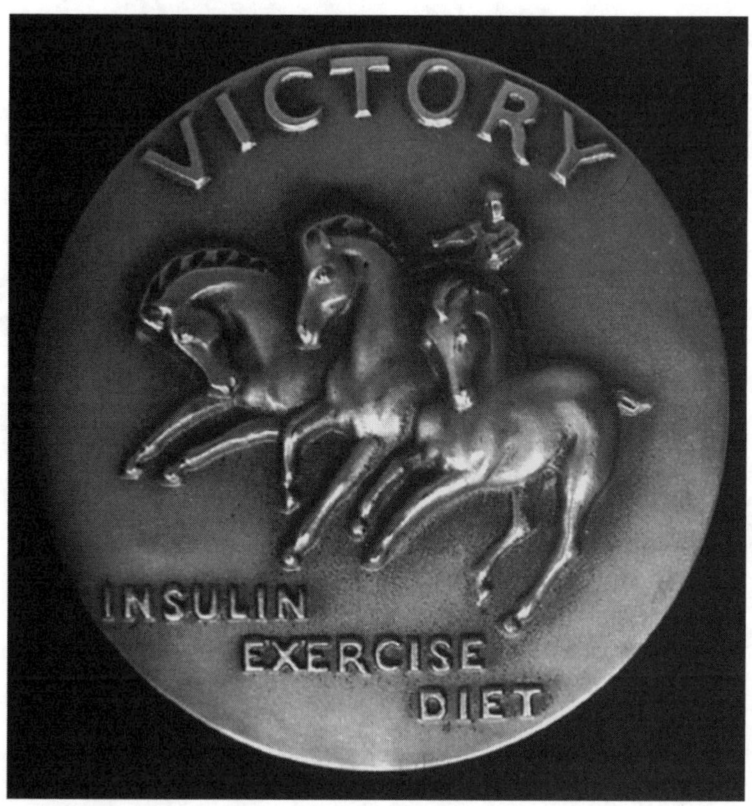

FIGURE 1.1 E.P. Joslin's "Victory" Medal.

Marble and Smith in 1936[13] may have been the first to suggest that hyperglycemia caused by heavy exercise in poorly controlled individuals with diabetes was the result of an exaggerated liver glucose output. Incorrectly, however, the authors suggested that high glucose levels were the consequence of unstable glycogen binding in the liver of diabetic patients. The true mechanisms for exaggerated glucose production and hyperglycemia during exercise would not be identified for another 4 decades (see below). In 1948, Errebo-Knudsen[14] used a number of advanced methodological techniques, such as expired gas sampling, Krogh's cycle ergometer, and blood and urine analysis, to confirm many of the previously observed responses to exercise in untreated individuals with type 1 diabetes. Several questions remained, however, concerning mechanisms of blood glucose regulation during exercise and the benefits of regular exercise on metabolic control in patients with type 1 and type 2 diabetes.

Exercise Sciences Period (1887 A.D. to present)

Although the great majority of research on the physiological and metabolic responses to both acute exercise and physical training in people with diabetes have been carried out since 1960, such studies originated in the 19th century. In 1887, Chaveau and Kaufmann[15] conducted what is generally considered to be the first experiment on the metabolic response to exercise. In their remarkable study, they measured oxygen uptake, carbon dioxide production, and glucose concentrations, as well as the flow in an artery and vein supplying blood to the facial muscles of a conscious mare. When the mare was fed hay, they observed a large increase in glucose uptake in the working muscle. This single observation was the starting point for future investigations of the regulation of glucose uptake during exercise—a topic that is now under intense investigation on a molecular level. Other early scientists, such as C. Bernard, O. Minkowski, J. von Mering, H.A. Krebs, and A. Krogh, among others, were instrumental in developing the theories suggesting that sugar could be formed in the liver of animals and secreted into the blood stream and metabolized with the aid of pancreatic secretions.

Much of what is currently known about the role of pancreatic hormones (i.e., insulin and glucagon) and diabetes in glucose homeostasis during exercise originated in studies conducted since the 1960s (many of which used animal models of diabetes). Using novel metabolic tracers for glucose and free fatty acids, B. Issekutz from Dalhousie University in Halifax, Nova Scotia, Canada, was able to quantify substrate turnover and muscle glycogenolysis in exercising depancreatized dogs.[16] This tracer methodology, also in use at the time by M. Vranic and colleagues at the University of Toronto,[17] helped to form our present understanding of the interaction among insulin, glucagon, and catecholamines in regulating hepatic glucose production and peripheral glucose utilization during exercise in both healthy and diabetic individuals (see Chapter 4). At the time, it was thought that insulin concentrations played a pivotal role in regulating glucose turnover during exercise in diabetes. Indeed, the influence of insulin concentrations on glucose production and disposal in diabetes was first demonstrated by Kawamori and Vranic in Toronto in the mid-1970s.[18] To illustrate the influence of exercise on the pharmacokinetics of subcutaneously injected insulin, this group and others also examined the effects of injected insulin on glucose homeostasis during exercise.[19–21] Such studies were the first to illustrate that the absorption of subcutaneously injected insulin was enhanced by physical exercise and that this could contribute to a relative hyperinsulinemia and hypoglycemia during and after exercise. Because of this research, it was felt by many diabetologists that altering the site of insulin injection to a non-working area would eliminate the risk of hypoglycemia. Shortly after this idea was proposed, however, F.M. Kemmer in Germany showed that this measure was often insufficient to limit hypoglycemia either during or after exercise.[22] Therefore, in the following decades, insulin and dietary strategies were developed and tested to combat what may be the most common deleterious influence of exercise—hypoglycemia. Chapter 20 deals specifically with the current recommendations based on many of these studies.

The 1970s were a flourishing period for the study of exercise metabolism and led to a renewed interest in evaluating the effects of exercise in the diabetic patient. Studies by J. Wahren and coworkers at Huddinge Hospital and the Karolinska Institute in Sweden[23] and M. Berger and colleagues in Germany[24] demonstrated that acute exercise in poorly controlled insulin-dependent diabetic patients is frequently associated with a further deterioration of metabolic control—findings that confirm the earlier observations of Külz and von Noorden. In addition, Wahren's group noted that exercise, 24 h after insulin withdrawal, increased plasma free fatty acid levels and ketogenesis and enhanced peripheral (leg) free fatty acid and ketone turnover. Thus, the metabolic responses to both insulin-treated and untreated diabetes were well known by the mid-1970s.

J. Wahren and L. Hagenfeldt at Huddinge Hospital in a collaborative effort with P. Felig at Yale University during the mid-1970s conducted pioneering studies in which arterial-venous differences across the working leg and measurement of blood flow were used to examine glucose utilization during exercise in humans. Wahren et al.[23] and, subsequently, Lyngsoe et al.[25] illustrated that net glucose uptake of the working leg in hyperglycemic, insulin-withdrawn diabetic patients was at least as great as that of control subjects. Also novel at the time was the observation that lactate production by the leg was elevated in diabetic subjects compared with control subjects, suggesting that hyperglycemia during exercise favored glucose utilization through the glycolytic pathway.

Other unique physiological and metabolic responses to exercise in patients with diabetes were described during the 1970s. For example, N.J. Christensen from the University of Copenhagen first reported that the plasma catecholamine response is greatly exaggerated during exercise in poorly controlled ketotic individuals with type 1 diabetes.[26] He also noted that this exaggerated catecholamine response was associated with an elevated heart rate, both at rest and during exercise, and that it could be attenuated with insulin treatment.

In addition to the above human studies, various animal models and experimental preparations were developed in the 1970s to examine the role of pancreatic hormones in glucose regulation during exercise.[27,28] For example, evidence that carbohydrate oxidation during exercise (muscle contraction) was dramatically reduced in severely insulin-deficient diabetes was demonstrated using an isolated rat hindlimb preparation by N. Ruderman's laboratory in Boston.[29] These investigators also noted that the activity of pyruvate dehydrogenase, a key regulatory enzyme for carbohydrate oxidation typically activated in contracting muscle, is diminished in diabetic control rats compared with nondiabetic control rats. In Toronto, Vranic's laboratory was concurrently developing the depancreatized dog model to investigate more precisely the hormonal control of substrate flux during exercise.[30] Studies with these animal models, carried out in these and other laboratories, have been key in elucidating many of the hormonal controls of metabolism and their pathophysiological alterations during exercise in individuals with diabetes.

Before 1980, the physiological adaptation to exercise training in individuals with type 1 diabetes was a focus of study for only a limited number of investigators. Initially, it was established by Costill et al.[31] and Saltin et al.[32] that the training adaptations in individuals with diabetes were qualitatively similar to those in healthy individuals.

The effect of exercise and, in particular, physical training on glucose homeostasis in what is currently classified as type 2 diabetes has only been actively investigated since the 1970s. Initially, it was observed by P. Björntorp and coworkers in Sweden that physically active men had much lower fasting plasma insulin concentrations after glucose ingestion than age- and weight-matched sedentary men. In a seminal study[33] (see Chapter 12), they compared glucose tolerance and plasma insulin levels in inactive and active nonobese middle-aged Swedish men. Several of the men in the active group had participated in physical activity since childhood and took part in the Vasaloppet, a cross-country skiing competition covering a distance of over 80 km. Glucose tolerance tests, carried out 2–5 days after a subject had last exercised, were clearly better in the athletes despite the 60–70% lower plasma insulin levels, indicating increased insulin sensitivity. Björntorp and colleagues also demonstrated in several different groups of patients, including a group of very obese individuals with glucose intolerance, that prolonged physical training is associated with a marked decrease in basal and glucose-stimulated circulating insulin levels.

The notion that exercise could be an integral component of therapy in patients with type 2 diabetes emanated from the Kroc Symposium: Exercise and Diabetes, mentioned earlier in this chapter. At this meeting, the first two articles presented, by B. Saltin and colleagues in Sweden[34] and by a group at the Joslin Research Laboratory in Boston,[35] demonstrated that regular physical activity might improve glucose tolerance in patients with type 2 diabetes. Both laboratories had started with the premise that type 2 diabetes is a disorder associated with insulin resistance and that exercise, by its ability to increase insulin sensitivity, might improve glucose tolerance in these patients. In addition, the Joslin group proposed that regular exercise might diminish the high risk for cardiovascular disease in these patients. Saltin et al.[34] investigated the influence of physical training on glucose tolerance in men with chemical diabetes (impaired glucose tolerance). They found that two weekly 60-min sessions of physical activity (calisthenics, walking, jogging, or recreational games) for periods ranging from 3 to 12 months increased maximal aerobic capacity, increased skeletal muscle glycolytic and mitochondrial enzyme activities, and improved oral glucose tolerance. Interestingly, the Joslin group, which studied patients with overt type 2 diabetes treated with diet alone, noted that the observed increase in glucose tolerance was transient. Thus, they found that 2 weeks after their patients had stopped training, a modest improvement in intravenous glucose tolerance observed 8 days earlier was totally lost. Despite this, strong arguments were made at the time that regular exercise would be beneficial for the patient with type 2 diabetes because it also was thought that exercise reduced the incidence of mortality from cardiovascular disease. However, these arguments were based primarily on studies of experimental animals and nondiabetic humans. As reviewed elsewhere in this book, evidence supporting (although not proving) this notion came later. Of historical note, within 5 years of the Kroc Symposium, the studies of the Swedish and Joslin groups were confirmed and extended. It was clearly shown that regular physical activity could improve both glucose tolerance and diminish risk factors for coronary heart disease in many patients with type 2 diabetes. Furthermore, in keeping with the premise of the original studies, the greatest improvements were observed in patients with hyperinsulinemia. In a particularly noteworthy study, J. Holloszy et al.[36] at Washington University in St. Louis, MO, were able to demonstrate that intensive physical training 5–6 days a week for a year could completely normalize glucose tolerance and correct insulin resistance in patients with mild type 2 diabetes.

Summary

The use of exercise to treat diabetes originated in ancient India, Rome, and Greece. However, modern-day interest in exercise and diabetes has principally evolved from the observations of clinicians and physiologists in the late 19th and early 20th centuries in Europe and North America. The physiological regulation of fuel utilization during exercise has been an area of intense research focus that has received considerable attention for well over a century. In the 1970s, a concentrated effort was made to elucidate the neuroendocrine control of glucose flux during exercise by using various animal models and human subjects with diabetes, and a renaissance in the investigation of exercise and diabetes occurred. These studies have had a profound effect on the ability of health care providers to deal with exercise in their patients with type 1 diabetes. For instance, they have provided the underpinning for current recommendations concerning the time and dosage of insulin administration and supplemental carbohydrate intake in relation to exercise to prevent hypoglycemia. In addition, the therapeutic benefits of exercise training for individuals with diabetes and insulin resistance have been shown by a number of well-designed studies, the first of which were initially carried out nearly 30 years ago.

References

1. Rollo J: An account of two cases of the diabetes mellitus: with remarks, as they arose during the progress of the cure. London, 1797

2. Stockvis BJ: Zur Pathologie und Therapie des Diabetes Mellitus. In *Verhandlungen des Congresses für Innere Medizin.* 1886, p. 126–159
3. Bouchardat M: De l'entrainement ou l'exercise forcé appliqué au traitement de la glucosurie. In *Annuaire de Thérapeutic de Metiére Médical Pour.* 1865, p. 291–336
4. Trousseau A: *Glucosuria: Saccharine Diabetes.* Lectures delivered at the Hotel Dieu, Paris. Vol. II, Lecture 64. Philadelphia, P. Blakiston, 1882, p. 307–31
5. Külz E: Die Erhöhung der Assimilationsgröße. In *Klinische Erfahrung über Diabetes Mellitus.* Fisher G, Ed. Jena, Germany, 1899, p. 279–85
6. von Noorden C: Abhängigkeit der Glykosurie von Muskelarbeit. In *Die Zuckerkrankheit und ihre Behandlung.* von Noorden C, Ed. Berlin, Verlag August Hirschwald, 1898, p. 77–78
7. von Noorden C: *Handbook der Pathologie des Stoffwechsels.* Berlin, 1907
8. Allen FM, Stillman E, Fitz R: Exercise. In *Total Dietary Regulation in the Treatment of Diabetes.* Monograph no. 11. New York, The Rockefeller Institute for Medical Research, 1919, p. 468–99
9. Hetzel KL, Long CNH: The metabolism of the diabetic individual during and after muscular exercise. *Proc R Soc London* 99:279–306, 1926
10. Lawrence RD: The effect of exercise on insulin action in diabetes. *BMJ* 1:648–50, 1926
11. Bürger M, Kramer KJ: Uber die durch Muskelarbeit hervorgerufene Steigerung der Insulinwirkung auf den Blutzuckergehalt beim normalen und gestörten Kohlenhydratstoffwechsel und ihre praktische und theoretische Bedeufung. *Klin Wochenschr* 7:745–50, 1928
12. Joslin EP, Root HF, White P: *The Treatment of Diabetes Mellitus.* Philadelphia, Lea & Febiger, 1959
13. Marble A, Smith RM: Exercise in diabetes mellitus. *Arch Int Med* 58:577–88, 1936
14. Errebo-Knudsen EO: *Diabetes Mellitus and Exercise.* Copenhagen, Denmark, C. Hamburgers Bogtrykkeri, 1948
15. Chaveau MA, Kaufmann M: Expériences pour la détermination du coefficient de l'activité nutritive et respiratoire des muscles in repos et en travail. *Compt Rend Ac Sciences (Paris)* 104:1126–32, 1887

16. Issekutz B Jr, Paul P, Miller HI: Metabolism in normal and pancreatectomized dogs during steady-state exercise. *Am J Physiol* 213:857–62, 1967
17. Vranic M, Wrenshall GA: Exercise, insulin and glucose turnover in dogs. *Endocrinology* 85:165–71, 1969
18. Kawamori R, Vranic M: Mechanism of exercise-induced hypoglycemia in depancreatized dogs maintained on long-acting insulin. *J Clin Invest* 59:331–37, 1977
19. Berger M, Halban PA, Assal JP, Offord RE, Vranic M, Renold AE: Pharmacokinetics of subcutaneously injected tritiated insulin: effects of exercise. *Diabetes* 28 (Suppl. 1):53–57, 1979
20. Koivisto VA, Felig P: Effects of leg exercise on insulin absorption in diabetic patients. *N Engl J Med* 298:79–83, 1978
21. Zinman B, Murray FT, Vranic M, Albisser AM, Leibel BS, McClean PA, Marliss EB: Glucoregulation during moderate exercise in insulin treated diabetics. *J Clin Endocrinol Metab* 45:641–52, 1977
22. Kemmer F, Berchtold P, Berger M, Starke A, Cuppers HJ: Exercise induced fall of blood glucose in insulin-treated diabetes unrelated to alteration of insulin mobilization. *Diabetes* 28:1131–37, 1979
23. Wahren J, Hagenfeldt L, Felig P: Splanchnic and leg exchange of glucose, amino acids, and free fatty acids during exercise in diabetes mellitus. *J Clin Invest* 55:1303–14, 1975
24. Berger M, Berchtold P, Cüppers HJ, Drost H, Kley HK, Müller WA, Wiegelmann W, Zimmermann-Telschow H, Gries FA, Krüskemper HL, Zimmermann H: Metabolic and hormonal effects of muscular exercise in juvenile type diabetics. *Diabetologia* 13:355–65, 1977
25. Lyngsoe J, Clausen JP, Trap-Jensen J, Sestoft L, Schaffalitzky de Muckadell O, Holst JJ, Nielsen SL, Rehfeld JF: Exchange of metabolites in the leg of exercising juvenile diabetic subjects. *Clin Sci Mol Med* 55:73–80, 1978
26. Christensen NJ: Abnormally high plasma catecholamines at rest and during exercise in ketotic juvenile diabetics. *Scand J Clin Lab Invest* 26:343–44, 1970
27. Berger M, Hagg SA, Ruderman NB: Glucose metabolism in perfused skeletal muscle: interaction of insulin and exercise on glucose uptake. *Biochem J* 146:231–38, 1975
28. Vranic M, Kawamori R, Wrenshall GA: The role of insulin and glucagon in regulating glucose turnover in dogs during exercise. *Med Sci Sports* 7:27–33, 1975

29. Berger M, Hagg SA, Goodman MN, Ruderman NB: Glucose metabolism in perfused skeletal muscle: effects of starvation, diabetes, fatty acids, acetoacetate, insulin and exercise on glucose uptake and disposition. *Biochem J* 158:191–202, 1976
30. Vranic M, Kawamori R, Pek S, Kovacevic N, Wrenshall G: The essentiality of insulin and the role of glucagon in regulating glucose utilization and production during strenuous exercise in dogs. *J Clin Invest* 57:245–56, 1976
31. Costill DL, Cleary P, Fink WJ, Foster C, Ivy JL, Witzmann F: Training adaptations in skeletal muscle of juvenile diabetics. *Diabetes* 28:818–22, 1979
32. Saltin B, Houston M, Nygaard E, Graham T, Wahren J: Muscle fiber characteristics in healthy man and patients with juvenile diabetes. *Diabetes* 28 (Suppl. 1):93–99, 1979
33. Björntorp P, Fahlen M, Grimby G, Gustafson A, Holm J, Renstrom P, Schersten T: Carbohydrate and lipid metabolism in middle-aged, physically well-trained men. *Metabolism* 21:1037–44, 1972
34. Saltin B, Lindgarde F, Houston M, Horlin R, Nygaard E, Gad P: Physical training and glucose tolerance in middle-aged men with chemical diabetes. *Diabetes* 28 (Suppl. 1):30–32, 1979
35. Ruderman NB, Ganda OP, Johansen K: The effect of physical training on glucose tolerance and plasma lipids in maturity-onset diabetes. *Diabetes* 28 (Suppl. 1):89–92, 1979
36. Holloszy JO, Schultz J, Kusnierkiewicz J, Hagberg JM, Ehsani AA: Effects of exercise on glucose tolerance and insulin resistance: brief review and some preliminary results. *Acta Med Scand Suppl* 711:55–65, 1986

Michael C. Riddell, PhD, is from York University, Toronto, Ontario, Canada. Neil Ruderman, MD, DPhil, is from the Boston University School of Medicine, Boston, MA. Michael Berger, MD, is from Heinrich-Heine University Düsseldorf, Düsseldorf, Germany. Mladen Vranic, MD, DSc, FRCP, FRSC, is from the University of Toronto, Ontario, Canada.

2

Diabetes and Exercise: The Risk-Benefit Profile Revisited

JOHN T. DEVLIN, MD, AND
NEIL RUDERMAN, MD, DPHIL

In the first edition of this book, titled *The Health Professional's Guide to Diabetes and Exercise,* we examined the important interrelationship between the benefits and risks of a physical training program. It was pointed out that each individual's unique characteristics (age, sex, and comorbid medical conditions, including diabetic complications, medications, psychosocial milieu, etc.) need to be carefully considered when a physician or other health care provider is formulating an exercise prescription. Thus, it is established that exercise target workloads need to be modified and carefully defined in the presence of coronary heart disease (CHD) (see Chapters 13 and 24), and the type of exercise may need to be limited in some patients with retinopathy (see Chapter 23) and neuropathy (see Chapters 22 and 27). However, given the demonstrated benefits of low to moderate–intensity exercise (including walking and household work), with its minimal associated risks, the benefits of exercise almost certainly outweigh the risks in the majority of people with diabetes. Furthermore, in diabetic patients without complications and in individuals at high risk for developing diabetes, the risk-to-benefit ratio for exercise is clearly diminished (see below). For this reason, the primary questions facing the health care provider are usually which types of exercise and how much should be recommended.

Since *The Health Professional's Guide to Diabetes and Exercise* was published in 1995, an increasing body of new research data has further demonstrated the numerous benefits of a physically active lifestyle. Thus, in patients with impaired glucose tolerance, it is now clear that progression to type 2 diabetes is substantially diminished by diet and exercise intervention (see Chapter 10). Likewise, in one of the studies in which this was demonstrated, a greater than 50% decrease in overall mortality and CHD mortality was observed after 12 years (see Chapter 12). In addition, well-designed, large cohort studies have shown significant (range ~35–55%) reductions in the risk of CHD in physically active individuals compared with sedentary individuals both in the presence (Table 2.1) and absence of diabetes (see Chapters 9 and 12). These findings have profound implications in that the risk of CHD is increased two- to threefold in men and three- to sevenfold in women with diabetes compared with nondiabetic individuals.

Other health benefits of an active lifestyle include reduced risk of hypertension, depression, and colon cancer. The Centers for Disease Control and Prevention (CDC) has estimated that 300,000 premature deaths each year can be attributed to overweight and physical inactivity, which are second only to tobacco as environmentally modifiable causes of mortality. Thus, if more people adopt an active lifestyle, the result could be a significant reduction in health care expenditures. For instance, the CDC estimates a potential savings of $29.2 billion in 1987 dollars, or $76.6 billion in 2000 dollars, if inactive Americans become

TABLE 2.1 Age-Adjusted Relative Risk of Cardiovascular Events According to Average Hours of Physical Activity per Week Over 14 Years in Women With Type 2 Diabetes

Exercise/Week (h)	Relative Risk
<1	1
1–1.9	0.93
2–3.9	0.82
4–6.9	0.54
≥7	0.52

Results are for 5,125 women in the Nurses Health Study. Of the 323 cardiovascular events, 225 were cases of CHD and 98 of stroke.[4]

physically active, based on an analysis of the 1987 National Medical Expenditures Survey data.[1]

Disturbing national trends in the U.S. were reported in the first U.S. Surgeon General's report on physical activity and health, commissioned by Donna Shalala (then Secretary of the U.S. Department of Health and Human Services) in 1994 and released during the Centennial Olympic Games in Atlanta[2] (see Chapter 8). The lay press has taken these statistics from the CDC and reported on the "diabetes epidemic" that our country is currently facing. During the 1990s, the prevalence of diabetes increased by 33%, largely because of a 58% increase in the prevalence of obesity (defined as a BMI ≥30 kg/m^2) over that time. Most alarming was the increased prevalence of diabetes in younger age-groups, including teenagers. In the 30- to 39-year-old age-group, the increase in obesity was 65% between 1991 and 1999 and was 10% between 1998 and 1999 alone. The trends are attributable to many factors, including a decreased requirement for physical labor in the workplace, a greater reliance on motorized transportation, and an increase in sedentary leisure-time activities, such as watching television, using the Internet, and playing video games.

The fact that these trends are especially strong in adolescents and young adults is of special concern because, according to the CDC, enrollment of high school students in physical education classes has declined from 42% in 1991 to 25% in 1995. In other words, the opportunity to educate the young about the benefits of a physically active lifestyle is being squandered.

As emphasized in the section titled Exercise and Diabetes Prevention (Chapters 8–12), individuals who have an increased risk of developing diabetes because of family history, obesity, ethnic background, a history of gestational diabetes, or impaired glucose tolerance (see Chapter 12 for a complete list) stand to gain the most from increases in their regular activity level. Available evidence strongly supports this contention, and it is anticipated that the U.S. multicenter Diabetes Prevention Program, which is scheduled for completion in 2002,[3] will provide definitive confirmation. In the interim, we strongly endorse the following recommendation of the Surgeon General's report: "People of all ages can improve the quality of their lives through a lifelong practice of moderate physical activity. A regular, preferably daily, regimen of at least 30–45 min of brisk walking, bicycling, or even working around the house or yard will reduce your risks."

References

1. The National Center for Chronic Disease Prevention and Health Promotion: Lower Direct Medical Costs Associated With Physical Activity. Available at http://www.cdc.gov/nccdphp/dnpa/pr-cost.htm
2. Physical Activity and Health: A Report of the Surgeon General. Available at http://www.cdc.gov/nccdphp/sgr/intro.htm
3. National Institute of Diabetes and Digestive and Kidney Diseases: Diabetes Prevention Program meets recruitment goals. Available at http://www.preventdiabetes.com
4. Hu FB, Stampfer MJ, Solomon C, Liu S, Colditz GA, Speizer FE, Willett WC, Manson JE: Physical activity and risk for cardiovascular events in diabetic women. *Ann Intern Med* 134:96–105, 2001

John T. Devlin, MD, is from the Maine Medical Center, Portland, ME. Neil Ruderman, MD, DPhil, is from the Boston University School of Medicine, Boston, MA.

Basic Considerations

3

Exercise Physiology and Adaptations to Training

JOHN L. IVY, PHD

Highlights

- Regularly performed exercise can be used for disease prevention and rehabilitation.
- A major component of a healthy lifestyle is physical fitness, and regularly performed exercise is required to remain physically fit.
- Both aerobic (with oxygen) and anaerobic (without oxygen) processes provide energy for muscle contraction during exercise.
- Skeletal muscles are composed of three basic muscle fiber types that have distinct contractile, biochemical, and morphological properties.
- A motor unit (a motor neuron and the muscle fibers it innervates) is composed of the same muscle fiber types, and its activation is exercise-intensity specific.
- The responses of the cardiovascular and pulmonary systems during exercise increase oxygen delivery to the exercising musculature.

- The cause of fatigue during exercise is determined by the type and intensity of exercise performed.
- Adaptations to exercise training follow the principles of specificity, overload, individuality, and reversibility.
- Adaptations to training optimize the physiological and metabolic systems being stressed and are specific to the systems being stressed.
- Excessive, prolonged intense exercise can result in an overtrained state in which there is an inability of the body to adapt and recover from exercise and a sudden decline in physical performance.
- Exercise training has been found to be effective in the prevention and treatment of impaired glucose tolerance and type 2 diabetes and may prove useful in their prevention.
- Improvements in glucose tolerance and type 2 diabetes appear to be manifested through physiological, biochemical, and morphological changes in insulin-regulatable tissue.

Physical activity can be defined as any form of body movement that results in an increase in metabolic demand.[1] Therefore, physical activity encompasses work-related tasks, normal daily activities, leisure-time pursuits, and recreational and competitive sports. Exercise may be considered the voluntary component of the overall physical activity performed. When a program of exercise is performed on a regular basis to achieve a goal such as improving cardiorespiratory fitness, it is referred to as physical training or exercise training. Generally, exercise training is considered in the context of athletic training, in which chronic exercise is performed to enhance athletic ability and improve physical performance. However, in actuality, most exercise training is performed for therapeutic purposes. It is used to promote physical fitness, reduce the risk of disease, rehabilitate orthopedic injuries, and strengthen muscles to prevent the recurrence of such injuries. It is also performed to rehabilitate from disease. Exercise training has been shown to reduce the risk of heart disease, lower blood pressure, slow bone mineral loss that occurs with advancing age, relieve lower back pain and stress, and be a major asset in the control of body weight. Recent evidence also suggests that regular exercise helps regulate carbohydrate metabolism and is beneficial in the treatment and management of both type 1 and type 2 diabetes.[2,3]

Physical Fitness

A major component of a healthy lifestyle is physical fitness. Physical fitness is the ability to perform the routine tasks of daily life with vigor and alertness, without undue fatigue, and to maintain sufficient energy to enjoy leisure-time pursuits and be able to respond to unforeseen emergencies.[4] Physical fitness is composed of three basic components: cardiorespiratory endurance, muscular fitness, and flexibility.

Cardiorespiratory Endurance

Cardiorespiratory endurance is the ability of the heart, lungs, and circulatory system to efficiently supply oxygen and nutrients to working muscles. One of the most valid measures of functional capacity of the cardiorespiratory system is maximum oxygen consumption ($\dot{V}O_{2max}$). $\dot{V}O_{2max}$ represents the maximum rate at which oxygen can be used by the body for energy production. As exercise intensity increases, oxygen uptake increases in direct proportion. Eventually, maximal oxygen delivery to the active muscle tissue is achieved, and oxygen uptake will plateau even with a continued increase in exercise intensity. Improvements in cardiorespiratory endurance are achieved by performing exercises that require rhythmic use of a large muscle mass. The exercises should be performed three to four times a week, a minimum of 15–20 min continuously at an intensity that elevates the heart rate and respiration but does not cause undue discomfort.[5] These types of exercises are normally referred to as aerobic exercises. Aerobic means requiring oxygen for energy production. Examples of aerobic exercises are brisk walking, jogging, cycling, swimming, rowing, aerobic dance, and cross-country skiing. Exercises of short duration that can be supported by the energy sources stored in the muscles and do not require oxygen are referred to as anaerobic exercises. Examples of anaerobic exercises are running, cycling, swimming at very fast speeds (sprinting), and weight lifting. Aerobic exercises are generally better in terms of overall health benefits and have fewer contraindications.

Muscle Fitness

Muscle fitness includes both muscle strength and muscle endurance. Muscle strength is the maximum force or tension that can be performed by a particular muscle group. Muscle contractions may be static or dynamic in nature, depending on the resistance encountered by the muscle. If the resistance is immovable, the muscle contraction is static or isometric; there is no change in the muscle length as tension develops. Dynamic contractions, in which the muscle changes length and there is visible joint movement, are concentric, eccentric, or isokinetic.[6] During concentric contraction, the force generated by the muscle is greater than the resistance, allowing the muscle to shorten and resulting in movement of the bony lever system. The muscle is also capable of exerting tension while lengthening. This is known as eccentric contraction and typically occurs when the muscles produce a braking force to decelerate rapidly moving body segments or to resist gravity, such as when lowering the body during a pull-up. It is the eccentric phase of a muscle contraction that causes muscle soreness. Sometimes the term "isotonic contraction" is used in the same context as "dynamic contraction." This is a misnomer. The word "isotonic" means same (iso) tension (tonic). However, tension produced by a muscle group fluctuates greatly when the resistance is constant throughout the range of motion of a joint (i.e., curling a barbell). This is due to the change in mechanical and physiological advantage brought about by a change in the muscle length and joint angle as the limb is moving. An isokinetic contraction is defined as a contraction in which the tension developed by the muscle while shortening or lengthening at a constant speed is maximal over the full range of motion. The speed of contraction is controlled mechanically so that the limb rotates at a set velocity. Electromechanical or hydraulic devices vary the resistance to match the muscular force produced at each point in the range of motion of a joint. Thus, the isokinetic devices allow the muscle groups to encounter variable maximum resistances throughout the movement. The isokinetic contraction is most commonly used for diagnostic tests of muscle strength and endurance and for rehabilitation of muscle groups after injury or surgery to a limb.

Muscle endurance is defined as the ability of a muscle group to exert submaximal force for extended periods. Muscle endurance can be assessed for both sustained (static) and repeated (dynamic) contractions. An exercise program of weight lifting and calisthenics is the most efficient way to improve muscle fitness.

Flexibility

Flexibility is the capacity of a joint to move smoothly through its full range of motion. Lack of flexibility is associated with musculoskeletal injury and lower back problems. Flexibility progressively decreases with aging owing to changes in the elasticity of the soft tissues of the body and a decrease in the physical activity level. Thus, flexibility exercises should be incorporated in all exercise training programs, particularly those of older people. A good time to perform these exercises is during the warm-up and cooldown phases of an exercise program. This will help prevent serious injury to the muscles and soft tissues around the muscles. When performing flexibility exercises, avoid bouncy, jerky movements. Slowly stretch the muscle until the muscle feels tight and then hold that position for 15–30 s. Repeat several times while gradually increasing the length the muscle is stretched.

Energy Systems

The energy for muscle contraction is derived directly from the breakdown of adenosine triphosphate (ATP) by the enzyme myosin ATPase. When acted on by myosin ATPase, a high-energy phosphate group (inorganic phosphate [P_i]) is split away from the ATP molecule, thereby releasing the energy necessary to drive muscle contraction (7.6 kcal/mol ATP). As the force and frequency of contraction increases, the rate of ATP breakdown increases. During muscle contraction, it is important that the ATP concentration of the muscle not decrease to any substantial degree because this would decrease the rate of free energy change and ultimately inhibit further contraction by the muscle. The free ATP concentration of the muscle, however, is quite limited and sufficient for a maximal contraction of only 2–3 s in length. To maintain the ATP concentration during contraction, the muscle relies on both anaerobic and aerobic metabolic processes. The proportion of energy provided by these processes is intensity related. The higher the intensity of the contraction, the greater the reliance on anaerobic energy production. Conversely, the lower the intensity of the contraction, the greater the reliance on aerobic energy production.

Anaerobic Energy Systems

The immediate and rapid replenishment of ATP during muscle contraction is supported by the breakdown of the high-energy phosphate compound creatine phosphate (PCr). Because both ATP and PCr are high-energy phosphate compounds, they are referred to as phosphagens, and the metabolic system in which these compounds are used for the liberation of energy for muscle contraction is referred to as the "phosphagen system." The end products of PCr hydrolysis are creatine and P_i. The energy released is immediately available and is biochemically coupled with the resynthesis of ATP, but the capacity to maintain levels of ATP from the energy derived from PCr is limited. The stores of ATP and PCr can only sustain the energy needs of the muscle during an all-out effort such as sprinting for ~8–12 s. Without this system, however, fast, powerful movements could not be performed.

A second anaerobic system in which ATP is produced within the muscle, anaerobic glycolysis, involves the breakdown of carbohydrate stored within the muscle cell (glycogen) to lactic acid. Glycolysis generates ATP when there is inadequate oxygen supplied to the muscle to meet metabolic demands. Unfortunately, this system of energy production is relatively inefficient, providing only three molecules of ATP from the anaerobic breakdown of one molecule of glucose derived from glycogen. A second limitation of this system is the production of lactic acid, which, if accumulated in high concentration, will interfere with muscle metabolism and contraction and adversely affect performance. However, anaerobic glycolysis, like the phosphagen system, is extremely important at the onset of exercise when oxygen availability is limited and during exercise of high intensity when the energy demand exceeds the energy-producing capability of the aerobic energy system.

Aerobic Energy System

For the muscles to continuously produce the force needed during long-term physical activity, they must have a steady supply of energy.

In the presence of oxygen, the muscle fiber is able to break down carbohydrates and fats, and protein if necessary, for generation of ATP. This process is referred to as aerobic metabolism or cellular respiration. As discussed, the anaerobic production of ATP is quite inefficient and inadequate for exercise lasting more than a few minutes. Consequently, aerobic metabolism is the primary method of energy production during endurance exercise.

Within each muscle fiber, there are special structures called mitochondria, which are capable of using fats and carbohydrates to produce large amounts of ATP. The reactions of the aerobic system can be divided into three main series: *1*) substrate preparation, *2*) Krebs cycle, and *3*) the electron transport chain. Substrate preparation can occur in the cytoplasm or mitochondria of the cell, depending on the substrate being used. Carbohydrates are broken down in the cytoplasm by glycolytic enzymes to form pyruvate before entry into a second series of reactions in the Krebs cycle of the mitochondria. Fatty acids are transported directly into the mitochondria by a membrane carrier and prepared to enter the Krebs cycle by a series of reactions called β-oxidation. Both reactions result in the formation of acetyl coenzyme A, which condenses with oxaloacetate to form citrate in the first reaction of the Krebs cycle. Citrate then enters a series of reactions controlled by oxidative enzymes, which result in the reformation of oxaloacetate and the liberation of CO_2 and hydrogen. The CO_2 produced diffuses into the blood and is carried to the lungs, where it is eliminated from the body. The hydrogen atom splits into a hydrogen ion (H^+) and an electron (e^-), which subsequently enters the electron transport chain of the mitochondria. Once in the electron transport chain, the e^- is transported to oxygen in a series of enzymatic reactions. At the final reaction of the electron transport chain, the e^- is reunited with the H^+ and combined with oxygen to form water. As the e^- is carried down the electron transport chain, energy is released, and ATP is resynthesized. For each pair of e^- carried down the electron transport chain, enough energy is released to produce three molecules of ATP.

The efficiency of aerobic energy production can be illustrated by comparing the ATP production from the breakdown of muscle glycogen to lactate during anaerobic glycolysis and the breakdown of muscle glycogen to CO_2 and H_2O during aerobic respiration. From one molecule of glucose derived from muscle glycogen, three molecules of ATP will be formed during anaerobic glycolysis. On the other hand, if the glucose is completely broken down to CO_2 and H_2O, 37 molecules of ATP will be formed. The obvious advantage of aerobic respiration over anaerobic processes is the efficiency with which ATP can be resynthesized. However, the rate of ATP production is limited by the availability of O_2, which must be transported from the lungs to the active muscle (Fig. 3.1).

Skeletal Muscle and Motor Units

Skeletal muscle is composed of two basic types of muscle fiber: slow-twitch (or type I fibers) and fast-twitch (or type II fibers).[7] The fast-twitch fibers can be subdivided into type IIa and type IIb. In general, the type I fibers have a high oxidative capacity and capillary density, have a relatively slow contraction and relaxation time, and are fatigue resistant. The type IIb fibers have a low oxidative capacity and capillary density, a high glycolytic capacity, a relatively fast contraction and relaxation time, and fatigue rapidly. The morphological and physiological characteristics of the type IIa fibers are intermediate to those of the type I and IIb fibers. Type IIa fibers have a high oxidative capacity and a high glycolytic capacity, a fast contraction and relaxation time, and are somewhat fatigue resistant (Fig. 3.2).

Muscle fibers of similar morphological and physiological characteristics are grouped into motor units. A motor unit is composed of a motor neuron and the muscle fibers it innervates. When a motor neuron is activated, all the muscle fibers within the motor unit will contract. However, like the three basic muscle fiber types, motor units differ with regard to speed and force of contraction, metabolic characteristics, and fatigability. Differences in contractile properties among motor units are due to differences in the motor neurons that innervate the muscle fibers as well as the contractile differences among the muscle fibers themselves.

Muscle Contraction

Muscle contraction is initiated by a neural impulse from a motor nerve. The impulse from the motor nerve causes the release of acetylcholine at the neuromuscular junction, resulting in the depolarization of the sarcolemma (plasma membrane) of the innervated muscle fibers. Depolarization spreads from the sarcolemma deep into the

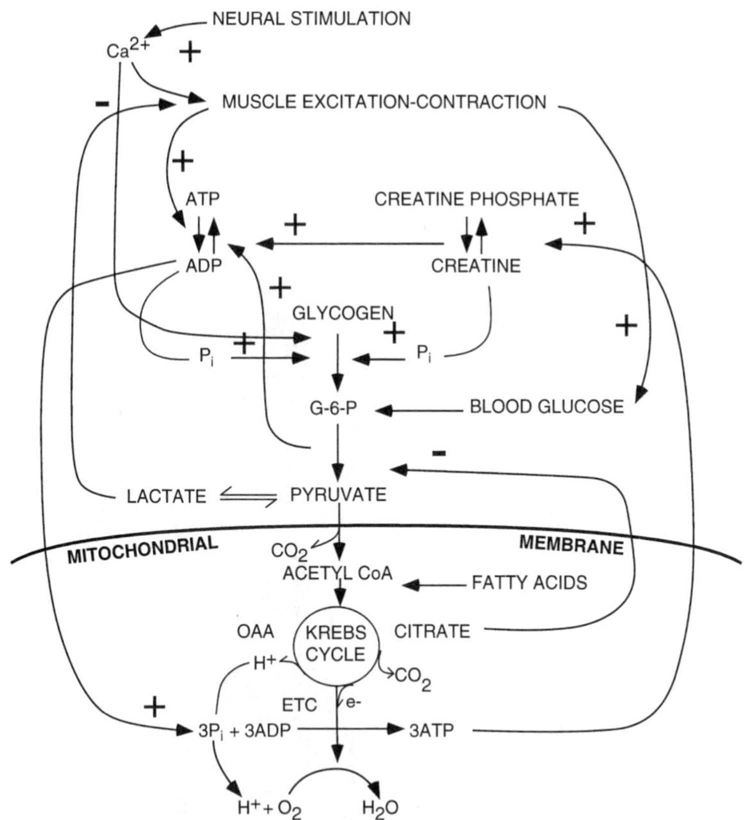

FIGURE 3.1 Energy systems responsible for replenishment of ATP to support muscle contraction. Neural stimulation results in the initiation of excitation and contraction of muscle, which in turn causes the hydrolysis of ATP to ADP and P_i. The immediate and rapid replenishment of ATP during muscle contraction is supported by the hydrolysis of PCr. A second system for rapid replenishment of ATP is glycolysis, which is activated by elevated levels of intracellular ADP and P_i. Glycolysis involves the incomplete breakdown of carbohydrates to lactate. High levels of intracellular lactate can cause muscle fatigue. Predominant sources of carbohydrate for glycolysis are muscle glycogen and blood glucose. Blood glucose uptake by muscle is stimulated by muscle contraction. The hydrolysis of PCr and glycolysis are anaerobic processes. A third source of ATP production is aerobic respiration. Aerobic respiration occurs in the mitochondria and requires the presence of oxygen (O_2). In the mitochondria, acetyl coenzyme A (acetyl CoA), produced from pyruvate or the β-oxidation of fatty acids, condenses with oxaloacetate (OAA) to form citrate. Citrate then enters a series of reactions, which result in the reformation of OAA and the liberation of carbon dioxide (CO_2) and hydrogen. The hydrogen atom is split into a proton (H^+) and electron (e^-), with the e^- entering the electron transport chain (ETC). Once in the ETC, the e^- is transported to O_2 in a series of enzymatic reactions. At the final reaction of the ETC, the e^- is reunited with the H^+ and combined with O_2 to form water. For each pair of e^- carried down the ETC, enough energy is released to produce three molecules of ATP. +, Activation of reaction; –, inhibition of reaction; G-6-P, glucose-6-phosphate.

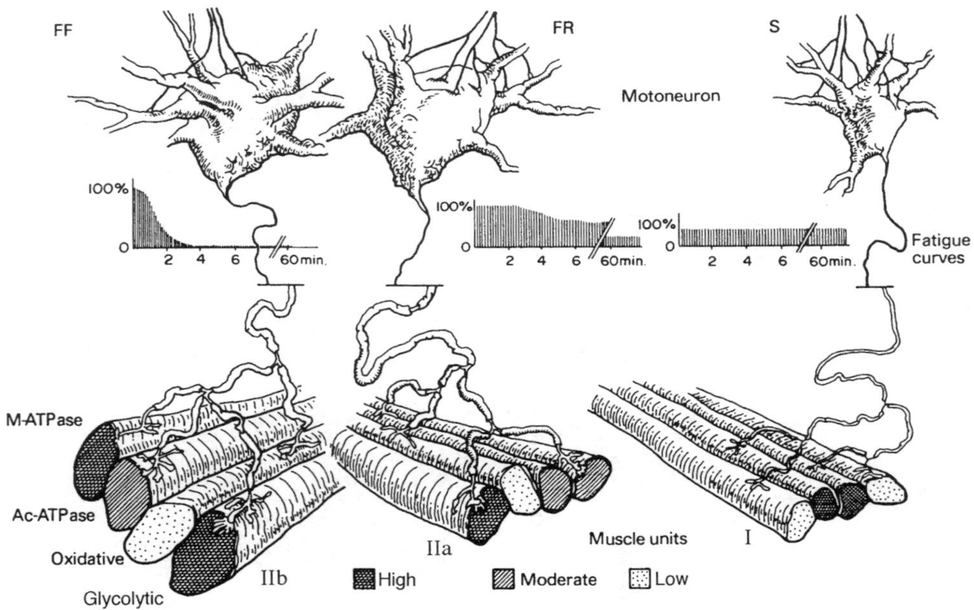

FIGURE 3.2 Three basic motor units found in human skeletal muscle. Axon diameter is directly related to conduction velocity. The muscle fibers (I, IIa, and IIb) have been stained for different biochemicals: myosin ATPase, acid ATPase, oxidative enzyme, and glycolytic enzyme. Note the differences in fatigue curves: FF, fast, fatigable; FR, fast, fatigue-resistant; S, slow, fatigue-resistant.

Modified from Edington and Edgerton.[48]

muscle fiber via the transverse tubules (T-tubules). The T-tubules connect with the sarcoplasmic reticulum, a system of channels that run in parallel with the major contractile proteins myosin and actin. At the junction where the T-tubule and sarcoplasmic reticulum meet, called the triad, calcium is stored in large quantity. Upon depolarization of this region, calcium is released into the cytoplasm where it binds with the regulatory protein troponin. This results in a conformational change in troponin and causes tropomyosin, a second regulatory protein, to shift its orientation along the actin filament, exposing myosin binding sites. With adenosine diphosphate ($ADP + P_i$) bound to myosin, myosin forms cross-bridges with actin. This causes the release of ADP and P_i and a conformational change in the myosin cross-bridge (Fig. 3.3). As the myosin cross-bridge changes position (the power stroke), it pulls the actin filament over the myosin filament, resulting in a shortening of the muscle fiber. ATP then binds to the myosin head, causing detachment of the myosin cross-bridge. ATP is then hydrolyzed by the enzyme myosin ATPase to form ADP + P_i, and the cross-bridge cycle is repeated in the presence of Ca^{2+} (Fig. 3.4).

Motor Unit Recruitment

The type, number, and frequency of motor unit recruitment[7] govern the force and speed of muscle contraction. Fiber recruitment is based on the size of the motor neuron, its threshold for activation, and its conduction velocity. Type I fiber motor units are innervated by small, low-threshold, slowly conducting motor nerves, whereas type II motor units are innervated by large, higher-threshold, fast-conducting motor nerves. In actuality, rather than discrete differences in motor neurons, there is a continuum of thresholds for activation. This allows for the systematic mobilization of motor units to accommodate the specific tension, speed, and metabolic requirements of the muscle contraction.[8] In general, type I motor units are recruited during low-intensity exercise. This is followed by activation of the more powerful, higher-threshold type II motor units as the muscle force requirements increase. When low-intensity activity is prolonged, type I motor units are initially recruited. As the exercise duration increases and the type I motor units start to fatigue, there is a progressive involvement of type II motor units, with the type IIa units being recruited before the type IIb

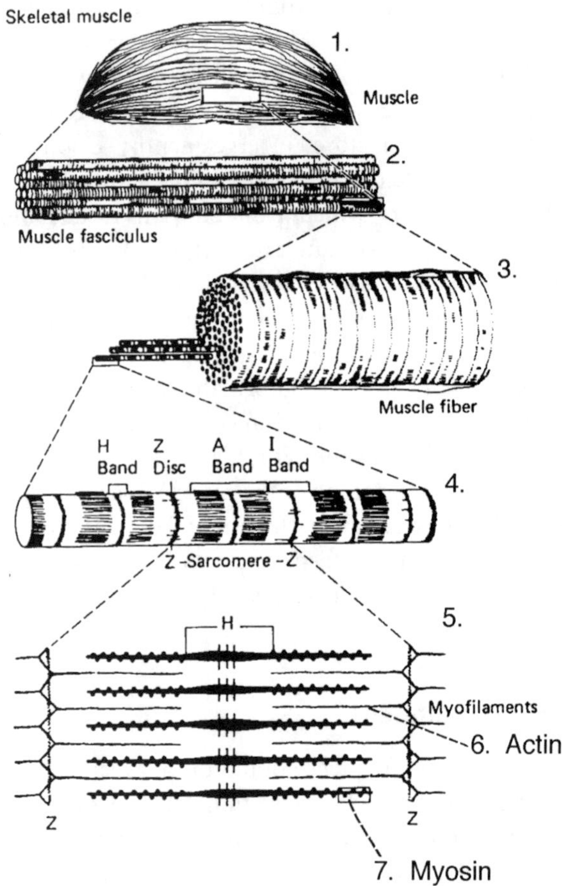

FIGURE 3.3 Organization of skeletal muscle. 1: Muscle; 2: fasciculus (muscle fiber bundles); 3: muscle fiber (muscle cell); 4: myofibril; 5: sarcomere (runs from Z-line to Z-line); 6: actin filament (attaches to Z-line); and 7: myosin filament.

Modified from Bloom and Fawcett.[49]

units. If the exercise is performed to exhaustion, practically all motor units may be recruited.

The differential control of the motor unit recruitment pattern is a major factor in determining success in various athletic activities. For example, weight lifters are capable of recruiting a high number of both type I and type II motor units in a synchronous pattern. This synchronous pattern of motor unit recruitment aids the weight lifter in

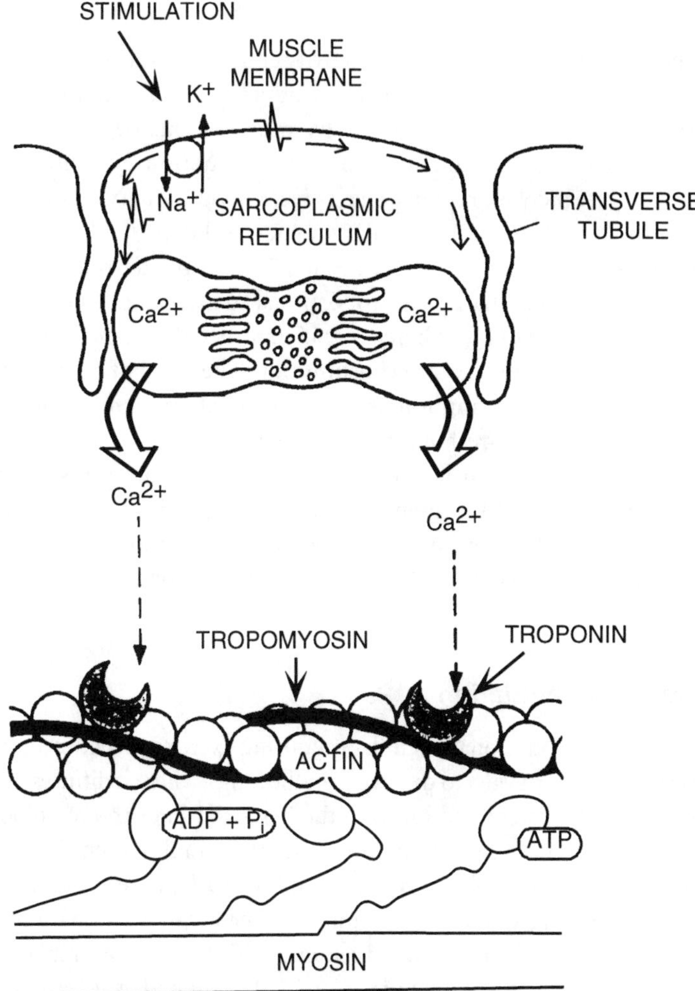

FIGURE 3.4 Excitation-contraction coupling of skeletal muscle. See text under MUSCLE CONTRACTION.

Modified from Fitts.[15]

generating high amounts of force quickly. Conversely, the endurance athlete recruits motor units asynchronously, depending heavily on the high oxidative type I and type IIa motor units. The asynchronous recruitment pattern is advantageous because it provides a recovery period for the motor units during the activity.

Cardiopulmonary Adjustments to Exercise

Along with an increase in physical activity comes an increased demand for oxygen to support aerobic energy production. This requires an increase in oxygen delivery to the active muscle tissue by the cardiopulmonary system. At the onset of exercise, pulmonary ventilation and heart rate increase rapidly. The increase in pulmonary ventilation is due to an increase in both the frequency and depth of breathing. During exercise, ventilation may be 20–25 times greater than at rest. The increase in ventilation is proportional to oxygen consumption up to ~60–70% $\dot{V}O_{2max}$. Thereafter, it becomes disproportionately greater than the rise in oxygen consumption. The point of delineation between oxygen consumption and pulmonary ventilation is referred to as the ventilatory threshold and is associated with the onset of blood lactate accumulation or lactate threshold.[9] The lactate threshold is important because it represents the maximal exercise intensity that can be sustained for a prolonged period of time. Typically, the majority of training performed by endurance athletes is at or around the lactate threshold[10] (Fig. 3.5).

Pulmonary Ventilation

The increase in pulmonary ventilation during exercise provides an increased supply of oxygen to the alveoli of the lungs, where it diffuses into the circulatory system and binds to the hemoglobin of the red blood cells. One gram of hemoglobin can transport 1.34 ml oxygen. In men, there are 15 g hemoglobin in each 100 ml blood. The value is less for women, averaging about 14 g/100 ml. The increase in pulmonary ventilation also results in an increased removal of CO_2 from the circulatory system. Generally, hemoglobin is 95–98% O_2 saturated as it leaves the lungs, even during maximal exercise. Therefore, oxygen consumption is not limited by pulmonary ventilation except in the case of lung disease or under conditions of low atmospheric pressure such as at high altitude.

Cardiac Function

Under normal conditions, cardiac output increases primarily to match the increased need for O_2 by the working muscles, and it is maximum cardiac output that determines $\dot{V}O_{2max}$. Cardiac output is the product of heart rate and stroke volume. Stroke volume is the amount of blood

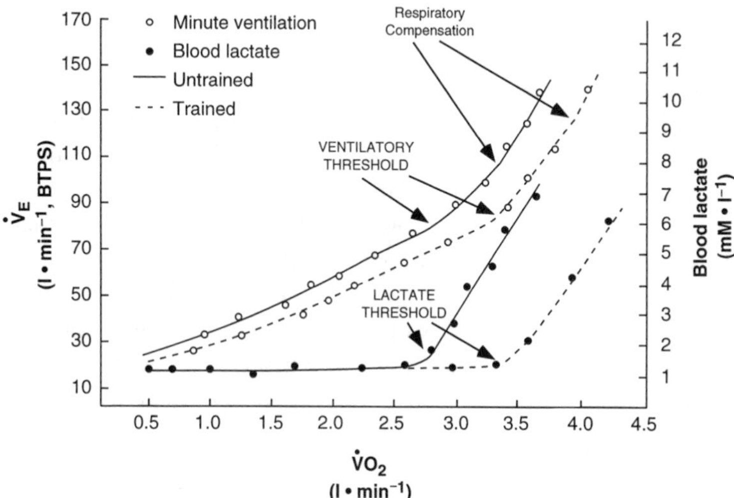

FIGURE 3.5 Pulmonary ventilation ($\dot{V}_E$) and blood lactate response to increasing workload expressed as oxygen consumption ($\dot{V}O_2$). The dashed line represents the extrapolation of the linear relationship between $\dot{V}_E$ and $\dot{V}O_2$ observed during submaximal exercise. Lactate threshold is the point at which blood lactate begins to increase above the resting value and generally corresponds with the ventilatory threshold or the point at which the relationship between ventilation and $\dot{V}O_2$ deviate from linearity. Respiratory compensation is a further increase in ventilation to counter the falling blood pH due to the rise in blood lactate.

Modified from McArdle et al.[50]

ejected from the heart per beat. At rest, cardiac output is ~5 l/min. Cardiac output increases directly with increasing exercise intensity to 20–40 l/min. The absolute value will vary with body size and aerobic conditioning.[11]

The increase in exercise heart rate is proportional to exercise intensity until near the point of exhaustion, when it begins to level off and maximum heart rate is obtained. When the rate of work is held constant at submaximal levels of exercise, heart rate increases fairly rapidly until it reaches a plateau. This is referred to as the steady-state heart rate, and it is the optimal heart rate for meeting the circulatory demands at that specific rate of work or exercise intensity. The concept of steady-state heart rate forms the basis for several physical fitness tests. Individuals in better physical condition, based on their cardiac endurance capacity, have lower steady-state heart rates at a standardized submaximal exercise intensity than individuals who are less fit.

Stroke volume also increases with an increase in physical activity. However, maximal stroke volume is thought to be reached at exercise intensities between 40 and 60% of $\dot{V}O_{2max}$. At this point, stroke volume plateaus, remaining essentially unchanged up to and including the point of exhaustion. Stroke volume is controlled by the volume of venous blood returned to the heart, ventricular capacity, ventricular contractility, and aortic artery pressure. The first two factors regulate the end diastolic volume, or the amount of blood accumulated in the ventricle during diastole. The last two factors influence the ability of the ventricle to empty, determining the force with which blood is ejected and the pressure against which it must flow in the arteries. The blood remaining in the ventricle after cardiac contraction is termed the end systolic volume. Therefore, stroke volume is equal to the end diastolic volume minus the end systolic volume.

Several mechanisms account for the increase in stroke volume during exercise, but the most important is an increase in venous return. This results in a greater left ventricular filling, placing more stretch on the ventricular wall and increasing the force of contraction. This is referred to as the Frank-Starling law. The increase in venous return is due to rapid redistribution of blood by sympathetic activation of arteries and arterioles in inactive areas of the body and a general sympathetic activation of the venous system. A second factor is the increased pumping action of the active muscles that assists in venous return. Also, there are greater differences in intra-abdominal and intrathoracic pressures because of increased breathing, which creates a more optimal flow gradient from the abdominal cavity to the thoracic cavity. An increase in stroke volume is also manifested by an increase in ventricular contractility, resulting from increased sympathetic nervous system activity. Aside from accelerating the heart rate during exercise, an increase in sympathetic activity can increase the strength of myocardial contraction two- to threefold.

Peripheral Changes

An essential response to increased physical activity is the redistribution of blood flow. This is necessary to provide sufficient oxygen to the working muscles. Blood is redirected through the action of the sympathetic nervous system and locally produced metabolites, away from areas where it is not essential, to those areas that are active during exercise. Only 15–20% of the resting cardiac output goes to muscle, but during exhaustive exercise, the muscles receive 80–85% of the cardiac output. This shift in blood flow to the muscles is accomplished primarily by reducing blood flow to the splanchnic area.

With aerobic-type exercise, systolic blood pressure increases in direct proportion to increased exercise intensity. Systolic blood pressure can exceed 200 mmHg at exhaustion. Increased systolic blood pressure results from the increased cardiac output that accompanies increasing rates of work. Its rise is necessary to drive the blood through the vasculature. Conversely, diastolic blood pressure decreases slightly or does not change during aerobic exercise. Increases in diastolic pressure of ≥15 mmHg are considered abnormal responses to aerobic exercise and are one of several indicators for immediately stopping a diagnostic exercise test.

Blood pressure responses to resistance exercise, such as weight lifting, can be quite high. Blood pressures in excess of 450/300 mmHg have been measured during intense resistance training.[12] This is partly due to an increase in intrathoracic pressure resulting from the use of the Valsalva maneuver. A Valsalva is performed when exhalation is attempted against a closed glottis.

The blood pressure response to the same absolute rate of energy expenditure is determined by the amount of muscle mass being used.[13] The greater the muscle mass involved, the lower the blood pressure; the lower the muscle mass involved, the higher the blood pressure. The use of a smaller muscle mass requires a greater percentage of available muscle fibers to be recruited at one time with a greater frequency of recruitment that results in a high intramuscular pressure. Coupled with a smaller vasculature, blood pressure must rise to overcome the high intramuscular pressure to deliver an adequate supply of blood to the active muscles.

During rest, the amount of oxygen extracted from the blood by the muscles is relatively small. At rest, arterial blood contains about 20 ml oxygen per 100 ml, whereas venous blood contains about 14 ml oxygen per 100 ml. The difference between these two values is referred to as the arterial-venous oxygen difference (a-vO_2diff). The value represents the extent to which oxygen is extracted from the blood by the tissues as it passes through the body. With increasing exercise intensity, the a-vO_2diff increases progressively. The a-vO_2diff can increase approximately threefold from rest to maximal levels of exercise. This reflects a decreasing venous oxygen content. The venous oxygen content can drop to values approaching zero in the active musculature, but the mixed venous blood in the right atrium of the heart rarely drops below 2–4 ml oxygen per 100 ml blood. This is due to the mixing of blood from the active tissues with blood from the inactive tissues as it returns to the heart.

Fatigue

Fatigue may be defined as the inability to maintain a given level of muscle force during sustained or repeated contractions. The causes of fatigue are generally exercise-intensity specific and appear to be due to either substrate depletion or metabolic by-product inhibition of muscle contractile activity. At the onset of exercise, there is a rise in the free intracellular ADP concentration of the muscle due to the hydrolysis of ATP. The rise in ADP stimulates the hydrolysis of PCr, resulting in an increase in P_i. The increase in P_i, as well as an increase in the cytosolic Ca^{2+} concentration of the muscle, signals an increase in glycogen breakdown through activation of the enzyme glycogen phosphorylase. The anaerobic metabolism of PCr and muscle glycogen as substrate for ATP resynthesis is used at the start of exercise and will continue to be used if the energy demand is higher than can be met by aerobic respiration. For the average man, the maximum rate of energy release from the phosphagens (ATP and PCr) is between 35 and 50 kcal/min. The maximum rate of energy release by anaerobic glycolysis is ~30 kcal/min. At exercise intensities lower than maximum, aerobic power (i.e., $\dot{V}O_{2max}$), the relative importance of blood glucose, and free fatty acids as substrates increase relative to the muscle PCr and glycogen stores. The lower the exercise intensity, the greater the percent contribution from aerobic respiration. The maximum rate of carbohydrate oxidation for an individual with a $\dot{V}O_{2max}$ of 35 l/min is 17 kcal/min, and for fat oxidation, it is ~10 kcal/min. From the above discussion, it can be seen that exercise of different intensities requires different energy systems and substrates.

Fatigue and Anaerobic Exercise

During exercise of maximum effort, such as sprinting, PCr utilization proceeds rapidly. The duration of this exercise intensity, however, is limited to seconds as a result of the low muscle PCr stores that cannot be replaced as rapidly as they are used. Studies of human thigh muscle and isolated muscle preparations have shown that exhaustion during repeated maximal contractions coincides with the depletion of PCr.[14]

During high-intensity exercise that lasts more than a few seconds, muscle glycogen becomes a primary source of energy for the synthesis of ATP. As with PCr use, the rate of hydrolysis of muscle glycogen is directly related to the intensity of the exercise. An increase in the rate of work results in an increase in muscle glycogen utilization. When the rate of muscle glycogen utilization is rapid, as during the mile run, lactic acid accumulates in the muscle. The accumulation of lactic acid can result in severe acidosis within the muscles and throughout the body. Such changes in pH have a negative effect on energy production and the contraction process within the muscle.[15] Substantial reductions in intracellular pH have been found to inhibit the activities of key glycolytic enzymes, thereby slowing the rate of ATP production via the glycolytic pathway. In addition, hydrogen ions will compete with calcium ions for binding to troponin, interfering with the interaction of myosin and actin and causing a decline in the contractile force of the muscle.

Fatigue and Aerobic Exercise

Under many circumstances, the cause of fatigue during aerobic exercise cannot be readily identified. However, for aerobic activities that require a substantial amount of carbohydrate for ATP production, the muscle glycogen concentration appears critical. Research has found that during aerobic activities that can be sustained from 60 to 90 min, fatigue is related to total muscle glycogen depletion or depletion within specific muscle fibers, such as the type II fibers.[16] At lower exercise intensities in which time to fatigue is ≥90 min, blood glucose can be taken up by the muscles at a rate fast enough to compensate for low muscle glycogen and meet the carbohydrate requirements for energy production. During exercises of this type, such as marathon running, fatigue appears because of a general depletion of the carbohydrate stores in the body. That is, fatigue is associated with a depletion of muscle glycogen and a low blood glucose level due to liver glycogen depletion. If carbohydrate is consumed during the exercise, the decline in blood glucose can be delayed, and exercise can be sustained for a considerably longer period of time.[17]

Exercise Training Adaptations

The adaptations to exercise training follow four principles: the principle of specificity, overload, individuality, and reversibility.[18] The principle of specificity implies that the biological adaptations to training are specific to the training program, and therefore, improvements are restricted to the energy systems, muscle groups, and other biological systems stressed during training. Skill activities are best improved when the training includes the muscle groups and simulates the movement patterns most often used during the actual execution of a particular skill.

Simply stated, the overload principle postulates that for a biological system to adapt, it must be stressed beyond its normal use. Continuous improvement, therefore, requires that the level of training increase as the system being trained improves. For example, if a continuous increase in muscle strength and hypertrophy are desired, the resistance against which the muscle works will have to be increased throughout the course of the training program. Overload can be increased by changing the intensity, duration, and/or frequency of the exercise.

The principle of individuality postulates that each individual adapts to a given training stimulus at his or her own rate. It suggests that training benefits are optimized when training programs consider the capacity for adaptability. In this manner, both over- and undertraining are prevented.

The reversibility principle states that training adaptations are transient and only maintained as long as training is continued. Once training ceases, there is a reversal of the physiological and metabolic functions associated with training. The rate of decline is system specific. For example, the declines in oxidative enzymes within skeletal muscle are detectable within days of detraining, whereas the major changes in the cardiovascular system are not detected for several weeks. Even the benefits of many years of training are transient and reversible.

Aerobic Training

After several weeks of endurance training, individuals are generally capable of exercising at higher workloads while maintaining sufficient energy production aerobically. They are capable of exercising for prolonged periods of time at exercise intensities that had previously resulted in early fatigue. They also demonstrate an increased ability to oxidize free fatty acids and to use carbohydrate stores more effectively during exercise. The adaptations that result in improved aerobic power and endurance reside both in the cardiorespiratory system and within the skeletal muscle. Aerobic power or $\dot{V}O_{2max}$ is limited by oxygen delivery to the active muscle tissue. Although aerobic exercise training stimulates adaptations in the respiratory system, it is the adaptations within the cardiovascular system that generally result in an improved aerobic power. Aerobic endurance, however, is increased primarily through biochemical and morphological adaptations in skeletal muscle.

Pulmonary Ventilation

With exercise training, there is a tendency for vital capacity to increase and residual volume to decrease, but these changes are minor and there is no significant change in total lung capacity. Pulmonary ventilation and ventilation rate, however, are lower after training when exercise is performed at the same submaximal standardized intensity. Exercise training generally results in a substantial increase in maximal pulmonary ventilation. For men, the increase can range from 120 l/min in the untrained state to 150 l/min in the trained state. Highly trained aerobic athletes may actually exceed pulmonary ventilations of 200 l/min. In addition, maximal pulmonary blood flow is increased, resulting in increased perfusion of the lungs. Along with the increase in maximal ventilation, the increased perfusion of the lungs provides a larger and more efficient surface area for gas exchange. Maximal ventilation, or the rate of gas exchange across the lungs, is not considered to be limiting for $\dot{V}O_{2max}$. Typically, hemoglobin oxygen binding is close to 100% at $\dot{V}O_{2max}$ before and after training. However, exceptions have been noted. Extremely highly trained individuals have been observed to have hemoglobin oxygen binding below 92% during maximal exercise, suggesting that $\dot{V}O_{2max}$ is limited by O_2 diffusion in the lungs.[19] These observations are rare, however, and $\dot{V}O_{2max}$ is generally considered to be limited by the cardiovascular system.

Cardiovascular Adaptations

As a result of endurance training, heart weight and volume increase. There may also be an increase in left ventricular septal and posterior wall thickness. Like skeletal muscle, cardiac muscle will undergo hypertrophy, and this hypertrophy is a normal adaptation to endurance training. The increase in chamber size allows for a greater end diastolic volume. An increase in chamber filling places a greater stretch on the cardiac muscle fibers, and this, in conjunction with an increase in ventricular wall thickness, will result in an increase in contractile force that can be generated by the heart during systole.

Resting heart rate decreases markedly as a result of endurance training. Heart rates of sedentary individuals average between 70 and 80 beats/min. Highly conditioned endurance athletes often have resting heart rates of ≤40 beats/min. After aerobic training, heart rate is reduced at the same absolute submaximal work rate. The reduction is proportional to the improvement in aerobic conditioning. Therefore, monitoring changes in submaximal exercise heart rate is a simple and easy means of monitoring improvement in aerobic conditioning.[20] The decrease in resting and submaximal exercise heart rate also indicates that the heart has become more efficient through training. That is, it requires less energy in the trained condition for the heart to do the same amount of work. Maximal heart rate shows little change with aerobic training. If it does change, it will generally decline slightly.

A major adaptation to endurance training is an increase in stroke volume. Stroke volume is increased at rest and during both submaximal and maximal exercise. In the untrained condition, resting stroke volume ranges from 55 to 75 ml and maximal stroke volume from 80 to 110 ml. After training, resting and maximal stroke volume may increase 40–60%. Exceptionally well-trained individuals have been reported to have resting stroke volumes of 100–120 ml and maximal stroke volumes of 160–220 ml.[21]

The increase in stroke volume is due in part to an increase in ventricular filling. This is a consequence of an increase in blood volume and ventricular chamber size. A longer diastole, due to a slower heart rate at rest and submaximal exercise, also contributes because this provides more time for adequate ventricular filling to occur. The net result is an increase in end diastolic volume. This increases the stretching of the ventricular walls and by the Frank-Starling law, results in an increased force of contraction during systole. An increase in rate of Ca^{2+} influx during depolarization of the myocardium as well as an increase in ventricular mass may also contribute to a more forceful contraction. Therefore, the increase in ventricular filling and force of contraction combines to increase stroke volume in the trained heart.

Resting cardiac output and cardiac output during a standardized submaximal exercise task are unchanged or slightly lower after aerobic training. With the reduction in heart rate under these conditions, cardiac output is maintained by an increase in stroke volume. Although the changes in submaximal cardiac output are minor after training, maximal cardiac output is increased significantly. This results from the increase in maximal stroke volume because maximal heart rate does not increase. Maximal cardiac output ranges from 15 to 20 l/min in untrained people, 20 to 30 l/min in trained people, and as much as 40 l/min or more in large, highly trained endurance athletes. The increase in $\dot{V}O_{2max}$ is directly related to the increase in cardiac output.

After aerobic training, muscle blood flow per gram of muscle is lower than in the untrained state during a standardized submaximal exercise task. However, recent animal research suggests that there is better redistribution of the muscle blood flow so that there is actually an increase around the most active muscle fibers.[22] That is, muscle blood flow is distributed differently among and within muscles after training so that the active high-oxidative fibers receive elevated blood flows and the inactive low-oxidative fibers received reduced flows. Blood flow to visceral tissues such as the kidney, spleen, and intestines is also increased. This is possible because of an increase in total blood volume. The increase in blood volume is due to both a greater plasma volume and red blood cell volume. The change in plasma volume, however, is greater than the change in red blood cell volume, so that the ratio of cell volume to total blood volume (hematocrit) decreases slightly.

Total muscle O_2 delivery for a standardized submaximal exercise intensity should decrease after training because of the decrease in total muscle blood flow. Since $\dot{V}O_2$ at a standardized submaximal exercise intensity is similar before and after training, the a-vO_2diff across the total musculature must be greater. The increased O_2 extraction may be related to the increase in muscle capillary density that occurs with training. This would maintain adequate capillary mean transit times in the active muscles and provide a greater capillary surface area for O_2 exchange. A redistribution of blood, as previously mentioned, and an increase in mitochondrial volume in the active muscles could also facilitate the increased O_2 extraction.

During exercise at $\dot{V}O_{2max}$, total muscle blood flow is increased after training, with little change in the amount of blood flow redirected from non-muscular organs. Thus, the increase in total cardiac output is quantitatively equal to the elevation in muscle blood flow that is due in part to an increase in total blood volume. As with submaximal exercise, it appears that the majority of increase in muscle blood flow during maximal exercise occurs in the active musculature.

With regard to the cardiovascular system, the overall effect of aerobic exercise training is to increase O_2 delivery to the active muscles. This occurs by increasing cardiac output, increasing blood flow in the active musculature, and providing better O_2 diffusion from the capillary to the muscle fiber by increasing the volume and surface area of the capillaries. Increases in maximal pulmonary ventilation and lung blood flow prevent the respiratory system from becoming rate-limiting for $\dot{V}O_{2max}$ (Fig. 3.6).

Cellular Adaptations of Skeletal Muscle

One of the major changes in skeletal muscle with exercise training is an increase in the number of capillaries around each muscle fiber. In the untrained state, the number of capillaries around type I fibers averages four per fiber, and the number around type II fibers averages about three per fiber. With aerobic training, the number of capillaries around each fiber has been seen to increase by 20–30% and parallels the increase in the oxidative capacity of the muscle.[21] The increase in capillarity allows for a greater exchange of gases, nutrients, waste products, and heat between the blood and active muscle tissue.

Another major morphological change with aerobic training is a shift in fiber type composition. In untrained individuals, type IIb fibers may compose 25–35% of the total type II fibers. After several weeks of training, there is an obvious decline in the number of low-oxidative type IIb fibers and an increase in moderate-oxidative type IIa fibers, suggesting that type IIb fibers are being converted to type IIa fibers.[23] Muscles of highly trained individuals may not show any type IIb fibers, but upon detraining for several weeks, type IIb fibers become apparent. The conversion of type II fibers to type I fibers by aerobic training has not been established. Short-term training studies have failed to identify this conversion. Cross-sectional studies, however, have found that the more successful endurance athletes have a higher percentage of type I fibers and that the percentage of type I fibers in these athletes is directly related to the number of years of training.[24] It therefore appears that if aerobic exercise training can

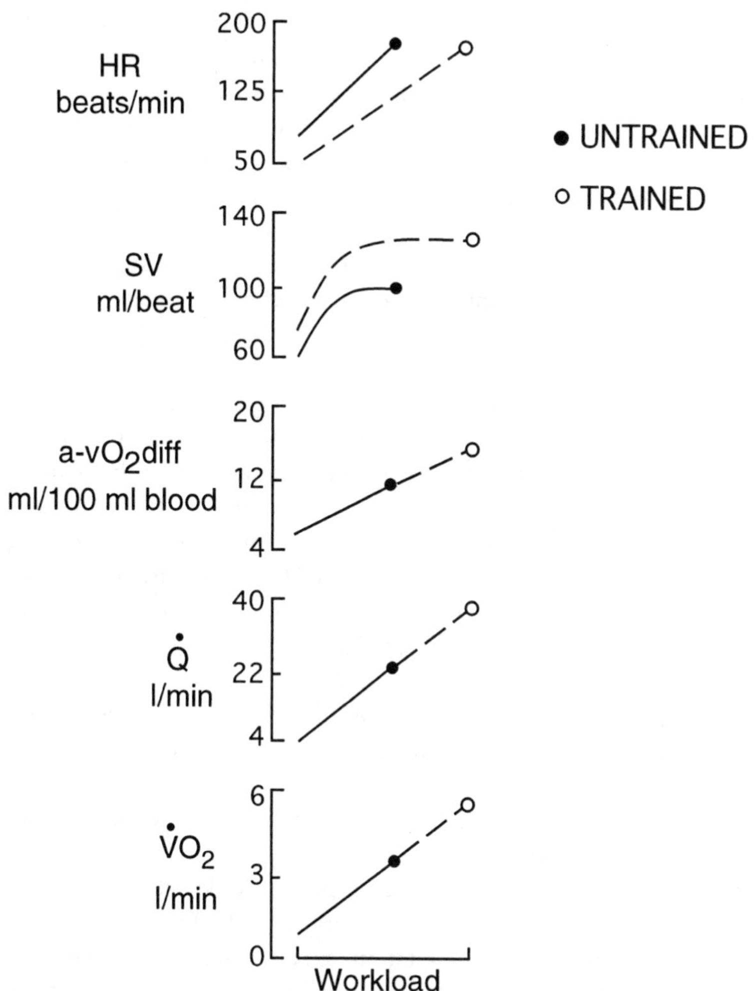

FIGURE 3.6 The effects of aerobic exercise training on the cardiovascular responses to increasing workloads to a maximum. Solid lines, submaximal responses in untrained subjects. Dashed lines, submaximal responses in trained subjects. HR, heart rate; SV, stroke volume; $\dot{Q}$, cardiac output; $\dot{V}O_2$, total-body oxygen consumption.

Modified from Rowell.[51]

cause the conversion of type II fibers to type I fibers, it occurs over many years of training.

Aerobic training has a substantial impact on the metabolic pathways of skeletal muscle.[25] The major adaptation is an increase in the size and number of mitochondria. Isolated mitochondrial preparations and muscle homogenates from trained muscle show an increased ability to oxidize pyruvate, fatty acids, and ketones. The ability for enhanced oxidation of substrate is associated with an increase in enzymes responsible for the activation, transport, and β-oxidation of long-chain fatty acids; the enzymes involved in ketone oxidation; the enzymes of the Krebs cycle; and the components of the electron transport chain. The mitochondria from trained muscle exhibit a high level of respiratory control and tightly coupled oxidative phosphorylation, indicating that these adaptations in the mitochondrial metabolic pathways are functional and are associated with an increased capacity for ATP production via oxidative phosphorylation. Other metabolic adaptations include an increase in the insulin-regulatable glucose transporter GLUT4 and an increase in hexokinase and glycogen synthase. These proteins control the rate of glucose uptake, phosphorylation, and storage, respectively. There is also an increase in the malate-aspartate shuttle, which is responsible for transferring the reducing equivalents (H_2) from cytoplasmic NADH formed during glycolysis into the mitochondria, where they enter the electron transport chain. If cytosolic NAD^+ is not replenished in this manner, then the NADH is oxidized in the cytoplasm by reducing pyruvate to form lactate. Thus, the increase in the rate of NAD^+ regeneration via the malate-aspartate shuttle is of significant importance in the control of lactate formation during exercise.

These biochemical adaptations of the skeletal muscle result in marked alterations in the metabolic response to exercise that requires a submaximal aerobic effort and are primarily responsible for the substantial improvements in aerobic endurance that follow aerobic training. The major metabolic adaptations are an increase in the workload that results in an accumulation of blood lactate, a sparing of stored carbohydrates, and an increase in fatty acid oxidation.

In the trained as opposed to the untrained state, blood lactate is lower at both the same absolute and relative (intensity based on a percentage of $\dot{V}O_{2max}$) workloads. Thus, the workload at which blood lactate starts to accumulate (the lactate threshold) is increased. A rise in blood lactate is secondary to an increase in lactate in the exercising muscles. Therefore, the increase in the lactate threshold is significant in that individuals are able to exercise at a higher relative exercise intensity for a given time period in the trained state compared with the untrained state.

Depletion of carbohydrate stores is directly associated with fatigue. Studies comparing individuals before and after training have demonstrated a reduced respiratory exchange ratio at the same relative workload. This indicates a reduced reliance on carbohydrate for fuel and an increase in fatty acid oxidation. Studies in which muscle biopsies were taken to evaluate the rate of muscle glycogen utilization during a standardized exercise bout clearly indicate that the rate of muscle glycogen utilization is slowed after training.[26] Although it has not been demonstrated directly in humans, rat studies indicate that training has a sparing effect on liver glycogen as well.[27] Thus, for the same absolute workload, the trained individual will have a slower rate of decline in both muscle and liver glycogen, which will also result in a reduced rate of decline in blood glucose. It is well documented that depletion of carbohydrate stores and the onset of hypoglycemia can be related to the development of fatigue. The increased reliance on fatty acid oxidation and the sparing of carbohydrate stores during prolonged exercise most likely play a major role in the increase in aerobic endurance after training.

Anaerobic Training

Anaerobic training can be divided into two major categories: *1*) sprint training, in which the training is of high intensity and short duration with adequate time to recover between intervals, and *2*) strength training, which requires work against a high resistance for short durations. Although they are both considered forms of anaerobic training, they result in substantially different neurological, physiological, and biochemical adaptations.[28]

Cardiovascular Adaptations

With anaerobic training such as high-resistance strength training and sprint workouts, there are few adaptations by the cardiovascular system. This is because there is little increase in venous return and therefore no volume overload on the heart. There are a few cardiovascular adaptations to strength training, however, because of the pressure overload that occurs from the increase in mean arterial blood pressure. Strength training can result in cardiac hypertrophy. The cardiac hypertrophy, however, is limited to an increase in ventricular wall thickness and not an increase in ventricular chamber size.[29] There is no change in maximal heart rate, stroke volume, cardiac output, or $\dot{V}O_{2max}$.

Neuronal Adaptations

During the first 2–3 months of strength training, the major gains in strength occur because of changes in the central and peripheral nervous systems.[30] Whether a motor unit will be activated depends on the algebraic sum of the excitatory and inhibitory impulses. Inhibitor mechanisms are in place to prevent the muscles from exerting more force than can be tolerated by the bones and connective tissues. When the tension of the tendon and internal connective tissue of a muscle becomes overly stressed, a reflex inhibition of motor neuron discharge occurs to prevent excessive motor unit recruitment. This process is referred to as autogenic inhibition, and it is activated when the tension on the tendon and connective tissue supporting the muscle exceeds a threshold level. With strength training, there is an increase in tendon, ligament, and internal connective tissue strength and a facilitation of motor unit recruitment by reducing autogenic inhibition. There also appears to be an increased coordination of motor unit recruitment and general neural trafficking that results in better synchronization of motor unit firing, which results in an increase in force development. Synchronization of motor unit firing also occurs with high-intensity training such as sprint training.

Myogenic Adaptations

After the first few months of strength training, there is generally a noticeable increase in muscle mass. This is due to hypertrophy of individual muscle fibers through increases in cytoplasmic volume, myofibrils, and filaments.[31] Muscle fiber hypertrophy is typically greatest in type II fibers. The increase in muscle mass may also be caused by hyperplasia, which is an increase in the number of muscle fibers. Although hyperplasia has not been directly demonstrated in humans, it has been demonstrated to occur in muscle of experimental animals taught to lift weights for rewards.[32] It has also been observed that the muscle fiber sizes of some body builders are the same as those of individuals of average size and muscle mass. Although strength training causes muscle hypertrophy and possibly hyperplasia, it does not appear to cause fiber type conversion.

The enzymatic changes that occur with strength training are small. There is a small increase in the activities of some glycolytic enzymes, such as phosphofructokinase, glycogen phosphorylase, and lactic dehydrogenase.[33] There may also be a decrease in aerobic enzyme activities due to a decreased mitochondrial density subsequent to an increase in myofibrils and cytoplasmic volume.

Myogenic training adaptations to high-intensity exercise are specific to the intensity and duration of the training and the energy requirements of the training.[18] Sprint training will result in elevations in ATP and PCr stores and increased anaerobic power. The activities of enzymes that catalyze the rapid replenishment of ATP and PCr, myokinase, and creatine kinase also increase. If the duration of exercise training results in high muscle and blood lactate accumulation, an increased tolerance to lactate will develop because of an increase in muscle proteins that buffer lactate. If type IIb fibers are recruited substantially, they may be converted to type IIa fibers. However, high-intensity exercise generally has little effect on muscle fiber type composition.

Overtraining

The stress of excessive, prolonged exercise training can result in a state of overtraining. Increases in psychological stress may also contribute to this condition. When the body is overtrained, there is an inability to adapt and recover from exercise, and a sudden decline in physical performance occurs. In the overtrained state, injuries and infections are more frequent, and there is a general feeling of despondency. Other characteristics associated with overtraining include a decrease in appetite, body weight loss, muscle tenderness, occasional nausea, sleep disturbance, elevated resting heart rate, and elevated blood pressure. Overtraining is not simply corrected by a few days of rest and dietary manipulation but generally requires weeks or even months of rest.

The etiology of overtraining is unknown, but one possibility is that it is associated with neuroendocrine alterations that affect the sympathetic nervous system.[34] It may also be linked to hormonal responses that control metabolism. During periods of intensified training, there are marked disturbances in endocrine function, such as an increase in the cortisol-to-testosterone ratio. This condition could effectively slow the anabolic processes of the body and inhibit recovery from exercise. Evidence of a reduced anabolic state during overtraining is an increase in blood urea levels and loss in muscle mass.[35] There is also substantial evidence that excessive training suppresses the immune system and increase susceptibility to infections. Numerous studies show that acute bouts of intense exercise temporarily impair the immune response and that successive days of intense training can augment this suppression.[36]

The early detection of overtraining has proven to be difficult because there are few consistent preliminary indicators. However, there are several possibilities that can be considered. As overtraining occurs, there appears to be a loss in neuromuscular coordination and reduced exercise efficiency. This reduced efficiency is revealed by an increase in oxygen consumption during a standardized submaximal exercise test. An abnormal resting electrocardiogram may also accompany overtraining. For example, individuals who show sudden decrements in physical performance often exhibit T-wave inversions. The most practical indicator of overtraining, however, may be changes in resting heart rate and heart rate at a standardized exercise intensity. With exercise training, heart rate at rest and during exercise declines. When overtraining becomes problematic, however, the resting and exercise heart rates start to rise above the normal trained heart rate response.

To avoid overtraining, an individual must have a good understanding of how his or her body tolerates the stresses of intense exercise and be willing to reduce the exercise load when feeling chronically fatigued and slow to recovery or when noticing signs of overtraining, such as an increase in resting heart rate. Exercise programs should have safeguards built in to avoid overtraining. These include using cyclic training procedures that vary training intensity sufficiently to allow for recovery from intense exercise sessions, the proper use of warm-up before and cool-down after exercise, and the incorporation of a competent nutritional plan.

The Role of Exercise in the Prevention and Treatment of Type 2 Diabetes

Despite years of advocating that physical activity is beneficial in the prevention of insulin resistance and type 2 diabetes, until recently, there was little scientific evidence to support this contention. In fact, the National Institutes of Health Consensus Development Conference on Diet and Exercise in Type 2 Diabetes in 1987 concluded that the impact of exercise on control of type 2 diabetes is small and ineffective. However, during the last decade, considerable evidence has accumulated from epidemiological studies, exercise training studies, and community health programs showing that increased physical activity can be an effective intervention for the prevention and treatment of insulin resistance and type 2 diabetes.

Exercise and the Prevention of Type 2 Diabetes

For individuals with normal insulin function, prolonged aerobic exercise training results in lower plasma insulin concentrations both during fasting and after glucose ingestion. Despite a markedly blunted insulin response to a glucose challenge, glucose tolerance is normal or improved, providing evidence that the effectiveness of insulin to control blood glucose is improved. Such results strongly suggest that regularly performed aerobic exercise can reduce the risk of insulin resistance and may prevent the development of impaired glucose tolerance and type 2 diabetes. This contention is strongly supported by epidemiological studies indicating that individuals who maintain a physically active lifestyle are much less likely to develop type 2 diabetes than individuals who have a sedentary lifestyle.[37,38] Furthermore, it was found that the protective effect of physical activity was strongest for individuals at highest risk for type 2 diabetes.[38] This included individuals who were overweight, had high blood pressure, and had a family history of type 2 diabetes. Reducing the risk of insulin resistance and type 2 diabetes by regularly performed exercise is also supported by several aging studies. Glucose tolerance generally deteriorates as an individual ages because of the development of insulin resistance. However, older individuals who vigorously train on a regular basis exhibit a greater glucose tolerance and lower insulin response to a glucose challenge than sedentary individuals of similar age and weight.[39] Older physically active individuals also demonstrate a similar glucose tolerance to that of young untrained individuals while maintaining a lower insulin response to an oral glucose load.

Exercise and the Treatment of Type 2 Diabetes

While the evidence is substantial that endurance exercise training can reduce the risk of glucose intolerance and type 2 diabetes, the evidence that exercise training is beneficial in the treatment of type 2 diabetes is not particularly strong. Many of the early studies investigating the effects of exercise training on type 2 diabetes could not demonstrate improvements in glucose tolerance or plasma insulin levels. The adequacy of the training programs in many of these studies, however, is questionable. More recent studies using prolonged, vigorous exercise training protocols have produced more favorable results. Holloszy et al.[40] found that 12 months of vigorous exercise training three to four times per week normalized the glucose tolerance while markedly lowering the plasma insulin response of patients classified as glucose intolerant or type 2 diabetic (Fig. 3.7). These findings are supported by Reitman et al.,[41] who reported that 6–10 weeks of intensive exercise training lowered the fasting plasma glucose level and improved the oral glucose tolerance of Pima Indians with recent-onset type 2 diabetes. Moreover, Dela et al.[42] found that exercise training significantly improved total-body insulin action and insulin-stimulated muscle glucose uptake in type 2 diabetic patients. The improvement in insulin-stimulated muscle glucose uptake was the result of increased muscle blood flow as well as an increase in glucose extraction. However, it should be considered that because exercise decreases insulin secretion to counter an improvement in insulin sensitivity, it is generally not effective as the sole treatment for type 2 diabetes in patients who have moderate to marked insulin deficiency.

Possible Mechanisms of Action

Adaptations that could contribute to an improvement in glucose intolerance and type 2 diabetes are an increase in the action of insulin on the peripheral tissues, an increased rate of liver glucose clearance, and a reduced rate of liver glucose production. Of the three, the most important is an increase in insulin action on peripheral tissue. Exercise training increases peripheral glucose clearance in the presence of insulin. This is due to both an increase in skeletal muscle blood flow and insulin action.[42] The increased skeletal muscle insulin action is associated with an increase in insulin-responsive glucose transporters (GLUT4) and enzymes that regulate the storage and oxidation of glu-

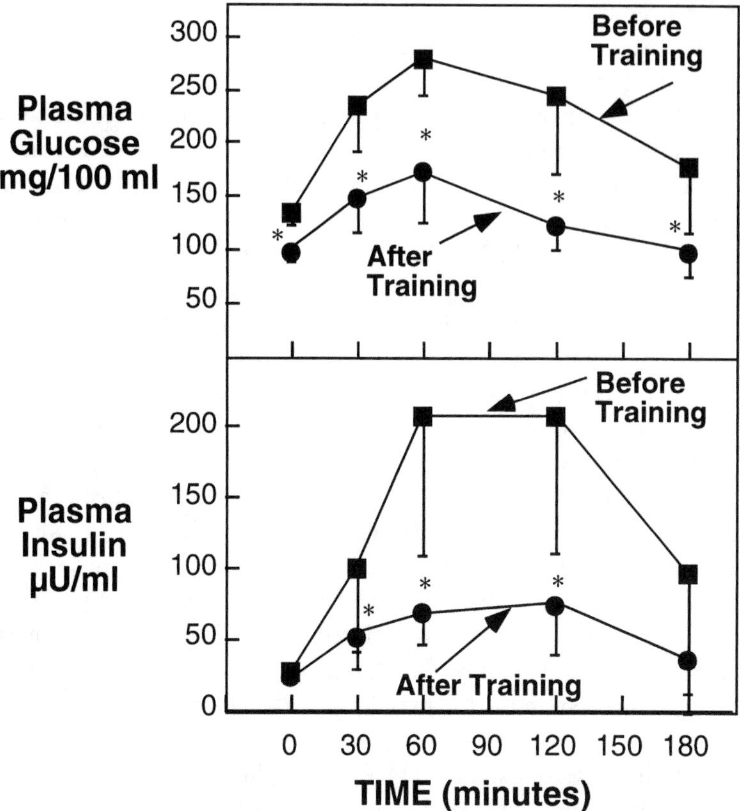

FIGURE 3.7 Values are means ± SE for five patients. Plasma glucose and insulin responses to a 100-g oral glucose load in patients with mild type 2 diabetes before and after 12 months of vigorous aerobic exercise training. The after-training glucose tolerance test was performed ~18 h after the patients' most recent bout of exercise. *Significant difference from the untrained state at the designated time.

Modified from Holloszy et al.[40]

cose in skeletal muscle. Changes in muscle morphology may also be important after training. As previously discussed, with aerobic exercise training, there is an increase in the conversion of type IIb fibers to type IIa fibers, as well as an increase in the muscle capillary density. Type IIa fibers have a greater capillary density and a higher concentration of glucose transporters, and they are more insulin responsive than type IIb fibers. Evidence has been provided that morphological changes in muscle, particularly the capillary density of the muscle, are associated with changes in fasting insulin concentrations and glucose tolerance. Furthermore, significant correlations between glucose clearance and muscle capillary density and fiber type have been found in humans during a euglycemic clamp[43] (Fig. 3.8).

Recently, an increase in intramuscular triglyceride stores has been associated with muscle insulin resistance.[44,45] This increase in intramuscular triglyceride is associated with abdominal obesity. Exercise training is effective in reducing abdominal fat stores, and as a consequence of a reduced adiposity, intramuscular triglyceride stores are reduced. Thus, another means by which exercise training may improve muscle insulin action is to reduce the fat stores of the body, particularly in the abdominal region.

An increase in muscle mass may also improve the insulin-resistant state by increasing glucose storage space. In support of this hypothesis is the finding that weight lifters have lower blood glucose and insulin responses to an oral glucose load than sedentary age-matched control subjects or endurance-trained athletes.[46] Also, Miller et al.[47] reported that the decline in the plasma insulin response to an oral glucose load following several months of weight training was significantly related to the increase in muscle mass achieved by the subjects. Such findings may be particularly pertinent to the elderly, who generally experience a large reduction in muscle mass as well as a deterioration in insulin sensitivity and glucose tolerance.

An increase in insulin-stimulated liver glucose tolerance after exercise training has not been documented. However, the liver does appear to become more sensitive to insulin, resulting in better control of liver glucose production. Exercise training may also improve control over liver glucose production by increasing insulin's control over blood free fatty acid concentration. An elevated blood free fatty acid level, which is associated with obesity and type 2 diabetes, stimulates gluconeogenesis, which, in turn, stimulates liver glucose production. An elevated blood free fatty acid level may also attenuate skeletal muscle glucose uptake and storage. Therefore, increased control over the blood free fatty acid concentration may serve to increase peripheral glucose clearance as well as reduce liver glucose production.

Summary

There is substantial evidence that exercise training can be used to prevent and treat impaired glucose tolerance and type 2 diabetes. The

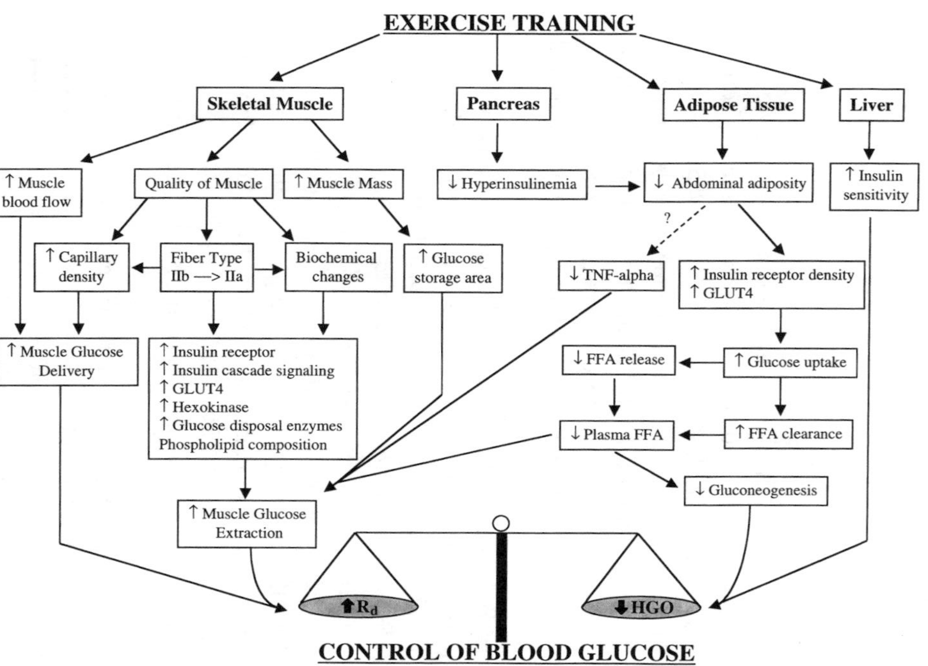

FIGURE 3.8 Mechanisms by which exercise training may improve insulin action and the control of blood glucose in glucose-intolerant and type 2 diabetic subjects. FFA, free fatty acid; HGO, hepatic glucose output; R_d, glucose uptake; TNF, tumor necrosis factor.

Modified from Ivy et al.[52]

mechanisms of action by which exercise training prevents or improves the insulin-resistant state involve alterations in body composition and biochemical, physiological, and morphological changes in skeletal muscle. Improvement in the response of the liver to insulin also may be of importance. These effects of exercise training, however, reverse rapidly if training is stopped.

References

1. Caspersen CJ, Powell KE, Christenson GM: Physical activity, exercise, and physical fitness: definitions and distinctions for health-related research. *Public Health Rep* 100:126–31, 1985
2. Kriska AM, Blair SN, Pereira MA: The potential role of physical activity in the prevention of non-insulin dependent diabetes mellitus: the epidemiological evidence. In *Exercise and Sport Sciences Reviews.* Vol. 22. Holloszy JO, Ed. Baltimore, MD, Williams and Wilkins, 1994, p. 121–43
3. Wallberg-Henriksson H: Exercise and diabetes mellitus. In *Exercise and Sport Sciences Reviews.* Vol. 20. Holloszy JO, Ed. Baltimore, MD, Williams and Wilkins, 1992, p. 339–68
4. Clarke HH: *Application of Measurement to Health and Physical Education.* Englewood Cliffs, NJ, Prentice-Hall, 1967, p. 14
5. American College of Sports Medicine: The recommended quantity and quality of exercise for developing and maintaining cardiorespiratory and muscular fitness in healthy adults (Position Statement). *Med Sci Sports Exerc* 22:265–74, 1994
6. Berger RA: *Applied Science Physiology*. Philadelphia, Lea & Febiger, 1982
7. Burke RE, Edgerton VR: Motor unit properties and selective involvement in movement. In *Exercise and Sport Sciences Reviews.* Vol. 3. Wilmore J, Krogh J, Eds. New York, Academic, 1975, p. 31–83
8. Henneman E, Mendell LM: Functional organization of motoneurone poll and its inputs. In *Handbook of Physiology*. Section 1, Vol. 2. Brooks VB, Ed. Bethesda, MD, American Physiology Society, 1981, p. 423–507
9. Ivy JL, Withers RT, VanHandel PJ, Elger DE, Costill DL: Muscle respiratory capacity and fiber type as determinants of the lactate threshold. *J Appl Physiol* 48:523–27, 1980

10. Farrell PA, Wilmore J, Coyle EF, Billing JE, Costill DL: Plasma lactate accumulation and distance running performance. *Med Sci Sports* 11:338–44, 1979
11. Åstrand PO, Cuddy TE, Saltin B, Stenberg J: Cardiac output during submaximal and maximal work. *J Appl Physiol* 19:268–74, 1964
12. MacDougall JD: Morphological changes in human skeletal muscle following strength training and immobilization. In *Human Muscle Power.* Jones NL, McCartney N, McComas AJ, Eds. Champaign, IL, Human Kinetics, 1986, p. 269–88
13. Lewis SF, Snell PG, Taylor WF, Hamra M, Granham RM, Pettinger WA, Blomqvist CG: Role of muscle mass and mode of contraction in circulatory responses to exercise. *J Appl Physiol* 58:146–51, 1985
14. Karlsson J: Lactate and phosphagen concentrations in working muscle of man. *Acta Physiol Scand Suppl* 358:1–72, 1971
15. Fitts RH: Mechanisms of muscular fatigue. In *Resource Manual for Guidelines for Exercise Testing and Prescription.* Blair SN, Painter P, Pate RR, Smith LK, Taylor CB, Eds. Philadelphia, Lea & Febiger, 1988, p. 76–82
16. Ahlborg B, Bergström J, Ekelund LG, Hultman E: Muscle glycogen and muscle electrolytes during prolonged physical exercise. *Acta Physiol Scand* 70:129–42, 1967
17. Coyle EF, Coggan AR, Hemmert MK, Ivy JL: Muscle glycogen utilization during prolonged strenuous exercise when fed carbohydrates. *J Appl Physiol* 61:165–72, 1986
18. Fox EL, Mathews DK: *The Physiological Basis of Physical Education and Athletics.* 3rd ed. New York, CBS College Publishing, 1981
19. Dempsey JA, Vidruk EH, Mitchell GS: Is the lung built for exercise? *Med Sci Sports Exerc* 18:143–55, 1986
20. Wilmore JH, Costill DH: *Training for Sport and Activity: the Physiological Basis of the Conditioning Process.* 3rd ed. Dubuque, IA, Brown, 1988
21. Saltin B, Rowell LB: Functional adaptations to physical activity and inactivity. *Fed Proc* 39:1506–13, 1980
22. Armstrong RB: Influence of exercise training on O_2 delivery to skeletal muscle. In *The Lung: Scientific Foundations.* Crystal RG, West JB, Eds. New York, Raven, 1991, p. 1517–24
23. Saltin B, Henriksson J, Nyaard E, Andersen P, Jansson E: Fiber types and metabolic potentials of skeletal muscles in sedentary man and endurance runners. In *The Marathon: Physiological,*

Medical, Epidemiological, and Psychological Studies. Ann N Y Acad Sci. Vol. 301. Milvy P, Ed. New York, 1977, p. 3–29

24. Coyle EF, Feltner ME, Kautz SA, Hamilton MT, Montain SJ, Baylor A, Abraham LD, Petrek GW: Physiological and biomechanical factors associated with elite endurance cycling performance. *Med Sci Sports Exerc* 23:93–107, 1991
25. Holloszy JO: Biochemical adaptations to exercise: aerobic metabolism. In *Exercise and Sport Sciences Reviews.* Vol. 1. Wilmore JH, Ed. New York, Academic, 1973, p. 44–71
26. Hermansen L, Hultman E, Saltin B: Muscle glycogen during prolonged severe exercise. *Acta Physiol Scand* 71:129–39, 1967
27. Fitts RH, Booth FW, Winder WW, Holloszy JO: Skeletal muscle respiratory capacity, endurance, and glycogen utilization. *Am J Physiol* 228:1029–33, 1975
28. Gollnick PD, Hermansen L: Biochemical adaptations to exercise: anaerobic metabolism. In *Exercise and Sport Sciences Reviews.* Vol. 1. Wilmore JH, Ed. New York, Academic, 1973, p. 1–43
29. Schaible TF, Scheur J: Cardiac adaptation to exercise. *Prog Cardiovasc Dis* 27:297–324, 1985
30. Sale DL: Influence of exercise and training on motor unit activation. In *Exercise and Sport Sciences Reviews.* Vol. 15. Pandolf KB, Ed. New York, MacMillan, 1987, p. 95–152
31. MacDougall JD, Tuxen D, Sale DG, Moroz JR, Sutton JR: Arterial blood pressure response to heavy resistance exercise. *J Appl Physiol* 58:785–99, 1985
32. Gonyea WJ, Sales DG, Gonyea FB, Mikesky A: Exercise induced increases in muscle fiber number. *J Appl Physiol* 55:137–41, 1986
33. Costill DL, Coyle EF, Fink WF, Lesmes GR, Witzmann FA: Adaptations in skeletal muscle following strength training. *J Appl Physiol* 46:96–99, 1979
34. Lehmann M, Foster C, Keul J: Overtraining in endurance athletes: a brief review. *Med Sci Sports Exerc* 25:854–62, 1993
35. Kuiper H, Keizer HA: Overtraining in elite athletes: review and directions for the future. *Sports Med* 6:72–92, 1988
36. Brahmi Z, Thomas JE, Park M, Park M, Dowdeswell IR: The effect of acute exercise on natural killer-cell activity of trained and sedentary human subjects. *J Clin Immunol* 5:321–28, 1985
37. Manson J, Rimm EB, Stampfer MJ, Colditz GA, Willett WC, Krolewski AS, Rosner B, Hennekens CH, Speizer FE: Physical ac-

tivity and incidence of non-insulin-dependent diabetes mellitus in women. *Lancet* 338:774–78, 1991

38. Helmrich SP, Ragland DR, Leung RW, Paffenbarger RS Jr: Physical activity and reduced occurrence of non-insulin-dependent diabetes mellitus. *N Engl J Med* 325:147–52, 1991
39. Seals DR, Hagberg JM, Allen WK, Hurley BF, Dalsky GP, Ehsani AA, Holloszy JO: Glucose tolerance in young and older athletes and sedentary men. *J Appl Physiol* 56:1521–25, 1984
40. Holloszy JO, Schultz J, Kusnierkiewic J, Hagberg JM, Ehsani AA: Effects of exercise on glucose tolerance and insulin resistance. *Acta Med Scand Suppl* 711:55–65, 1986
41. Reitman JS, Vasquez B, Dimes I, Nauglesparan M: Improvement of glucose homeostasis after exercise training in non-insulin-dependent diabetes. *Diabetes Care* 7:434–41, 1984
42. Dela F, Larsen JJ, Mikines KJ, Ploug T, Petersen LN, Galbo H: Insulin-stimulated muscle glucose clearance in patients with NIDDM: effects of one-legged physical training. *Diabetes* 44: 1010–20, 1995
43. Lillioja S, Young AA, Cutler CL, Ivy JL, Abbott WGH, Zawadzki JK, Yki-Järvinen H, Christin L, Secomb TW, Bogardus C: Skeletal muscle capillary density and fiber type are possible determinants of in vivo insulin resistance in man. *J Clin Invest* 80:415–24, 1987
44. Goodpaster BH, Thaete FL, Simoneau JA, Kelly DE: Subcutaneous abdominal fat and thigh muscle composition predict insulin sensitivity independently of visceral fat. *Diabetes* 46:1579–85, 1997
45. Pan DA, Lillioja S, Milner MR, Kriketos AD, Baur LA, Bogardus C, Storlien LH: Skeletal muscle lipid composition is related to adiposity and insulin action. *J Clin Invest* 96:2802–08, 1995
46. Cüppers HJ, Erdmann D, Schubert H, Berchtold P, Berger M: Glucose tolerance, serum insulin, serum lipids and athletes. In *Diabetes and Exercise.* Berger M, Christacopoulus P, Wahren J, Eds. Bern, Han Huber, 1982, p. 115–65
47. Miller WJ, Sherman WM, Ivy JL: Effects of strength training on glucose tolerance and post-glucose insulin response. *Med Sci Sports Exerc* 16:539–43, 1984
48. Edington DW, Edgerton VR: *The Biology of Physical Activity.* Boston, MA, Houghton Mifflin, 1976
49. Bloom W, Fawcett DW: *A Textbook of Histology.* Philadelphia, Saunders, 1975

50. McArdle WD, Katch FI, Katch VL: *Exercise Physiology, Energy, Nutrition, and Human Performance.* 3rd ed. Philadelphia, Lea & Febiger, 1991
51. Rowell LB: *Human Circulation: Regulation During Physical Stress.* New York, Oxford, 1986
52. Ivy JL, Zderic TW, Fogt DL: Prevention and treatment of non-insulin-dependent diabetes mellitus. In *Exercise and Sport Sciences Reviews.* Vol. 27. Holloszy JO, Ed. New York, Oxford University Press, 1999, p. 1–35

John L. Ivy, PhD, is from the University of Texas, Austin, TX.

4

Fuel Metabolism During Exercise in Health and Diabetes

DAVID H. WASSERMAN, PhD,
STEPHEN N. DAVIS, MD,
AND BERNARD ZINMAN, MD

Highlights

- Energy requirements of exercise require increased fuel mobilization and utilization.
- Changes in glucagon and insulin levels stimulate the release of glucose from the liver during moderate-intensity exercise.
- Catecholamines and insulin are important in the mobilization of glycogen stored in muscle and lipids stored in adipose tissue.
- High-intensity exercise results in a disproportionate increase in carbohydrate metabolism and hyperglycemia.
- Glucose uptake and oxidation by the working muscle is increased because of acceleration in the rate of insulin-independent processes.
- The exercise response in subjects with type 1 diabetes is highly variable depending on many factors, including the absorptive state, insulinization, and the type of exercise.

- Subjects with type 1 diabetes who are over-insulinized risk becoming hypoglycemic during exercise, whereas those who are under-insulinized risk undergoing a worsening of the diabetic state.
- Impaired counterregulation may contribute to the incidence of exercise-induced hypoglycemia in people with diabetes.
- Over-insulinization of type 1 diabetic subjects during exercise can result from mismatching of insulin dose with needs, accelerated insulin absorption from its subcutaneous depot, and increased insulin action.
- Deleterious effects of too little insulin in subjects with type 1 diabetes can be amplified by an accelerated counterregulatory hormone response.
- Weight loss and improved glucose tolerance resulting from regular exercise is beneficial in the treatment of type 2 diabetes.
- Nutritional state, form of insulin therapy, fitness, and presence of macrovascular/microvascular complications must be considered when prescribing exercise to the individual with diabetes.

Increased metabolic demands during exercise require an increase in fuel mobilization from sites of storage and an increase in fuel oxidation within the working muscle. The increment in fuel metabolism is controlled by a precise endocrine response. The importance of the endocrine system is apparent in individuals with type 1 diabetes because the normal endocrine response to exercise is often lost. When a person with type 1 diabetes undertakes exercise with too little circulating insulin, an excessive counterregulatory hormone response may ensue, and the already elevated blood glucose and ketone body levels can increase further. On the other hand, too much insulin can attenuate the exercise-induced increase in hepatic glucose production, and lipolysis and, as a result, hypoglycemia may ensue. Modification of insulin therapy in anticipation of exercise can be used to avoid states of under- or over-insulinization. In addition, increased carbohydrate ingestion may be used to compensate for the hypoglycemic effects of inappropriately high circulating insulin. In contrast to individuals with type 1 diabetes, individuals with type 2 diabetes treated with diet do not have the same risk of metabolic deterioration with exercise. However, the use of oral hypoglycemic agents can increase the frequency of exercise-induced hypoglycemia in this population. It is important to note that the presence of advanced diabetic complications can limit exercise in people with type 1 and type 2 diabetes. In this chapter, we describe the regulation of fuel metabolism during exercise and the means by which this regulation is affected by diabetes. For the purpose of conciseness, many older citations have been excluded, and the reader is referred to comprehensive discussions in earlier reviews.[1,2]

Physiology of Fuel Metabolism During Exercise

Individuals with type 1 diabetes must overcome obstacles in metabolic regulation during each acute bout of exercise to enjoy the benefits of regular exercise. The metabolic adaptations to moderate-intensity exercise in the nondiabetic individual are designed to meet the energy needs of the working muscle while at the same time maintaining glucose homeostasis. To understand the difficulty individuals with type 1 diabetes face and address possible approaches by which defects in fuel metabolism can be corrected, it is necessary to understand the normal means by which the regulation of fuel utilization is intended to occur. This section describes the utilization of fuels during exercise and provides an overview of the central role hormones play in regulating these processes.

The metabolic response to exercise will vary in accordance with factors such as nutritional state, age, general health, and work capacity. Variables that influence the metabolic response to exercise in the general population are summarized in Table 4.1. The precise mix of fuels used will always be a function of the exercise duration and intensity. During the transition from rest to exercise, the working muscle shifts from using mainly nonesterified fatty acids (NEFAs) to a blend of NEFAs, blood glucose, and muscle glycogen. During the initial stages of exercise, muscle glycogen is the chief source of energy. With increasing exercise duration, the contributions of circulating glucose and particularly NEFAs become of increasing importance as

TABLE 4.1 Factors That Influence the Hormonal and Metabolic Response to Acute Exercise

General population (including individuals with diabetes)

- Exercise intensity, duration, and type
- Fitness level
- Nutritional state
- Temporal relationship to meal
- Calories and content of meal
- Environmental factors

Factors specific to individuals with diabetes

- Temporal relationship to insulin or oral hypoglycemic agents
- If insulin is used, temporal relationship to last treatment, type of insulin, site of administration, or mode of delivery
- Metabolic control
- Presence of complications

muscle glycogen gradually depletes. In addition, the origin of the blood glucose shifts from hepatic glycogenolysis to the gluconeogenic pathway. The greater reliance on gluconeogenesis is facilitated by adaptations that increase the gluconeogenic precursor supply to the liver and the use of these precursors within the liver.

Fuel mobilization and utilization during exercise is governed by changes in hormone levels and sympathetic nerve activity. Generally, arterial insulin levels decrease, and arterial glucagon, cortisol, epinephrine, and norepinephrine levels increase. Usually, the magnitude of these changes is greater with increasing exercise duration and intensity. Ascribing metabolic effects to hormone action based on concentration changes in peripheral blood can, to some extent, be misleading, particularly for the pancreatic hormones and norepinephrine because their levels at the liver and synaptic cleft, respectively, will not necessarily be reflected.[1] The events that lead to the exercise-induced hormone responses remain to be fully elucidated. The endocrine response may be triggered by the stimulation of afferents from the working muscle, subtle deviations in blood glucose, and/or feed forward mechanisms originating in the hypothalamus.[1]

Regulation of Hepatic Glucose Production

Despite the increase in muscle glucose uptake, arterial glucose levels change little during moderate-intensity exercise because the sum of increments in hepatic glycogenolysis and gluconeogenesis is similar to this increase. The importance of the close tracking of glucose utilization by hepatic glucose production is illustrated by the precipitous fall in circulating glucose that would otherwise result. Glucose utilization may rise by 3 mg · kg^{-1} · min^{-1} in response to just moderate-intensity exercise. If the liver did not respond to exercise, blood glucose would decrease at a rate of ~1.5 mg/dl every minute, and overt hypoglycemia would be present in 30 min.

Studies in healthy humans[3] and dogs[1] have shown that the fall in insulin and rise in glucagon are the major determinants of glucose production during moderate-intensity exercise. The fall in insulin is necessary for the full increase in hepatic glycogenolysis, whereas the rise in glucagon is required for the full increment in both hepatic glycogenolysis and gluconeogenesis.[1] When the rise in glucagon and fall in insulin are both prevented during exercise by somatostatin infusion and these hormones are replaced to basal levels, plasma glucose levels fall by ~25–50 mg/dl over the course of an hour.[1] Although changes in glucagon and insulin are individually important, the interaction of these hormones is a component of the stimulus. The exercise-induced glucagon rise increases glucose production fourfold when insulin is allowed to fall compared with when it is maintained at basal levels. Hence, during exercise, as is the case at rest, a fall in insulin sensitizes the liver to the effects of glucagon.

In contrast to the importance of glucagon and insulin during moderate-intensity exercise, epinephrine plays only a minor role in regulating hepatic glucose production. The majority of the literature indicates that epinephrine is unimportant for the increase in hepatic glucose production, at least during moderate-intensity exercise with a duration <120 min.[1] Studies conducted in humans who were adrenalectomized for treatment of Cushing's disease or bilateral pheochromocytoma show that these patients have a normal increase in glucose production during 60 min of moderate-intensity exercise.[4] The rise in epinephrine, however, may be more important to the increase in glucose toward the latter stages of prolonged exercise (>120 min).[1] Because epinephrine stimulates glucose production during prolonged exercise when gluconeogenesis is high and coincides with the increase in arterial lactate, it can be speculated that the effect of epinephrine is to facilitate gluconeogenic precursor mobilization from peripheral sites.

Sympathetic innervation of the liver has been proposed to be important in the stimulation of hepatic glucose production during exercise. This suggestion is based on two premises.[1] First, increases in phosphorylase a activity and hepatic glycogenolysis occur with direct hepatic nerve stimulation. Second, the exercise-induced increase in glucose production is more rapid than changes in arterial glucagon, insulin, and epinephrine levels. Despite the circumstantial evidence that seems to implicate the sympathetic nerves, no role during exercise has been demonstrated. In fact, even hepatic norepinephrine spillover, an index of sympathetic activation, is not increased by moderate-intensity exercise in the dog.[5] Studies using a pharmacological blockade of the sympathetic response or adrenergic receptors have failed to demonstrate a stimulatory role of the catecholamines in control of glucose production in normal subjects.[1] The demonstration that human subjects receiving liver transplants have a normal increase in glucose production with exercise further supports the lack of the role of hepatic sympathetic innervation.[6] These human studies are consistent with findings in animal models.[1]

The role of glucocorticoids has generally been considered to be small within a single bout of exercise because the effects of these hormones generally take hours to be manifested. Nevertheless, evidence suggests that they may play a role in the increase in intrahepatic gluconeogenic efficiency during prolonged exercise. Transgenic mice carrying a gene consisting of an intact phosphoenolpyruvate carboxykinase (PEPCK) promoter (including the glucocorticoid response element) linked to a reporter gene for bovine growth hormone (bGH) exhibit nearly a fivefold increase in hepatic bGH mRNA in response to exercise.[7] However, transgenic mice with a deletion in the PEPCK gene glucocorticoid regulatory element show no change. This observation is supported by the finding that the exercise-induced increase in PEPCK mRNA is attenuated in adrenalectomized mice, and dexamethasone corrects the impairment.[7]

The response of the liver to high-intensity exercise and the regulation of this response may be different than that outlined above for exercise of lesser intensities. The main identifiable difference in glucoregulation is that the increase in hepatic glucose production no longer matches but, in fact, exceeds the rise in glucose utilization. This results in an increase in arterial glucose levels that extends into the post-exercise state. Because a single bout of high-intensity exercise can only be sustained for a short interval, it is likely that the added glucose released by the liver originates from liver glycogen. In a practical sense, activities such as basketball and soccer may consist of repeated bouts of high-intensity exertion, which, if not preceded by caloric intake and if extended for a prolonged period, may draw on glucose derived from the gluconeogenic pathway. It has been hypothesized that during high-intensity exercise, there may be a shift in the control of glucose production away from the pancreatic hormones to the catecholamines.[8] This is based on two observations. First, peripheral blood norepinephrine and epinephrine can increase by 10- to 20-fold, whereas the increase in the glucagon-to-insulin ratio in peripheral blood is considerably less.[8] Second, when high-intensity exercise is superimposed on a preexisting pancreatic clamp, hepatic glucose production increases normally even though the increase in glucagon is blunted and the fall in insulin is absent.[9] Nevertheless, all studies that have attempted to directly assess the role of catecholamines in stimulating hepatic glucose production during heavy exercise (<80% maximum O_2 uptake) have been negative.[8,10,11] Interpretation of adrenergic blocker studies in humans has been difficult because of the lack of specificity of these pharmacological agents. However, a recent dog study showed that a complete blockade of α- and β-adrenergic receptors specifically at the liver had no effect on high-intensity exercise that resulted in a twofold increase in hepatic norepinephrine spillover.[12]

Regulation of Fat Mobilization

Moderate-intensity exercise is typically associated with a 10-fold increase in fat oxidation. This is due to increased energy expenditure coupled with greater fatty acid availability. Lipolysis, as assessed by the increase in arterial glycerol concentration and by isotopic techniques, increases with the onset of moderate-intensity exercise.[13] Arterial NEFA levels, however, increase gradually. The slower time course for the rise in plasma NEFA levels reflects an increase in the clearance of this fuel by the working muscle.[13] The increase in fatty acid availability is due largely to an increase in lipolysis from adipose tissue triglycerides. In addition, the percentage of released fatty acids that are re-esterified is decreased by 50%,[13] presumably because of alterations in blood flow that facilitate the delivery of fatty acids from adipose tissue to working muscles.

The balance between factors that stimulate (β-adrenergic mechanism) hormone-sensitive lipase and those that inhibit it (primarily insulin) regulates adipose tissue lipolytic activity.[2] Circulating NEFAs are reduced during exercise by a β-adrenergic blockade due to a suppression of lipolysis. The exercise-induced increase in NEFA levels is retained in the absence of the normal epinephrine response to exercise, suggesting that norepinephrine released from sympathetic nerves is an important stimulus.[2] The mechanism by which catecholamines stimulate lipolysis is related not only to an increase in sympathetic nerve activity, but also to an increased efficacy of β-adrenergic stimulation.[14] Adipocytes taken from human subjects after exercise have an increased lipolytic responsiveness to catecholamines, which is mediated through a β-adrenergic mechanism.[14] This effect occurs without an increase in catecholamine binding to the β-adrenergic receptor, suggesting that the effects of exercise are on a step distal to ligand binding. Prevention of the exercise-induced fall in insulin with an exogenous infusion of the hormone also attenuates the increase in arterial NEFA levels.[2] Because this is accompanied by a diminished increase in circulating glycerol levels, it is likely that the fall in insulin increases NEFA levels, at least in part, by stimulating lipolysis. Nevertheless, the possibility of a decrease in re-esterification resulting from the exercise-induced fall in insulin cannot be excluded.

In contrast to the importance of NEFA mobilization from adipose tissue during moderate-intensity exercise, its role during high-intensity exercise is considerably less. Despite the increased adrenergic drive that is present during high-intensity work, the arterial NEFA levels in plasma decrease. A diminished lipolytic response and increased rate of re-esterification both could lead to a decrease in NEFA availability. Stimulation of adipocyte α_2-adrenergic receptors is negatively coupled with adenylate cyclase and decreases lipolysis. The decrease in NEFA mobilization during high-intensity exercise may be due to stimulation of α_2-adrenergic receptors by the high epinephrine concentrations that occur under these conditions.[15] Increased re-esterification of NEFA due to excessive lactate levels during high-intensity exercise has been proposed as a possible reason for the decrease in NEFA availability. This is consistent with the observation that blood glycerol levels may still rise during heavy exercise, even when NEFAs are not increased. It is also possible that the increased blood glycerol levels are due to release from triglycerides within the working muscle, and the

NEFAs that are liberated in the process are oxidized locally within the muscle.

With regard to the possible role of intramuscular triglyceride stores during exercise, there is a large body of evidence that suggests these stores may represent an important metabolic substrate.[16] Estimates of the oxidation of intramuscular fat stores calculated indirectly using whole-body isotopic methods suggest that intramuscular fats provide >50% of the total fat oxidized during exercise[17] and muscle contraction.[18] This issue is still far from resolved because results obtained using muscle biopsies or arteriovenous differences generally cannot account for such a large contribution of muscle fat stores during exercise.[19]

Ketogenesis is increased with prolonged exercise because of elevated mobilization of NEFAs from adipose tissue and delivery to the liver, the extraction of NEFAs by the liver, and the conversion of NEFAs to ketone bodies within the liver.[20] The rate that the liver releases ketone bodies is unimportant when considering ketone bodies as a direct fuel for the working muscle in healthy humans. The significance of hepatic ketogenesis rests with the fact that it is a reflection of the energy state of the liver. It is a marker of fat oxidation—a key pathway in providing energy to fuel gluconeogenesis. Acute and chronic circumstances requiring accelerated gluconeogenic rates are characterized by high ketogenic rates. It has been shown that inhibiting fat oxidation pharmacologically reduces the exercise-induced increase in glucose production in depancreatized dogs, which are heavily reliant on gluconeogenesis.[21]

Few studies have assessed the role of potential hormonal and neural effectors in the control of ketogenesis during exercise. Any hormone or neurotransmitter that regulates hepatic NEFA delivery, hepatic NEFA extraction, or intrahepatic fat oxidation may play a role. Of these, hepatic NEFA delivery and ketone body output are particularly well correlated during rest and exercise.[2] Therefore, factors that stimulate NEFA mobilization, such as a fall in insulin or the β-adrenergic effects of the catecholamines, may stimulate ketogenesis. The exercise-induced rise in glucagon stimulates fat oxidation in the liver and is necessary for the full increase in ketogenesis observed during exercise.[2] This stimulatory effect of glucagon occurs even though hepatic NEFA uptake is unaffected, indicating that glucagon stimulates ketogenic processes with the liver.

Regulation of Muscle Glycogenolysis

Muscle glycogen is an important local fuel during the early stages of exercise. As exercise duration progresses, glycogen stores decline in working muscle. With prolonged exercise, glycogenolysis is also stimulated in inactive muscle fibers. In these muscles, glycogen is metabolized to lactate and then released from the muscle and delivered to the liver, where it is used in the gluconeogenic pathway. Increasing work intensities accelerate the rate of glycogen breakdown in contracting muscle. Glycogen breakdown is regulated by the rate-limiting enzyme glycogen phosphorylase. Phosphorylase is phosphorylated by phosphorylase kinase, creating the active form of the enzyme, phosphorylase a. The enzyme is dephosphorylated to its inactive form, phosphorylase b, by phosphorylase phosphatase. Studies using a β-adrenergic blockade indicate that the catecholamines play a major role in the mobilization of muscle glycogen during exercise.[22] Studies in the isolated hindlimb indicate that in addition to epinephrine, contraction per se can stimulate muscle glycogenolysis, even in the absence of catecholamines.[23] Intracellular cAMP levels mediate the activation of phosphorylase a and the stimulation of muscle glycogenolysis by catecholamines. It appears that contraction causes the events by the release of calcium from the muscle sarcoplasmic reticulum.

Regulation of Muscle Glucose Uptake

In contrast to muscle NEFA utilization, which is determined primarily by the availability of NEFAs, muscle glucose uptake is closely regulated by hormonal and non-hormonal mechanisms. Kinetic analyses of glucose uptake, conducted in vivo[24] and in vitro,[25] generally indicate that the maximal velocity (V_{max}) for this process is increased by exercise without affecting the Michaelis-Menton constant (K_m). The K_m for glucose oxidation by the working limb is the same as that for glucose uptake, implying that both processes are controlled at the same step.[24] Prior exercise increases GLUT4 in plasma membranes prepared from skeletal muscle, reflecting an increase in translocation.[26] GLUT4 recruited by muscle contraction is derived from a pool that is distinct from the GLUT4 source deployed by insulin stimulation.[27]

The exercise-stimulated increases in GLUT4 translocation to the sarcolemma and muscle blood flow result in increases in muscle glucose permeability and delivery. Whereas exercise leads to an increase in hexokinase II expression, the enzyme that catalyzes glucose phosphorylation, it does not appear to be adequate to accommodate the increase in glucose flux into the muscle cell caused by the increased rates of glucose delivery and transport.[28–30] The consequence is a greater role for glucose phosphorylation in the control of muscle glucose uptake during exercise.[31,32]

An increase in glucose utilization and a seemingly paradoxical fall in circulating insulin levels characterize exercise. Therefore, exercise must stimulate insulin-independent glucose uptake, increase insulin action, or both. Exercise does, in fact, appear to stimulate both insulin-independent glucose uptake and insulin action. Muscle contraction stimulates muscle glucose uptake in vitro in the absence of insulin.[33] Studies conducted in vivo are somewhat less clear because different model systems give different estimates of insulin-dependent and -independent mechanisms.[1] In the insulin-deficient depancreatized dog, a model of poorly controlled diabetes, the exercise-induced increment in glucose metabolic clearance rate is small, indicating that insulin-independent mechanisms are minimal. In contrast, in a model system characterized by insulin deficiency but largely normal circulating NEFA and glucose levels (acute somatostatin-induced insulinopenia), the exercise-induced increase in glucose uptake and oxidation occurs primarily by insulin-independent processes. Finally, indirect estimates obtained by using multiple insulin clamps indicate that the glucose uptake and carbohydrate oxidation responses are insulin independent. Taken together, it seems that in a physiological setting, the increase in glucose metabolism can occur to a large extent via insulin-independent processes. Under conditions characterized by the metabolic abnormalities present in diabetes (e.g., elevated NEFA levels), factors antagonistic to glucose uptake are present. Insulin becomes essential to glucose uptake during exercise in the insulin-deficient diabetic state to overcome this antagonism.[1]

In addition to activation of insulin-independent mechanisms for muscle glucose uptake, exercise is well known to increase muscle sensitivity to insulin (Fig. 4.1). The mechanism(s) by which exercise enhances insulin action may include the following: *1*) an increased blood flow to the working muscle, *2*) increased transendothelial insulin transport, *3*) indirect effects mediated by the insulin-induced suppression of NEFA levels, *4*) potentiation by adenosine, and *5*) an undefined insulin receptor or post–insulin receptor modification.

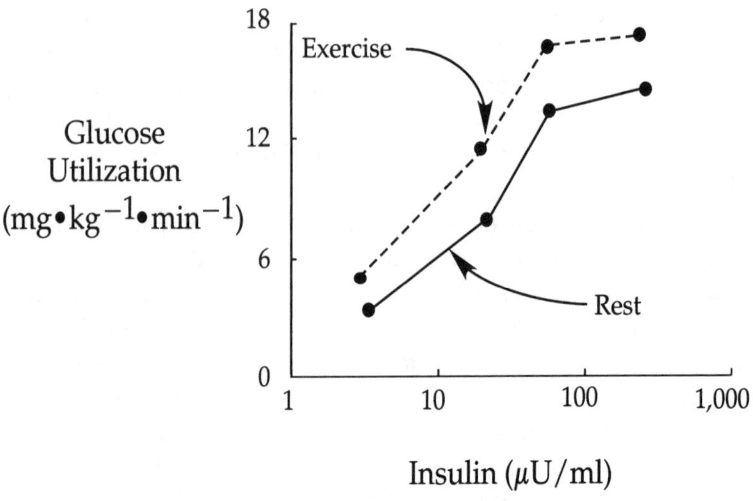

FIGURE 4.1 Exercise increases an individual's sensitivity to insulin. Data were obtained from hyperinsulinemic-euglycemic insulin clamps conducted during rest and exercise in healthy subjects. Insulin infusion rates were 0, 0.5, 1.0, 2.0, and 15 mU · kg^{-1} · min^{-1}.

The potential importance of the muscle "metabolic state" in the regulation of glucose uptake is evident from the excessive increments in glucose uptake that occur under conditions in which oxygen availability is limited, such as during anemia, when breathing a hypoxic gas mixture, or during severe exercise.[1] The high rates of glucose uptake during exercise in anemia or while breathing a hypoxic gas mixture occur even though insulin levels are no higher and catecholamine levels, which may be antagonistic to glucose uptake, are elevated. The link between muscle glucose uptake and the metabolic state may relate to the accumulation of adenosine monophosphate (AMP) and the activation of AMP kinase.[34] The ability of hypoxia and the muscle metabolic state to increase glucose uptake may be particularly important in individuals with diabetes and cardiovascular impairments.

Postexercise State

The metabolic demands of exercise lead to adaptations that persist into the postexercise state. As is the case during exercise, the more persistent metabolic effects after exercise are also controlled, in large part, by glucoregulatory hormones. For this reason, individuals with type 1 diabetes may experience a derangement in metabolism long after the cessation of exercise. The hormone concentrations present during exercise are generally restored toward basal shortly after exercise. Exercise that results in significant changes in circulating glucose levels, however, will have more persistent effects on hormone levels. For example, the hyperglycemia that is associated with high-intensity exercise will result in postexercise hyperinsulinemia, and the fall in glucose that occurs during prolonged exercise can lead to a persistent elevation in counterregulatory hormone levels. Exercise, in many ways, simply accelerates the transition of the body into a more fasted state. Liver and muscle glycogen stores progressively deplete, and hepatic gluconeogenesis is accelerated. The extent of this effect depends on work intensity and duration. Muscle glycogen depletion is a potent stimulus for glycogen synthesis and facilitates the initial repletion of muscle stores in the postexercise state.[35–37]

The repletion of muscle glycogen after exercise occurs in two phases.[36] In the first phase, glucose uptake is elevated, glycogen synthase activity is elevated, and muscle glycogen is rapidly restored. This phase occurs immediately after the cessation of exercise and is notable in that it does not require insulin. In the second phase, muscle glycogen returns to near-normal levels and glucose uptake requires insulin. The second phase is characterized by a marked and persistent increase in insulin action. This model for postexercise muscle glycogen resynthesis is consistent with findings obtained using ^{13}C nuclear magnetic resonance spectroscopy after contraction of the human gastrocnemius.[37] These experiments showed that muscle glycogen synthesis is predominantly insulin independent the first hour after the cessation of contraction but insulin dependent after this interval. An increase in insulin binding to muscle is not necessary for the increase in insulin action after exercise,[36] indicating that postreceptor events are responsible. The added insulin-stimulated glucose disposal after exercise is due solely to an increase in nonoxidative glucose metabolism.[36] As expected, GLUT4 is the primary means by which glucose enters the cell in the postexercise state. Although GLUT4 null mice have normal fed, fasted, and postexercise muscle glycogen content, the restoration of glycogen following a glucose load after exercise was markedly slowed.[38] It is possible that overexpression of GLUT1 could compensate for any shortage of GLUT4 in the plasma membrane because mice overexpressing this protein have increased muscle glycogenesis in the postexercise state.[39] The duration of these alterations in muscle glucose metabolism is probably longer after more extensive glycogen-depleting exercise and can be protracted by an absence of dietary carbohydrate.[35] Glycogen repletion to pre-exercise levels requires ~24 h in humans maintained on a high-carbohydrate diet but may take as long as 8–10 days if carbohydrate is absent from the diet.[35]

In addition to the well-known adaptations in skeletal muscle, prior exercise can lead to persistent effects on splanchnic tissue. Studies in a dog model that provides access to gut and liver in vivo show that prior exercise increases the intestinal absorption of an intraduodenal glucose load[40] and increases the intrinsic capacity of the liver to consume glucose.[41] Whether the effect on liver glucose uptake, like the effect on muscle glucose uptake, is related to an increase in insulin action is unknown. Studies using ^{13}C magnetic resonance spectroscopy showed that ingestion of 1 g/kg glucose or sucrose immediately after completion of prolonged moderate-intensity exercise caused liver glycogen resynthesis to increase by ~0.7 and ~1.3 $mg \cdot kg^{-1} \cdot min^{-1}$, respectively, over a period of 4 h of postexercise recovery.[42] There was no liver glycogen resynthesis over the same period when a placebo was ingested. The ability to replenish liver glycogen after exercise may be functionally important in the performance of subsequent exercise because there is a significant positive correlation between liver glycogen content and exercise endurance.[42] It has been suggested that supplementation of a glucose load with glutamine after exercise may serve to preferentially enhance liver glycogen resynthesis.[43]

Exercise and Type 1 Diabetes

It is apparent from the preceding discussion that the prevailing insulin level is an important determinant of the metabolic response to exercise. In accordance with metabolic needs, the release of insulin from the β-cells of the pancreas is spontaneously regulated in nondiabetic subjects. The inability of type 1 diabetic subjects to regulate the delivery of insulin into the blood in a similar fashion can seriously compromise their ability to meet the requirements of exercise. Given our current insulin treatment regimens, it is extremely difficult to duplicate the normal metabolic responses seen in nondiabetic individuals. Frequently, insulin delivery is mismatched to insulin needs, and the risk of hypoglycemia or exacerbated hyperglycemia can result. The following sections address the problems of over- and under-insulinization in type 1 diabetes. Figure 4.2 summarizes the potential repercussions of too much or too little insulin.

The results of the Diabetes Control and Complications Trial (DCCT), an assessment of the effects of glucose control on the long-term complications of diabetes, demonstrate conclusively that tight glucose control prevents the advent and/or delays the progression of microvascular complications. Whereas the DCCT findings provide a firm basis for advocating tight metabolic control in individuals with type 1 diabetes, the move toward more rigorous control creates an added risk of hypoglycemia and is exemplified by the third panel of Fig. 4.2.

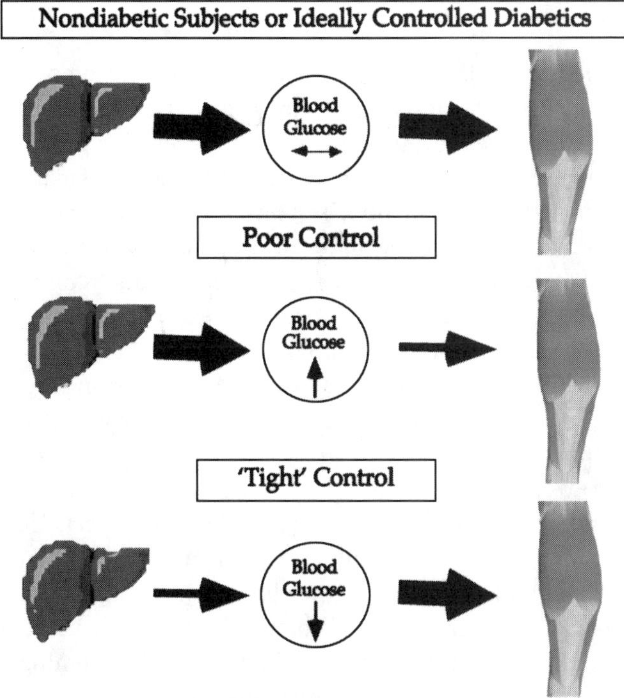

FIGURE 4.2 Scheme illustrating blood glucose response to exercise determined by a balance between liver glucose output and muscle glucose uptake. This balance is a function of diet, therapy, parameters related to exercise modality, and characteristics of the subject.

Over-Insulinization

All diabetic patients treated with subcutaneous insulin injections are over-insulinized at times. If this occurs during exercise, the increases in the release of glucose from the liver and NEFAs from adipose tissue that normally occur with exercise are inhibited. Because muscle glucose utilization increases with exercise, the attenuation of hepatic glucose production leads to a fall in circulating glucose. If the exercise period is sufficiently long, hypoglycemia will eventually result. Because exercise is one of the main causes of hypoglycemia in well-controlled type 1 diabetic subjects, the implementation of treatment regimens designed to achieve tight control requires an understanding of the factors that can increase the risk of hypoglycemia during exercise. Three factors make the person with type 1 diabetes vulnerable to becoming over-insulinized and hypoglycemic during exercise:

1. The failure of plasma insulin to decrease as it does in nondiabetic subjects with the onset and during exercise can result in relative over-insulinization. As a result, a dose of insulin appropriate at rest may be excessive during exercise. Although the fall in insulin is essential to the metabolic response to exercise in nondiabetic subjects, this may not be uniformly true for individuals with type 1 diabetes receiving a peripheral infusion. In studies conducted in postabsorptive type 1 diabetic subjects exercising during a constant basal infusion of insulin, glucose levels have been shown both to remain constant[44] and to fall.[45] A reduction in premeal insulin dose may be more important for exercise conducted in the postprandial state (see below).[46]
2. The exercise-induced increase in insulin action may lead to a relative over-insulinization in type 1 diabetic subjects if a compensatory decrease in insulin dosage is not made. Because the exercise-induced increase in insulin action can persist for many hours after exercise, type 1 diabetic subjects who have not made appropriate adjustments in insulin dosage risk becoming hypoglycemic long after the cessation of exercise.
3. The absorption of subcutaneously injected insulin can be accelerated by exercise.[44] Injecting away from the site of contraction can minimize this effect. The effect of exercise on insulin absorption can be increased even further if insulin is injected into the muscle

as opposed to the subcutaneous region of the working limb.[47] Thus, extra care must be taken to avoid inadvertent injection into skeletal muscle. Even though precautions need to be made to minimize inappropriately rapid insulin absorption, it is important to realize that hypoglycemia can result even when insulin mobilization is not accelerated.

Prevention of Hypoglycemia Resulting From Over-Insulinization

Counterregulation

The mechanism for relative or absolute over-insulinization during exercise is discussed above, and its role in the pathogenesis of exercise-related hypoglycemia is well recognized.[48] Recently, an additional mechanism was proposed that suggests that impaired counterregulatory responses may also contribute to exercise-related hypoglycemia. Many similarities exist in the homeostatic neuroendocrine responses to exercise and hypoglycemia. In both exercise and hypoglycemia, stress, increased glucagon secretion, reduced insulin release, and activation of the sympathetic nervous system with resultant elevation of epinephrine and norepinephrine concentrations provide acute defense against hypoglycemia. Typically, neuroendocrine counterregulatory responses are amplified when a normal individual exercises during a hypoglycemic condition.[49] Additionally, counterregulatory responses are activated by minimal decreases in glycemia during exercise (≅5–10 mg/dl)[1] compared with glycemic reductions of ≅20 mg/dl at rest.[50] Based on these findings, it is apparent that glucose homeostasis is protected even more vigorously during exercise than during rest. Recent studies, however, have demonstrated that neuropathic complications of diabetes[51] and prior glycemic control[52] can independently reduce neuroendocrine counterregulatory responses to exercise. Bottini et al.[51] reported that levels of norepinephrine and epinephrine are reduced two- and fivefold, respectively, when patients with classic diabetic autonomic neuropathy exercise. Schneider et al.[52] also demonstrated that catecholamine responses are diminished when intensively treated type 1 diabetic patients (with no clinical evidence of diabetic autonomic neuropathy) exercise. These two reports clearly indicate that counterregulatory responses during exercise in diabetic patients can be compromised. This latter finding is similar to the scenario that occurs in intensively treated diabetic patients who develop defects in counterregulatory responses to hypoglycemia.[53] Following the initial observation by Heller and Cryer,[54] several other laboratories have confirmed that antecedent hypoglycemia can blunt counterregulatory responses to subsequent hypoglycemia.[53] Based on the above substantive body of information, there is a consensus that the increased prevalence of hypoglycemia occurring in intensively treated diabetic patients is due in part to compromised counterregulatory responses that have been blunted by recent prior hypoglycemia.

In response to the findings arising from hypoglycemia studies, recent work has investigated whether prior hypoglycemia can also diminish counterregulatory responses to subsequent exercise. To date, the majority of information supports a blunting effect by antecedent hypoglycemia on subsequent neuroendocrine and metabolic response to exercise. Davis et al.[55] demonstrated in healthy individuals that two 2-h episodes of hypoglycemia (52 ± 1 mg/dl) can substantially reduce neuroendocrine responses to next-day exercise. Similarly, a subsequent study[56] determined that two episodes of prior exercise can also blunt counterregulatory responses to next-day hypoglycemia. Taken together, the above two studies indicate that a vicious cycle may be created in patients with diabetes, whereby an episode of prior hypoglycemia may reduce counterregulatory responses during subsequent exercise, thereby predisposing the individual to hypoglycemia. This in turn could further blunt counterregulatory responses to any future episodes of exercise and/or hypoglycemia. Although studies in healthy dogs also support the finding that prior exercise could blunt counterregulatory responses to subsequent neuroglycopenia,[57] studies in type 1 diabetic humans (albeit under differing experimental conditions) have not observed blunted exercise-related neuroendocrine responses after prior hypoglycemia.[58] At this time, work has just started investigating the possible role of blunted counterregulatory responses in the pathogenesis of exercise-related hypoglycemia. Clearly, further studies will be required to fully elucidate the mechanisms responsible for this troublesome clinical problem.

Therapeutic Measures

There are many ways to manipulate the timing and amount of insulin administration and food intake to best avoid hypoglycemia, and many different options have been studied. It is clear that a reduction in insulin dose in anticipation of exercise decreases the risk of hypoglycemia. This is particularly important in the postprandial state because the extra insulin needed to minimize the glycemic excursion in response to feeding can create insulin levels that, while normal for meal ingestion, are excessive when exercise is added. Type 1 diabetic subjects maintained on intensive insulin therapy using either multiple subcutaneous injections or continuous subcutaneous insulin infusions (CSIIs) can become hypoglycemic over the course of 45 min of moderate-intensity exercise conducted 2 h after an insulin injection and 90 min after a standard meal.[59] Hypoglycemia was avoided by reducing the insulin dose by 30–50%. This is consistent with the finding that insulin-infused subjects who exercise 30 min after breakfast exhibit a rapid fall in circulating glucose if the insulin infusion rate is increased to simulate the normal insulin response.[46] The fall in plasma glucose is avoided, however, if insulin is lowered by ~70% below the elevated postprandial insulin infusion rate. It may not be necessary to reduce the insulin dose if the duration between subcutaneous injection and exercise is long enough and insulin levels are in decline.[60] This may effectively recreate the decrease in insulin normally present during exercise.

More prolonged exercise may require a greater reduction in insulin dosage. Individuals with type 1 diabetes are able to exercise in the postabsorptive state for nearly 3 h without becoming hypoglycemic if the insulin dose is reduced by 80% compared with 90 min when the dosage is reduced by 50%.[61] Furthermore, the glucose-lowering effect of insulin during heavy exercise is greater than that during moderate-intensity exercise of similar duration.[62,63] Naturally, the magnitude of the glucose fall that can be tolerated by an individual before hypoglycemia ensues will depend on the glycemia at the onset of exercise. Nevertheless, if the primary objective of insulin therapy is tight glucose control, the margin of error in estimating an exercise insulin dose should be considered small.

Because exercise is often spontaneous, it is not always possible to anticipate the need to decrease the insulin dosage. In these instances, glucose ingestion takes on added importance as a means of preventing hypoglycemia. The effectiveness of an oral carbohydrate load will depend, in large part, on its intestinal absorption kinetics. The absorption and metabolic availability can be expedited if the ingested carbohydrate is in the form of simple sugars. Therefore, these readily absorbable substrates are most suitable for ingestion during exercise or in the postexercise state if the individual is in immediate risk of developing hypoglycemia. It has been suggested, on the other hand, that a slowly absorbed carbohydrate might be more useful in decreasing the risk of delayed-onset hypoglycemia, which can occur hours after the cessation of exercise.[64] This is of particular importance if exercise is performed in the late afternoon or evening because hypoglycemia may occur during sleep. A possible inhibitory effect of exercise on food absorption from the gut has been a concern. However, gastrointestinal glucose absorption does not appear to be a limitation because the majority of ^{13}C-glucose contained in an oral glucose load consumed during moderate-intensity exercise can be accounted for by the $^{13}CO_2$ content of the expired air of nondiabetic and well-controlled type 1 diabetic subjects.[65]

Selection of the ideal quantity of calories necessary to avoid hypoglycemia can be determined by many of the factors summarized in Table 4.1. Exercise intensity and duration are of particular importance. High-intensity exercise leads to the less efficient use of oral glucose compared with moderate- or light-intensity exercise because the availability of glucose from the gut does not increase proportionally to the metabolic demands.[66] The amount of ingested glucose can be reduced if exercise is initiated under hyperglycemic conditions. Based on assumptions regarding the size of the body glucose pool, it can be estimated that a 70-kg individual requires ~5 g less of ingested glucose for every 50 mg/dl increment above the target blood glucose level. Although ways to estimate the amount of added glucose needed during exercise have been suggested and are clearly useful,[67] it is impossible to precisely identify the amount needed for each individual. Variability exists not only between people but also within a given subject depending on the time that exercise is performed.[68] The potential variability between and within subjects is exemplified by the results from one study that showed that in a group of eight type 1 diabetic subjects, three different types of responses to exercise after breakfast and lunch could be identified.[68] In the majority of these subjects, exercise reduced the glycemic excursion after both meals. In two subjects, however, exercise lowered the glycemic response after lunch only, and in a third subject, exercise had no effect on glycemia. Considerable variation in the postexercise glycemic response is also observed.[69,70] Making recommendations on how to adjust insulin and diet for exercise that are broadly applicable to the type 1 diabetic population is clearly not feasible. Recommendations for treatment modification need to be tailored to the specific exercise response of each individual. It is equally important to emphasize that whereas therapeutic strategies must be specific to the individual, the vast majority of physically active individuals with diabetes can be adequately controlled by a variety of insulin/diet options and should not feel bound to a single regimen. With the widespread use of self-monitoring of blood glucose, blood glucose concentrations are easy to obtain, and patients should be encouraged to document responses to particular activities.

Under-Insulinization

Subjects with type 1 diabetes in poor control are hyperglycemic, hyperlipidemic, and ketotic. Although glucose fluxes may be normal or accelerated, the mechanisms responsible for the metabolic changes are different in individuals with and without type 1 diabetes. A greater fraction of the glucose released by the liver is gluconeogenic in origin under insulin-deficient conditions.[71] Muscle glucose utilization occurs even when insulin levels are deficient because the mass-action effect of hyperglycemia overcomes the lack of insulin-stimulated glucose uptake.[71] Nevertheless, a smaller percentage of glucose used in poorly controlled type 1 diabetic subjects is fully oxidized because of impaired pyruvate dehydrogenase activity. Type 1 diabetic subjects not meticulously controlled may also have diminished glycogen stores and increased lipid stores within the muscle. This may in turn result in a decrease and an increase, respectively, in the use of these intramuscular stores during moderate-intensity exercise.[72,73] The metabolic demands of heavy exercise may be adequate to override deficits in metabolic control and hormone changes during high-intensity exercise (~80% maximum oxygen uptake) because substrate utilization has been shown to be similar in subjects with type 1 diabetes and in normal control subjects.[73]

Exercise in the insulin-deficient state can result in a further deterioration of metabolic control. Exercise in type 1 diabetic patients deprived of insulin for 18–48 h results in an exacerbation of the hyperglycemia and ketosis already present in these individuals.[74] The rise in blood glucose is due to an impairment in the exercise-induced increase in glucose utilization accompanied by a normal increase in hepatic glucose production. The added increase in hepatic ketone body output during exercise in poorly controlled type 1 diabetic patients is, in part, secondary to an unrestrained increase in lipolysis and possibly to an increase in intrahepatic ketogenic efficiency.[20] Heavy exercise in some instances can be more deleterious to metabolic control than moderate-intensity exercise of the same duration. Even well-controlled type 1 diabetic subjects receiving a CSII may have an increase in blood glucose and NEFA levels after high-intensity exercise.[75] This is probably due to a failure of insulin to rise as it would normally after heavy exercise in nondiabetic subjects.

In well-controlled type 1 diabetic subjects free of autonomic neuropathies, the counterregulatory hormone response to exercise is similar to the response in nondiabetic subjects, provided that hypoglycemia does not occur. In the nondiabetic state, the counterregulatory system is sensitized to changes in glucose during exercise because both the counterregulatory hormone threshold and the magnitude of the counterregulatory hormone response are increased.[76] Although this efficient counterregulation may be sustained in some patients with type 1 diabetes, it seems to be defective in others.[52] In contrast to well-controlled people with type 1 diabetes, type 1 diabetic subjects in poor control have increased counterregulatory hormone responses,[74] all of which may contribute to the deleterious metabolic effect of exercise in these individuals. As is the case in the nondiabetic state, glucagon probably contributes to the increased hepatic glucose and ketone body outputs present in poorly controlled type 1 diabetes.[2] The role of glucagon during exercise in type 1 diabetes is summarized with regard to metabolic control in Table 4.2. The β-adrenergic effects of the catecholamines play a minor role in controlling hepatic metabolism in

TABLE 4.2 Role of Glucagon During Exercise in Diabetes

Too little insulin
- Glucagon response is exaggerated
  - Increased hepatic glucose output
  - Increased ketogenesis

Too much insulin
- Glucagon response is reduced
  - Decreased hepatic glucose output
  - Increased risk of hypoglycemia

nondiabetic control subjects but may be of greater significance in type 1 diabetes. Application of a specific hepatic adrenergic blockade in a diabetic dog model, however, did not affect the exercise-induced increase in hepatic glucose production, suggesting that sympathetic drive does not have a direct effect on this variable at the liver.[77] The potent effects of the catecholamines in stimulating fuel mobilization from muscle (glycogen) and adipose tissue (triglycerides) and delivery to the liver (lactate, alanine, glycerol, and NEFA) may be more important in poorly controlled type 1 diabetic subjects because this process provides precursors for gluconeogenesis and ketogenesis to the liver. Thus, catecholamines may act indirectly in control of liver metabolism by providing substrates. The metabolic actions of the catecholamines during exercise in type 1 diabetic subjects are summarized with respect to metabolic control in Table 4.3.

Exercise and Type 2 Diabetes

Although type 2 is the predominant form of diabetes, the metabolic response to exercise in this population has not received a corresponding degree of attention. This syndrome is often characterized by obesity, hyperinsulinemia, and hypertension, and treatment may consist of dietary prescriptions, oral hypoglycemic agents, lipid-lowering agents, and/or insulin. However, the use of exercise as a therapeutic modality may be particularly beneficial because it has a positive impact on insulin resistance, the fundamental abnormality of this metabolic state.

TABLE 4.3 Role of Catecholamines During Exercise in Diabetes

Too little insulin

- Catecholamine response is exaggerated
  - Increased lipolysis
  - Increased free fatty acids and ketones
  - Impaired glucose utilization

Too much insulin

- In the absence of advanced autonomic neuropathy and prior stress, hypoglycemia causes an increased catecholamine response, leading to the metabolic responses described above and the prevention of more severe hypoglycemia.

Obese type 2 diabetic patients maintained on diet therapy alone or diet and sulfonylurea therapy with postabsorptive plasma glucose in excess of 200 mg/dl and normal basal insulin show a fall in glycemia of ~50 mg/dl during a 45-min exercise session.[78] The fall in glucose under these conditions is due to an attenuated rise in hepatic glucose production. Obese type 2 diabetic patients with just mild hyperglycemia (<150 mg/dl) also exhibit a fall in blood glucose in response to 45 min of moderate-intensity exercise, but blood glucose fell less (~20 mg/dl) in these subjects than in the more hyperglycemic subjects.[79] The response to exercise in nonobese type 2 diabetic subjects with mild hypoglycemia is essentially the same as the response in those who are obese.[80] Subjects with type 2 diabetes in whom glyburide treatment was withheld for 1 week had a plasma glucose of ~200 mg/dl before exercise and exhibited an ~15% fall in response to exercise. The glycemic response and the contribution of muscle glycogen, plasma glucose, and fats to fuel needs in these individuals were the same as those in anthropometrically matched nondiabetic control subjects at 50 and 70% maximum oxygen uptake.[81] This finding is supported by the demonstration that high-intensity intermittent exercise performed in postprandial type 2 diabetic subjects[82] has the same plasma glucose and insulin-lowering effect as moderate-intensity exercise of an equivalent caloric requirement.[83] These studies indicate that high-intensity exercise is as useful as moderate-intensity exercise in improving metabolic control in type 2 diabetic subjects.

It is important to note that although type 2 diabetic subjects are insulin resistant, they are not resistant to the stimulatory effects of exercise on glucose utilization. Type 2 diabetic subjects retain the capacity to translocate GLUT4 to the sarcolemma in response to exercise. The reduced rise in glucose production could be due to the failure of insulin to fall as it does in control subjects and/or to the hepatic effects of hyperglycemia present in these subjects.

During 3 h of moderate-intensity exercise in type 2 diabetic subjects with moderate fasting hyperglycemia (140 mg/dl) and hyperinsulinemia (23 μU/ml), plasma glucose falls by ~40 mg/dl.[84] Moreover, a decrease in the elevated insulin levels is also present. One study[85] showed that a single session of glycogen-depleting exercise significantly increases insulin sensitivity in the liver and in muscle 12–16 h later in type 2 diabetic subjects. Prior exercise reduced basal hepatic glucose production and accentuated the suppressive effects of a low-dose insulin infusion on this variable. Peripheral insulin sensitivity was increased, as reflected by an enhanced rate of nonoxidative glucose disposal and increased glycogen synthase activity. Studies that illustrate how exercise can lower circulating glucose levels and increase insulin sensitivity in type 2 diabetic subjects emphasize the potential importance of exercise as a therapy in this population.

Subjects with type 2 diabetes maintained on diet therapy alone should be able to exercise with no more caution than the individual with normal glucose tolerance provided there are no major vascular or neurological complications. There may be a tendency for hypoglycemia during prolonged exercise when oral hypoglycemic agents (sulfonylureas) are used. Glibenclamide adds to the hypoglycemic action of prolonged moderate-intensity exercise by increasing plasma insulin and preventing the normal rise in hepatic glucose production in postabsorptive type 2 diabetic subjects.[86] Experimental use of the free fatty acid oxidation inhibitor methylpalmoxirate has been shown to impair total hepatic glucose production in exercising depancreatized dogs.[21] If such compounds are used for therapeutic purposes, the tendency for hypoglycemia during exercise will be enhanced. In addition, chronic use of fatty acid oxidation inhibitors may lead to accumulation of esterified fat in the liver and to hypertrophy of the myocardium. Clearly, more work is necessary to fully understand the full spectrum of the effects of fatty acid oxidation inhibitors. Regardless of the course of treatment, future studies should ascertain more precisely the metabolic response to exercise as a function of the therapeutic regimen.

For many patients with type 2 diabetes, weight loss is an important aspect of their therapy. For this reason, these individuals may be maintained on a low-calorie diet combined with exercise. Although calorie restriction is usually necessary to lose weight, it is also important that enough calories be provided for a subject to exercise safely. Diets containing <400 kcal/day have been associated with cardiac arrhythmias and sudden death. An individual participating in an exercise program should probably be kept on a diet containing no less than 800 kcal/day. It seems that low-calorie diets can be used without affecting exercise tolerance provided that the diet contains enough carbohydrate (at least 35% of the total calories) to maintain normal muscle glycogen levels.

Although many type 2 diabetic patients are reliant on exogenous insulin, most of the data concerning the exercise response in patients receiving insulin have been derived from studies of patients with type 1 diabetes. Although there may be certain discrepancies, the practical considerations that apply when planning a therapeutic regimen for individuals with type 1 diabetes will probably apply to those with type 2 diabetes who are receiving insulin.

Practical Considerations for Adapting Therapy to Physical Activity

Individuals with type 2 diabetes not treated with insulin and without extensive vascular or neurological complications can generally exercise with no more concern than nondiabetic individuals of equal cardiovascular fitness. On the other hand, type 1 or type 2 diabetic patients taking insulin should take a number of precautions. Table 4.4 presents some general guidelines for patients taking insulin.[87] It is impossible, however, to give precise guidelines for diet and insulin therapy that will be suitable for all type 1 diabetic individuals who wish to be physically active. Moreover, the metabolic demands associated with exercise vary depending on the type of exercise. Nevertheless, some general strategies can be applied to help prevent the problems associated with exercise. Frequent self-monitoring of blood glucose should be conducted so that immediate risks of hypoglycemia or hyperglycemia can be identified. In addition, self-monitoring of blood glucose provides feedback that will form the basis for implementing therapy for subsequent exercise. If, before exercise, blood glucose readings are below ~90 mg/dl, the risk of hypoglycemia is great, and exercise should not be initiated without the ingestion of glucose. If fasting blood glucose is greater than ~250–300 mg/dl and ketone bodies are present in the urine, patients are generally advised to administer more insulin and delay exercising. In addition to pre-exercise evaluation, blood glucose monitoring should be performed during and after exercise with the primary purpose of minimizing the risk of hypoglycemia. It is important to consider not only the absolute glycemic levels when monitoring blood glucose but also the rate at which any change in glycemia may occur. For example, a glucose level that is stable at 100 mg/dl may reflect a safe situation, whereas a glucose level that is 100 mg/dl is indicative of an imbalance between glucose production and utilization if the preceding glucose measurement was 150 mg/dl. The latter situation would require further attention (i.e., glucose ingestion).

TABLE 4.4 Prevention of Hypoglycemia or Hyperglycemia During Exercise

Before exercise

1. Estimate intensity, duration, and the energy expenditure of exercise.
2. Eat a meal 1–3 h before exercise.
3. Administer insulin correctly.
   a. Administer insulin >1 h before exercise.
   b. Decrease the dose of insulin that has peak activity coinciding with the exercise period.
4. Assess metabolic control.
   a. If blood glucose is <5 mmol/l (90 mg/dl), extra calories before exercise will likely be required.
   b. If blood glucose is 5–15 mmol/l (90–270 mg/dl), extra calories may not be required.
   c. If blood glucose is >15 mmol/l (270 mg/dl), delay exercise and measure urine ketones.
      i. If urine ketones are negative, exercise can be performed, and extra calories are not required.
      ii. If urine ketones are positive, take insulin and delay exercise until ketones are negative.
5. Do not use an exercising extremity as an injection site.

During exercise

1. Monitor blood glucose during long sessions.
2. Always replace fluid losses adequately.
3. If required, use supplemental carbohydrate feedings (30–40 g for adults, 15–25 g for children) every 30 min during extended periods of exercise.

After exercise

1. Monitor blood glucose, including overnight, if amount of exercise is not habitual.
2. Adjust insulin therapy to decrease immediate and delayed insulin action (intensive therapy regimes provide increased flexibility in adjusting insulin).
3. If required, increase calorie intake for 12–24 h after activity, depending on the intensity and duration of exercise and risk of hypoglycemia.

Adapted from Tsui and Zinman.[87]

The need to reduce the insulin dose before exercise and avoid administrating the insulin in the region of the working muscles was emphasized in a previous section. The precise size of any reduction in insulin depends on many variables that will vary from person to person and with different exercise parameters (i.e., work intensity and duration). Individuals maintained on intermediate- and short-acting insulin may decrease or omit the short-acting insulin, depending on the circumstances. Alternatively, the intermediate-acting dose could be reduced but supplemented with added short-acting insulin later in the day. People relying on CSII with the intention of exercising in the postprandial state should reduce the premeal bolus. An advantage of using an insulin pump is that it eliminates much of the variability in circulating insulin levels that occurs because of exercise-induced changes in insulin absorption from subcutaneous depots. The reason for variability in insulin levels is that with a pump, the insulin depot is in the device and not in a subcutaneous depot where it is subject to changes in the absorption profile.

Aside from considerations relating to modifications in insulin delivery and glucose ingestion, such as type of exercise, duration of exercise, and time of exercise, several other considerations are necessary. Exercise that requires repetitive recruitment of large muscle groups, such as running or walking, cycling, or swimming, causes large and sustained increases in oxygen uptake and is appropriate for obtaining long-term cardiovascular adaptations. A work intensity that elicits an increase to ~50% of an individual's maximum oxygen uptake and an exercise duration of >20 min is sufficiently rigorous to obtain exercise-related adaptations. Exercise of extended duration, however, increases the risk of hypoglycemia and should be undertaken with appropriate precautions. Competitive sports frequently require high-intensity exertion. This type of exercise is important not only because of its contribution to fitness but also because it is an important part of the socialization of, in particular, children and young adults. Because of the integral role of strenuous exercise, it is important to understand glucoregulation during this type of exercise. The time of day that an individual exercises should be considered. The risk of hypoglycemia appears to be lowest if an individual engages in exercise in the morning before the prebreakfast insulin dose.[88] Insulin levels are usually lowest at this time. Late afternoon or early evening exercise can be hazardous if sufficient precautions are not taken to minimize the risk of hypoglycemia during sleep. Adapting insulin and diet therapy to regular exercise can be achieved if the time of day for exercise and the exercise parameters are consistent. Although this may be a reasonable objective for some adults, the spontaneity of exercise in children and the variety of different sports in which they may participate make this goal difficult to obtain.

Conclusions

Exercise should be encouraged in people with diabetes for the same reasons it should be encouraged in the general population. Regular exercise can decrease risk factors for cardiovascular disease and is felt by many to improve the general quality of life. Physical activity can improve metabolic control in type 2 diabetic subjects and even alleviate symptoms of the syndrome altogether. Evidence that the adaptations to regular exercise improve glucose control in subjects with type 1 diabetes is, however, lacking. Although the benefits of regular physical activity in diabetic and nondiabetic populations are generally similar, the individual with type 1 diabetes faces a number of challenges in preparation for, during, and after each session that are unique to the diabetic syndrome. Exercise-induced changes in insulin and counterregulatory hormone levels control the mobilization of fuels from various storage sites. In people with type 1 diabetes, the normal endocrine response to exercise is lost, resulting in derangements in fuel metabolism. Exercise can lead to profound hypoglycemia if insulin levels are excessive or to an exacerbated diabetic state (e.g., hyperglycemia or ketosis) if insulin levels are deficient. There a number of strategies that must be considered to safely adapt insulin therapy and diet to accommodate daily exercise. Because the most serious and frequent metabolic problem is hypoglycemia during and after exercise, adjustments in therapy for the type 1 diabetic subject involve a reduction in insulin dose in anticipation of exercise and/or the ingestion of readily absorbable carbohydrate. The value and appropriateness of an exercise program for the individual with type 1 diabetes is judged by the extent to which the beneficial adaptive effects of regular exercise exceed the risks of a single exercise session.

The results of the DCCT have emphasized the importance of tight glucose control in deterring the complications of diabetes and should lead to an increase in the number of individuals who make tight control an objective of their therapy. With this, the onus is on the patient and health care providers to understand the factors that contribute to hypoglycemia during exercise and develop strategies to avoid it. Research in the area of exercise and diabetes has progressed to the point where a knowledgeable patient can adjust therapy in anticipation of exercise of predetermined length and intensity and minimize the risk of hypoglycemia. Children rarely set out with a precise agenda and frequently become involved in recreation after administration of insulin, at which time they become committed to a given dose. Further research needs to be conducted to develop means of minimizing the risk of hypoglycemia during exercise when it is not anticipated and the option to reduce the insulin dose is no longer present. Furthermore, most of our understanding of exercise in the individual with diabetes is obtained from experiments designed to look at the effects of moderate-intensity exercise. Exercise is often conducted in high-intensity bursts. More research needs to be focused on means to accommodate participation in competitive sports so that children and adults with type 1 diabetes who wish to engage in recreational activities can do so safely.

References

1. Wasserman DH: Control of glucose fluxes during exercise in the postabsorptive state. In *Annual Review of Physiology*. Palo Alto, CA, Annual Reviews, 1995, p. 191–218
2. Wasserman DH, Cherrington AD: Regulation of extrahepatic fuel sources during exercise. In *Handbook of Physiology*. Rowell LB, Shepherd JT, Eds. Columbia, MD, Bermedica Production, 1996, p. 1036–74
3. Hirsch IB, Marker JC, Smith LJ, Spina R, Parvin CA, Holloszy JO, Cryer PE: Insulin and glucagon in the prevention of hypoglycemia during exercise in humans. *Am J Physiol* 260:E695–704, 1991
4. Howlett K, Galbo H, Lorentsen J, Bergeron R, Zimmerman-Belsing T, Bulow J, Feldt-Rasmussen U, Kjaer M: Effect of adrenaline on glucose kinetics during exercise in adrenalectomised humans. *J Physiol* 519:911–21, 1999
5. Coker RH, Krishna MG, Lacy DB, Zinker B, Wasserman DH: Sympathetic drive to liver and nonhepatic splanchnic tissue during prolonged exercise is increased in diabetes. *Metabolism* 46:1327–32, 1997
6. Kjaer M, Keiding S, Engfred K, Rasmussen K, Sonne B, Kirkegard P, Galbo H: Glucose homeostasis during exercise in humans with a liver or kidney transplant. *Am J Physiol* 268:E636–44, 1995
7. Friedman JE: Role of glucocorticoids in activation of hepatic PEPCK gene transcription during exercise. *Am J Physiol* 266:E560–66, 1994
8. Marliss EB, Purdon C, Halter JB, Sigal RJ, Vranic M: *Glucoregulation During and After Intense Exercise in Control and Diabetic Subjects*. London, Smith-Gordon, 1992
9. Sigal RJ, Fisher SF, Halter JB, Vranic M, Marliss EB: The roles of catecholamines in glucoregulation in intense exercise as defined by the islet cell clamp technique. *Diabetes* 45:148–56, 1995

10. Kjaer M, Engfred K, Fernandez A, Secher N, Galbo H: Regulation of hepatic glucose production during exercise in humans: role of sympathoadrenergic activity. *Am J Physiol* 265:E275–83, 1993
11. Sigal RJ, Purdon C, Bilinski D, Vranic M, Halter JB, Marliss EB: Glucoregulation during and after intense exercise: effects of beta-blockade. *J Clin Endocrinol Metab* 78:359–66, 1994
12. Coker RH, Krishna MG, Lacy DB, Bracy DP, Wasserman DH: Role of hepatic alpha- and beta-adrenergic receptor stimulation on hepatic glucose production during heavy exercise. *Am J Physiol* 273:E831–38, 1997
13. Wolfe RR, Klein S, Carraro F, Weber JM: Role of triglyceride-fatty acid cycle in controlling fat metabolism in humans during and after exercise. *Am J Physiol* 258:E382–89, 1990
14. Wahrenberg H, Engfeldt P, Bolinder J, Arner P: Acute adaptation in adrenergic control of lipolysis during physical exercise in humans. *Am J Physiol* 253:E383–90, 1987
15. Stich V, DeGliesezinski I, Crampes F, Suljkovicova H, Galitzky J, Riviere D, Hejnova J, Lafontan M, Berlan M: Activation of antilipolytic alpha2-adrenergic receptors by epinephrine during exercise in human adipose tissue. *Am J Physiol* 277:R1076–83, 1999
16. Horowitz JF, Klein S: Lipid metabolism during endurance exercise. *Am J Clin Nutr* 72 (Suppl.):558S–563S, 2000
17. Martin WH, Dalsky GP, Hurley BF: Effect of endurance training on plasma free fatty acid turnover and oxidation during exercise. *Am J Physiol* 265:E708–14, 1993
18. Dyck DJ, Bonen A: Muscle contraction increases palmitate esterification and oxidation and triacylglycerol oxidation. *Am J Physiol* 275:E888–96, 1998
19. Bergman BC, Butterfield GE, Wolfel EE, Casazza GA, Lopaschuk GD, Brooks GA: Evaluation of exercise and training on muscle lipid metabolism. *Am J Physiol* 276:E106–17, 1999
20. Wahren J, Sato Y, Ostman J, Hagenfeldt L, Felig P: Turnover and splanchnic metabolism of free fatty acids and ketones in insulin-dependent diabetics during exercise. *J Clin Invest* 73:1367–76, 1984
21. Shi Z, Giacca A, Yamatani K, Fisher SJ, Lickley H, Vranic M: Effects of subbasal insulin infusion on resting and exercise-induced glucose turnover in depancreatized dogs. *Am J Physiol* 264:E334–41, 1993

22. Chasiostis D, Sahlin K, Hultman E: Regulation of glycogenolysis in human muscle at rest and during exercise. *J Appl Physiol* 53: 708–15, 1982
23. Richter EA, Ruderman NB, Gavras H, Belur E, Galbo H: Muscle glycogenolysis during exercise: dual control by epinephrine and contractions. *Am J Physiol* 242:E25–32, 1982
24. Zinker BA, Bracy D, Lacy DB, Jacobs J, Wasserman DH: Regulation of glucose uptake and metabolism during exercise: an in vivo analysis. *Diabetes* 42:956–65, 1993
25. Nesher R, Karl I, Kipnis D: Dissociation of effects of insulin and contraction on glucose transport in rat epitrochlearis muscle. *Am J Physiol* 249:C226–32, 1985
26. Kennedy JW, Hirshman MF, Gervino EV, Ocel JV, Forse RA, Hoenig SJ, Aronson D, Goodyear LJ, Horton ES: Acute exercise induces GLUT4 translocation in skeletal muscle of normal human subjects and subjects with type 2 diabetes. *Diabetes* 48:1192–97, 1999
27. Coderre L, Kandror KV, Vallega G, Pilch PF: Identification and characterization of an exercise-sensitive pool of glucose transporters in skeletal muscle. *J Biol Chem* 270:27584–88, 1995
28. O'Doherty RM, Bracy DP, Osawa H, Wasserman DH, Granner DK: Rat skeletal muscle hexokinase II mRNA and activity are increased by a single bout of acute exercise. *Am J Physiol* 266:E171–78, 1994
29. O'Doherty RM, Bracy DP, Granner DK, Wasserman DH: Hexokinase II gene transcription is increased by acute exercise in rat skeletal muscle. *J Appl Physiol* 81:789–93, 1996
30. Koval JA, DeFronzo RA, O'Doherty RM, Printz RL, Ardehali H, Granner DK, Mandarino LJ: Regulation of hexokinase II activity and expression in human muscle by moderate exercise. *Am J Physiol* 274:E304–08, 1998
31. Halseth A, Bracy D, Wasserman D: Overexpression of hexokinase II increases insulin- and exercise-stimulated muscle glucose uptake in vivo. *Am J Physiol* 276:E70–77, 1999
32. Halseth AE, Bracy DP, Wasserman DH: Limitations to exercise- and maximal insulin-stimulated muscle glucose uptake in vivo. *J Appl Physiol* 85:2305–13, 1998
33. Richter EA: Glucose utilization. In *Handbook of Physiology*. Rowell LB, Shepherd JT, Eds. New York, Oxford University, 1996, p. 912–51

34. Hayashi T, Hirshman MF, Kurth EJ, Winder WW, Goodyear LJ: Evidence for 5′-AMP activated protein kinase mediation of the effect of muscle contraction on glucose transport. *Diabetes* 47: 1369–73, 1998
35. Hultman E, Bergstrom J, Roch-Norland AE: Glycogen storage in human skeletal muscle. In *Muscle Metabolism During Exercise.* Pernow BSB, Ed. New York, Plenum, 1971, p. 273–88
36. Garetto LP, Richter EA, Goodman MN, Ruderman NB: Enhanced muscle glucose metabolism after exercise in the rat: the two phases. *Am J Physiol* 246:E471–75, 1984
37. Price TB, Rothman DL, Taylor R, Avison MJ, Shulman GI, Shulman RG: Human muscle glycogen resynthesis after exercise: insulin-dependent and -independent phases. *J Appl Physiol* 76:104–11, 1994
38. Ryder JW, Kawano Y, Galuska D, Fahlman RF, Wallberg-Henriksson H, Charron MJ, Zierath JR: Postexercise glucose uptake from glycogen synthesis in skeletal muscle from GLUT4-deficient mice. *FASEB J* 13:2246–56, 1999
39. Ren JM, Barucci N, Marshall BA, Hansen P, Muekler M, Shulman GI: Transgenic mice overexpressing GLUT1 protein in muscle exhibit increased muscle glycogenesis after exercise. *Am J Physiol* 278:E588–92, 2000
40. Hamilton KS, Gibbons FK, Bracy DP, Lacy DB, Cherrington AD, Wasserman DH: Effect of prior exercise on the partitioning of an intestinal glucose load between splanchnic bed and skeletal muscle. *J Clin Invest* 98:125–35, 1996
41. Galassetti P, Coker RH, Lacy DB, Cherrington AD, Wasserman DH: Prior exercise increases net hepatic glucose uptake during a glucose load. *Am J Physiol* 276:E1022–29, 1999
42. Casey A, Mann R, Banister K, Fox J, Morris PG, MacDonald IA, Greenhaff PL: Effect of carbohydrate ingestion on glycogen resynthesis in human liver and skeletal muscle, measured by 13C MRS. *Am J Physiol* 278:E65–75, 2000
43. Bowtell JL, Gelly K, Jackman ML, Patel A, Simeoni M, Rennie MJ: Effect of oral glutamine on whole body carbohydrate storage during recovery from exhaustive exercise. *J Appl Physiol* 86:1770–77, 1999
44. Zinman B, Murray FT, Vranic M, Albisser AM, Leibel BS, Mc Clean PA, Marliss EB: Glucoregulation during moderate exercise in insulin-treated diabetics. *J Clin Endocrinol Metab* 45:641–52, 1977

45. Simonson DC, Koivisto VA, Sherwin RS, Ferrannini E, Hendler R, DeFronzo RA: Adrenergic blockade alters glucose kinetics during exercise in insulin-dependent diabetics. *J Clin Invest* 73:1648–58, 1984
46. Nelson JD, Poussier P, Marliss EB, Albisser AM, Zinman B: Metabolic response of normal man and insulin-infused diabetics to postprandial exercise in type 1 diabetics. *Am J Physiol* 242:E309–16, 1982
47. Frid A, Ostman J, Linde B: Hypoglycemia risk during exercise after intramuscular injection of insulin in thigh in IDDM. *Diabetes Care* 13:473–77, 1990
48. Sonnenberg GE, Kemmer FW, Berger M: Exercise in type I (insulin-dependent) diabetic patients treated with continuous subcutaneous insulin infusion: prevention of exercise-induced hypoglycaemia. *Diabetologia* 33:696–703, 1990
49. Sotsky M, Shilo S, Shamoon H: Regulation of counterregulatory hormone secretion in man during exercise and hypoglycemia. *J Clin Endocrinol Metab* 68:9–16, 1989
50. Amiel SA, Sherwin RS, Simonson D, Tamborlane WV: Effect of intensive insulin therapy on glycemic thresholds for counterregulatory hormone release. *Diabetes* 37:901–07, 1988
51. Bottini P, Boschetti E, Pampanelli S, Ciofetta M, Sindaco PD, Scionti L, Brunetti P, Bolli GB: Contribution of autonomic neuropathy to reduce plasma adrenaline responses to hypoglycemia in IDDM: evidence for a nonselective defect. *Diabetes* 46:814–23, 1997
52. Schneider SH, Vitug A, Ananthakrishnan R, Khachadurian AK: Impaired adrenergic response to prolonged exercise in type 1 diabetes. *Metabolism* 40:1219–25, 1991
53. Dagogo-Jack S, Craft S, Cryer PE: Hypoglycemia-associated autonomic failure in insulin-dependent diabetes mellitus: recent antecedent hypoglycemia reduces autonomic responses to, symptoms of, and defense against subsequent hypoglycemia. *J Clin Invest* 91:819–28, 1993
54. Heller SR, Cryer PE: Reduced neuroendocrine and symptomatic responses to subsequent hypoglycemia after one episode of hypoglycemia in nondiabetic humans. *Diabetes* 40:223–26, 1991
55. Davis SN, Galassetti P, Wasserman DH, Tate D: Effects of antecedent hypoglycemia on subsequent counterregulatory responses to exercise. *Diabetes* 49:73–81, 2000

56. Galassetti P, Tate D, Mann S, Costa F, Wasserman DH, Davis SN: Effect of antecedent exercise on counterregulatory responses to subsequent hypoglycemia (Abstract). *Diabetes* 49 (Suppl. 1): A112, 2000
57. Kozlowski S, Brzezinska K, Nazar K: Diminished adrenergic response to 2-deoxy-D-glucose after prolonged exhausting physical exercise in dogs. *Acta Physiol Pol* 30:331–35, 1979
58. Rattarasarn C, Dagogo-Jack S, Zachwieja JJ, Cryer PE: Hypoglycemia-induced autonomic failure in IDDM is specific for stimulus of hypoglycemia and is not attributable to prior autonomic activation. *Diabetes* 43:809–18, 1994
59. Schiffrin A, Parikh S: Accommodating planned exercise in type 1 diabetic patients on intensive treatment. *Diabetes Care* 8:337–43, 1985
60. Trovati M, Anfossi G, Vitali S, Mularoni E, Massucco P, DeFacis R, Carta Q: Postprandial exercise in type 1 diabetic patients on multiple daily insulin injection regimen. *Diabetes Care* 11:107–10, 1988
61. Kemmer FW, Berger M: Therapy and better quality of life: the dichotomous role of exercise in diabetes mellitus. *Diabetes Metab Rev* 2:53–68, 1986
62. Zander E, Bruns W, Wulfert P, Besch W, Lubs D, Chlup R, Schulz B: Muscular exercise in type 1 diabetics. I. Different metabolic reactions during heavy muscular work: independence on actual insulin availability. *Exp Clin Endocrinol* 82:78–90, 1983
63. Hubinger A, Ridderskamp I, Lehmann E: Metabolic response to different forms of physical exercise in type 1 diabetics and the duration of the glucose lowering effect. *Eur J Clin Invest* 15:197–205, 1985
64. Nathan DM, Madnek SF, Delahanty L: Programming pre-exercise snacks to prevent post-exercise hypoglycemia in intensively treated insulin-dependent diabetics. *Ann Int Med* 102:483–86, 1985
65. Krzentowski G, Pirnay F, Pallikarakis N, Luyckx AS, Lacroix M, Mosora F, Lefebvre PJ: Glucose utilization during exercise in normal and diabetic subjects: the role of insulin. *Diabetes* 30:983–89, 1981
66. Pirnay F, Crielaard JM, Pallikarakis N, Lacroix M, Mosora F, Luyckx A, Lefebvre PJ: Fate of exogenous glucose during exercise of different intensities in humans. *J Appl Physiol* 43:258–61, 1982
67. Riddell MC, Bar-Or O, Ayub BV, Calvert RE, Heigenhauser GJ: Glucose ingestion matched with total carbohydrate utilization

attenuates hypoglycemia during exercise in adolescents with IDDM. *Int J Sport Nutr* 9:24–34, 1999

68. Caron D, Poussier P, Marliss EB, Zinman B: The effect of postprandial exercise on meal-related glucose intolerance in insulin-dependent diabetic individuals. *Diabetes Care* 5:364–69, 1982
69. Campaigne BN, Wallberg-Henricksson H, Gunnarsson R: Glucose and insulin responses in relation to insulin dose and caloric intake 12 h after physical exercise in men with IDDM. *Diabetes Care* 10:716–21, 1987
70. Hernandez JM, Moccia T, Fluckey JD, Ulbrecht JS, Farrell PA: Fluid snacks to avoid late onset postexercise hypoglycemia. *Med Sci Sports Exerc* 32:904–10, 2000
71. Wahren J, Hagenfeldt L, Felig P: Splanchnic and leg exchange of glucose, amino acids, and free fatty acids during exercise in diabetes mellitus. *J Clin Invest* 55:1303–14, 1975
72. Standl E, Lotz N, Dexel TH, Janka H, Kolb H: Muscle triglycerides in diabetic subjects. *Diabetologia* 18:463–69, 1980
73. Raguso CA, Coggan AR, Gastaldelli A, Sidossis LS, Bastyr EJ, Wolfe RR: Lipid and carbohydrate metabolism in IDDM during moderate and intense exercise. *Diabetes* 44:1066–74, 1995
74. Berger M, Berchtold P, Kuppers HJ, Drost H, Kley HK, Muller WA, Wiegelmann W, Zimmerman-Telschow H, Gries FA, Kruskemper HL, Zimmerman H: Metabolic and hormonal effects of muscular exercise in juvenile type diabetics. *Diabetologia* 13: 355–65, 1977
75. Mitchell TH, Abraham G, Schiffrin A, Leiter A, Marliss EB: Hyperglycemia after intense exercise in IDDM subjects during continuous subcutaneous insulin infusion. *Diabetes Care* 11:311–17, 1988
76. Wasserman DH, Zinman B: Exercise in individuals with IDDM (Technical Review). *Diabetes Care* 17:924–37, 1994
77. Coker RH, Lacy DB, Williams PE, Wasserman DH: Hepatic adrenergic receptors do not mediate the increase in endogenous glucose production during exercise in the alloxan-diabetic dog. *Am J Physiol* 278:444–51, 2000
78. Minuk HL, Vranic M, Hanna AK, Albisser AM, Zinman B: Glucoregulatory and metabolic response to exercise in obese noninsulin-dependent diabetes. *Am J Physiol* 240:E458–64, 1981
79. Giacca A, Groenewoud Y, Tsui E, McClean P, Zinman B: Glucose production, utilization, and cycling in response to moderate ex-

ercise in obese subjects with type 2 diabetes and mild hyperglycemia. *Diabetes* 47:1763–70, 1998
80. Martin IK, Katz A, Wahren J: Splanchnic and muscle metabolism during exercise in NIDDM patients. *Am J Physiol* 269:E583–90, 1995
81. Kang J, Kelley DE, Robertson RJ, Goss FL, Suminski RR, Utter AC, DaSilva SG: Substrate utilization and glucose turnover during exercise of varying intensities in individuals with NIDDM. *Med Sci Sports Exerc* 31:82–89, 1999
82. Larsen JJS, Dela F, Madsbad S, Galbo H: The effect of intense exercise on postprandial glucose homeostasis in type II diabetic patients. *Diabetologia* 42:1282–92, 1999
83. Larsen JJ, Dela F, Kjaer M, Galbo H: The effect of moderate exercise on postprandial glucose homeostasis in NIDDM patients. *Diabetologia* 40:447–53, 1997
84. Koivisto V, DeFronzo R: Exercise in the treatment of type II diabetes. *Acta Endocrinol* 262 (Suppl.):107–16, 1984
85. Devlin JT, Hirshman M, Horton ED, Horton ES: Enhanced peripheral and splanchnic insulin sensitivity in NIDDM men after single bout of exercise. *Diabetes* 36:434–39, 1987
86. Larsen JJ, Dela F, Madsbad S, Vibe-Peterson J, Galbo H: Interaction of sulfonylurea and exercise on glucose homeostasis in type 2 diabetic patients. *Diabetes Care* 22:1647–54, 1999
87. Tsui EYL, Zinman B: Exercise and diabetes: new insights and therapeutic goals. *Endocrinologist* 5:263–71, 1995
88. Ruegemer JJ, Squires RW, Marsh HM, Haymond MW, Cryer PE, Rizza RA, Miles JM: Differences between prebreakfast and late afternoon glycemic responses to exercise in IDDM. *Diabetes Care* 13:104–10, 1990

David H. Wasserman, PhD, and Stephen N. Davis, MD, are from the Vanderbilt University School of Medicine, Nashville, TN. Bernard Zinman, MD, is from the University of Toronto, Toronto, Ontario, Canada.

5

Signal Transduction and Glucose Transport in Muscle

LAURIE J. GOODYEAR, PHD, AND
EDWARD S. HORTON, MD

Highlights

- Physical exercise can lower blood glucose concentrations in people with type 2 diabetes and make the contracting muscles more sensitive to insulin.
- Glucose transport is rate-limiting for glucose utilization with exercise.
- The GLUT4 glucose transporter is responsible for the majority of exercise-stimulated and insulin-stimulated glucose transport in skeletal muscle. With exercise and insulin, GLUT4 moves from inside the muscle to the cell surface (translocation).
- The intracellular signals that lead to GLUT4 translocation are distinct for exercise and insulin.
- Insulin signaling to GLUT4 translocation requires a complex series of steps that involves phosphatidylinositol 3-kinase.
- Exercise signaling to GLUT4 translocation is poorly understood, but recent evidence suggests a role for

AMP-activated protein kinase (AMPK), a metabolic fuel sensor.

- The finding that there are different signaling proteins leading to exercise- and insulin-stimulated GLUT4 translocation provides a molecular explanation for the ability of exercise to result in normal or near-normal activation of glucose transport in insulin-resistant individuals.
- The signaling molecules that mediate the ability of exercise to make the contracting muscles more sensitive to insulin in the postexercise period have not been defined.
- AMPK, or AMPK "downstream" substrates, may be good targets for pharmacological agents designed to improve glucose homeostasis in people with type 2 diabetes.

Physical exercise is a clinically important modality to decrease blood glucose concentrations in patients with diabetes. Part of the mechanism through which exercise results in lower blood glucose concentrations involves an increase in the rate of glucose transport into the contracting skeletal muscles. In addition to the acute effects of exercise in increasing glucose transport, the period after exercise is characterized by an increase in insulin sensitivity (defined as a decrease in the concentration of insulin required to achieve a submaximal rate of glucose transport). These effects of exercise on muscle glucose transport and insulin sensitivity provide important health benefits for all people and are likely to be a critical underlying mechanism for the reduced risk of diabetes in individuals who exercise regularly. In recent years, there have been significant advances in our scientific understanding of the basis for these important effects of exercise, although the precise mechanisms that mediate these phenomena are still not fully understood.

The Glucose Transport System in Skeletal Muscle

Under normal physiological conditions, glucose transport is the rate-limiting step in glucose utilization[1] (Fig. 5.1). Glucose transport occurs primarily by facilitated diffusion, an energy-independent process that uses a carrier protein for transport of a substrate across a membrane. The glucose transporter carrier proteins in mammalian tissues are a family of structurally related proteins that are expressed in a tissue-specific manner.[2] GLUT4 is the predominant isoform present in human, rat, and mouse skeletal muscle. The GLUT1 isoform has considerably lower levels of expression in skeletal muscle than GLUT4,[3,4] and there is some evidence that GLUT1 may be important in the regulation of basal rates of glucose transport.[5] GLUT5 is also expressed in skeletal muscle and is thought to primarily function as a fructose transporter with a low capacity to transport glucose.[6]

The contraction of muscle fibers that occurs when an individual exercises and stimulation by insulin are considered the major physiological mediators of glucose transport activity in muscle. The combination of exercise and insulin can have additive or partially additive effects on glucose transport,[7–9] suggesting that at some level, there are different mechanisms leading to the activation of transport by these stimuli. Numerous other factors, including catecholamines, hypoxia, growth factors, and corticosteroids, are also known to regulate glucose

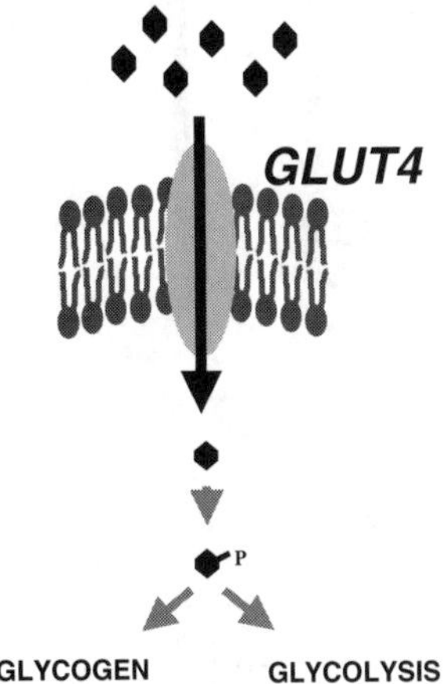

FIGURE 5.1 Skeletal muscle glucose transport system.

transport in skeletal muscle. Glucose transport in skeletal muscle follows saturation kinetics, and most reports have shown that exercise and insulin increase glucose transport through an increase in the maximal velocity of transport (V_{max}), without an appreciable change in the substrate concentration at which glucose transport is half-maximal (K_m).[10–13] This increase in transport V_{max} may occur through an increase in the rate that each carrier protein transports glucose (transporter turnover number), an increase in the number of functional glucose transporter proteins present in the plasma membrane, or both.

GLUT4 Translocation

Exercise results in the movement of glucose transporter proteins from an intracellular compartment to the surface of the cell,[14] and this "translocation" is considered to be the major mechanism by which exercise increases glucose uptake in skeletal muscle (Fig. 5.2). Sciatic nerve stimulation resulting in contraction of hindlimb skeletal muscles

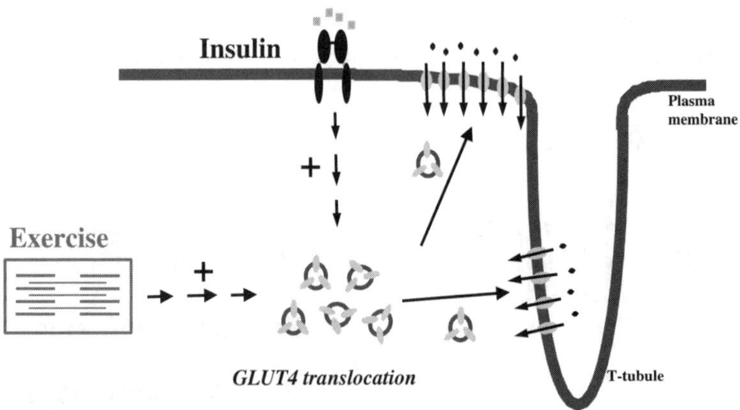

FIGURE 5.2 GLUT4 translocation in skeletal muscle. In the basal (resting) state, the majority of GLUT4 glucose transporters are sequestered within the muscle fibers in small tubulo-vesicular organelles. In response to exercise and insulin, the GLUT4-rich vesicles translocate to both the cell surface plasma membranes and the transverse tubules (T-tubules), allowing for transport of glucose into the muscle fibers. This translocation is the major mechanism by which exercise and insulin increase glucose transport in skeletal muscle.

in situ also increases the number of plasma membrane glucose transporters in the rat.[14] The exercise-induced translocation of glucose transporters is due to an increase in the plasma membrane content of the GLUT4 isoform, because a single session of exercise does not alter the abundance of plasma membrane GLUT1[15–17] or GLUT5.[18] The absolute requirement for GLUT4 in mediating glucose transport with exercise has been demonstrated in genetically manipulated mice that do not express GLUT4 in skeletal muscle (GLUT4 "knockout" mice). In these animals, a bout of treadmill running exercise does not stimulate glucose transport.[5] A significant percentage of the GLUT4 that is translocated to the cell surface with exercise associates with nonjunctional transverse tubules,[19] which may function to optimize delivery of fuel to the interior of the muscle fibers. The majority of the work done in this area comes from studies using subcellular fractionation of skeletal muscle, although subsequent studies using immunocytochemical analysis of skeletal muscle sections by electron microscopy,[20] or labeling of cell surface GLUT4 protein using a membrane-impermeable *bis*-mannose photolabel,[21,22] have confirmed that muscle contractions increase plasma membrane GLUT4 protein.

As mentioned above, insulin is the other major physiological regulator of glucose transport in skeletal muscle, and insulin also works to stimulate this process by causing GLUT4 translocation.[15,17,23,24] Because blood flow is increased during exercise, it is conceivable that the exercise-induced recruitment of GLUT4 to the plasma membrane is due to increased delivery of insulin to the working muscles. However, when a perfusion system is used to contract hindlimb skeletal muscles in situ in the total absence of insulin, plasma membrane GLUT4 is increased to a similar extent to that which occurs with exercise in vivo.[24–27] Thus, contraction can recruit GLUT4 to the plasma membrane in rat skeletal muscle independent of insulin, a finding that supports earlier reports showing that insulin is not required for muscle contraction to increase glucose uptake in skeletal muscle.[28–30]

Exercise and insulin can have additive or partially additive effects on glucose transport,[7–9,12] which may be due to an additive effect on GLUT4 recruitment to the plasma membrane.[22,27] Interestingly, some studies suggest that there are two distinct intracellular locations or "pools" of glucose transporters in skeletal muscle—one that responds to exercise and one that responds to insulin.[15,31,32] Initially, these studies showed that insulin, but not exercise, decreased glucose transporters from an intracellular microsomal membrane fraction. Subsequently, modifications of one of these methods led to the isolation of a novel intracellular membrane fraction that is sensitive to exercise,[19,33] giving further support to the hypothesis that there are separate pools of glucose transporters in skeletal muscle. Although there are different sedimentation coefficients for the insulin- and exercise-sensitive fractions, there appears to be little difference in the major protein composition of these fractions,[33] and the exact intracellular locations of the putative exercise- and insulin-stimulated GLUT4 pools have not yet been elucidated.

GLUT4 within the muscle fibers is located in small tubulovesicular organelles.[20,23] Most studies in adipose cells suggest that there is a low rate of continuous recycling of GLUT4 in the basal state and that insulin acts primarily through increasing transporter exocytosis. It is not known if the exercise-induced recruitment of GLUT4 also occurs through the regulation of vesicular exocytosis in skeletal muscle. Several proteins that are involved in regulated endocytosis or exocytosis in other tissues have also been identified as components of GLUT4-containing vesicles in skeletal muscle.[33–37] Insulin-responsive amino peptidase (IRAP) (formally gp160/vp165)[33] and vesicle-associated membrane protein-2 (VAMP-2)[34] translocate to the plasma membrane in response to physical exercise in skeletal muscle, similar to the effects of insulin. In contrast, insulin, but not exercise, results in the redistribution of Rab4,[37] a small GTP-binding protein that has also been implicated in the regulation of GLUT4 translocation in adipose cells.[38,39] The studies of Rab4 suggest that there may be distinct exercise- and insulin-stimulated GLUT4-containing vesicles that use different molecular "switches" for mobilization.

Glucose Transport and Insulin Sensitivity After Exercise

After a bout of physical activity, glucose utilization continues to remain elevated in the previously exercised muscles, primarily functioning to restore muscle glycogen concentrations. Once exercise ceases, there is a relatively slow reversal of the increase in blood flow and glucose transport, and glucose transport can remain elevated for periods of up to 1 h after the cessation of exercise. In addition, for a prolonged period of time, these muscles will be more sensitive to the actions of insulin on a range of metabolic processes, including glucose transport.

This was first demonstrated in the rat, in which using the perfused rat hindlimb model, the previously exercised muscles were more insulin sensitive for glucose uptake, even when the effects of the exercise session per se were no longer present.[40] In humans, there is also a well-characterized increase in insulin-stimulated whole-body glucose utilization after exercise,[41–44] an effect that is predominantly mediated by an increase in muscle glucose uptake.[45,46] Thus, exercise has two different effects on muscle glucose uptake: an increase in glucose uptake in skeletal muscle during and shortly after exercise and a more prolonged increase in the sensitivity of muscle glucose uptake to insulin.

Studies in both rats[47] and humans[45,46] demonstrate that the increase in insulin sensitivity with exercise is restricted to the working muscle, signifying that changes in systemic factors are not the cause of the increase in insulin sensitivity to stimulate muscle glucose uptake. However, when rat epitrochlearis muscles are removed from animals and contracted in the test tube by applying electrical stimulation, there are no systemic factors present and no changes in insulin sensitivity.[48] Based on this finding and an additional report,[49] it has been proposed that a factor released into the circulation during contractile activity is necessary for the postexercise increase in insulin sensitivity. Because there is an increase in insulin sensitivity to stimulate glucose transport in muscles of the perfused rat hindlimb after electrical stimulation,[47] it might be the paracrine action of a neurotrophic factor that initiates the events leading to the increase in insulin sensitivity after exercise.[50]

The duration of the increase in muscle insulin sensitivity after exercise depends on the intensity and duration of the exercise session and the rate of carbohydrate metabolism and glycogen resynthesis in the period after exercise. Compared with rats fed a carbohydrate-rich diet after exercise, carbohydrate-deprived animals have a more prolonged increase in insulin sensitivity to stimulate glucose transport.[51] Alternatively, if previously exercised muscles are incubated under conditions that favor enhanced glucose transport (e.g., high glucose and low insulin), exercise-induced increases in insulin sensitivity will be reduced.[52] This decrease in insulin sensitivity is not mediated by the glucose transport and phosphorylation steps, because the exercise-induced increase in insulin sensitivity is not reversed when muscles are incubated in high concentrations of the non-metabolized glucose analogue 2-deoxyglucose.[52] Importantly, enhanced insulin sensitivity can persist after glycogen resynthesis is complete, suggesting that muscle glycogen resynthesis and muscle glycogen concentrations are not the only factors responsible for the enhanced insulin action after exercise.[51]

Signaling Mechanisms Mediating Glucose Transport

The studies summarized in the previous sections clearly demonstrate that physical exercise can increase the rate of glucose transport in skeletal muscle and that the translocation of GLUT4 from an intracellular location to the plasma membrane and transverse tubules is necessary to increase transport in response to these stimuli. Another major goal has been to elucidate the cellular signals that lead to GLUT4 translocation in skeletal muscle. Elucidating these signals has been quite difficult, and we are only now beginning to understand how contracting muscle fibers regulate signal transduction processes in general and how these signals may regulate glucose transport.

Exercise Effects on Insulin-Signaling Molecules

Because both exercise and insulin increase glucose uptake through the translocation of GLUT4, several studies have determined whether these two stimuli share common signaling intermediaries. In contrast to our limited but emerging knowledge of exercise signaling, much more is known about the signaling components involved in insulin action. In skeletal muscle, insulin stimulation results in the rapid phosphorylation of tyrosine residues of the insulin receptor and the insulin receptor substrates 1 and 2 (IRS-1 and IRS-2). Phosphorylated IRS-1 and IRS-2 can then bind and activate phosphatidylinositol 3-kinase (PI 3-kinase).[53,54] Inhibition of PI 3-kinase by pharmacological blockade using wortmannin has shown that PI 3-kinase is an essential molecule for insulin-stimulated GLUT4 translocation[22] and glucose transport.[22,55–58] In contrast to these effects of insulin, exercise and contraction of hindlimb muscles in situ have no effect on tyrosine phosphorylation of the insulin receptor and IRS-1 or PI 3-kinase activity.[54] Furthermore, wortmannin does not inhibit glucose transport in isolated rat muscle incubated and contracted in vitro.[22,55,56] A study of knockout mice that do not express insulin receptors in skeletal muscles has shown that exercise can increase glucose transport normally, whereas insulin-stimulated muscle glucose transport is fully inhibited.[59] Likewise, IRS-2 knockout mice have normal rates of exercise-stimulated glucose transport.[60] Thus, while exercise and insulin both recruit GLUT4 to the plasma membrane and activate glucose transport, proximal insulin-signaling events are not necessary for exercise to increase GLUT4 translocation or glucose transport in skeletal muscle.

Calcium and Other Putative Signaling Mechanisms

Elucidating the specific molecular signaling mechanisms that result in exercise-induced glucose transport is complicated by the fact that during contraction, the muscle fibers are exposed to numerous metabolic and mechanical stimuli. A shift in the AMP/ATP ratio, changes in cell pH, and changes in the intracellular concentration of calcium and other metabolites could act as second messengers for the regulation of glucose transport with exercise. The increase in cytoplasmic calcium concentrations that occurs with muscle contraction has long been considered a critical mediator or initiator of contraction-stimulated glucose transport.[61] Some isoforms of protein kinase C (PKC) are examples of calcium-dependent signaling intermediaries, and early studies demonstrated that PKC is activated by muscle contraction.[62,63] Thus, it will be important to determine which, if any, PKC isoforms are involved in regulating contraction-stimulated glucose transport.

There is also evidence that the increase in glucose transport with muscle contraction could be mediated by an autocrine or paracrine factor. Nitric oxide is one example, being a molecule that is produced in a variety of tissues, occurring through the activation of different isoforms of nitric oxide synthase (NOS).[64] Nitric oxide has been reported to be released from isolated extensor digitorum longus muscles from the rat incubated at rest, and prior electrical stimulation used to generate contractile activity further increases nitric oxide release.[65] Exercise can activate NOS in gastrocnemius muscles,[66] providing additional evidence that nitric oxide production in skeletal muscle increases during exercise. During the last few years, it has been proposed that nitric oxide mediates exercise-stimulated glucose transport in skeletal muscle.[67,68] Exogenously administered nitric oxide, which is generated from the nitric oxide donor sodium nitroprusside, stimulates glucose transport in isolated skeletal muscles[68–70] by increasing GLUT4 translocation.[70] In studies in which rats were first exercised on a treadmill[67] or had hindlimb muscles contracted via nerve stimulation[68] followed by isolation of muscles and measurement of glucose transport, one group showed that NOS inhibition blocked exercise/contraction-stimulated glucose transport. In contrast, other groups showed that when muscles are isolated and then contracted in vitro in the presence of a NOS inhibitor, there is normal activation of contraction-stimulated glucose transport.[70,71] Thus, there is still considerable controversy as to whether nitric oxide plays a significant role in exercise-stimulated glucose transport.

Mitogen-Activated Protein Kinase Signaling

During the past several years, there has been extensive investigation among signal transduction researchers of the three parallel mitogen-activated protein (MAP) kinase cascades. These pathways, known as the MAP kinase pathway (also called extracellular signal–regulated protein kinase or ERK), the c-Jun NH_2-terminal kinase (JNK) pathway (also stress-activated protein kinase or SAPK), and the p38 kinase pathway, are activated by a variety of growth factors and/or environmental stresses.[72–74] Exercise activates the ERK signaling cascade in both rat[75] and human[76] skeletal muscle, but inhibition of MAP kinase signaling using a pharmacological blockade (PD98059) has no effect on contraction-stimulated glucose transport in vitro[77] or in the perfused hindlimb.[78] The JNK and p38 kinase signaling cascades are also stimulated by physical exercise in both rat and human skeletal muscle.[75,79–81] It is not known if these signaling cascades mediate the effects of contraction on carbohydrate metabolism, although one report has suggested that JNK signaling is involved in the regulation of insulin-stimulated glycogen synthesis in skeletal muscle.[82] To date, it has not been possible to directly determine if there is a role for JNK signaling in exercise-stimulated glucose transport because specific inhibitors to the JNK signaling cascade are not currently available. However, there are compounds that have been used to block p38 kinase signaling in vitro. Unfortunately, experiments using these agents have not provided a consensus as to whether p38 kinase signaling is involved in contraction-stimulated glucose transport.[83,84] Thus, at this point, it is clear that the ERK signaling cascade is not involved in the regulation of glucose transport in response to exercise in skeletal muscle, whereas much more work will be required to understand any putative role of JNK or p38 kinase signaling in this process. It is also important to recognize that because these signaling cascades have been implicated in the regulation of gene transcription in other cell types, activation of these pathways by each individual exercise session may function to regulate more chronic adaptations with training.

AMP-Activated Protein Kinase

The 5′AMP-activated protein kinase (AMPK) has recently been proposed to be an important mediator of exercise-stimulated glucose transport in skeletal muscle. AMPK is a heterotrimeric protein consisting of α, β, and γ subunits.[85] The α subunit is considered the catalytic subunit containing the kinase domain, and skeletal muscle expresses the two isoforms of the α subunit that have been identified (α1 and α2). Interestingly, in comparison to all other tissues, the highest expression level of the α2 isoform is found in skeletal muscle. AMPK has been proposed to act as a fuel gauge in mammalian cells.[85] When the cell senses low fuel (decreased ATP and/or decreased creatine phosphate), AMPK appears to function to switch off ATP-consuming pathways and switch on alternative pathways for ATP regeneration.

Exercise will alter the fuel status of skeletal muscle, and depending on the intensity of the contractions, there will be significant decreases in both creatine phosphate and ATP concentrations. Thus, exercise should be a potent stimulus for the activation of AMPK in working skeletal muscles. Studies using treadmill running exercise in rats[86,87] and contraction of rat hindlimb muscles[88] provided the first evidence that these in vivo stimuli increase AMPK activity. Subsequent studies have demonstrated that contraction of isolated rat skeletal muscles in vitro in the absence of systemic factors increases AMPK activity,[89,90] and the greater the force production generated by contraction, the greater the increase in AMPK.[91] In humans, moderate-intensity cycle exercise (70% VO_{2max}) has now been shown to increase AMPK activity in the vastus lateralis muscle.[92]

The hypothesis that AMPK mediates contraction-stimulated glucose transport has come primarily from studies using 5-aminoimidazole-4-carboxamide ribonucleoside (AICAR). AICAR is a compound that is taken up into skeletal muscle and metabolized by adenosine kinase to form ZMP, the monophosphorylated derivative that mimics the effects of AMP on AMPK.[89,93] AICAR infusion enhances insulin-stimulated glucose transport in the perfused rat hindlimb skeletal muscle.[93] The ability of AICAR to stimulate glucose transport in the presence of insulin is similar to the additive effects of contraction plus insulin that were discussed above. AICAR also increases glucose transport in rat epitrochlearis muscles incubated in vitro in the total absence of insulin.[89,94] Similar to contraction-stimulated transport, AICAR-stimulated transport is not inhibited by wortmannin.[89,94] In addition, the increase in glucose transport with the combination of maximal AICAR plus maximal insulin treatments is partially additive, whereas there is no additive effect on glucose transport with the combination of AICAR plus contraction.[89,94] Infusion of rats in vivo with AICAR (and glucose to maintain euglycemia) also increased glucose transport by more than twofold in soleus, medial, and lateral gastrocnemius muscles.[94] Interestingly, circulating lactate levels were increased ~10-fold in response to the AICAR infusion, which may reflect the effects of AICAR to inhibit hepatic gluconeogenesis along with a greatly enhanced rate of glycolysis in the muscle.[93] Thus, AICAR and contraction appear to share a similar, insulin-independent signaling mechanism, consistent with the hypothesis that AMPK is an intermediary in the signaling cascade leading to contraction-stimulated glucose transport.

The studies discussed above support a role for AMPK in regulating glucose transport, but clearly much more work is needed in this area. In fact, one report suggests a dissociation of glucose transport and AMPK activity in contracting skeletal muscle.[95] In this study, contraction did not increase AMPK activity in soleus muscles that had high glycogen levels, but contraction did have some effect on increasing glucose transport. Furthermore, recent generation of a transgenic mouse expressing an inactive (dominant-negative) AMPK protein has suggested that AMPK may only be part of the mechanism leading to contraction-stimulated glucose transport. Glucose transport in response to electrically stimulated contractions of hindlimb muscles was reduced by only 30% in these mice (M.J. Birnbaum, personal communication). Much more work on the role of AMPK in contraction-stimulated glucose transport and insulin sensitivity is necessary to understand the precise role of this important signaling molecule in skeletal muscle. However, at this time, it appears that although AMPK is important in regulating exercise-stimulated glucose transport, there are additional signaling molecules that contribute to the stimulation of GLUT4 translocation in contracting muscle.

Signals Mediating Postexercise Insulin Sensitivity

Earlier in this chapter, it was clearly established that exercise per se does not activate proximal signaling molecules.[54,96] On the other hand, it is not inconceivable that the postexercise period is characterized by modulation of some aspects of insulin signaling, especially under conditions in which insulin concentrations are increased. Several years ago, it was hypothesized that the underlying molecular mechanism for the changes in insulin action involved enhanced insulin signaling in the exercised muscles. Paradoxically, however, there was a small decrease in maximally insulin-stimulated insulin receptor and IRS-1 tyrosine phosphorylation after contraction of rat hindlimb in situ.[54] Furthermore, there was a distinct blunting of insulin-stimulated PI 3-kinase activity assayed in anti–IRS-1 immune complexes.[54] Similarly, in humans, it was shown that there is a 50% decrease in IRS-1–associated PI 3-kinase activity in the muscle from the prior exercised leg. Thus, the lack of enhancement in insulin-stimulated IRS-1–associated PI 3-kinase activity after exercise is consistent in both humans[45] and rat[97] skeletal muscle.

In contrast to this report, a more recent study in rats[98] and our own observations in mice[59] suggest that immediately after treadmill exercise, the increase in insulin responsiveness to stimulate muscle glucose transport is associated with an increase in insulin-stimulated PI 3-kinase activity found in a general phosphotyrosine protein immunoprecipitate. However, this enhanced activation by insulin is not associated with a greater increase in IRS-1–associated PI 3-kinase, similar to the studies described above. This suggests that there is another yet unidentified tyrosine phosphorylated protein that is activated by exercise. Elucidating this protein may provide important insight into understanding the cellular mechanism that regulates enhanced postexercise insulin action.

Summary and Future Directions

It is now well established that physical exercise and insulin can increase the rate of glucose transport in skeletal muscle and that GLUT4 translocation from an intracellular location to the plasma membrane and transverse tubules is necessary to increase transport with these stimuli (Fig. 5.3). Although exercise and insulin are similar in this respect, there are several lines of evidence to suggest that the underlying mechanisms

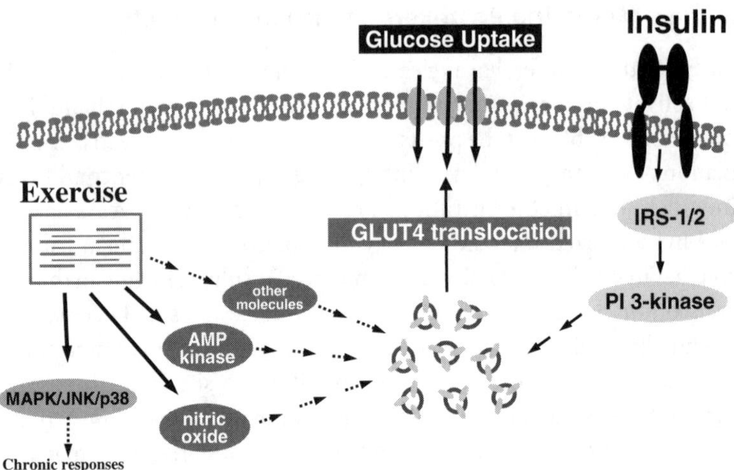

FIGURE 5.3 Exercise and insulin signaling in skeletal muscle. Exercise and insulin use distinct signaling mechanisms leading to GLUT4 translocation. PI 3-kinase is necessary for insulin-stimulated GLUT4 translocation and glucose transport but not for exercise-stimulated translocation and transport. Exercise is now known to activate a number of intracellular signaling molecules, some of which are likely to lead to the chronic adaptations to exercise and others to the regulation of glucose transport. There is good evidence of the role of AMPK in exercise signaling to GLUT4 translocation, although more studies are needed to definitively prove this hypothesis. Nitric oxide and other molecules not yet defined may also play a part in this response.

leading to insulin- and exercise-stimulated GLUT4 translocation are distinct. For example, contraction of isolated skeletal muscle in vitro can stimulate GLUT4 translocation in the absence of insulin, the combination of contraction and insulin can have additive or partially additive effects on glucose transport, and some studies suggest there are different intracellular pools of glucose transporters. Furthermore, in the insulin-resistant Zucker (*fa/fa*) rat[99,100] and in human patients with type 2 diabetes,[101,102] insulin-stimulated GLUT4 translocation is impaired,[99,102] but exercise-stimulated GLUT4 translocation is normal,[100] suggesting that exercise might be able to bypass defects in insulin signaling. All of these findings provide evidence that exercise and insulin stimulate GLUT4 translocation and glucose transport by different mechanisms. A major challenge has been to elucidate the molecules or cascade of molecules that signal GLUT4 to translocate by this insulin-independent, exercise-stimulated signaling pathway.

Over the last few years, AMPK has emerged as an important molecule for the regulation of multiple metabolic processes in skeletal muscle in response to exercise. Exercise and muscle contraction increase AMPK activity, perhaps functioning to increase ATP regeneration in contracting muscle by enhancing the rate of glucose transport. Determining the downstream substrate(s) for AMPK in mediating the putative effects of the enzyme on glucose transport is an important goal for future studies. Although the study of AMPK in skeletal muscle is an exciting area of investigation that should lead to a better understanding of the important effects of exercise in regulating glucose homeostasis, it appears that there are other signaling mechanisms that contribute to glucose transport regulation during exercise. Ultimately, work in this area will elucidate the molecular mechanisms that enable exercise to have these beneficial effects on glucose transport in skeletal muscle.

Acknowledgments

Studies from L.J.G.'s laboratory were supported by grants from the National Institute of Arthritis Musculoskeletal and Skin Diseases (AR42238 and AR45670) and the American Diabetes Association.

References

1. Kubo K, Foley JE: Rate-limiting steps for insulin-mediated glucose uptake into perfused rat hindlimb. *Am J Physiol* 250:E100–02, 1986
2. Bell GI, Burant CF, Takeda J, Gould GW: Structure and function of mammalian facilitative sugar transporters. *J Biol Chem* 268: 19161–64, 1993
3. Klip A, Paquet MR: Glucose transport and glucose transporters in muscle and their metabolic regulation. *Diabetes Care* 13:228–42, 1990
4. Kayano T, Burant CF, Fukumoto H, Gould GW, Fan Y, Eddy RL, Byers MG, Shows TB, Seino S, Bell GI, Fan YS: Human facilitative glucose transporters: isolation, functional characterization, and gene localization of cDNAs encoding an isoform (GLUT5) expressed in small intestine, kidney, muscle, and adipose tissue and an unusual glucose transporter pseudogene-like sequence (GLUT6). *J Biol Chem* 265:13276–82, 1990
5. Zisman A, Peroni OD, Abel ED, Michael MD, Mauvais-Jarvis F, Lowell BB, Wojtaszewski JF, Hirshman MF, Virkamaki A, Goodyear LJ, Kahn CR, Kahn BB: Targeted disruption of the

glucose transporter 4 selectively in muscle causes insulin resistance and glucose intolerance. *Nat Med* 6:924–28, 2000

6. Burant CF, Takeda J, Brot-Laroche E, Bell GI, Davidson NO: Fructose transporter in human spermatozoa and small intestine is Glut-5. *J Biol Chem* 267:14523–26, 1992
7. Garetto LP, Richter EA, Goodman MN, Ruderman NB: Enhanced muscle glucose metabolism after exercise in the rat: the two phases. *Am J Physiol* 246:E471–75, 1984
8. Wallberg-Henriksson H, Constable SH, Young DA, Holloszy JO: Glucose transport into rat skeletal muscle: interaction between exercise and insulin. *J Appl Physiol* 65:909–13, 1988
9. Zorzano A, Balon TW, Goodman MN, Ruderman NB: Additive effects of prior exercise and insulin on glucose and AIB uptake by rat muscle. *Am J Physiol* 251:E21–26, 1986
10. Narahara HT, Ozand P, Cori CF: Studies of tissue permeability. VII. The effect of insulin on glucose penetration and phosphorylation in frog muscle. *J Biol Chem* 235:3370–78, 1960
11. Holloszy JO, Narahara HT: Changes in permeability to 3-methylglucose associated with contraction of isolated frog muscle. *J Biol Chem* 240:3493–3500, 1965
12. Nesher R, Karl IE, Kipnis DM: Dissociation of effects of insulin and contraction on glucose transport in rat epitrochlearis muscle. *Am J Physiol* 249:C226–32, 1985
13. Hansen P, Gulve E, Gao J, Schluter J, Mueckler M, Holloszy J: Kinetics of 2-deoxyglucose transport in skeletal muscle: effects of insulin and contractions. *Am J Physiol* 268:C30–35, 1995
14. Hayashi T, Wojtaszewski JF, Goodyear LJ: Exercise regulation of glucose transport in skeletal muscle. *Am J Physiol* 273:E1039–51, 1997
15. Douen AG, Ramlal T, Cartee GD, Klip A: Exercise modulates the insulin-induced translocation of glucose transporters in rat skeletal muscle. *FEBS Lett* 261:256–60, 1990
16. Goodyear LJ, Hirshman MF, Horton ES: Exercise induced translocation of skeletal muscle glucose transporters. *Am J Physiol* 261:E795–99, 1991
17. Goodyear LJ, Hirshman MF, Smith RJ, Horton ES: Glucose transporter number, activity and isoform content in plasma membranes of red and white skeletal muscle. *Am J Physiol* 261:E556–61, 1991

18. Hundal HS, Darakhshan F, Kristiansen S, Blakemore SJ, Richter EA: GLUT5 expression and fructose transport in human skeletal muscle. *Adv Exp Med Biol* 441:35–45, 1998
19. Roy D, Marette A: Exercise induces the translocation of GLUT4 to transverse tubules from an intracellular pool in rat skeletal muscle. *Biochem Biophys Res Commun* 223:147–52, 1996
20. Rodnick KJ, Slot JW, Studelska DR, Hanpeter DE, Robinson LJ, Geuze HJ, James DE: Immunocytochemical and biochemical studies of GLUT4 in rat skeletal muscle. *J Biol Chem* 267:6278–85, 1992
21. Wilson CM, Cushman SW: Insulin stimulation of glucose transport activity in rat skeletal muscle: increase in cell surface GLUT4 as assessed by photolabelling. *Biochem J* 299:755–59, 1994
22. Lund S, Holman GD, Schmitz O, Pedersen O: Contraction stimulates translocation of glucose transporter GLUT4 in skeletal muscle through a mechanism distinct from that of insulin. *Proc Natl Acad Sci U S A* 92:5817–21, 1995
23. Hirshman MF, Goodyear LJ, Wardzala LJ, Horton ED, Horton ES: Identification of an intracellular pool of glucose transporters from basal and insulin-stimulated rat skeletal muscle. *J Biol Chem* 265:987–91, 1990
24. Goodyear LJ, King PA, Hirshman MF, Thompson CM, Horton ED, Horton ES: Contractile activity increases plasma membrane glucose transporters in absence of insulin. *Am J Physiol* 258:E667–72, 1990
25. Etgen GJ Jr, Memon AR, Thompson GA Jr, Ivy JL: Insulin- and contraction-stimulated translocation of GTP-binding proteins and GLUT4 protein in skeletal muscle. *J Biol Chem* 268:20164–69, 1993
26. Brozinick JT Jr, Etgen GJ Jr, Yaspelkis BB, Ivy JL: The effects of muscle contraction and insulin on glucose-transporter translocation in rat skeletal muscle. *Biochem J* 297:539–45, 1994
27. Gao J, Ren J, Gulve EA, Holloszy JO: Additive effect of contractions and insulin on GLUT-4 translocation into the sarcolemma. *J Appl Physiol* 77:1597–1601, 1994
28. Ploug T, Galbo H, Richter EA: Increased muscle glucose uptake during contractions: no need for insulin. *Am J Physiol* 247: E726–31, 1984
29. Richter EA, Ploug T, Glabo H: Increased muscle glucose uptake after exercise: no need for insulin during exercise. *Diabetes* 34: 1041–48, 1985

30. Wallberg-Henriksson H, Holloszy JO: Activation of glucose transport in diabetic muscle: responses to contraction and insulin. *Am J Physiol* 249:C233–37, 1985
31. Douen AG, Ramlal T, Klip A, Young DA, Cartee GD, Holloszy JO: Exercise-induced increase in glucose transporters in plasma membranes of rat skeletal muscle. *Endocrinology* 124:449–54, 1989
32. Douen AG, Ramlal T, Rastogi S, Bilan PJ, Cartee GD, Vranic M, Holloszy JO, Klip A: Exercise induces recruitment of the "insulin-responsive glucose transporter": evidence for distinct intracellular insulin- and exercise-recruitable transporter pools in skeletal muscle. *J Biol Chem* 265:13427–30, 1990
33. Coderre L, Kandror KV, Vallega G, Pilch PF: Identification and characterization of an exercise-sensitive pool of glucose transporters in skeletal muscle. *J Biol Chem* 270:27584–88, 1995
34. Kristiansen S, Hargreaves M, Richter EA: Exercise-induced increase in glucose transport, GLUT-4, and VAMP-2 in plasma membrane from human muscle. *Am J Physiol* 270:E197–201, 1996
35. Volchuk A, Mitsumoto Y, He L, Liu Z, Habermann E, Trimble W, Klip A: Expression of vesicle-associated membrane protein 2 (VAMP-2)/synaptobrevin II and cellubrevin in rat skeletal muscle and in a muscle cell line. *Biochem J* 304:139–45, 1994
36. Mastick CC, Aebersold R, Lienhard GE: Characterization of a major protein in GLUT4 vesicles. *J Biol Chem* 269:6089–92, 1994
37. Sherman LA, Hirshman MF, Cormont M, Le Marchand-Brustel Y, Goodyear LJ: Differential effects of insulin and exercise on Rab4 distribution in rat skeletal muscle. *Endocrinology* 137:266–73, 1996
38. Cormont M, Tanti J-F, Zahraoui A, Van Obberghen E, Tavitian A, Le Marchand-Brustel Y: Insulin and okadaic acid induce Rab4 redistribution in adipocytes. *J Biol Chem* 268:19491–97, 1993
39. Shibata H, Omata W, Suzuki Y, Tankaka T, Kojima I, Tanaka S: A synthetic peptide corresponding to the Rab4 hypervariable carboxyl-terminal domain inhibits insulin action on glucose transport in rat adipocytes. *J Biol Chem* 271:9704–09, 1996
40. Richter EA, Garetto LP, Goodman MN, Ruderman NB: Muscle glucose metabolism following exercise in the rat: increased sensitivity to insulin. *J Clin Invest* 69:785–93, 1982
41. Bogardus C, Thuillex P, Ravussin E, Vasquez B, Narimiga M, Ashar S: Effect of muscle glycogen depletion on in vivo insulin action in man. *J Clin Invest* 72:1605–10, 1983

42. Devlin JT, Hirshman MF, Horton ES, Horton ED: Enhanced peripheral and splanchnic insulin sensitivity in NIDDM men after single bout of exercise. *Diabetes* 36:434–39, 1987
43. Mikines KJ, Sonne B, Farrell PA, Tronier B, Galbo H: Effect of physical exercise on sensitivity and responsiveness to insulin in humans. *Am J Physiol* 254:E248–59, 1988
44. Perseghin G, Price TB, Petersen KF, Roden M, Cline GW, Gerow K, Rothman DL, Shulman GL: Increased glucose transport-phosphorylation and muscle glycogen synthesis after exercise training in insulin-resistant subjects. *N Engl J Med* 335:1357–62, 1996
45. Wojtaszewski JF, Hansen BF, Kiens B, Richter EA: Insulin signaling in human skeletal muscle: time course and effect of exercise. *Diabetes* 46:1775–81, 1997
46. Richter EA, Mikines KJ, Galbo H, Kiens B: Effect of exercise on insulin action in human skeletal muscle. *J Appl Physiol* 66:876–85, 1989
47. Richter EA, Garreto LP, Goodman MN, Ruderman NB, Garetto LP: Enhanced muscle glucose metabolism after exercise: modulation by local factors. *Am J Physiol* 246:E476–82, 1984
48. Cartee GD, Holloszy JO: Exercise increases susceptibility of muscle glucose transport to activation by various stimuli. *Am J Physiol* 258:E390–93, 1990
49. Gao J, Gulve EA, Holloszy JO: Contraction-induced increase in muscle insulin sensitivity: requirement for a serum factor. *Am J Physiol* 266:E186–92, 1994
50. Richter EA: Glucose utilization. In *Exercise: Regulation and Integration of Multiple Systems.* Rowell LB, Shepherd JT, Eds. New York, Oxford University Press, 1996, p. 912–51
51. Cartee GD, Young DA, Sleeper MD, Zierath J, Wallberg-Henriksson H, Holloszy JO: Prolonged increase in insulin-stimulated glucose transport in muscle after exercise. *Am J Physiol* 256:E494–99, 1989
52. Gulve EA, Cartee GD, Zierath J, Corpus VM, Holloszy JO: Reversal of enhanced muscle glucose transport after exercise: roles of insulin and glucose. *Am J Physiol* 259:E685–91, 1990
53. Folli F, Saad MJA, Backer JM, Kahn CR, Saad MJ: Insulin stimulation of phosphatidylinositol 3-kinase activity and association with insulin receptor substrate 1 in liver and muscle of the intact rat. *J Biol Chem* 267:22171–77, 1992

54. Goodyear LJ, Giorgino F, Balon TW, Condorelli G, Smith RJ: Effects of contractile activity on tyrosine phosphoproteins and phosphatidylinositol 3-kinase activity in rat skeletal muscle. *Am J Physiol* 268:E987–95, 1995
55. Lee AD, Hansen PA, Holloszy JO: Wortmannin inhibits insulin-stimulated but not contraction-stimulated glucose transport activity in skeletal muscle. *FEBS Lett* 361:51–54, 1995
56. Yeh JI, Gulve EA, Rameh L, Birnbaum MJ: The effects of wortmannin on rat skeletal muscle: dissociation of signaling pathways for insulin- and contraction-activated hexose transport. *J Biol Chem* 270:2107–11, 1995
57. Le Marchand-Brustel Y, Gautier N, Cormont M, Van Obberghen E: Wortmannin inhibits the action of insulin but not that of okadaic acid in skeletal muscle: comparison with fat cells. *Endocrinology* 136:3564–70, 1995
58. Wojtaszewski JFP, Hansen BF, Urso B, Richter EA: Wortmannin inhibits both insulin- and contraction-stimulated glucose uptake and transport in rat skeletal muscle. *J Appl Physiol* 81:1501–09, 1996
59. Wojtaszewski JF, Higaki Y, Hirshman MF, Michael MD, Dufresne SD, Kahn CR, Goodyear LJ: Exercise modulates postreceptor insulin signaling and glucose transport in muscle-specific insulin receptor knockout mice. *J Clin Invest* 104:1257–64, 1999
60. Higaki Y, Wojtaszewski JFP, Hirshman MF, Withers DJ, Towery H, White MF, Goodyear LJ: Insulin receptor substrate-2 is not necessary for insulin- and exercise-stimulated glucose transport in skeletal muscle. *J Biol Chem* 274:20791–95, 1999
61. Holloszy JO, Constable SH, Young DA: Activation of glucose transport in muscle by exercise. *Diabetes Metab Rev* 1:409–24, 1986
62. Richter EA, Cleland PJF, Rattigan S, Clark MG, Cleland PJ: Contraction-associated translocation of protein kinase C in rat skeletal muscle. *FEBS Lett* 217:232–36, 1987
63. Cleland PJ, Appleby GJ, Rattigan S, Clark MG: Exercise-induced translocation of protein kinase C and production of diacylglycerol and phosphatidic acid in rat skeletal muscle in vivo: relationship to changes in glucose transport. *J Biol Chem* 264:17704–11, 1989
64. Moncada S, Higgs A: The L-arginine-nitric oxide pathway. *N Engl J Med* 329:2002–12, 1993

65. Balon TW, Nadler JL: Nitric oxide release is present from incubated skeletal muscle preparations. *Am J Physiol* 77:2519–21, 1994
66. Roberts CK, Barnard RJ, Jasman A, Balon TW: Acute exercise increases nitric oxide synthase activity in skeletal muscle. *Am J Physiol* 277:E390–94, 1999
67. Roberts CK, Barnard RJ, Scheck SH, Balon TW: Exercise-stimulated glucose transport in skeletal muscle is nitric oxide dependent. *Am J Physiol* 273:E220–25, 1997
68. Balon TW, Nadler JL: Evidence that nitric oxide increases glucose transport in skeletal muscle. *J Appl Physiol* 82:359–63, 1997
69. Young ME, Radda GK, Leighton B: Nitric oxide stimulates glucose transport and metabolism in rat skeletal muscle in vitro. *Biochem J* 322:223–28, 1997
70. Etgen GJ Jr, Fryburg DA, Gibbs EM: Nitric oxide stimulates skeletal muscle glucose transport through a calcium/contraction- and phosphatidylinositol-3-kinase-independent pathway. *Diabetes* 46:1915–19, 1997
71. Higaki Y, Hirshman MF, Fujii N, Goodyear LJ: Nitric oxide increases glucose uptake through a mechanism that is distinct from the insulin and contraction pathways in rat skeletal muscle. *Diabetes* 50:241–47, 2001
72. Cano E, Mahadevan LC: Parallel signal processing among mammalian MAPKs. *Trends Biochem Sci* 20:117–22, 1995
73. Davis RJ: MAPKs: new JNK expands the group. *Trends Biochem Sci* 19:470–73, 1994
74. Marshall CJ: Specificity of receptor tyrosine kinase signaling: transient versus sustained extracellular signal-regulated kinase activation. *Cell* 80:179–85, 1995
75. Goodyear LJ, Chung P-Y, Sherwood D, Dufresne SD, Moller DE: Effects of exercise and insulin on mitogen-activated protein kinase signaling pathways in rat skeletal muscle. *Am J Physiol* 271:E403–08, 1996
76. Aronson D, Violan MA, Dufresne SD, Zangen D, Fielding RA, Goodyear LJ: Exercise stimulates the mitogen-activated protein kinase pathway in human skeletal muscle. *J Clin Invest* 99:1251–57, 1997
77. Hayashi T, Hirshman MF, Dufresne SD, Goodyear LJ: Skeletal muscle contractile activity in vitro stimulates mitogen-activated protein kinase signaling. *Am J Physiol* 277:C701–07, 1999

78. Wojtaszewski JF, Lynge J, Jakobsen AB, Goodyear LJ, Richter EA: Differential regulation of MAP kinase by contraction and insulin in skeletal muscle: metabolic implications. *Am J Physiol* 277:E724–32, 1999
79. Boppart MD, Asp S, Wojtaszewski JF, Fielding RA, Mohr T, Goodyear LJ: Marathon running transiently increases c-Jun NH2-terminal kinase and p38 activities in human skeletal muscle. *J Physiol (Lond)* 526:663–69, 2000
80. Aronson D, Boppart MD, Dufresne SD, Fielding RA, Goodyear LJ: Exercise stimulates c-Jun NH_2 kinase activity and c-Jun transcriptional activity in human skeletal muscle. *Biochem Biophys Res Commun* 251:106–10, 1998
81. Boppart MD, Aronson D, Gibson L, Roubenoff R, Abad LW, Bean J, Goodyear LJ, Fielding RA: Eccentric exercise markedly increases c-Jun NH_2-terminal kinase activity in human skeletal muscle. *J Appl Physiol* 87:1668–73, 1999
82. Moxham CM, Tabrizchi A, Davis RJ, Malbon CC: Jun N-terminal kinase mediates activation of skeletal muscle glycogen synthase by insulin in vivo. *J Biol Chem* 271:30765–73, 1996
83. Fukuwatari T, Boppart MD, Hirshman MF, Goodyear LJ: Insulin does not increase p38 MAP kinase activity or phosphorylation in rat skeletal muscle (Abstract). *Diabetes* 49 (Suppl. 1): A15, 2000
84. Somwar R, Perreault M, Kapur S, Taha C, Sweeney G, Ramlal T, Kim DY, Keen J, Cote CH, Klip A, Marette A: Activation of p38 mitogen-activated protein kinase alpha and beta by insulin and contraction in rat skeletal muscle: potential role in the stimulation of glucose transport. *Diabetes* 49:1794–1800, 2000
85. Hardie DG, Carling D, Carlson M: The AMP-activated/SNF1 protein kinase subfamily: metabolic sensors of the eukaryotic cell? *Annu Rev Biochem* 67:821–55, 1998
86. Winder WW, Hardie DG: Inactivation of acetyl-CoA carboxylase and activation of AMP-activated protein kinase in muscle during exercise. *Am J Physiol* 270:E299–304, 1996
87. Rasmussen BB, Winder WW: Effect of exercise intensity on skeletal muscle malonyl-CoA and acetyl-CoA carboxylase. *J Appl Physiol* 83:1104–09, 1997
88. Vavvas D, Apazidis A, Saha AK, Gamble J, Patel A, Kemp BE, Witters LA, Ruderman NB: Contraction-induced changes in

acetyl-CoA carboxylase and 5′-AMP-activated kinase in skeletal muscle. *J Biol Chem* 272:13255–61, 1997

89. Hayashi T, Hirshman MF, Kurth EJ, Winder WW, Goodyear LJ: Evidence for 5′ AMP-activated protein kinase mediation of the effect of muscle contraction on glucose transport. *Diabetes* 47: 1369–73, 1998
90. Hayashi T, Hirshman MF, Fujii N, Habinowski SA, Witters LA, Goodyear LJ: Metabolic stress and altered glucose transport: activation of AMP-activated protein kinase as a unifying coupling mechanism. *Diabetes* 49:527–31, 2000
91. Ihlemann J, Ploug T, Hellsten Y, Galbo H: Effect of tension on contraction-induced glucose transport in rat skeletal muscle. *Am J Physiol* 277:E208–14, 1999
92. Fujii N, Hayashi T, Hirshman MF, Smith JT, Habinowski SA, Kaijser L, Mu J, Ljungqvist O, Birnbaum MJ, Witters LA, Thorell A, Goodyear LJ: Exercise induces isoform-specific increase in 5′AMP-activated protein kinase activity in human skeletal muscle. *Biochem Biophys Res Commun* 273:1150–55, 2000
93. Merrill GF, Kurth EJ, Hardie DG, Winder WW: AICA riboside increases AMP-activated protein kinase, fatty acid oxidation, and glucose uptake in rat muscle. *Am J Physiol* 273:E1107–12, 1997
94. Bergeron R, Russell RR III, Young LH, Ren JM, Marcucci M, Lee A, Shulman GI: Effect of AMPK activation on muscle glucose metabolism in conscious rats. *Am J Physiol* 276:E938–44, 1999
95. Derave W, Ai H, Ihlemann J, Witters LA, Kristiansen S, Richter EA, Ploug T: Dissociation of AMP-activated protein kinase activation and glucose transport in contracting slow-twitch muscle. *Diabetes* 49:1281–87, 2000
96. Lund S, Pryor PR, Ostergaard S, Schmitz O, Pedersen O, Holman GD: Evidence against protein kinase B as a mediator of contraction-induced glucose transport and GLUT4 translocation in rat skeletal muscle. *FEBS Lett* 425:472–74, 1998
97. Lowell BB: Fat metabolism: slimming with leaner enzyme. *Nature* 382:585–86, 1996
98. Hickey MS, Tanner CJ, O'Neill DS, Morgan LJ, Dohm GL, Houmard JA: Insulin activation of phosphatidylinositol 3-kinase in human skeletal muscle in vivo. *J Appl Physiol* 83:718–22, 1997
99. King PA, Horton ED, Hirshman MF, Horton ES: Insulin resistance in obese Zucker rat (fa/fa) skeletal muscle is associated

with a failure of glucose transporter translocation. *J Clin Invest* 90:1568–75, 1992

100. King PA, Betts JJ, Horton ED, Horton ES: Exercise, unlike insulin, promotes glucose transporter translocation in obese Zucker rat muscle. *Am J Physiol* 265:R447–52, 1993
101. Kennedy JW, Hirshman MF, Gervino EV, Ocel JV, Forse RA, Hoenig SJ, Aronson D, Goodyear LJ, Horton ES: Acute exercise induces GLUT4 translocation in skeletal muscle of normal human subjects and subjects with type 2 diabetes. *Diabetes* 48: 1192–97, 1999
102. Zierath JR, Krook A, Wallberg-Henriksson H: Insulin action in skeletal muscle from patients with NIDDM. *Mol Cell Biochem* 182:153–60, 1998

Laurie J. Goodyear, PhD, and Edward S. Horton, MD, are from the Joslin Diabetes Center, Brigham and Women's Hospital, and Harvard Medical School, Boston, MA.

6

Psychological Benefits of Exercise

S. TZIPORAH COHEN, BA, AND
ALAN M. JACOBSON, MD

Highlights

- Exercise can have important effects on mental health for individuals with and without psychiatric disorders.
- Regular exercise can have an antidepressant effect in patients with mild to moderate depressive disorders.
- Aerobic exercise can reduce anxiety levels acutely, and regular exercise may have a role in reducing chronic anxiety in individuals with anxiety disorders.
- Emotionally healthy individuals who exercise regularly report improved mood, sense of well-being, and self-esteem.
- Rarely, exercise may have negative psychological effects, such as exercise addiction.
- It is not known how often or for how long individuals should exercise to achieve optimal psychological benefit.
- Adherence to exercise regimens is problematic; 50% of those beginning an exercise program will drop out.

- Little is known about predicting adherence to exercise programs.
- Patients with diabetes, like healthy individuals, can benefit emotionally as well as physically from regular exercise.

Although the physical benefits of regular exercise are well known, important psychological effects need to be considered. These include possible benefits for *1*) individuals with psychiatric disorders, *2*) emotionally healthy individuals, and *3*) individuals who may be at risk for future psychiatric disorders.

Initial interest in the effects of exercise on mental health was spurred by the finding of an inverse relationship between an individual's level of physical fitness and the presence of psychopathology; more physically fit individuals generally showed lower degrees of psychopathology.[1] Although only a cross-sectional association, subsequent studies examined whether exercise was effective in actually lowering the degree of psychopathology in affected individuals.

An increasing number of studies have now examined the effects of exercise on psychological functioning, looking for effects on anxiety, depression, self-esteem and self-concept, and general sense of well-being. Most of these studies have looked at aerobic exercise, such as running or aerobics classes, and have involved nonclinical as well as clinical populations. A few have looked at nonaerobic exercise, such as weight training or yoga. In this chapter, we briefly summarize some of these findings and address some important clinical issues in the use of exercise in the treatment of emotional distress. Although these studies were not done in diabetic populations, their findings are likely to be useful for and applicable to individuals with diabetes.

Effects of Exercise on Individuals With Psychiatric Disorders

The effects of exercise on mood and anxiety disorders have been fairly well established. Regular exercise has an antidepressant effect in patients with mild to moderate unipolar depressive disorders.[2–4] This effect is seen with both aerobic and nonaerobic forms of exercise and thus seems to be independent of any change in aerobic fitness. Preliminary evidence shows that exercise may be as effective as some psychotherapies in treating depression.[5,6] Another study showed positive effects of exercise on hospitalized depressed patients, with regular aerobic exercise having an antidepressant effect.[7] A meta-analysis of 15 studies examining depressed patients found a statistically significant decrease in depression scores in exercisers versus nonexercisers.[8] Importantly, however, exercise has not been evaluated in severely depressed patients, e.g., those with severe psychomotor retardation or psychotic symptoms. In the studies cited above, patients were excluded if they were psychotic or thought to have a high suicide risk. There is no evidence that exercise alone is adequate to treat severe depression, and exercise should not be used in place of traditional therapies, but rather as an adjunct.

Aerobic exercise apparently has an anxiolytic effect as well. Studies measuring anxiety generally focus on either trait anxiety (the general predisposition of an individual to respond across many situations with high levels of anxiety) or state anxiety (the more specific measure of an individual's anxiety at a particular moment).[9,10] In studies that measured state anxiety, aerobic exercise 20–40 min in duration resulted in decreased anxiety for up to 4 h after exercise.[9,11] One study also suggested that aerobic exercise can be beneficial for patients with panic disorders.[12] At least two meta-analyses examining the effect of aerobic exercise on anxiety found a significant decrease in state and trait anxiety in the exercisers, although the effects were limited to men.[9,13] As in the depression studies, this decrease in anxiety has been shown to be independent of any increase in aerobic fitness.[14]

Effects of Exercise in Emotionally Healthy Individuals

A few studies suggest that exercise may reduce normal feelings of depression and anxiety among individuals without a history of psychiatric illness. In one study of healthy adults without psychiatric disorders, 10 weeks of regular aerobic exercise (walking or running for 1 h, three times per week) decreased state and trait anxiety, tension, depressive feelings, and fatigue in exercisers compared with a control group.[15] A more recent study comparing similar aerobic exercise to yoga and a wait-list control group showed aerobic exercise to be associated with reduced depression and anxiety. In addition, the subjects in the exercise and yoga groups reported improved mood, self-confidence, and life satisfaction and better family relationships and sex lives.[16] In a study of college students, regular exercise was associated with decreased anger, fatigue, hostility, and inertia, as well as improved sleep.[17] Even in studies where no objective difference was seen, the majority of subjects reported "feeling better" and experiencing feelings of "exhilaration" after exercise—evidence of a possible effect that is not picked up by traditional measures.[18] In general, however, exercise has less of a psychological effect on emotionally healthy individuals than on individuals with psychiatric disorders such as depression or anxiety.[8] It is important to remember that exercise does not make psychologically normal people supernormal, much as antidepressants do not make nondepressed individuals euphoric.

In addition to having beneficial effects on specific symptoms of anxiety and depression, research indicates that exercise is associated with an improved sense of well-being, self-esteem, and self-efficacy.[10,19,20] A meta-analysis of 37 studies of the effect of exercise on self-concept (defined as how one sees oneself, including variables such as self-esteem, self-image, self-awareness, and self-ideal) found a significant increase in self-concept scores of exercisers versus nonexercisers.[8]

If exercise improves well-being in healthy individuals and reduces symptoms in patients with psychiatric disorders, could exercise prevent or slow the onset of psychiatric disorders? One theory suggests that the acute decrease in depression and anxiety after exercise might prevent the development of chronic depression or anxiety.[21] Unfortunately, no studies have examined this intriguing hypothesis, and no evidence exists to suggest exercise can prevent the onset of depressive or anxiety disorders.

Negative Effects of Exercise

Exercise may have negative psychological consequences in some individuals. A small subgroup of individuals may begin to exercise compulsively, becoming, in effect, addicted to exercise. Morgan[22] describes such an addiction as "present if the person feels compelled to exercise daily and feels unable to live without it and when deprived of exercise, experiences withdrawal symptoms including anxiety, irritability, and depression." Such individuals may continue to exercise despite serious injury or interference with social and occupational activities.[23]

Exercise compulsion is often seen in individuals with eating disorders, especially anorexia nervosa. Exercise may begin as a way to decrease hunger and increase weight loss and may progress to an addiction in its own right. These individuals become "obligate exercisers." Some researchers have proposed that obligatory exercise is actually a variant of anorexia nervosa, and they have reported that many of these individuals, even if they do not have the hallmark weight loss and fear of fatness, share many of the obsessive characteristics, as well as character, style, and background, of anorexic patients.[24]

A few studies have tried to identify personality traits that would predict individuals at risk for becoming addicted to exercise, but only one study was able to find any correlation.[25] This study found that weight pre-occupation in men and women and obsessive-compulsiveness in men were strongly related to excessive exercising. Because this is only one study, more research needs to be done to determine which individuals are at risk for developing an exercise addiction, although individuals who are excessively weight conscious may be one group at risk.

Another negative effect of exercise is the "staleness syndrome," characterized by mood and sleep disturbances and often resembling depression.[21] Because this is almost exclusively seen in serious athletes in intensive training, it will not be discussed here. Despite these occasional detrimental effects, exercise is still a safe, low-risk activity, even for individuals with symptoms of depression or anxiety. Among patients with bulimic or anorexic symptoms, however, there is a theoretical risk that exercise prescriptions may promote obligate and dangerous regimens. Table 6.1 summarizes the psychological benefits and potential side effects of exercise.

TABLE 6.1 Potential Psychological Benefits and Side Effects of Exercise

Benefits	Side Effects
Antidepressant effect	Compulsive exercising
Anxiolytic effect	Exercise addiction
Increased sense of well-being	"Staleness syndrome"
Enhanced self-esteem	

Clinical Issues

Does exercise have a therapeutic index or a dose-response curve in terms of psychological benefit? Some of the transient benefits of exercise, such as a decrease in state anxiety or an improvement in well-being, may be seen after just a single exercise session. In most studies, subjects exercised three times per week, but no studies have examined exactly how many exercise sessions per week are necessary for long-lasting psychological benefit.[26] Also, as the number of exercise sessions per week increases, so might the rates of injury—an important factor in prescribing an exercise regimen.

Adherence is an issue when prescribing any medical or psychiatric treatment, and exercise is no exception. Although some of the symptoms of depression (fatigue, anhedonia, and psychomotor retardation) may make it difficult for patients to initiate and maintain an exercise regimen, adherence rates to exercise programs are similar between psychiatric and nonpsychiatric populations.[2] Approximately 50% of patients continue to exercise regularly after the end of a formal training program.[2] To state this differently, half of the individuals beginning an exercise program will drop out, usually after only a few weeks. This is a major detriment in using exercise as a treatment for any benefit, whether physical or psychological. Unfortunately, while a few studies have sought to examine predictors of successful exercise initiation and maintenance, little definitive information is available to predict outcome.[27,28] Tailored advice, found to enhance diet change and smoking cessation, does not seem to enhance exercise adherence.[29]

Whether adherence to exercise programs is more problematic in patients with diabetes is not clear. Given the regimen complexities posed by taking insulin and the weight-related issues for obese patients, adherence may be more difficult in these individuals than among those without a concomitant illness. There is also no research to indicate whether exercise promotes or impedes adherence to other elements of the diabetic treatment program. With the increasing incidence of obesity and type 2 diabetes in adolescents and young adults, exercise is clearly warranted for both prevention and early intervention in young individuals. There is little research on this group of diabetic patients. As with other health promotion behaviors, exercise programs for young individuals must be developed within a social context, i.e., parents and schools are critical for successful implementation.

Exercise, in general, is not contraindicated in patients on psychiatric medications, although certain issues must be taken into account. Patients on antipsychotic medications, such as haloperidol or chlorpromazine, can safely exercise; however, the sedation and Parkinsonian-like side effects of these medications can interfere with motivation to exercise and with coordination.[30] Antidepressants are commonly prescribed for moderate to severe depression, and again, patients taking these drugs can safely exercise. However, orthostatic hypotension secondary to the use of certain antidepressants can make exercise dangerous and thus should be monitored. This is an especially important problem among the elderly and among diabetic patients with signs of autonomic neuropathy. It is generally recommended that only light exercise be attempted during adjustment to a new medication and during the initial titration to therapeutic dosage.[2] Once patients are on full doses and are not experiencing certain side effects (orthostatic hypotension, hypertension), they can participate in a full-intensity exercise program appropriate for their level of physical fitness.

Summary

In summary, the majority of studies have found beneficial effects of exercise on psychosocial functioning. Exercise can help reduce depression and anxiety, as well as give individuals an improved sense of well-being. Although negative effects of exercise, such as exercise addiction, can occur, exercise is generally a safe method for improving psychological health. Table 6.2 summarizes our clinical recommendations for prescribing exercise to patients as part of a mental health treatment plan.

TABLE 6.2 Clinical Recommendations

- Include regular exercise (30–60 min, three times/week) as part of the treatment plan for mild to moderately depressed or anxious patients if no contraindications are present.
- For patients on psychotropic medications, defer regular exercise until adjustment to medication is complete and no serious side effects are present.
- Recognizing that adherence is a long-term issue in maintaining regular exercise routines, refer patients to organized exercise programs/classes and provide active follow-up and encouragement.

Acknowledgments

This research was supported by National Institutes of Health Grants DK-27845 and DK-42315 and a donation from Herbert Graetz.

References

1. Morgan WP: Physical fitness and emotional health: a review. *Am Correct Ther J* 23:124–27, 1969
2. Martinsen EW: Benefits of exercise for the treatment of depression. *Sports Med* 9:380–89, 1990
3. Paluska SA, Schwenk TL: Physical activity and mental health: current concepts. *Sports Med* 29:167–80, 2000
4. Blumenthal JA, Babyak MA, Moore KA, Craighead WE, Herman S, Khatri P, Waugh R, Napolitano MA, Forman LM, Appelbaum M, Doraiswamy PM, Krishnan KR: Effects of exercise training on older patients with major depression. *Arch Intern Med* 159:2349–56, 1999
5. Klein MH, Greist JH, Gurman AS, Neimeyer RA, Lesser DP, Bushnell NJ, Smith RE: A comparative outcome study of group psychotherapy vs. exercise treatments for depression. *Int J Ment Health* 13:148–77, 1985
6. Greist JH, Klein MH, Eischens RR, Faris J, Gurman AS, Morgan WP: Running as treatment for depression. *Compr Psychiatry* 20: 41–54, 1979
7. Martinsen EW, Medhus A, Sandvik L: Effects of aerobic exercise on depression: a controlled study. *Br Med J* 291:109, 1985
8. McDonald DG, Hodgdon JA: *Psychological Effects of Aerobic Fitness Training: Research and Theory.* New York, Springer-Verlag, 1991
9. Landers DM, Petruzzello SJ: Physical activity, fitness and anxiety. In *Physical Activity, Fitness, and Health: International Proceedings and Consensus Statement.* Bouchard C, Shepard RG, Stephens T, Eds. Champaign, IL, Human Kinetics, 1994, p. 868–82
10. Scully D, Kremer J, Meade MM, Graham R, Dudgeon K: Physical exercise and psychological well being: a critical review. *Br J Sports Med* 32:111–20, 1998
11. Morgan WP: Reduction of state anxiety following acute physical activity. In *Exercise and Mental Health.* Morgan WP, Goldston SE, Eds. Washington, DC, Hemisphere Publishing, 1987, p. 105–09
12. Broocks A, Bandelow B, Pekrun G, George A, Meyer T, Bartmann U, Hillmer-Vogel U, Ruther E: Comparison of aerobic exercise,

clomipramine, and placebo in the treatment of panic disorder. *Am J Psychiatry* 155:603–09, 1998

13. Petruzello SJ, Landers DM, Hatfield BD, Kubitz KA, Salazar W: A meta-analysis on the anxiety-reducing effects of acute and chronic exercise: outcomes and mechanisms. *Sports Med* 11:143–82, 1991
14. Martinsen EW, Hoffart A, Solberg Y: Aerobic and non-aerobic forms of exercise in the treatment of anxiety disorders. *Stress Med* 5:115–20, 1989
15. Blumenthal JA, Williams RS, Needels TL, Wallace AG: Psychological changes accompany aerobic exercise in healthy middle-aged adults. *Psychosom Med* 44:529–36, 1982
16. Blumenthal JA, Emery CF, Madden DJ, George LK, Coleman RE, Riddle MW, McKee DC, Reasoner J, Williams RS: Cardiovascular and behavioral effects of aerobic exercise training in healthy older men and women. *J Gerontol* 44:M147–57, 1989
17. Brown RS: Exercise as an adjunct to the treatment of mental disorders. In *Exercise and Mental Health.* Morgan WP, Goldston SE, Eds. Washington, DC, Hemisphere Publishing, 1987, p. 131–37
18. Ismail AH: Psychological effects of exercise in the middle years. In *Exercise and Mental Health.* Morgan WP, Goldston SE, Eds. Washington, DC, Hemisphere Publishing, 1987, p. 111–16
19. McAuley E: Physical activity and psychosocial outcomes. In *Physical Activity, Fitness, and Health: International Proceedings and Consensus Statement.* Bouchard C, Shepard RG, Stephens T, Eds. Champaign, IL, Human Kinetics, 1994, p. 551–68
20. Sonstroem RJ, Morgan WP: Exercise and self-esteem: rationale and model. *Med Sci Sports Exerc* 21:329–37, 1989
21. Raglin JS: Exercise and mental health: beneficial and detrimental effects. *Sports Med* 9:323–29, 1990
22. Morgan WP: Negative addiction in runners. *Physical Sports Med* 7:57–70, 1979
23. Polivy J: Physical activity, fitness, and compulsive behaviors. In *Physical Activity, Fitness, and Health: International Proceedings and Consensus Statement.* Bouchard C, Shepard RG, Stephens T, Eds. Champaign, IL, Human Kinetics, 1994, p. 883–96
24. Yates A, Leehey K, Shisslak CM: Running: an analogue of anorexia? *N Engl J Med* 308:251–55, 1983
25. Davis C, Brewer H, Ratusny D: Behavioral frequency and psychological commitment: necessary concepts in the study of excessive exercising. *J Behav Med* 16:611–27, 1993

26. Ekkekakis P, Petruzzello SJ: Acute aerobic exercise and affect: current status, problems and prospects regarding dose-response. *Sports Med* 28:337–74, 1999
27. Marcus BH, Dubbert PM, Forsyth LH, McKenzie TL, Stone EJ, Dunn AL, Blair SN: Physical activity behavior change: issues in adoption and maintenance. *Health Psychol* 19 (Suppl. 1):32–41, 2000
28. Frederick CM, Morrison C, Manning T: Motivation to participate, exercise affect and outcome behaviors toward physical activity. *Percept Mot Skills* 82:691–701, 1996
29. Bull FC, Jamrozik K, Blanksby BA: Tailored advice on exercise: does it make a difference? *Am J Prev Med* 16:230–39, 1999
30. Martinsen EW: Exercise and medications in the psychiatric patient. In *Exercise and Mental Health.* Morgan WP, Goldston SE, Eds. Washington, DC, Hemisphere Publishing, 1987

S. Tziporah Cohen, BA, and Alan M. Jacobson, MD, are from the Joslin Diabetes Center, Boston, MA.

7

Determinants of the Response to Regular Physical Activity: Genetic Versus Environmental Factors

TUOMO RANKINEN, PhD, ERIC RAVUSSIN, PhD, AND CLAUDE BOUCHARD, PhD

Highlights

- There are marked interindividual differences in responsiveness to exercise training; in a group of subjects following an identical training program, some show no or only minor changes, whereas others show marked improvements in risk factor levels.

- Age, sex, and race do not seem to contribute to these interindividual differences. Pretraining phenotype levels are strong determinants of training responses for some phenotypes, such as blood pressure and heart rate, but have little effect on others, such as VO_{2max} and HDL cholesterol.

- Training response phenotypes are characterized by significant familial aggregation, suggesting the contribution of genetic factors and a shared environment.

- There is no evidence that some subjects are "general non-responders" (i.e., an individual may be a non-responder to one phenotype but a high-responder to another phenotype). Thus, effectiveness of a training program should be evaluated using several response indicators.

Modern lifestyle in industrialized countries is characterized by growing sedentarism and low levels of physical activity. This lifestyle persists despite the fact that beneficial effects of regular exercise on risk factors for several chronic diseases have been increasingly recognized and that a physically active lifestyle is often defined as the cornerstone of primary and secondary prevention for chronic diseases such as cardiovascular disease, hypertension, type 2 diabetes, and obesity.[1,2]

The effects of exercise training on risk factors or morbidities are usually evaluated in terms of average changes in a group of individuals subjected to an exercise program. This method is a useful way to emphasize the general trend observed in a given population, but it neglects an important feature—the interindividual variation in response to the exercise protocol. In a group of subjects following an identical training program, some individuals exhibit profound changes in risk factors (high-responders), whereas others show little change (low-responders).[3] For example, in the HERITAGE Family Study, 742 healthy sedentary subjects (483 white subjects from 99 families and 259 black subjects from 105 families) followed an identical endurance training program for 20 weeks.[4] The mean increase in VO_{2max} (an indicator of aerobic fitness level) in response to training was 384 ml/min (~16%) with a standard deviation of ~200 ml/min. As shown in Fig. 7.1, the responses ranged from no change up to increases of >1,000 ml/min.[5] Because all the subjects completed the same supervised training program, the variability in the improvement in VO_{2max} was not due to differences in the exercise program or compliance but to differences in trainability. Similar patterns of variation in responsiveness have been shown for other phenotypes of the metabolic syndrome, such as blood lipids[6] and blood pressure.[7,8]

These data emphasize that the effects of regular physical activity should be evaluated not only in terms of mean changes, but also in terms of response heterogeneity. This individual variability has been described as a normal biological phenomenon that may reflect genetic

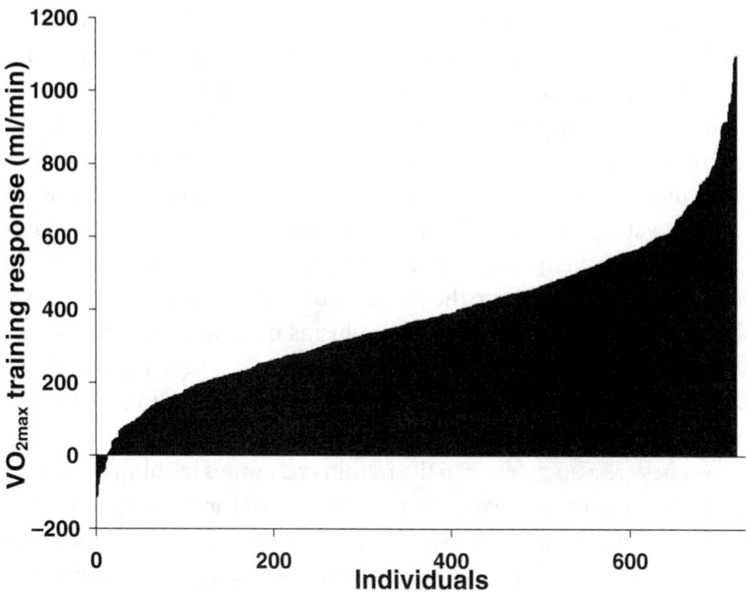

FIGURE 7.1 Distribution of VO_{2max} training responses in the HERITAGE Family Study.

Modified from Bouchard and Rankinen.[3]

diversity.[9] This hypothesis has been tested in training studies with pairs of monozygotic (MZ) twins and nuclear families. In pairs of MZ twins, the VO_{2max} response to standardized training in a series of experiments showed six to nine times more variance between genotypes (i.e., between pairs of twins) than within genotypes (i.e., within pairs of twins).[10] For example, in 10 pairs of male MZ twins submitted to a standardized endurance training program for 20 weeks, the gain in absolute VO_{2max} had almost eight times more variance between pairs than within pairs of twins. The intrapair resemblance for changes in VO_{2max} was high, with an intraclass correlation reaching 0.77.[10,11] Similarly, in the HERITAGE Family Study, there was 2.5 times more variance in VO_{2max} training response between families than within families.[12] Taken together, these results indicate that some families experience a greater beneficial response to training than others. The heritability of the VO_{2max} training response, which includes both genetic and nongenetic causes of familial aggregation, reached 47%.

One goal of the HERITAGE Family Study is to identify the genes and mutations that contribute to the interindividual differences in responsiveness to exercise training. However, because the risk factor responses to training are multifactorial (influenced by various environmental and genetic factors) and polygenic (genetic effect contributed by mutations at several genes) traits, the identification of the DNA sequence variation underlying these genetic effects represents a major challenge. Furthermore, gene–gene and gene–environment interaction effects further complicate the picture. So far, few candidate genes have been tested. For example, polymorphisms in skeletal muscle-specific creatine kinase[13] and Na,K-ATPase $\alpha 2$[14] genes have been reported to be associated with training-induced changes in VO_{2max}. Similarly, polymorphisms in the endothelial nitric oxide synthase and angiotensinogen genes are associated with the training responses in submaximal exercise blood pressure levels.[15,16] It is obvious that candidate gene studies alone will not be sufficient to elucidate the genetics of adaptation to regular physical activity. A wide range of study designs and techniques, such as case-control and association studies, family studies, genome-wide linkage scans, gene expression studies, and animal experimentation (transgenic, crossbreeding, congenics, and gene targeting), will be needed. The first genome-wide scan for the VO_{2max} training response was only recently published.[17] Thus, the search for relevant genes and mutations has barely begun, and much work remains to be done.

The contribution of environmental factors to the interindividual variation in training response is less clear at the moment. Data from the HERITAGE Family Study indicate that age, sex, and ethnic origin are not major determinants of human responsiveness to regular physical activity. On the other hand, in selected cases, the level of risk factors before the training program explains a considerable proportion of the variation in training response.[3] For example, baseline systolic blood pressure measured during submaximal exercise explained one-third of the variation in its training response in the HERITAGE cohort, i.e., subjects with higher initial levels showed greater reduction following the training program. However, the initial phenotype level had no effect on VO_{2max} and HDL cholesterol training responses.[3] Contribution of other environmental factors, such as diet, to the interindividual variability in responsiveness to exercise training has not yet been systematically addressed.

As discussed elsewhere in this book (see Chapters 3 and 8–12), there is a considerable amount of data supporting the beneficial effects of a physically active lifestyle or exercise training on diabetes and its risk factors. However, data on interindividual differences in responsiveness to regular exercise in diabetic subjects are still missing. It is likely that a similar level of variability exists among diabetic subjects as in asymptomatic sedentary individuals. Interestingly, patients with type 2 diabetes have a higher prevalence of type IIb skeletal muscle fibers and a lower muscle capillary density.[18,19] Furthermore, the number of type IIb fibers is increased in first-degree relatives of patients with type 2 diabetes.[20] Skeletal muscle metabolic properties or fiber type composition may contribute to the interindividual variation in responsiveness to exercise training. However, this hypothesis needs to be tested in standardized and controlled exercise training studies in diabetic and asymptomatic individuals.

In summary, there is marked heterogeneity in responsiveness to regular physical activity, with some individuals being high-responders and others being low-responders. It is therefore important to recognize that a failure to normalize a patient's risk factor level with an exercise program is not necessarily only due to noncompliance. On the other hand, it is equally important to understand that there are few individuals who do not respond at all to exercise training. Even if a diabetic patient's blood glucose concentration does not decrease in response to training, it is likely that the exercise program has beneficial effects on other risk factors. The effectiveness of a training program should therefore be evaluated in a broad perspective, and patients should be encouraged to engage in a physically active lifestyle when it is medically safe for them to do so.

References

1. Bouchard C, Shephard R, Stephens T, Eds. *Physical Activity, Fitness, and Health: International Proceedings and Consensus Statement*. Champaign, IL, Human Kinetics, 1994
2. U.S. Department of Health and Human Services: *Physical Activity and Health: A Report of the Surgeon General*. Atlanta, GA, U.S. Dept. of Health and Human Services, Centers for Disease Control and Prevention, National Center for Chronic Disease Prevention and Health Promotion, 1996

3. Bouchard C, Rankinen T: Individual differences in response to regular physical activity. *Med Sci Sports Exerc.* 33:S446–51, 2001
4. Skinner JS, Wilmore KM, Krasnoff JB, Jaskolski A, Jaskolska A, Gagnon J, Province MA, Leon AS, Rao DC, Wilmore JH, Bouchard C: Adaptation to a standardized training program and changes in fitness in a large, heterogeneous population: the HERITAGE Family Study. *Med Sci Sports Exerc* 32:157–61, 2000
5. Bouchard C, Daw EW, Rice T, Perusse L, Gagnon J, Province MA, Leon AS, Rao DC, Skinner JS, Wilmore JH: Familial resemblance for VO_{2max} in the sedentary state: the HERITAGE Family Study. *Med Sci Sports Exerc* 30:252–58, 1998
6. Leon AS, Rice T, Mandel S, Despres JP, Bergeron J, Gagnon J, Rao DC, Skinner JS, Wilmore JH, Bouchard C: Blood lipid response to 20 weeks of supervised exercise in a large biracial population: the HERITAGE Family Study. *Metabolism* 49:513–20, 2000
7. Rankinen T, Bouchard C: Genetics and blood pressure response to exercise, and its interactions with obesity. *Preventive Cardiology.* In press
8. Wilmore JH, Stanforth PR, Gagnon J, Rice T, Mandel S, Leon AS, Rao DC, Skinner JS, Bouchard C: Heart rate and blood pressure changes with endurance training: the HERITAGE Family Study. *Med Sci Sports Exerc* 33:107–16, 2001
9. Bouchard C: Individual differences in the response to regular exercise. *Int J Obes Relat Metab Disord* 19:S5–S8, 1995
10. Bouchard C, Dionne FT, Simoneau JA, Boulay MR: Genetics of aerobic and anaerobic performances. *Exerc Sport Sci Rev* 20:27–58, 1992
11. Prud'homme D, Bouchard C, Leblanc C, Landry F, Fontaine E: Sensitivity of maximal aerobic power to training is genotype-dependent. *Med Sci Sports Exerc* 16:489–93, 1984
12. Bouchard C, An P, Rice T, Skinner JS, Wilmore JH, Gagnon J, Perusse L, Leon AS, Rao DC: Familial aggregation of VO_{2max} response to exercise training: results from the HERITAGE Family Study. *J Appl Physiol* 87:1003–08, 1999
13. Rivera MA, Dionne FT, Simoneau JA, Perusse L, Chagnon M, Chagnon Y, Gagnon J, Leon AS, Rao DC, Skinner JS, Wilmore JH, Bouchard C: Muscle-specific creatine kinase gene polymorphism and VO_{2max} in the HERITAGE Family Study. *Med Sci Sports Exerc* 29:1311–17, 1997

14. Rankinen T, Perusse L, Borecki I, Chagnon YC, Gagnon J, Leon AS, Skinner JS, Wilmore JH, Rao DC, Bouchard C: The Na^+K^+-ATPase α2 gene and trainability of cardiorespiratory endurance: the HERITAGE Family Study. *J Appl Physiol* 88:346–51, 2000
15. Rankinen T, Rice T, Pérusse L, Chagnon YC, Gagnon J, Leon AS, Skinner JS, Wilmore JH, Rao DC, Bouchard C: NOS3 Glu298Asp genotype and blood pressure response to endurance training: the HERITAGE Family Study. *Hypertension* 36:885–89, 2000
16. Rankinen T, Gagnon J, Perusse L, Chagnon Y, Rice T, Leon A, Skinner J, Wilmore J, Rao D, Bouchard C: AGT M235T and ACE ID polymorphisms and exercise blood pressure in the HERITAGE Family Study. *Am J Physiol Heart Circ Physiol* 279:H368–74, 2000
17. Bouchard C, Rankinen T, Chagnon YC, Rice T, Perusse L, Gagnon J, Borecki I, An P, Leon AS, Skinner JS, Wilmore JH, Province M, Rao DC: Genomic scan for maximal oxygen uptake and its response to training in the HERITAGE Family Study. *J Appl Physiol* 88:551–59, 2000
18. Lillioja S, Bogardus C: Insulin resistance in Pima Indians: a combined effect of genetic predisposition and obesity-related skeletal muscle cell hypertrophy. *Acta Med Scand Suppl* 723:103–19, 1988
19. Marin P, Andersson B, Krotkiewski M, Bjorntorp P: Muscle fiber composition and capillary density in women and men with NIDDM. *Diabetes Care* 17:382–86, 1994
20. Nyholm B, Qu Z, Kaal A, Pedersen SB, Gravholt CH, Andersen JL, Saltin B, Schmitz O: Evidence of an increased number of type IIb muscle fibers in insulin-resistant first-degree relatives of patients with NIDDM. *Diabetes* 46:1822–28, 1997

Tuomo Rankinen, PhD, Eric Ravussin, PhD, and Claude Bouchard, PhD, are from the Pennington Biomedical Research Center, Baton Rouge, LA.

Exercise and Diabetes Prevention

8

Physical Activity in the Prevention of Type 2 Diabetes: The Epidemiological Evidence Across Ethnicity and Race

ANDREA KRISKA, PhD, AND ED HORTON, MD

Highlights

- Physical activity has the potential to prevent and/or delay progression to type 2 diabetes in many individuals.
- The level of physical activity recommended is relatively feasible for individuals of all ages, income groups, races, and ethnic backgrounds.
- The major thrust of these recommendations is to encourage sedentary individuals to increase their levels of moderate physical activity, such as walking, for 20–30 min throughout the day (on most days of the week).
- Physical activity that is incorporated into an individual's lifestyle has the potential for being maintained over the years, and maintenance of adequate physical activity levels appears to be necessary to exert a lasting impact on type 2 diabetes.

The fact that a physically active lifestyle is important in the prevention of many chronic diseases and conditions is well accepted. As stated in the 1996 U.S. Surgeon General's Report on Physical Activity and Health,[1] physically active individuals appear to have a lower risk of various diseases and health conditions, such as type 2 diabetes, cardiovascular disease, hypertension, and obesity, than sedentary individuals. Detailed examples of the potential benefits of physical activity with regard to health status and the prevention of chronic diseases will be provided in the following chapters in this section. Not only will it become clear that physical activity has the potential to prevent and/or delay progression to type 2 diabetes (and possibly coronary heart disease) in many individuals, but it will also be evident that the level of physical activity recommended is feasible for individuals of all ages and ethnic backgrounds.

The Prevalence of Sedentary Behavior

One of the most upsetting statistics in public health today is the extremely high number of individuals who continue to lead a sedentary lifestyle.[1] As cars, elevators, and TV sets replace human effort, the addition of physical activity into a typical day has become less of an automatic occurrence and more of a planned behavior.

National U.S. surveys of physical activity, such as the Behavioral Risk Factor Surveillance System (BRFSS), indicate that >25% of U.S. adults do not engage in any leisure-time physical activity.[1] Unfortunately, the prevalence of sedentary behavior is even higher in U.S. minority populations. For example, results of the Third National Health and Nutrition Examination Survey (NHANES III) (1988–1991) demonstrated that the age-adjusted prevalence of reporting no leisure-time physical activity over the past month in individuals ≥20 years was higher for non-Hispanic black and Mexican-American men and women than for their non-Hispanic white counterparts.[2] Similar trends[1] were noted in two other national physical activity surveys of adults: the National Health Interview Survey (NHIS) (1985, 1990, and 1991) and the BRFSS (1986–1991, 1992, and 1994).

What Is the Physiological and Epidemiological Evidence That Physical Activity Can Play a Role in Preventing Type 2 Diabetes?

It is physiologically plausible that physical activity can play a role in preventing type 2 diabetes (as discussed in detail in Chapters 10–12). In general, active individuals have better insulin and glucose profiles than their inactive counterparts, whereas complete inactivity, with detraining and bed rest, results in a deterioration of these metabolic parameters. Most convincingly, exercise training studies have found that physical activity improves insulin action or, in other words, decreases insulin resistance. Physical activity has also been shown to be inversely related with obesity and central fat distribution (particularly visceral obesity). (Studies demonstrating that physical training can reduce both of these parameters are thoroughly discussed in Chapters 11 and 12.) In summary, it appears that physical activity may reduce the risk for type 2 diabetes both directly, by improving insulin sensitivity, and indirectly, by producing beneficial changes in body mass and composition.[3,4]

The epidemiological evidence that physical activity plays a significant role in the prevention of type 2 diabetes is also quite convincing.[5,6] From observational studies to clinical trials, in a variety of populations and age-groups, physical activity appears to reduce the risk of developing type 2 diabetes (see Chapter 9 for a thorough discussion of these various studies).

Currently, the most convincing of all of the epidemiological evidence are three intervention studies in which a decreased progression to overt type 2 diabetes development was observed at follow-up in adult Swedish men, Chinese men and women, and Finnish men and women with impaired glucose intolerance at baseline.[7–9] The Swedish (Malmo) study was a nonrandomized feasibility trial of diabetes prevention in which physical activity was an integral part of the intervention. Among 47- to 49-year-old men with impaired glucose intolerance at baseline, those men who elected not to participate in the treatment program developed twice as much diabetes at the 5-year follow-up than those who participated.[7] The Chinese study identified individuals with impaired glucose tolerance from a city-wide health screening in Da Qing and randomized them by clinic into one of four groups: exercise only, diet only, diet plus exercise, and a control group. The exercise only arm of the trial fared as well as the diet and/or the diet plus exercise arm in preventing diabetes.[8] Interestingly, the decrease in diabetes development in this study occurred without a significant change in BMI and was evident in both initially lean and overweight participants. The Finnish Diabetes Prevention Study recently demonstrated a 58% reduction in diabetes in individuals who participated in the lifestyle intervention arm of the study (physical activity and dietary intervention) compared with the control group. Chapter 10 contains details on the results of this important study.

How Feasible Is It to Raise Physical Activity Levels Across Ethnicity and Race?

Although maximal is better from a physiological point of view,[10] it is well recognized that a sedentary individual will most likely not undergo a high-intensity activity exercise regimen.[11] In contrast, evidence is mounting regarding compliance to moderate levels of activity, which are easier to fit into an individual's lifestyle and are relatively less likely to result in injury.[12] These issues were the focus of an expert panel that was brought together in early 1993 by the U.S. Centers for Disease Control and Prevention and the American College of Sports Medicine to review the pertinent scientific evidence and to develop a clear, concise public health message regarding physical activity. One of the most important concerns identified at this meeting was the public misconception that, to gain health benefits from physical activity, an individual must engage in vigorous, continuous exercise.[11]

The outcome of this meeting was a major revamping of the national public health recommendations for physical activity. The old exercise prescription was a structured inflexible series of criteria designed for athletes. As with any prescription, the patient had to follow it religiously or else the effort "didn't count." Exercise meant high levels of intensity and was associated with gyms, exercise equipment, and sweat.

This type of physical activity recommended in the old exercise prescription was also relatively costly, limiting participation to those who could afford it. In fact, the relatively lower rates of exercise participation in underserved and minority groups were thought to be in part due to these differences in income and socioeconomic status.[13,14] Evidence in support of this is also provided by three national surveys

(NHIS, BRFSS, and NHANES III), in which the prevalence of physical inactivity was found to be greater among individuals with lower income and lower levels of education.[1] Affordability, whether in regard to exercise equipment, facilities, or child care, is a very real issue that serves as a barrier to exercise participation.

The old exercise prescription was also inflexible with regard to time demands, requiring large blocks of time designated throughout the week for the exercise routine. This time demand was shown to be a consistent barrier to exercise in most people, especially those from underserved and minority populations. Taking time out to focus on yourself and temporarily removing yourself from the obligations of family and work to exercise is often not acceptable in many minority subgroups. Exercising for the sake of exercise is an indulgence that only the wealthy can afford.

Physical activity, as defined by the new set of recommendations, can be more easily incorporated into the daily routine of all individuals, regardless of income or race. The major thrust of these recommendations[11] is to encourage sedentary individuals across ethnicity, race, and income groups to increase their levels of moderate, feasible physical activity, such as walking, for 20–30 min throughout the day (on most days of the week) (see Chapter 11). Few individuals have large blocks of free time, but many are able to fit one or more short bouts of activity in throughout a day. The types of physical activity recommended are much more flexible and realistic for underserved and minority individuals. In fact, physical activity, as defined by the new set of recommendations, can be custom fit into the lives of minority men, women, and children in a manner that makes sense to their lifestyle and life demands.

Most importantly, physical activity that is incorporated into an individual's lifestyle has the potential of being maintained for years, as suggested by a 10-year follow-up study of older women who participated in a 3-year clinical trial of walking. Not only were the women who were originally randomized to the walking intervention group more active at the end of the trial, but they maintained higher physical activity levels than control women 10 years after the clinical trial had ended.[15]

Maintenance of adequate levels of physical activity is a key concern in patients with type 2 diabetes and other chronic diseases. A substantial part of the improvement in glucose tolerance and insulin resistance due to exercise is believed to be the result of the cumulative effects of the frequent lowering of blood glucose levels and the increase in insulin sensitivity that accompanies each individual session of exercise.[16] As noted in Chapters 14 and 31, much of the effect of exercise in decreasing insulin resistance is short lived and is lost after only a few days of inactivity.[16–18] Likewise, regularity of increased physical activity is certainly required to produce the beneficial changes in body composition that may independently affect insulin resistance (as discussed in Chapter 11). For these reasons, it appears that adequate physical activity levels must be maintained over the years to exert a lasting impact on type 2 diabetes and the cardiovascular complications that arise from the disease (see Chapters 9, 11, and 12).

As already noted, compared with high-intensity sports and recreation, moderate-intensity activities, such as walking, are much more likely to be maintained over the years by people of different ethnicities and races. However, from a public health point of view, to maximize the likelihood that a walking regimen will be maintained, environmental and policy changes will need to create a more favorable "active" environment in schools, communities, and workplaces. Individuals are easily discouraged from exercising if they do not have a safe, accessible, convenient place in which to be active.

Are Moderate-Intensity Activities Such as Walking Enough to Prevent Diabetes?

The new public health recommendations call for an increase in moderate levels of physical activity, such as walking, for ~30 min on most days. This averages to be ~150 min of moderate activity per week, which was also the goal of the 1982 clinical trial of walking in older women mentioned earlier (Fig. 8.1). The Walking Women Follow-up Study suggests that this activity goal can be maintained over a long period of time. However, is this level of physical activity sufficient to prevent type 2 diabetes?

Examination of two of the three completed clinical trials in type 2 diabetes, the Malmo and Da Qing studies,[7,8] reveals that they both had set their exercise goals at around 150 min/week of moderate-intensity activities such as walking (Fig. 8.1). The Finnish Diabetes Prevention Study had recommended 30 min a day or about 210 min/week of moderate-intensity activities (see Chapter 10). Interestingly, all three

How Much Physical Activity Is Enough?

Study		Exercise Goal
Surgeon General's Report	→	30 min on most days or 150 min/week
Walking Women Follow-up (Kriska)	→	7 miles or 140–150 min/week

How Much Physical Activity Is Enough to Reduce the Risk of Developing Type 2 Diabetes?

Study		Exercise Goal		
Malmo Feasibility Study (Eriksson)	→	60-min sessions, two times/week	→	120 min/week
Da Qing Study (Pan)	→	20 min of walking per day	→	140 min/week
Diabetes Prevention Program (DPP)	→	150 min of brisk walking	→	150 min/week

FIGURE 8.1 Physical activity recommendations for exercise goals.

of these studies demonstrated a significant decrease in the progression to type 2 diabetes in the activity intervention groups, suggesting that this prescribed level of activity (150–210 min/week of moderate-intensity activity) was sufficient to prevent or delay progression to diabetes in many individuals.

In the U.S., a randomized, multicenter clinical trial of type 2 diabetes prevention is currently underway in which physical activity (150 min/week of moderate-intensity activity similar to that of a brisk walk) and dietary modification compose one of the treatment arms of the study.[19] With over 3,200 individuals participating in this study, half of whom were recruited from U.S. minority subgroups, this trial should provide valuable information regarding the issue of diabetes prevention across ethnicity and race.[19]

References

1. *Physical Activity and Health: A Report of the Surgeon General.* U.S. Department of Health and Human Services, Centers for Disease Control and Prevention, National Center for Chronic Disease Prevention and Health Promotion, President's Council on Physical Fitness and Sports, 1996

2. Crespo CJ, Keteyian SJ, Heath GW, Sempos CT: Leisure time physical activity among US adults: results from the Third National Health and Nutrition Examination Survey. *Arch Intern Med* 156:93–98, 1996
3. Ivy JL, Zderic TW, Fogt DL: The prevention and treatment of non-insulin-dependent diabetes mellitus. *Exerc Sports Sci Rev* 27: 1–35, 1999
4. Albright A, Franz M, Hornsby G, Kriska A, Marrerro D, Ullrich I, Verity L: Exercise and type 2 diabetes (Position Stand). *Med Sci Sports Exerc* 32:1345–60, 2000
5. Kriska AM: Physical activity and the prevention of type 2 diabetes. In *Physical Activity and Fitness Research Digest.* Series 2, no. 10. Washington, DC, President's Council on Physical Fitness and Sports, 1997
6. Kriska A: Physical activity and the prevention of type 2 diabetes mellitus: how much for how long? *Sports Med* 29:147–51, 2000
7. Eriksson KF, Lindgärde F: Prevention of type 2 (non-insulin-dependent) diabetes mellitus by diet and physical exercise. *Diabetologia* 34:891–98, 1991
8. Pan X, Li G, Hu Y, Wang JX, Yang WY, An ZX, Hu ZX, Lin J, Xiao JZ, Cao HB, Liu PA, Jiang XG, Jiang YY, Wang JP, Zheng H, Zhang H, Bennett PH, Howard BV: Effects of diet and exercise in preventing NIDDM in people with impaired glucose tolerance: the Da Qing IGT and Diabetes Study. *Diabetes Care* 20:537–44, 1997
9. Tuomilehto J, Lindstrom J, Eriksson JG, Valle TT, Hamalainen H, Ilanne-Parikka P, Keinanen-Kiukaanniemi S, Laakso M, Louheranta A, Rastas M, Salminen V, Uusitupa M, for the Finnish Diabetes Prevention Group: Prevention of type 2 diabetes mellitus by changes in lifestyle among subjects with impaired glucose tolerance. *N Engl J Med* 344:1343–50, 2001
10. Holloszy JO, Schultz J, Kusnierkiewicz J, Hagberg JM, Ehsani AA: Effects of exercise on glucose tolerance and insulin resistance. *Acta Med Scand* 711 (Suppl.):55–65, 1986
11. Pate RR, Pratt M, Blair SN, Haskell WL, Macera CA, Bouchard C, Buckner D, Caspersen CJ, Ettinger W, Heath GW, King A, Kriska AM, Leon AS, Marcus BH, Morris J, Paffenbarger R, Patrick K, Pollock M, Rippe JM, Sallis J, Wilmore JH: Physical activity and public health: recommendation from the Centers for Disease

Control and Prevention and the American College of Sports Medicine. *JAMA* 273:402–07,1995

12. Pollock ML, Carroll JF, Graves JE, Leggett SH, Braith RW, Limacher M, Hagberg JM: Injuries and adherence to walk/jog and resistance training programs in the elderly. *Med Sci Sports Exerc* 23:1194–200, 1991
13. Clark DO: Racial and educational differences in physical activity among older adults. *Gerontologist* 35:472–80, 1995
14. Ford E, Merritt R, Heath G, Powell K, Washburn R, Kriska A, Haile G: Physical activity behaviors in lower and higher socioeconomic status populations. *Am J Epidemiol* 133:1246–56, 1991
15. Pereira MA, Kriska AM, Day RD, Cauley JA, LaPorte RE, Kuller LH: A randomized walking trial in postmenopausal women: effects on physical activity and health 10 years later. *Arch Intern Med* 158:1695–1701, 1998
16. Schneider SH, Amorosa LF, Khachadurian AK, Ruderman NB: Studies on the mechanism of improved glucose control during regular exercise in type 2 diabetes. *Diabetologia* 26:355–60, 1984
17. Heath G, Gavin J, Hinderlites J, Hagberg J, Bloomfield S, Holloszy J: Effects of exercise and lack of exercise on glucose tolerance and insulin sensitivity. *J Appl Physiol* 55:512–17, 1983
18. Koivisto VA, Yki-Jarvinen H, DeFronzo RA: Physical training and insulin sensitivity. *Diabetes Metab Rev* 1:445–81, 1986
19. Diabetes Prevention Program Research Group: The Diabetes Prevention Program: design and methods for a clinical trial in the prevention of type 2 diabetes. *Diabetes Care* 22:623–34, 1999

Andrea Kriska, PhD, is from the University of Pittsburgh, Pittsburgh, PA. Ed Horton, MD, is from the Joslin Diabetes Center, Boston, MA.

9

Reduction in Risk of Coronary Heart Disease and Diabetes

PATRICK J. SKERRETT, MS,
AND JOANN E. MANSON, MD, DrPH

Highlights

Reduction in Risk of Coronary Heart Disease

- Increased physical activity improves the cardiovascular risk factor profile; its effects include reducing adiposity, blood pressure, dyslipidemia, and platelet adhesiveness, as well as enhancing fibrinolysis.
- Increased physical activity may also reduce coronary heart disease risk independently of favorable alterations in traditional coronary risk factors.
- The estimated reduction in the risk of coronary heart disease with the maintenance of an active, compared with a sedentary, lifestyle is estimated to be 35–55%.

Reduction in Risk of Type 2 Diabetes

- Physical activity improves insulin sensitivity and glycemic control among nondiabetic individuals, as well as among those with impaired glucose tolerance or overt type 2 diabetes.

- The addition of exercise to caloric restriction facilitates loss of adipose tissue, assists in maintenance of reduced body weight, and may independently improve insulin sensitivity.
- The potential reduction in the risk of type 2 diabetes associated with an active, compared with a sedentary, lifestyle is 30–50%.

A sedentary lifestyle should be considered an important modifiable risk factor for both cardiovascular disease (CVD) and diabetes in the general population.[1] Although the proportion of U.S. adults considered to be sedentary has declined from an estimated 40% in the early 1970s to ~25% by the early 1990s, >60% of U.S. adults are not regularly active.[1] Older individuals, who are at increased risk of CVD and type 2 diabetes, are less likely to be physically active than younger individuals, and women tend to be less active than men.[2] Racial and ethnic minorities also tend to have low rates of physical activity.[3] Physical activity favorably influences a variety of known cardiovascular risk factors, including obesity, hypertension, dyslipidemia, and fibrinolysis. It also improves insulin sensitivity and glycemic control among individuals with impaired glucose tolerance (IGT) or overt type 2 diabetes and among nondiabetic individuals.[4]

Among patients with diabetes, atherosclerotic disease (including coronary heart disease [CHD], stroke, hypertension, and peripheral vascular disease) is a major cause of morbidity and mortality.[5] Age-adjusted rates of CHD are two to three times higher among diabetic men and three to seven times higher among diabetic women than among their counterparts without diabetes.[6] Therefore, increased physical activity among individuals at increased risk of glucose intolerance or those who have diabetes may be particularly important on two fronts—in the prevention of CVD and in the prevention and/or control of diabetes.

In this chapter, we summarize the currently available evidence concerning the role of increased physical activity in the primary prevention of CHD and diabetes. Because type 1 and type 2 diabetes have different etiologies and because exercise is unlikely to be relevant to the primary prevention of type 1 diabetes, this chapter will focus on type 2 diabetes.

Reduction in Risk of CHD

Observational Evidence

Observational epidemiological studies of exercise and CHD consistently demonstrate a lower risk among more physically active individuals than among their less-active peers. An early meta-analysis of 27 prospective cohort studies that assessed the association between physical activity and CHD estimated an increased relative risk of CHD of 1.9 (95% confidence interval [CI] 1.6–2.2) for people with sedentary occupations compared with people with more active occupations and a relative risk of 1.6 (95% CI 1.2–2.2) for people who were recreationally sedentary compared with people with greater recreational activity.[7] Across studies, differences in the magnitude of the association depended on methodological features. Studies with high quality scores (i.e., those with detailed assessments of physical activity and adequate control for potential confounding by other lifestyle or dietary factors) tended to demonstrate a stronger risk reduction with physical activity than methodologically weaker studies. In a separate review, the maintenance of an active lifestyle was estimated to reduce the risk of myocardial infarction by 35–55% when compared with a sedentary lifestyle.[8]

More recent long-term prospective studies of men and women also consistently demonstrate an inverse association between regular physical activity and risk of CHD.[9–16] These apparent benefits also apply to moderate-intensity activities such as brisk walking, which has been found to be associated with a reduced risk of CHD in women[15] and men,[14] as well as with a reduced risk of type 2 diabetes.[17] Adopting a more active lifestyle, even late in life, is related to a reduction in CHD.[18] Physical activity is also associated with a decreased risk of stroke in men[19,20] and women,[21] primarily because of its beneficial effects on body weight, blood pressure, serum cholesterol, and glucose tolerance.

When interpreting the inverse association between physical activity and CHD reported in observational studies, both the possibility that unmeasured or unknown factors may influence the selection and participation of study subjects (selection bias) and the possibility that unmeasured or unknown third factors may be responsible for the association (confounding bias) must be considered. However, the consistency of the results across studies supports a causal association, as does the biological plausibility due to the known salutary effects of increased physical activity on the coronary risk factor profile (see BIOLOGICAL MECHANISMS below).

Intervention Studies

Large-scale randomized trials of sufficient duration are generally able to minimize, if not eliminate, the biases inherent in observational study designs. Although no large-scale randomized trials of physical activity and CHD are available to date, numerous trials of moderate size and duration have been conducted among healthy individuals, those at high risk of developing CVD, and those with existing CVD. Despite differences in design, these trials generally demonstrate that increased physical activity has a positive impact on coronary risk factors and clinical coronary events.[22] The ideal intensity, frequency, and duration of physical activity, however, have yet to be determined.

Biological Mechanisms

Reductions in risk of CHD associated with increased physical activity are likely due to a host of physiological and metabolic changes produced by physical activity. One such important change is weight loss. In a randomized trial of 52 obese men, individuals assigned to exercise-induced weight loss had a significantly greater reduction in total fat and the ratio of visceral to subcutaneous fat than those assigned to diet-induced weight loss.[23] Other studies such as the Pound of Prevention Study, which included 1,044 women and men taking part in a 3-year community weight prevention project, have found physical activity to be a strong determinant of successful weight loss.[24] In addition, independent of its effects on adiposity, physical activity has beneficial effects on dyslipidemia[25,26] and resting blood pressure.[27] It also favorably influences fibrinolysis.[28] Other mechanisms may also be at work. Physical activity improves functional work capacity and myocardial oxygen demand[29] and reduces the adrenergic response to stress.[30,31] Among a group of 3,331 middle-aged Japanese men, engaging in continuous physical activity for at least 30 min on 1 or more days per week was associated with significant beneficial changes in a number of CHD risk factors, including higher levels of HDL cholesterol and significantly lower tricep, scapula, and iliac subcapsular fat thickness.[32] The benefits accrued in a dose-response fashion, with the greatest improvements observed among men exercising three or more times per week.

The cardiovascular benefits of exercise are also supported by animal studies. Among primates fed an atherogenic diet over an 18-month period, those undergoing moderate conditioning exercise showed a substantial reduction in the severity of atherosclerosis compared with primates without exercise.[33] This inverse association could not be explained fully by alterations in plasma lipids, glucose, or blood pressure, suggesting an independent anti-atherogenic effect of physical activity. For a summary of the potential beneficial effects of physical activity on coronary risk factors and atherosclerosis, see Chapter 10, Tables 1 and 2 and Chapter 12, Figure 1 and Table 2.

Impact of Inactivity on CHD

Because of the high prevalence of physical inactivity, the proportion of CHD deaths in the U.S. attributable to a sedentary lifestyle has been estimated to be 34.6% (Table 9.1). This attributable risk (i.e., the excess rate of CHD deaths that can be related to physical inactivity) is larger than that for any other coronary risk factor except high serum cholesterol. Based on a cost-effectiveness analysis estimating the health and economic implications of a physical activity program in the prevention of CHD, the cost per quality-adjusted life-year was found to be lower for physical activity than for any other coronary risk factor intervention (Table 9.1).[34]

TABLE 9.1 Selected Risk Factors for CHD, by Prevalence, Population Attributable Risk, and Cost-Effectiveness: U.S.

Risk Factor	Prevalence (%)	Attributable Risk (%)	Cost-Effectiveness
Physical inactivity	58.0	34.6	$11,313 per QALY
Hypertension	18.0	28.9	$25,000 per QALY
Smoking	25.5	25.0	$21,947 total lifetime benefits of quitting
Obesity	23.0	32.1	Not available
Elevated serum cholesterol (≥200 mg/dl)	37.0	42.7	$28,000 per QALY

Percentages for attributable risk cannot be summed because they are calculated independently for each risk factor. QALY, quality-adjusted life-year. Cost-effectiveness data for physical inactivity and hypertension are from Hatziandreu EI, Koplan JP, Weinstein MC, Caspersen CJ, Warner KE: A cost-effectiveness analysis of exercise as a health-promotion activity. *Am J Public Health* 78:1417–21, 1988. Cost-effectiveness data for smoking are from Weinstein MC, Stanson WB: Cost-effectiveness of interventions to prevent or treat coronary heart disease. *Annu Rev Public Health* 6:41–63, 1985. Cost-effectiveness data for elevated serum cholesterol are from Oster G, Colditz GA, Kelly NL: The economic costs of smoking and benefits of quitting for individual smokers. *Prev Med* 13:377–89, 1984.

Modified from Ref. 34.

Reduction in Risk of Type 2 Diabetes

Observational Evidence

Relatively few epidemiologic studies have examined the potential beneficial effects of physical activity on the development of type 2 diabetes. Support for the benefits of exercise in relation to type 2 diabetes risk has been provided by descriptive studies of societies undergoing a transition from traditional lifestyle patterns to more Westernized patterns, examinations of migrants from traditional to more urbanized environments, comparisons of active rural versus more sedentary urban populations, case-control studies, retrospective cohort studies, and prospective studies of active compared with sedentary individuals.

Cross-Cultural and Migrant Studies

In Melanesian and Indian Fijian men, the age-standardized prevalence of type 2 diabetes among men classified as sedentary was more than twice the rate than among those classified as exercising moderately to heavily.[35] A similar association was observed among Hindu and Muslim Asian Indians, African-origin Creoles, and Chinese Mauritians of both sexes after controlling for potential confounders such as BMI, central adiposity, age, and family history of diabetes.[36] Among migrants from Tokelau Island (an atoll in the Pacific Ocean) to urban New Zealand, prevalence and incidence of type 2 diabetes increased significantly more than it did for nonmigrants between 1968 and 1982.[37] Not all such ecological studies, however, have demonstrated a significant association between glucose tolerance and physical activity.[38,39]

Cross-Sectional Studies

Studies comparing the most sedentary individuals in a population with the most active individuals at a single point in time generally show an inverse association between physical activity and prevalence of IGT or type 2 diabetes. For example, in the Zutphen Elderly Study, among 389 men aged 70–89 years who were free of diagnosed diabetes, IGT was found in 12.6%. Men in the highest quartile of self-reported weekly physical activity had significantly lower insulin levels during the glucose tolerance test than less active men.[40] In the San Luis Valley Diabetes Study, which included 219 Hispanic and non-Hispanic white women and men with IGT, higher levels of physical activity were associated with lower insulin areas.[41] Among 916 middle-aged African-American men and women surveyed in the Pitt County Study, those who were moderately active were less likely to have type 2 diabetes (odds ratio [OR] 0.35; 95% CI 0.12–0.98) after adjustment for age, sex, education, BMI, and waist-to-hip ratio.[42] In the Rotterdam Study, an ongoing population-based cohort study of chronic diseases in the elderly, >1,000 men and women aged 55–75 years who were not known to have type 2 diabetes underwent an oral glucose tolerance test and had their physical activity assessed by a self-administered questionnaire. A total of 118 subjects were diagnosed with type 2 diabetes, and another 153 were found to have IGT. Vigorous physical activities such as bicycling and sports were inversely associated with type 2 diabetes; similar associations were observed for IGT, but they did not reach statistical significance.[43]

Case-Control Studies

A case-control study conducted among men aged 50–59 years serving in the Japanese Self-Defense Forces, 38 of whom had IGT and 60 of whom were control subjects, showed that individuals with a high level of physical fitness in their 30s were substantially less likely to have IGT (OR 0.31; 95% CI 0.11–0.68) after adjustment for parental history of diabetes and BMI.[44]

Retrospective Cohort Studies

In a retrospective cohort study of 5,398 female college alumnae aged 20–70 years, women who did not engage in vigorous athletic activities during their college years had a 3.4-fold increased risk of developing type 2 diabetes compared with women who trained regularly.[45] Another retrospective cohort study of 1,282 athletes who had represented Finland in the Olympics and other international competitions found that former endurance athletes had a substantially lower risk of type 2 diabetes than did 777 referents (OR 0.24; 95% CI 0.07–0.81).[46]

Prospective Cohort Studies

Prospective observational studies have consistently shown a marked reduction in type 2 diabetes risk among physically active individuals compared with their sedentary peers (Table 9.2). Despite differences in study populations and assessments of physical activity, the available

TABLE 9.2 Association Between Physical Activity and Risk of Type 2 Diabetes: Prospective Studies

Study	Population	Incident Cases; Duration	Comparison Groups	Relative Risk (95% CI)	Potential Confounding Factors Controlled in Analysis
Alumni Health Study[47]	5,990 men aged 39–68 years free of type 2 diabetes	202 cases; 14 years	Each 500 kcal/week increase in physical activity	0.94 (0.90–0.98)	Age, parental history of diabetes, BMI, history of hypertension
Nurses' Health Study[92]	87,253 women aged 34–59 years free of type 2 diabetes, CVD, and cancer	1,303 cases; 8 years	Vigorous exercise at least weekly versus less than weekly	0.67 (0.60–0.75)	Age
				0.84 (0.75–0.95)	Age, family history of diabetes, BMI, smoking, alcohol consumption, hypertension, high serum cholesterol
Physicians' Health Study[48]	21,271 men aged 40–84 years free of type 2 diabetes, CVD, and cancer	285 cases; 4.9 years	Vigorous exercise at least weekly versus less than weekly	0.64 (0.51–0.82)	Age
				0.71 (0.54–0.94)	Age, BMI, smoking, alcohol consumption, hypertension, high serum cholesterol
British Regional Heart Study[93]	7,577 men aged 40–59 years free of type 2 diabetes	194 cases; 12.8 years	Moderate activity versus inactivity	0.4 (0.2–0.7)	Age and BMI; further adjustment for prevalent CHD, alcohol intake, smoking, systolic blood pressure, HDL cholesterol, heart rate, and uric acid had little effect on risk estimates

Honolulu Heart Program[94]	6,815 men aged 45–68 years free of type 2 diabetes	381 cases; 6 years	Highest quintile of physical activity (calculated from time spent per day in different activity levels weighted by estimated O_2 consumption) versus lower four quintiles	0.55 (0.41–0.75)	Age
				0.49 (0.34–0.72)	Age, parental history of diabetes, BMI, subcapsular–to–triceps skinfold ratio, systolic blood pressure, triglycerides, glucose, hematocrit
Kuopio Ischemic Heart Disease Risk Factor Study[95]	897 men aged 42–60 years free of type 2 diabetes	46 cases; 4.2 years	Leisure time physical activity with an intensity of ≥5.5 METs for at least 40 min/week versus less activity	0.44 (0.22–0.88)	Age, parental history of diabetes, BMI, triglycerides, baseline blood glucose, alcohol consumption
Malmo Preventive Trial[96]	4,637 men aged 48 years free of type 2 diabetes	116 cases; 6 years	Men with type 2 diabetes versus men without type 2 diabetes at baseline	16% lower physical activity index	
Northeastern Finland Cohort[97]	891 men and women aged 35–63 years free of type 2 diabetes	118 cases; 10 years	Total weekly leisure time physical activity calculated from self-reports. For men, low (0–1,100 kcal/week) versus high (>1,900 kcal/week) activity; for women, low (0–900 kcal/week) versus high (>1,500 kcal/week) activity	Men: 1.54 (0.83–2.84) Women: 2.64 (1.28–5.44)	Age, parental history of diabetes, BMI, triglycerides, baseline blood glucose, alcohol consumption

(*continued*)

TABLE 9.2 (*Continued*)

Study	Population	Incident Cases; Duration	Comparison Groups	Relative Risk (95% CI)	Potential Confounding Factors Controlled in Analysis
Nurses' Health Study*[17]	70,102 women aged 40–65 years free of type 2 diabetes, CVD, and cancer	1,419 cases; 8 years	At least 21.8 MET hours per week of physical activity (highest quintile) versus ≤2.0 (lowest quintile)	0.74 (0.62–0.89)	Age, parental history of diabetes, BMI, smoking, menopausal status, alcohol consumption, history of hypertension, history of high cholesterol
			Among women who did not perform vigorous activities, at least 10.0 MET hours per week of walking (highest quintile) versus ≤0.5 (lowest quintile)	0.74 (0.59–0.93)	
Aerobics Center Longitudinal Study[98]	8,633 men aged 30–79 years free of type 2 diabetes	149 cases; 6.1 years	Men with lowest 20% of cardiorespiratory fitness based on treadmill test versus men with highest 40%	2.6 (1.6–4.2)	Age, parental diabetes, fitness level, BMI, high blood pressure, high LDL and total cholesterol, high triglycerides, alcohol consumption, current smoking, years of follow-up

Osaka Health Survey[99]	6,013 men aged 35–60 years free of type 2 diabetes, IGT, and hypertension	444 cases; 10 years	Physical activity at least once per week versus less often Vigorous physical activity on weekends versus sedentary	0.75 (0.61–0.93) 0.55 (0.35–0.88)	Age, parental history of diabetes, BMI, smoking, blood pressure, alcohol consumption
Iowa Women's Health Study[100]	34,257 women aged 55–69 years free of type 2 diabetes	1,997 cases; 12 years	Any physical activity versus no physical activity Physical activity index	0.69 (0.63–0.77) Low: 1.0 (referent) Moderate: 0.75 (0.67–0.84) High: 0.58 (0.51–0.66)	Age, parental history of diabetes, smoking, alcohol consumption, education, energy intake, whole grain intake, and Keys' score; further adjustment for BMI and waist-to-hip ratio somewhat attenuated the risk reductions
British Regional Heart Study†[101]	5,159 men aged 40–59 years free of CHD and type 2 diabetes	196 cases; 16.8 years	Versus no physical activity	Light: 0.65 (0.41–1.03) Moderate: 0.48 (0.28–0.83) Moderately vigorous to vigorous: 0.46 (0.27–0.79)	Age, smoking, alcohol use, social class, BMI, and pre-existing CHD; further adjustment for insulin, diastolic blood pressure, lipids, and γ-glutamyltransferase slightly weakened these associations

*Updated analysis of Ref. 92 based on detailed physical activity questionnaires from 1986 onward; †updated analysis of Ref. 93 with 4 additional years of follow-up and excluding men with CHD at baseline. MET, metabolic equivalent.

prospective studies show reductions in the risk of type 2 diabetes ranging from 15 to 60%, with most showing reductions between 30 and 50%. Women and men appear to benefit in a similar fashion from physical activity, as do younger and older individuals. In some studies, risk reductions with physical activity were more pronounced among overweight individuals than among lean individuals.[47,48] Moderate activity appears to yield similar benefits as vigorous activity. For example, after 8 years of follow-up among >70,000 female nurses aged 40–65 years who did not have diabetes, cardiovascular disease, or cancer at baseline, the relative risk of developing type 2 diabetes declined significantly across increasing quintiles of moderate physical activity (relative risks of 1.0, 0.95, 0.80, 0.81, and 0.74, respectively; *P* for trend, 0.01) after adjusting for age, BMI, and other risk factors.[17] In addition, equivalent energy expenditures from walking and vigorous activity resulted in comparable magnitudes of risk reduction.

These prospective studies controlled for age, BMI, and several other potential confounding variables. Furthermore, most were conducted in populations that were relatively homogeneous in educational attainment and socioeconomic status, thereby minimizing selection and confounding biases. However, it is possible that selection factors and residual confounding by related lifestyle factors may have influenced these results, highlighting the importance of randomized clinical trials.

Intervention Studies

Intervention studies have routinely shown the benefits of physical activity for people with diabetes. A single bout of exercise can increase the sensitivity of skeletal muscle to insulin and increase rates of whole-body glucose disposal, effects that can last for several hours after the completion of exercise.[49] Regular physical activity, either alone or combined with dietary therapy, has been shown to improve insulin sensitivity, glycemic control, and the metabolic profile among a range of populations.[50–54] Trials of physical activity in the prevention of type 2 diabetes are more limited. Currently, published data are available from a completed feasibility study, two completed randomized trials, and an ongoing trial.

In a nonrandomized feasibility study among Swedish men aged 47–49 years at baseline, the effects of a structured diet and exercise regimen on 181 men with IGT and 41 men with newly diagnosed type 2 diabetes were compared with no intervention in a control group of 79 individuals with IGT and 114 healthy individuals.[55] In the intervention group, BMI decreased significantly and oxygen uptake increased significantly after 5 years, whereas in the nonintervention groups, BMI increased and oxygen uptake decreased. Among subjects with IGT, glucose tolerance improved in 75.8% of individuals in the intervention group, whereas 10.6% developed type 2 diabetes; in the nonintervention group, glucose tolerance deteriorated among 67.1% of participants with IGT, and 28.6% developed type 2 diabetes. In the intervention group, the relative risk of type 2 diabetes was 0.37 (95% CI 0.20–0.68; $P < 0.003$). Among subjects with type 2 diabetes at baseline, after 5 years of treatment and follow-up, 53.8% no longer had glucose levels diagnostic for diabetes.

In the Da Qing IGT and Diabetes Study, a large-scale screening project in northern China, 577 men and women aged ≥25 years identified as having IGT were randomly assigned to a control group or one of three interventions—diet only, exercise only, or diet plus exercise.[56] Participants assigned to exercise were encouraged to increase their daily physical activity by 1 or more units, with a unit defined as 30 min of mild-intensity activity (walking), 20 min of moderate-intensity activity (brisk walking or doing laundry), 10 min of strenuous activity (slow running or climbing stairs), or 5 min of very strenuous activity (jumping rope or playing basketball). After 6 years, the cumulative incidence of diabetes was 67.7% in the control group, 43.8% in the diet-only group, 41.1% in the exercise-only group, and 46.0% in the diet-plus-exercise group (*P* for trend, <0.05). Similar reductions in rate of development of diabetes were observed in both lean (BMI <25 kg/m^2) and overweight (BMI ≥25 kg/m^2) individuals. In a proportional hazards analysis adjusted for differences in baseline BMI and fasting glucose, the reductions in risk of developing type 2 diabetes were 0.69 for diet alone, 0.53 for exercise alone, and 0.62 for diet and exercise.

The Finnish Diabetes Prevention Study randomized 522 overweight (mean BMI 31 kg/m^2) middle-aged men and women with IGT to either general advice on healthy lifestyle modifications (control group) or individualized counseling aimed at reducing weight and intake of total and saturated fat and increasing physical activity and intake of dietary fiber. After a mean 3.2 years of follow-up, statistically significant differences were observed in mean weight loss, decreased consumption of fat, increased consumption of vegetables, and increased physical activity in the intervention group compared with the control group. The cumulative incidence of diabetes was 11% (95% CI 6–15) in the control group and 23% (17–29) in the intervention group, or a 58% reduction in risk of diabetes.[57]

In the U.S., the Diabetes Prevention Program is a multicenter trial that began in 1996. When enrollment closed in June 1999, 3,819 subjects aged ≥25 years with IGT and BMI ≥24 kg/m^2 had been randomized. Of these, ~20% are over age 60 years, and ~45% are from minority populations.[58] The study has three arms—intensive lifestyle intervention, drug therapy with metformin combined with standard advice on diet and exercise, and placebo plus standard advice on diet and exercise. (A fourth arm designed to test troglitazone plus standard medical advice on diet and exercise was discontinued in 1998.) The goals of the intensive lifestyle intervention include achieving and maintaining a 7% reduction in weight and performing at least 150 min per week of moderate-intensity physical activity (equivalent to ~700 kcal/week), such as walking or bicycling.[59] The trial is expected to be completed in 2002.

The available data from these trials point to the feasibility of sustained modification of dietary changes and increased physical activity. They also suggest that such changes may help prevent, or at least postpone, the onset of type 2 diabetes. At present, however, data are limited regarding the optimal intensity, frequency, and duration of exercise for reducing the occurrence of type 2 diabetes. According to estimates derived from prospective studies, the potential reduction in the risk of type 2 diabetes associated with regular moderate and/or vigorous exercise compared with a sedentary lifestyle is 30–50%.

The benefits of the interventions in these trials may extend beyond the prevention of type 2 diabetes. Increased physical activity and healthier eating patterns are integral components of recommendations made for the prevention of CVD, many forms of cancer, and other chronic diseases. This overlap is important given that individuals with IGT or type 2 diabetes tend to have higher levels of CVD risk factors, and such strategies could help control this important comorbidity.

Biological Mechanisms

Several biologically plausible mechanisms could explain the possible role of physical activity in preventing type 2 diabetes. First, exercise is associated with a lower BMI, which in turn is associated with a lower risk of type 2 diabetes. Studies among nondiabetic individuals suggest that exercise alone or in addition to caloric restriction facilitates the loss of adipose tissue and helps maintain reduced body weight.[60] Obesity (in particular, central adiposity) has been linked to glucose intolerance, hyperinsulinemia, hypertension, and dyslipidemia; insulin resistance has been identified as a mediating factor.[61–63] In addition, exercise appears to have independent effects on insulin sensitivity and glucose metabolism.[4,49,64] These mechanisms are discussed in detail in Chapters 4 and 14.

Reduction in Risk of CHD Among Individuals With Type 2 Diabetes

Declines in CVD Mortality Are Less Pronounced Among Individuals With Diabetes

Over the last 4 decades in the U.S., we have witnessed substantial declines in mortality from diseases of the heart, from an age-adjusted rate of 370 per 100,000 for men and 194 per 100,000 for women in 1965 to 173 per 100,000 for men and 95 per 100,000 for women in 1997.[65] This dramatic and encouraging decline has resulted from both reductions in cardiovascular risk factors and improvements in the diagnosis and treatment of CVD.[66] These overall reductions in mortality, however, are not apparent among people with diabetes. In a comparison of 10,649 individuals who participated in the First National Health and Nutrition Examination Survey (NHANES I) between 1971 and 1975 and 9,233 individuals who participated in the NHANES I Epidemiologic Follow-up Survey between 1982 and 1984, Gu et al.[67] found a 36.4% age-adjusted decline in CHD among men without diabetes compared with a 13.1% decline among men with diabetes. For women, CHD mortality declined 27% among individuals without diabetes and increased 23% among those with diabetes. Several studies have also documented that patients with diabetes who develop clinical CVD have a worse prognosis for survival[68–70] and are more likely to die after an acute myocardial infarction[71–74] than those without diabetes.

One possible explanation for this disparity may be the extra burden of traditional and nontraditional CHD risk factors observed among people with diabetes. In the Atherosclerosis Risk In Communities

Study, for example, after adjusting for traditional CHD risk factors, levels of albumin, fibrinogen, von Willebrand factor, factor VIII activity, and leukocyte count were significant predictors of CHD among people with diabetes.[75] These associations could indicate common pathophysiological pathways for both diabetes and CHD. They may also reflect inflammation or microvascular injury underlying both atherosclerosis and diabetes.

Evidence From Observational and Intervention Studies

Few data are available concerning the benefits of physical activity in preventing CHD among individuals with diabetes. Physical activity improves insulin sensitivity and glycemic control among lean nondiabetic individuals as well as among obese individuals and patients with type 2 diabetes. In type 1 diabetes, exercise also increases skeletal muscle sensitivity to insulin and reduces insulin requirements; glycemic control does not appear to be favorably altered,[76] perhaps because of associated increases in caloric intake.[77] The effects of long-term exercise among patients with type 1 diabetes remain inconclusive. The sparse follow-up data available suggest that type 1 diabetic patients who participate in physical activity early in life may experience fewer macrovascular complications, as well as less nephropathy and neuropathy, than nonparticipants.[78,79] Studies in patients with mild type 2 diabetes have demonstrated the benefits of exercise in increasing insulin sensitivity and glucose tolerance, as well as inducing favorable changes in blood lipids.[80–82] Exercise as an adjunct to diet regimens produces greater weight loss and higher maintenance rates in obese nondiabetic individuals[83–85] and type 2 diabetic patients.[86] However, benefits of exercise, when added to weight loss, have not been consistently reported in all studies.[87,88] Methodological differences between studies, such as the intensity of the applied exercise regimens, compliance, and differing degrees of control of food intake, may explain the observed inconsistencies.[85] No randomized clinical trials have been conducted to assess reductions in clinical CHD events induced by increased physical activity in type 2 diabetic patients. Based on the available evidence, however, physical activity may play an important role in the reduction of CHD among diabetic as well as nondiabetic individuals.[89]

With regard to overall mortality, physical activity appears to offset some of the excess mortality observed among patients with diabetes. In a 12-year follow-up of ~7,000 men who participated in the Malmo Preventive Trial of diet and exercise, similar rates of mortality were observed among individuals with IGT, assigned to increased physical activity and dietary counseling, and those without IGT (6.5 vs. 6.2 per 1,000 person-years). In contrast, men with IGT assigned to routine treatment had a mortality rate of 14.0 per 1,000 person-years.[90] These data suggest that physical activity and dietary modifications may reduce mortality in individuals at high risk of premature death due to IGT. Data from the Aerobics Center Longitudinal Study support these findings. Among 1,263 men with type 2 diabetes who were followed for an average of 11.7 years, those in the lowest physical fitness group (assessed by a maximal treadmill exercise test) had a twofold higher risk of all-cause mortality than more fit men after adjustment for age, baseline CVD, fasting plasma glucose level, cholesterol level, overweight, current smoking, hypertension, and parental history of CVD.[91] In addition, men who reported being physically inactive had a 1.7-fold higher adjusted risk of dying than men who reported being physically active.

Summary

The currently available epidemiological evidence indicates a substantial reduction in the risk of CHD and type 2 diabetes with the maintenance of an active, compared with a sedentary, lifestyle. The estimated risk reductions are 35–55% for CHD and 30–50% for type 2 diabetes. The activity must be regular and ongoing because the possible benefits fade within a short period after a return to inactivity. Clinician counseling and prescription of regular physical activity should represent a major goal in the primary prevention of CHD and type 2 diabetes. This responsibility is of paramount importance, particularly in light of the high prevalence of physical inactivity and the high incidence of atherosclerotic diseases and diabetes in the U.S. and throughout the world.

References

1. U.S. Department of Health and Human Services: *Physical Activity and Health: A Report of the Surgeon General.* Washington, DC, U.S. Department of Health and Human Services, Centers for Disease Control and Prevention, 1996

2. Eyler AA, Brownson RC, King AC, Brown D, Donatelle RJ, Heath G: Physical activity and women in the United States: an overview of health benefits, prevalence, and intervention opportunities. *Women Health* 26:27–49, 1997
3. Crespo CJ, Smit E, Andersen RE, Carter-Pokras O, Ainsworth BE: Race/ethnicity, social class and their relation to physical inactivity during leisure time: results from the Third National Health and Nutrition Examination Survey, 1988–1994. *Am J Prev Med* 18:46–53, 2000
4. Borghouts LB, Keizer HA: Exercise and insulin sensitivity: a review. *Int J Sports Med* 21:1–12, 2000
5. Gu K, Cowie CC, Harris MI: Mortality in adults with and without diabetes in a national cohort of the U.S. population, 1971–1993. *Diabetes Care* 21:1138–45, 1998
6. Barrett-Connor EL, Cohn BA, Wingard DL, Edelstein SL: Why is diabetes mellitus a stronger risk factor for fatal ischemic heart disease in women than in men? The Rancho Bernardo Study. *JAMA* 265:627–31, 1991
7. Berlin JA, Colditz GA: A meta-analysis of physical activity in the prevention of coronary heart disease. *Am J Epidemiol* 132:612–28, 1990
8. Manson JE, Tosteson H, Ridker PM, Satterfield S, Hebert P, O'Connor GT, Buring JE, Hennekens CH: The primary prevention of myocardial infarction. *N Engl J Med* 326:1406–16, 1992
9. Eaton CB, Medalie JH, Flocke SA, Zyzanski SJ, Yaari S, Goldbourt U: Self-reported physical activity predicts long-term coronary heart disease and all-cause mortalities: twenty-one-year follow-up of the Israeli Ischemic Heart Disease Study. *Arch Fam Med* 4:323–29, 1995
10. Folsom AR, Arnett DK, Hutchinson RG, Liao F, Clegg LX, Cooper LS: Physical activity and incidence of coronary heart disease in middle-aged women and men. *Med Sci Sports Exerc* 29:901–09, 1997
11. Leon AS, Myers MJ, Connett J: Leisure time physical activity and the 16-year risks of mortality from coronary heart disease and all-causes in the Multiple Risk Factor Intervention Trial (MRFIT). *Int J Sports Med* 18 (Suppl. 3):S208–15, 1997
12. Rosengren A, Wilhelmsen L: Physical activity protects against coronary death and deaths from all causes in middle-aged men:

evidence from a 20-year follow-up of the primary prevention study in Goteborg. *Ann Epidemiol* 7:69–75, 1997

13. Dorn JP, Cerny FJ, Epstein LH, Naughton J, Vena JE, Winkelstein W Jr, Schisterman E, Trevisan M: Work and leisure time physical activity and mortality in men and women from a general population sample. *Ann Epidemiol* 9:366–73, 1999
14. Hakim AA, Curb JD, Petrovitch H, Rodriguez BL, Yano K, Ross GW, White LR, Abbott RD: Effects of walking on coronary heart disease in elderly men: the Honolulu Heart Program. *Circulation* 100:9–13, 1999
15. Manson JE, Hu FB, Rich-Edwards JW, Colditz GA, Stampfer MJ, Willett WC, Speizer FE, Hennekens CH: A prospective study of walking as compared with vigorous exercise in the prevention of coronary heart disease in women. *N Engl J Med* 341:650–58, 1999
16. Sherman SE, D'Agostino RB, Silbershatz H, Kannel WB: Comparison of past versus recent physical activity in the prevention of premature death and coronary artery disease. *Am Heart J* 138:900–07, 1999
17. Hu FB, Sigal RJ, Rich-Edwards JW, Colditz GA, Solomon CG, Willett WC, Speizer FE, Manson JE: Walking compared with vigorous physical activity and risk of type 2 diabetes in women: a prospective study. *JAMA* 282:1433–39, 1999
18. Wannamethee SG, Shaper AG, Walker M: Changes in physical activity, mortality, and incidence of coronary heart disease in older men. *Lancet* 351:1603–08, 1998
19. Lee IM, Paffenbarger RS Jr: Physical activity and stroke incidence: the Harvard Alumni Health Study. *Stroke* 29:2049–54, 1998
20. Lee IM, Hennekens CH, Berger K, Buring JE, Manson JE: Exercise and risk of stroke in male physicians. *Stroke* 30:1–6, 1999
21. Hu FB, Stampfer MJ, Colditz GA, Ascherio A, Rexrode KM, Willett WC, Manson JE: Physical activity and risk of stroke in women. *JAMA* 283:2961–67, 2000
22. Stefanick ML: Exercise and weight loss. In *Clinical Trials in Cardiovascular Disease: A Companion Guide to Braunwald's Heart Disease.* Hennekens CH, Ed. Philadelphia, Saunders, 1999, p. 375–91
23. Ross R, Dagnone D, Jones PJ, Smith H, Paddags A, Hudson R, Janssen I: Reduction in obesity and related comorbid conditions after diet-induced weight loss or exercise-induced weight

loss in men: a randomized, controlled trial. *Ann Intern Med* 133:92–103, 2000

24. Sherwood NE, Jeffery RW, French SA, Hannan PJ, Murray DM: Predictors of weight gain in the Pound of Prevention Study. *Int J Obes Relat Metab Disord* 24:395–403, 2000
25. Stefanick ML, Mackey S, Sheehan M, Ellsworth N, Haskell WL, Wood PD: Effects of diet and exercise in men and postmenopausal women with low levels of HDL cholesterol and high levels of LDL cholesterol. *N Engl J Med* 339:12–20, 1998
26. Prabhakaran B, Dowling EA, Branch JD, Swain DP, Leutholtz BC: Effect of 14 weeks of resistance training on lipid profile and body fat percentage in premenopausal women. *Br J Sports Med* 33:190–95, 1999
27. Kelley GA, Kelley KS: Aerobic exercise and resting blood pressure in women: a meta-analytic review of controlled clinical trials. *J Womens Health Gend Based Med* 8:787–803, 1999
28. Lindahl B, Nilsson TK, Jansson JH, Asplund K, Hallmans G: Improved fibrinolysis by intense lifestyle intervention: a randomized trial in subjects with impaired glucose tolerance. *J Intern Med* 246:105–12, 1999
29. Maskin CS: Aerobic exercise training in cardiopulmonary disease. In *Cardiopulmonary Exercise Testing: Physiologic Principles and Clinical Applications.* Weber KT, Janicki JS, Eds. Philadelphia, Saunders, 1986, p. 317–32
30. Cooksey JD, Reilly P, Brown S, Bomze H, Cryer PE: Exercise training and plasma catecholamines in patients with ischemic heart disease. *Am J Cardiol* 42:372–76, 1978
31. Spina RJ, Turner MJ, Ehsani AA: Beta-adrenergic-mediated improvement in left ventricular function by exercise training in older men. *Am J Physiol* 274:H397–404, 1998
32. Hsieh SD, Yoshinaga H, Muto T, Sakurai Y: Regular physical activity and coronary risk factors in Japanese men. *Circulation* 97:661–65, 1998
33. Kramsch DM, Aspen AJ, Abramowitz BM, Kreimendahl T, Hood WB Jr: Reduction of coronary atherosclerosis by moderate conditioning exercise in monkeys on an atherogenic diet. *N Engl J Med* 305:1483–89, 1981
34. Public health focus: physical activity and the prevention of coronary heart disease. *MMWR Morb Mortal Wkly Rep* 42:669–72, 1993

35. Taylor R, Ram P, Zimmet P, Raper LR, Ringrose H: Physical activity and prevalence of diabetes in Melanesian and Indian men in Fiji. *Diabetologia* 27:578–82, 1984
36. Dowse GK, Zimmet PZ, Gareeboo H, George K, Alberti MM, Tuomilehto J, Finch CF, Chitson P, Tulsidas H: Abdominal obesity and physical inactivity as risk factors for NIDDM and impaired glucose tolerance in Indian, Creole, and Chinese Mauritians. *Diabetes Care* 14:271–82, 1991
37. Ostbye T, Welby TJ, Prior IA, Salmond CE, Stokes YM: Type 2 (non-insulin-dependent) diabetes mellitus, migration and Westernisation: the Tokelau Island Migrant Study. *Diabetologia* 32: 585–90, 1989
38. King H, Taylor R, Koteka G, Nemaia H, Zimmet P, Bennett PH, Raper LR: Glucose tolerance in Polynesia: population-based surveys in Rarotonga and Niue. *Med J Aust* 145:505–10, 1986
39. Jarrett RJ, Shipley MJ, Hunt R: Physical activity, glucose tolerance, and diabetes mellitus: the Whitehall Study. *Diabet Med* 3:549–51, 1986
40. Feskens EJ, Loeber JG, Kromhout D: Diet and physical activity as determinants of hyperinsulinemia: the Zutphen Elderly Study. *Am J Epidemiol* 140:350–60, 1994
41. Regensteiner JG, Shetterly SM, Mayer EJ, Eckel RH, Haskell WL, Baxter J, Hamman RF: Relationship between habitual physical activity and insulin area among individuals with impaired glucose tolerance: the San Luis Valley Diabetes Study. *Diabetes Care* 18:490–97, 1995
42. James SA, Jamjoum L, Raghunathan TE, Strogatz DS, Furth ED, Khazanie PG: Physical activity and NIDDM in African-Americans: the Pitt County Study. *Diabetes Care* 21:555–62, 1998
43. Baan CA, Stolk RP, Grobbee DE, Witteman JC, Feskens EJ: Physical activity in elderly subjects with impaired glucose tolerance and newly diagnosed diabetes mellitus. *Am J Epidemiol* 149: 219–27, 1999
44. Takemura Y, Kikuchi S, Inaba Y, Yasuda H, Nakagawa K: The protective effect of good physical fitness when young on the risk of impaired glucose tolerance when old. *Prev Med* 28:14–19, 1999
45. Frisch RE, Wyshak G, Albright TE, Albright NL, Schiff I: Lower prevalence of diabetes in female former college athletes compared with nonathletes. *Diabetes* 35:1101–05, 1986

46. Kujala UM, Kaprio J, Taimela S, Sarna S: Prevalence of diabetes, hypertension, and ischemic heart disease in former elite athletes. *Metabolism* 43:1255–60, 1994
47. Helmrich SP, Ragland DR, Leung RW, Paffenbarger RS Jr: Physical activity and reduced occurrence of non-insulin-dependent diabetes mellitus. *N Engl J Med* 325:147–52, 1991
48. Manson JE, Nathan DM, Krolewski AS, Stampfer MJ, Willett WC, Hennekens CH: A prospective study of exercise and incidence of diabetes among US male physicians. *JAMA* 268:63–67, 1992
49. Goodyear LJ, Kahn BB: Exercise, glucose transport, and insulin sensitivity. *Annu Rev Med* 49:235–61, 1998
50. Raz I, Hauser E, Bursztyn M: Moderate exercise improves glucose metabolism in uncontrolled elderly patients with non-insulin-dependent diabetes mellitus. *Isr J Med Sci* 30:766–70, 1994
51. Yamanouchi K, Shinozaki T, Chikada K, Nishikawa T, Ito K, Shimizu S, Ozawa N, Suzuki Y, Maeno H, Kato K, Oshida Y, Sato Y: Daily walking combined with diet therapy is a useful means for obese NIDDM patients not only to reduce body weight but also to improve insulin sensitivity. *Diabetes Care* 18:775–78, 1995
52. Honkola A, Forsen T, Eriksson J: Resistance training improves the metabolic profile in individuals with type 2 diabetes. *Acta Diabetol* 34:245–48, 1997
53. Agurs-Collins TD, Kumanyika SK, Ten Have TR, Adams-Campbell LL: A randomized controlled trial of weight reduction and exercise for diabetes management in older African-American subjects. *Diabetes Care* 20:1503–11, 1997
54. Dunstan DW, Puddey IB, Beilin LJ, Burke V, Morton AR, Stanton KG: Effects of a short-term circuit weight training program on glycaemic control in NIDDM. *Diabetes Res Clin Pract* 40:53–61, 1998
55. Eriksson KF, Lindgarde F: Prevention of type 2 (non-insulin-dependent) diabetes mellitus by diet and physical exercise: the 6-year Malmo Feasibility Study. *Diabetologia* 34:891–98, 1991
56. Pan XR, Li GW, Hu YH, Wang JX, Yang WY, An ZX, Hu ZX, Lin J, Xiao JZ, Cao HB, Liu PA, Jiang XG, Jiang YY, Wang JP, Zheng H, Zhang H, Bennett PH, Howard BV: Effects of diet and exercise in preventing NIDDM in people with impaired glucose tolerance: the Da Qing IGT and Diabetes Study. *Diabetes Care* 20: 537–44, 1997

57. Tuomilehto J, Lindstrom J, Eriksson JG, Valle TT, Hamalainen H, Ilanne-Parikka P, Keinanen-Kiukaanniemi S, Laakso M, Louheranta A, Rastas M, Salminen V, Uusitupa M, for the Finnish Diabetes Prevention Study Group: Prevention of type 2 diabetes mellitus by changes in lifestyle among subjects with impaired glucose tolerance. *N Engl J Med* 344:1343–50, 2001
58. National Institute of Diabetes and Digestive and Kidney Diseases: Diabetes prevention program meets recruitment goals: http://www.preventdiabetes.com/recruitment_pressrelease.htm
59. The Diabetes Prevention Program: Design and methods for a clinical trial in the prevention of type 2 diabetes. *Diabetes Care* 22:623–34, 1999
60. Grundy SM, Blackburn G, Higgins M, Lauer R, Perri MG, Ryan D: Physical activity in the prevention and treatment of obesity and its comorbidities: evidence report of independent panel to assess the role of physical activity in the treatment of obesity and its comorbidities. *Med Sci Sports Exerc* 31:1493–1500, 1999
61. Reaven GM: Banting Lecture 1988: Role of insulin resistance in human disease. *Diabetes* 37:1595–1607, 1988
62. Kaplan NM: The deadly quartet: upper-body obesity, glucose intolerance, hypertriglyceridemia, and hypertension. *Arch Intern Med* 149:1514–20, 1989
63. Sheehan MT, Jensen MD: Metabolic complications of obesity: pathophysiologic considerations. *Med Clin North Am* 84:363–85, 2000
64. Kelley DE, Goodpaster BH: Effects of physical activity on insulin action and glucose tolerance in obesity. *Med Sci Sports Exerc* 31:S619–23, 1999
65. National Center for Health Statistics: *Vital Statistics of the United States.* Hyattsville, MD, National Center for Health Statistics, 1965–1997
66. Hunink MG, Goldman L, Tosteson AN, Mittleman MA, Goldman PA, Williams LW, Tsevat J, Weinstein MC: The recent decline in mortality from coronary heart disease, 1980–1990: the effect of secular trends in risk factors and treatment. *JAMA* 277:535–42, 1997
67. Gu K, Cowie CC, Harris MI: Diabetes and decline in heart disease mortality in US adults. *JAMA* 281:1291–97, 1999

68. Stone PH, Muller JE, Hartwell T, York BJ, Rutherford JD, Parker CB, Turi ZG, Strauss HW, Willerson JT, Robertson T, Braunwald E, Jaffee AS: The effect of diabetes mellitus on prognosis and serial left ventricular function after acute myocardial infarction: contribution of both coronary disease and diastolic left ventricular dysfunction to the adverse prognosis: the MILIS Study Group. *J Am Coll Cardiol* 14:49–57, 1989
69. Singer DE, Moulton AW, Nathan DM: Diabetic myocardial infarction: interaction of diabetes with other preinfarction risk factors. *Diabetes* 38:350–57, 1989
70. Smith JW, Marcus FI, Serokman R: Prognosis of patients with diabetes mellitus after acute myocardial infarction. *Am J Cardiol* 54:718–21, 1984
71. Abbott RD, Donahue RP, Kannel WB, Wilson PW: The impact of diabetes on survival following myocardial infarction in men vs women: the Framingham Study. *JAMA* 260:3456–60, 1988
72. Donahue RP, Goldberg RJ, Chen Z, Gore JM, Alpert JS: The influence of sex and diabetes mellitus on survival following acute myocardial infarction: a community-wide perspective. *J Clin Epidemiol* 46:245–52, 1993
73. Miettinen H, Lehto S, Salomaa V, Mahonen M, Niemela M, Haffner SM, Pyorala K, Tuomilehto J: Impact of diabetes on mortality after the first myocardial infarction: the FINMONICA Myocardial Infarction Register Study Group. *Diabetes Care* 21: 69–75, 1998
74. Vaccarino V, Parsons L, Every NR, Barron HV, Krumholz HM: Impact of history of diabetes mellitus on hospital mortality in men and women with first acute myocardial infarction: the National Registry of Myocardial Infarction 2 Participants. *Am J Cardiol* 85:1486–89, 2000
75. Saito I, Folsom AR, Brancati FL, Duncan BB, Chambless LE, McGovern PG: Nontraditional risk factors for coronary heart disease incidence among persons with diabetes: the Atherosclerosis Risk in Communities (ARIC) Study. *Ann Intern Med* 133:81–91, 2000
76. Wasserman DH, Zinman B: Exercise in individuals with IDDM. *Diabetes Care* 17:924–37, 1994
77. Devlin JT: Effects of exercise on insulin sensitivity in humans. *Diabetes Care* 15:1690–93, 1992

78. LaPorte RE, Dorman JS, Tajima N, Cruickshanks KJ, Orchard TJ, Cavender DE, Becker DJ, Drash AL: Pittsburgh Insulin-Dependent Diabetes Mellitus Morbidity and Mortality Study: physical activity and diabetic complications. *Pediatrics* 78:1027–33, 1986
79. Kriska AM, LaPorte RE, Patrick SL, Kuller LH, Orchard TJ: The association of physical activity and diabetic complications in individuals with insulin-dependent diabetes mellitus: the Epidemiology of Diabetes Complications Study: VII. *J Clin Epidemiol* 44:1207–14, 1991
80. Ruderman NB, Ganda OP, Johansen K: The effect of physical training on glucose tolerance and plasma lipids in maturity-onset diabetes. *Diabetes* 28 (Suppl. 1):89–92, 1979
81. Ruderman N, Apelian AZ, Schneider SH: Exercise in therapy and prevention of type II diabetes: implications for blacks. *Diabetes Care* 13:1163–68, 1990
82. Saltin B, Lindgarde F, Houston M, Horlin R, Nygaard E, Gad P: Physical training and glucose tolerance in middle-aged men with chemical diabetes. *Diabetes* 28 (Suppl. 1):30–32, 1979
83. Pavlou KN, Krey S, Steffee WP: Exercise as an adjunct to weight loss and maintenance in moderately obese subjects. *Am J Clin Nutr* 49:1115–23, 1989
84. Pavlou KN, Whatley JE, Jannace PW, DiBartolomeo JJ, Burrows BA, Duthie EA, Lerman RH: Physical activity as a supplement to a weight-loss dietary regimen. *Am J Clin Nutr* 49 (Suppl. 5): 1110–14, 1989
85. Wing RR: Physical activity in the treatment of the adulthood overweight and obesity: current evidence and research issues. *Med Sci Sports Exerc* 31:S547–52, 1999
86. Wing RR, Epstein LH, Paternostro-Bayles M, Kriska A, Nowalk MP, Gooding W: Exercise in a behavioural weight control programme for obese patients with type 2 (non-insulin-dependent) diabetes. *Diabetologia* 31:902–09, 1988
87. Van Dale D, Saris WH, Schoffelen PF, Ten Hoor F: Does exercise give an additional effect in weight reduction regimens? *Int J Obes* 11:367–75, 1987
88. Phinney SD, LaGrange BM, O'Connell M, Danforth E Jr: Effects of aerobic exercise on energy expenditure and nitrogen balance during very low calorie dieting. *Metabolism* 37:758–65, 1988

89. Schneider SH, Vitug A, Ruderman N: Atherosclerosis and physical activity. *Diabetes Metab Rev* 1:513–53, 1986
90. Eriksson KF, Lindgarde F: No excess 12-year mortality in men with impaired glucose tolerance who participated in the Malmo Preventive Trial with diet and exercise. *Diabetologia* 41:1010–16, 1998
91. Wei M, Gibbons LW, Kampert JB, Nichaman MZ, Blair SN: Low cardiorespiratory fitness and physical inactivity as predictors of mortality in men with type 2 diabetes. *Ann Intern Med* 132:605–11, 2000
92. Manson JE, Rimm EB, Stampfer MJ, Colditz GA, Willett WC, Krolewski AS, Rosner B, Hennekens CH, Speizer FE: Physical activity and incidence of non-insulin-dependent diabetes mellitus in women. *Lancet* 338:774–78, 1991
93. Perry IJ, Wannamethee SG, Walker MK, Thomson AG, Whincup PH, Shaper AG: Prospective study of risk factors for development of non-insulin dependent diabetes in middle aged British men. *BMJ* 310:560–64, 1995
94. Burchfiel CM, Sharp DS, Curb JD, Rodriguez BL, Hwang LJ, Marcus EB, Yano K: Physical activity and incidence of diabetes: the Honolulu Heart Program. *Am J Epidemiol* 141:360–68, 1995
95. Lynch J, Helmrich SP, Lakka TA, Kaplan GA, Cohen RD, Salonen R, Salonen JT: Moderately intense physical activities and high levels of cardiorespiratory fitness reduce the risk of non-insulin-dependent diabetes mellitus in middle-aged men. *Arch Intern Med* 156:1307–14, 1996
96. Eriksson KF, Lindgarde F: Poor physical fitness, and impaired early insulin response but late hyperinsulinaemia, as predictors of NIDDM in middle-aged Swedish men. *Diabetologia* 39:573–79, 1996
97. Haapanen N, Miilunpalo S, Vuori I, Oja P, Pasanen M: Association of leisure time physical activity with the risk of coronary heart disease, hypertension and diabetes in middle-aged men and women. *Int J Epidemiol* 26:739–47, 1997
98. Wei M, Gibbons LW, Mitchell TL, Kampert JB, Lee CD, Blair SN: The association between cardiorespiratory fitness and impaired fasting glucose and type 2 diabetes mellitus in men. *Ann Intern Med* 130:89–96, 1999
99. Okada K, Hayashi T, Tsumura K, Suematsu C, Endo G, Fujii S: Leisure-time physical activity at weekends and the risk of type 2

diabetes mellitus in Japanese men: the Osaka Health Survey. *Diabet Med* 17:53–58, 2000

100. Folsom AR, Kushi LH, Hong CP: Physical activity and incident diabetes mellitus in postmenopausal women. *Am J Public Health* 90:134–38, 2000
101. Wannamethee SG, Shaper AG, Alberti KG: Physical activity, metabolic factors, and the incidence of coronary heart disease and type 2 diabetes. *Arch Intern Med* 160:2108–16, 2000

Patrick J. Skerrett, MS, is from Brigham and Women's Hospital and Harvard Medical School, Boston, MA, and JoAnn E. Manson, MD, DrPH, is from Brigham and Women's Hospital, Harvard Medical School, and the Harvard School of Public Health, Boston, MA.

10

Primary Prevention of Type 2 Diabetes by Lifestyle Modification: Convincing Evidence From the Finnish Diabetes Prevention Study

JOHAN ERIKSSON, MD, PHD,
JAANA LINDSTRÖM, MSC,
MATTI UUSITUPA, MD, PHD, AND
JAAKKO TUOMILEHTO, MD, MPOLSC, PHD,
FOR THE FINNISH DIABETES PREVENTION STUDY GROUP

Highlights

- The incidence of type 2 diabetes is increasing rapidly worldwide. Physical inactivity and obesity are the main environmental determinants of the disease.
- Based on epidemiological data, it has been estimated that the risk of type 2 diabetes may be reduced by 50% when controlling obesity and increasing physical activity.
- Until recently, it was not proven scientifically if type 2 diabetes could be prevented by lifestyle intervention in high-risk subjects.
- The main objective of the Finnish Diabetes Prevention Study was to find out whether the onset of type 2 diabetes could be prevented by lifestyle intervention in high-risk individuals.

- A total of 522 middle-aged overweight subjects with impaired glucose tolerance (IGT) were randomized into an intervention or control group. The intervention goals were as follows: reduction in weight of ≥5%, total fat intake <30% of energy consumed, saturated fat intake <10% of energy consumed, fiber intake of 15 g/1,000 kcal, and moderate exercise for ≥30 min/day.
- The overall incidence of type 2 diabetes was reduced 58% by the lifestyle intervention program.
- Our findings emphasize the importance of modest weight reduction (5–10%) combined with exercise in the prevention of type 2 diabetes.
- An optimal exercise program for individuals with IGT should include components that improve cardiorespiratory fitness, muscular strength, and endurance.
- The primary prevention of type 2 diabetes is possible by a nonpharmacological intervention. To reduce the burden of type 2 diabetes, such an intervention is necessary as part of routine preventive care.

The incidence of type 2 diabetes is increasing rapidly worldwide.[1] The disease results in genetically predisposed individuals who have been exposed to environmental risk factors.[2] Although the genetic basis of type 2 diabetes is still unidentified, it is understood that a large proportion of the world's population carries diabetes susceptibility genes, demonstrated by the high prevalence of type 2 diabetes among elderly people.[3] At present, there is unequivocal evidence that obesity and physical inactivity are the main environmental determinants of the disease.[4–11]

Primary prevention of type 2 diabetes has been increasingly emphasized over the past 10–20 years.[4–9,12] The main justification for prevention of type 2 diabetes is the potential for prevention or postponement of long-term complications related to the disease. Based on epidemiological data, it has been estimated that the risk of type 2 diabetes may be reduced by 50–75% by controlling obesity and by 30–50% by increasing physical activity.[13] Until recently, it was not proven scientifically if type 2 diabetes could be prevented by lifestyle intervention in high-risk subjects. This lack of evidence is mainly due to the lack of studies assessing the potential for prevention, which is both surprising and unfortunate. Only recently have carefully designed controlled trials been initiated to provide the answer to this important question.[14,15]

Past Experiences From Studies on Primary Prevention of Type 2 Diabetes

Even though primary prevention of diabetes was first proposed about 80 years ago[16] and more recently stressed by the World Health Organization Study Group,[12] there are few studies assessing the value of measures aimed at reducing obesity and increasing physical activity in people with an increased risk of developing type 2 diabetes. Some previous intervention studies have used drugs, and these studies will not be considered here. An intervention program using lifestyle intervention alone is a natural way of preventing type 2 diabetes. The increased prevalence and incidence of the disease in most populations is primarily due to the adaptation to a sedentary lifestyle and excessive food intake—changes that have taken place during the last decades.

Unfortunately, none of the previously published lifestyle intervention studies[12,17,18] were properly designed to give an unequivocal answer to the question of whether primary prevention of type 2 diabetes is possible by lifestyle modification. Nevertheless, they have consistently provided suggestive evidence in favor of this. We will briefly discuss some of these results here.

The feasibility of diet and exercise treatment in 217 men with impaired glucose tolerance (IGT) was assessed in the Malmö study.[17] The effect of increased exercise and balanced diet was compared with a control group who did not receive any formal intervention. The reference group consisted of men who, after the initial screening, were referred to other clinics for care, but the group assignment of study subjects was not done at random. By the end of the 5-year study period, 11% of men in the intervention group and 21% in the control group had developed diabetes. Thus, the incidence in the intervention group was reduced 50% compared with that in the reference group. This study is important in demonstrating the feasibility of carrying out a diet and exercise program for 5 years, and furthermore, it suggests that the incidence of type 2 diabetes can be reduced by 50% within a 5-year period.

More recently, data on the preventive effect of diet and exercise were reported from a cluster-randomized clinical trial on 577 subjects with IGT in Da-Qing, China.[18] The cumulative 6-year incidence of type 2 diabetes was notably lower in the three (diet, exercise, and diet and exercise combined) intervention groups (41–46%) than in the control group (68%).

There are currently two ongoing randomized intervention trials that deal with lifestyle intervention in subjects with IGT: The Finnish Diabetes Prevention Study (DPS) and the U.S. Diabetes Prevention Program (DPP).[15] Results on the incidence of diabetes from the former trial have been recently disclosed,[19] whereas the latter will probably report their results in 2002.

The Finnish Diabetes Prevention Study

The main objective of the Finnish DPS was to find out whether the onset of type 2 diabetes could be prevented or delayed by lifestyle intervention in high-risk individuals with IGT. IGT is a category between normoglycemia and manifest diabetes and is defined based on a 2-h glucose concentration after an oral glucose load (75 g), with the range being 7.8–11.0 mmol/l (plasma glucose). IGT is the most common abnormality in glucose homeostasis; in various populations, ~15% of adults aged ≥30 years have IGT.[20–23] IGT is one of the first abnormalities leading to type 2 diabetes that can be conveniently identified using the oral glucose tolerance test. A large proportion of people with IGT will subsequently develop diabetes.[24] Thus, people with IGT serve as an important high-risk group when determining actions to prevent the development of type 2 diabetes. People with IGT were recruited into this trial because of their high predicted progression to diabetes, which increased the power of the study.

A total of 522 middle-aged (mean age 55 ± 7 years), overweight (mean BMI 31 ± 5 kg/m^2) subjects with IGT (mean fasting plasma glucose 6.1 ± 0.7 mmol/l, mean 2-h plasma glucose 8.9 ± 1.5 mmol/l) were randomized into either the intervention or control group in five study centers in Finland. The subjects in the intervention group were given detailed advice on how to achieve the intervention goals, which were as follows: reduction in weight of ≥5%, total fat intake <30% of energy consumed, saturated fat intake <10% of energy consumed, fiber intake of 15 g/1,000 kcal, and moderate exercise for ≥30 min/day. Frequent use of whole-grain products, vegetables, berries and fruit, low-fat milk and meat products, soft margarines, and vegetable oils rich in monounsaturated fatty acids was recommended. The dietary advice was individually designed and based on 3-day food records completed four times per year. The subjects in the intervention group had seven sessions with a nutritionist during the first year of the study and one session every 3 months thereafter.

The exercise programs differed slightly between the study centers according to local situations and facilities. Group counseling and group meetings were used to motivate people to exercise. As a part of the lifestyle intervention program, subjects were advised to increase their everyday physical activity. Endurance exercise (walking, jogging, swimming, aerobic ball games, and cross-country skiing) was recommended to increase aerobic capacity and cardiorespiratory fitness. Supervised, progressive, individually tailored circuit-type resistance training sessions were also organized to improve the functional capacity and strength of the large muscle groups. Compliance was monitored by exercise questionnaires every 3 months.

To avoid being unethical, the individuals in the control group were also given health promotion advice. They were given routine verbal and written information, but no specific individual dietary propositions were given, and no individual exercise programs were offered. Only general advice to increase physical activity was provided. The control group received health behavior advice at randomization and subsequently at each annual follow-up visit.

We monitored the health-related behavior of the study subjects before the randomization and subsequently at each annual follow-up visit. At baseline, both groups were similar with regard to the amount and type of fat used, fiber intake, and exercise habits. Success in achieving the intervention goals was estimated from the food records and exercise questionnaires collected at the annual follow-up examination. After the first year, the proportion of subjects in the intervention group who succeeded in achieving a specific target varied from 25% (fiber intake target) to 86% (exercise target) (Table 10.1).

Weight, waist circumference, and all other indicators of overweight/adiposity were reduced significantly more in the intervention

TABLE 10.1 Success in Achieving Intervention Goals by Group at the 1-Year Examination

Intervention Goal	Intervention Group (%)	Control Group (%)	*P*
Weight reduction ≥5%	43	13	0.001
Fat intake <30% of energy consumed	47	26	0.001
Saturated fat intake <10% of energy consumed	26	11	0.001
Fiber intake >15 g/1,000 kcal	25	12	0.001
Exercise >4 h/week*	86	71	0.001

*Self-reported exercise frequency, category 2 or higher in a four-category variable: *1)* "I read, watch TV, and work in the household, performing tasks that don't strain me physically"; *2)* "I walk, cycle, or exercise otherwise lightly at least 4 h per week"; *3)* "I exercise to maintain my physical condition by running, jogging, skiing, doing gymnastics, swimming, playing ball games, etc., for at least 3 h per week"; *4)* "I exercise competitively several times a week by running, orienteering, skiing, playing ball games, or participating in other sports that require heavy exertion."

group than in the control group at both the 1-year and 2-year follow-up examinations (Table 10.2). The mean values of fasting glucose, 2-h post-challenge glucose and insulin, and blood pressure were reduced at a more statistically significant rate in the intervention group than in the control group.

At the 1-year and 2-year examinations, there was a statistically significant difference between the groups in health-related behavior: the subjects in the intervention group had started to use more soft margarine and vegetable oil and spent more time on physical activities than the control group subjects ($P < 0.001$).

A total of 86 incident cases of diabetes were diagnosed among the 522 subjects randomized into the DPS. Of them, 27 occurred in the intervention group and 59 in the control group (Table 10.3). The average conversion rate from IGT to diabetes was 5.5% per year in the control group and 2.6% per year in the intervention group during the 4-year follow-up period. The absolute risk of diabetes was 18/1,000 person-years in the intervention group and 43/1,000 person-years in the control group.

The risk of diabetes was reduced by 58% ($P = 0.0002$) in the intervention group during the entire trial. The lifestyle intervention reduced the incidence of diabetes in men by 63% ($P = 0.0099$) and women by 54% ($P = 0.0076$).

TABLE 10.2 Changes in Some Clinical and Metabolic Variables During the Intervention

	Intervention Group (n = 256)	Control Group (n = 250)	P*
Change from baseline to year 1			
Weight (kg)	−4.2 ± 5.1 (−4.8 to −3.6)	−0.8 ± 3.7 (−1.3 to −0.3)	0.0001
Waist circumference (cm)	−4.4 ± 5.2 (−5.1 to −3.9)	−1.3 ± 4.8 (−1.9 to −0.7)	0.0000
Fasting plasma glucose (mmol/l)	−0.2 ± 0.7 (−0.3 to −0.1)	0.0 ± 0.7 (−0.1 to 0.1)	0.0000
2-h plasma glucose (mmol/l)	−0.9 ± 1.9 (−1.1 to −0.7)	−0.3 ± 2.2 (−0.6 to 0.0)	0.0026
Fasting serum insulin (μU/ml)	−2 ± 9 (−3 to −1)	−1 ± 7 (−2 to 0)	0.1369
2-h serum insulin (μU/ml)	−29 ± 64 (−37 to −21)	−11 ± 51 (−18 to −4)	0.0013
Serum total cholesterol (mmol/l)	−0.1 ± 0.7 (−0.2 to 0)	−0.1 ± 0.7 (−0.2 to 0)	0.6232
Serum HDL cholesterol (mmol/l)	0.05 ± 0.19 (0.03 to 0.07)	0.02 ± 0.17 (0 to 0.04)	0.0604
Serum triglycerides (mmol/l)	−0.19 ± 0.56 (−0.25 to −0.14)	−0.01 ± 0.66 (−0.09 to 0.07)	0.0010
Systolic blood pressure (mmHg)	−5 ± 14 (−7 to −3)	−1 ± 15 (−3 to 1)	0.0066
Diastolic blood pressure (mmHg)	−5 ± 9 (−6 to −4)	−3 ± 9 (−4 to −2)	0.0163
Change from baseline to year 2			
Weight (kg)	−3.5 ± 5.5 (−4.2 to −2.8)	−0.8 ± 4.4 (−1.4 to −0.2)	0.0001
Waist circumference (cm)	−4.2 ± 5.2 (−4.9 to −3.5)	−1.3 ± 5.4 (−2.0 to −0.6)	0.0000
Fasting plasma glucose (mmol/l)	−0.1 ± 0.7 (−0.2 to 0.0)	0.2 ± 0.8 (0.1 to 0.3)	0.0001
2-h plasma glucose (mmol/l)	− 0.8 ± 2.1 (−1.1 to −0.5)	0.0 ± 2.5 (−0.3 to 0.3)	0.0002
Fasting serum insulin (μU/ml)	−2 ± 6 (−3 to −1)	−1 ± 6 (−2 to 0)	0.0699
2-h serum insulin (μU/ml)	−29 ± 69 (−39 to −19)	−12 ± 44 (−18 to −6)	0.0037
Serum total cholesterol (mmol/l)	−0.1 ± 0.8 (−0.2 to 0)	0.0 ± 0.7 (−0.1 to 0.1)	0.1834
Serum HDL cholesterol (mmol/l)	0.10 ± 0.18 (0.08 to 0.12)	0.07 ± 0.18 (0.05 to 0.09)	0.2003
Serum triglycerides (mmol/l)	−0.20 ± 0.58 (−0.27 to −0.13)	0.00 ± 0.82 (−0.10 to 0.10)	0.0026
Systolic blood pressure (mmHg)	−5 ± 14 (−7 to −3)	0 ± 15 (−2 to 2)	0.0005
Diastolic blood pressure (mmHg)	−5 ± 9 (−6 to −4)	−3 ± 9 (−4 to −2)	0.0125

Data are means ± SD (95% confidence interval). *Two-tailed t test for difference between groups.

TABLE 10.3 Cumulative Incidence of Diabetes During the Lifestyle Intervention in the Intervention and Control Groups

Year	Intervention Group			Control Group		
	Cumulative Number of Diabetic Cases	Cumulative Incidence (%)	95% Confidence Interval	Cumulative Number of Diabetic Cases	Cumulative Incidence (%)	95% Confidence Interval
1	5	1.9	0.2–3.6	16	6.1	3.–9.0
2	15	6.3	3.2–9.2	37	14.4	9.9–18.6
3	22	9.1	5.4–12.6	51	20.9	15.5–25.9
4	24	10.9	6.4–15.2	53	23.0	16.9–28.6
5	27	20.0	8.8–29.8	57	34.4	21.9–44.9
6	27	20.0	8.8–29.8	59	42.6	26.0–55.5

Discussion

This study provides convincing evidence that type 2 diabetes can be prevented by lifestyle intervention in middle-aged women and men at high risk for type 2 diabetes. The overall incidence of diabetes was reduced by 58% in this trial, which had a median duration of 3 years. The observed effect of the intervention can be considered conservative for two reasons. First, the results were analyzed using the intention-to-treat principle, although it was clearly known that some subjects in the intervention group did not follow the recommended diet and exercise advice. Second, because of ethical reasons, all subjects allocated to the control group also received general health advice at baseline and at annual follow-up visits. Thus, subjects in the control group likely also benefited from the advice provided, which notion is supported by the fact that many subjects in the control group also achieved targets set for the intervention group. Thus, the impact of lifestyle changes is even larger than shown by our comparison between the intervention and control groups. Indeed, in both groups, none of the subjects who achieved all five lifestyle targets have thus far developed diabetes.

The average weight reduction achieved was relatively modest in absolute terms, yet the reduction of diabetes incidence in the intervention group was remarkable. Normal weight (BMI <25 kg/m^2) is often hard to achieve in obese subjects. Our findings emphasize the importance of a modest weight reduction of 5–10% in the prevention of diabetes.

Our physical exercise counseling included components that improve both cardiorespiratory fitness and muscular strength. We propose that an optimal exercise program for individuals with IGT should include components that improve cardiorespiratory fitness, muscular strength, and endurance. It is unlikely that the type of physical activity performed matters. Sports, household or yard work, and occupational activities are probably all beneficial, at least in increasing energy expenditure. We have collected data on the type and amount of physical activity in our study, and we will be able to analyze these data in more detail in the future.

The Da Qing IGT and Diabetes Study attempted to find out whether diet intervention or exercise intervention was more efficient and whether a combination of the two would bring additional benefits, but it failed to reveal any major differences in outcome between the different types of intervention.[18] This is in keeping with the Swedish study.[17] Furthermore, neither of these studies was based on individual random allocation of study subjects, and therefore, no conclusive inferences can be drawn from their results. In the DPS, we did not try to separate these interventions, but tried to achieve the largest changes possible on an individual basis while trying not to force the subjects to follow a rigid scheme. Also, in some people at high risk for diabetes, diet may be the primary problem, whereas in others, it is physical inactivity. However, in the majority of cases, multiple lifestyle changes may be needed simultaneously. Furthermore, in promoting a healthy lifestyle, it may not be possible to restrict the action to one single measure; once health promotion is successful, people tend to pay attention to several components of their lifestyles simultaneously.

The lifestyle intervention in the DPS not only improved glucose tolerance but also reduced the levels of several other cardiovascular risk factors. In the future, the DPS will continue follow-up of study subjects with respect to diabetes and cardiovascular end points as well as long-term effects of the intervention on diet and physical activity. It is commonly argued that changing the lifestyle of obese and sedentary people is difficult, but we think such pessimism may not be justified. The reasonably low dropout rate (8%) in our study also indicates that subjects with IGT are willing to participate in a demanding intervention program if one is available.

In conclusion, there was a marked and statistically significant difference in the cumulative incidence of diabetes between the intervention group and the control group. The risk reduction was 58%, and a significant difference was already visible after 2 years of intervention. Thus, the correction of an unhealthy lifestyle is not only feasible, but the benefits can be obtained without a major delay. The public health implications of these results are wide. The primary prevention of type 2 diabetes is possible by a nonpharmacological intervention that can be implemented in the primary health care setting. It is necessary that such an intervention become part of routine preventive care to reduce the burden of type 2 diabetes, which is reaching epidemic proportions in many countries. At the same time, it is also necessary to develop national programs for the primary prevention of type 2 diabetes that include not only the high-risk strategy but also the population strategy.

Acknowledgements

This study was supported by the Finnish Academy (grants 8473/2298, 40758/5767, 38387/54175), Ministry of Education, Novo Nordisk Foundation, Yrjö Jahnsson Foundation, and Finnish Diabetes Research Foundation.

The Finnish Diabetes Prevention Study Group includes the following: Jaakko Tuomilehto, MD, MPolSc, PhD; Jaana Lindström, MSc; Johan Eriksson, MD, PhD; Timo Valle, MD; Helena Hämäläinen, MD, PhD; Pirjo Ilanne-Parikka, MD, PhD; Sirkka Keinänen-Kiukaanniemi, MD, PhD; Mauri Laakso, MD; Anne Louheranta, MS; Merja Rastas, MS; Virpi Salminen, MS; Matti Uusitupa, MD, PhD; Timo Lakka, MD, PhD; Sirkka Aunola, PhD; Zygimantas Cepaitis, Dipl. Eng; Vladislav Moltchanov, PhD; Martti Hakumäki, MD, PhD; Marjo Mannelin, MS; Vesa Martikkala, MS; and Jouko Sundvall, MS.

References

1. King H, Aubert RE, Herman WH: Global burden of diabetes, 1995–2025. *Diabetes Care* 21:1414–31, 1998
2. Neel JV: Diabetes mellitus: a “thrifty” genotype rendered detrimental by progress? *Am J Hum Genet* 14:353–62, 1962
3. Stengård J, Tuomilehto J, Pekkanen J: Diabetes mellitus, impaired glucose tolerance and mortality among elderly men: The Finnish cohorts of the Seven Countries Study. *Diabetologia* 35:760–65, 1992
4. King H, Dowd JE: Primary prevention of type 2 (non-insulin-dependent) diabetes mellitus. *Diabetologia* 33:3–8, 1990
5. Tuomilehto J, Wolf E: Primary prevention of diabetes mellitus. *Diabetes Care* 10:238–48, 1987
6. Tuomilehto J, Tuomilehto-Wolf E, Zimmet P, Alberti K, Knowler W: Primary prevention of diabetes mellitus. In *International Textbook of Diabetes Mellitus.* Alberti K, Zimmet P, DeFronzo R, Keen H, Eds. Chichester, U.K., Wiley, 1997, p. 1799–1827
7. Hamman RF: Genetic and environmental determinants of non-insulin-dependent diabetes mellitus (NIDDM). *Diabetes Metab Rev* 8:287–338, 1992
8. Zimmet PZ: Primary prevention of diabetes mellitus. *Diabetes Care* 11:258–62, 1988

9. Stern MP: Primary prevention of type II diabetes mellitus. *Diabetes Care* 14:399–410, 1991
10. Ohlson LO, Larsson B, Björntorp P, Eriksson H, Svardsudd K, Welin L, Tibblin G, Wilhelmsen L: Risk factors for type 2 (non-insulin-dependent) diabetes mellitus: thirteen and one-half years of follow-up of the participants in a study of Swedish men born in 1913. *Diabetologia* 31:798–805, 1988
11. Manson JE, Rimm EB, Stampfer MJ, Colditz GA, Willett WC, Krolewski AS, Rosner B, Hennekens CH, Speizer FE: Physical activity and incidence of non-insulin-dependent diabetes mellitus in women. *Lancet* 338:774–78, 1991
12. WHO Study Group: *Primary Prevention of Diabetes Mellitus.* Geneva, World Health Org., 1994 (Tech. Rep. Ser., no. 844)
13. Manson JE, Spelsberg A: Primary prevention of non-insulin-dependent diabetes mellitus. *Am J Prev Med* 10:172–84, 1994
14. Eriksson J, Lindström J, Valle T, Aunola S, Hamalainen H, Ilanne-Parikka P, Keinanen-Kiukaanniemi S, Laakso M, Lauhkonen M, Lehto P, Lehtonen A, Louheranta A, Mannelin M, Martikkala V, Rastas M, Sundvall J, Turpeinen A, Viljanen T, Uusitupa M, Tuomilehto J: Prevention of type II diabetes in subjects with impaired glucose tolerance: the Diabetes Prevention Study (DPS) in Finland: study design and 1-year interim report on the feasibility of the lifestyle intervention programme. *Diabetologia* 42:793–801, 1999
15. The Diabetes Prevention Program Research Group: The Diabetes Prevention Program: design and methods for a clinical trial in the prevention of type 2 diabetes. *Diabetes Care* 22:623–34, 1999
16. Joslin E: The prevention of diabetes mellitus. *JAMA* 76:79–84, 1921
17. Eriksson KF, Lindgärde F: Prevention of type 2 (non-insulin-dependent) diabetes mellitus by diet and physical exercise: the 6-year Malmö feasibility study. *Diabetologia* 34:891–98, 1991
18. Pan XR, Li GW, Hu YH, Wang JX, Yang WY, An ZX, Hu ZX, Lin J, Xiao JZ, Cao HB, Liu PA, Jiang XG, Jiang YY, Wang JP, Zheng H, Zhang H, Bennett PH, Howard BV: Effects of diet and exercise in preventing NIDDM in people with impaired glucose tolerance: The Da Qing IGT and Diabetes Study. *Diabetes Care* 20:537–44, 1997
19. Tuomilehto J, Lindstrom J, Eriksson JG, Valle TT, Hamalainen H, Ilanne-Parikka P, Keinanen-Kiukaanniemi S, Laakso M, Louheranta

A, Rastas M, Salminen V, Uusitupa M, for the Finnish Diabetes Prevention Study Group: Prevention of type 2 diabetes mellitus by changes in lifestyle among subjects with impaired glucose tolerance. *N Engl J Med* 344:1343–50, 2001

20. King HG, Rewers M: Global estimates for prevalence of diabetes mellitus and impaired glucose tolerance in adults: WHO Ad Hoc Diabetes Reporting Group. *Diabetes Care* 16:157–77, 1993
21. Harris MI, Flegal KM, Cowie CC, Eberhardt MS, Goldstein DE, Little RR, Wiedmeyer HM, Byrd-Holt DD: Prevalence of diabetes, impaired fasting glucose, and impaired glucose tolerance in U.S. adults: The Third National Health and Nutrition Examination Survey, 1988–1994. *Diabetes Care* 21:518–24, 1998
22. DECODE Study Group: Will new diagnostic criteria for diabetes mellitus change the phenotype of patients with diabetes? Reanalysis of European epidemiological data. *Br Med J* 317:371–75, 1998
23. Qiao Q, Nakagami T, Tuomilehto J, Borch-Johnsen K, Balkau B, Iwamoto Y, Tajima N, for the DECODA Study Group and International Diabetes Epidemiology Group: Comparison of the fasting and the 2-h glucose criteria for diabetes in different Asian cohorts. *Diabetologia* 43:1470–75, 2000
24. Valle T, Tuomilehto J, Eriksson J: Epidemiology of NIDDM in Europids. In *International Textbook of Diabetes Mellitus.* Alberti K, Zimmet P, DeFronzo R, Keen H, Eds. Chichester, U.K., Wiley, 1997, p. 125–42

Johan Eriksson, MD, PhD, Jaana Lindström, MSc, and Jaakko Tuomilehto MD, MPolSc, PhD, are from the National Public Health Institute, Helsinki, Finland. Matti Uusitupa, MD, PhD, is from University of Kuopio, Kuopia, Finland.

11

Regional Body Fat Distribution, the Insulin Resistance-Dyslipidemic Syndrome, and the Risk of Type 2 Diabetes and Coronary Heart Disease

JEAN-PIERRE DESPRÉS, PHD, CHARLES COUILLARD, PHD, JEAN BERGERON, MD, AND BENOÎT LAMARCHE, PHD

Highlights

- Visceral adipose tissue accumulation is an important factor to consider in the evaluation of health risks associated with obesity.
- The simultaneous presence of hyperinsulinemia, hyperapolipoprotein B, and small, dense LDL particles is associated with a 20-fold increase in the risk of ischemic heart disease.
- A simple and inexpensive screening test to identify a high-risk form of abdominal obesity is to determine if the patient has the following: a waist circumference ≥90 cm and triglyceride levels ≥2.0 mmol/l.
- Improvements in the metabolic risk profile resulting from endurance exercise training are more related to the volume of exercise than to its intensity.

- From a public health standpoint, the greatest benefit would be to transform our largely sedentary population into moderately active individuals.

The prevalence of obesity is unfortunately increasing,[1,2] and a report of the World Health Organization[3] emphasized the worldwide trend for an increased prevalence for overweight and obesity in numerous countries. This phenomenon is a source of concern because an excess of body fat has been associated with several complications, such as hypertension, diabetes, and dyslipidemia, as well as with an increased risk of cerebral and vascular diseases.[4–9]

The objective of the present chapter is to review the health hazards of obesity, paying particular attention to metabolic risk factors for coronary heart disease (CHD). Pathophysiological aspects of insulin resistance and dyslipidemia commonly found among obese patients will be discussed, with a section on the potential role of regular physical activity as an approach to improve metabolic parameters and reduce the risk of type 2 diabetes and CHD.

Metabolic Complications of Obesity: The Importance of Visceral Adipose Tissue

Although it is commonly accepted that overweight or obese patients are frequently characterized by hypertension, diabetes, dyslipidemia, and cerebral and vascular diseases,[4–7,10] this is not the case in every obese patient.[11] For instance, some very obese patients have a fairly normal metabolic risk factor profile, whereas some moderately overweight individuals are characterized by severe insulin resistance, a marked dyslipidemic state, and hypertension, and they may develop type 2 diabetes or premature CHD. Thus, obesity is not only heterogeneous in terms of its etiology, but also with respect to its related metabolic complications.[6–8,10–15] In 1947, the French physician Jean Vague was the first to discover that body fat topography was more important than excess fatness in the evaluation of the obese patient.[16] At such an early time, Vague had already suggested that upper-body obesity, a condition that he described as android or male type obesity, was commonly accompanied by hypertension, diabetes, or clinical signs of CHD, whereas he noted that the typical female pattern of body fat deposition, which he referred to as gynoid obesity, was seldom associated with complications.[16,17] However, it took a few decades before these pioneering clinical observations received support from large epidemiological studies.

Waist-to-Hip Circumference Ratio

In the early 1980s, an American group led by Ahmed Kissebah[10] and a Swedish team conducted by Per Björntorp[18] almost simultaneously reported that a high proportion of abdominal fat was associated with alterations in glucose tolerance as well as with increased fasting insulin and triglyceride (TG) levels. One year later, results from the prospective study of men and women of Göthenburg confirmed that a high proportion of abdominal fat, crudely assessed by an increased ratio of waist-to-hip circumferences, was also predictive of an increased risk of ischemic heart disease (IHD)[19,20] (this association being completely independent from the concomitant variation in the level of total body fat). In 1985, the same group also reported that a high waist-to-hip ratio (WHR) combined with an elevated BMI was associated with a more than 30-fold increase in the risk of developing diabetes (Fig. 11.1).[21] These studies provided epidemiologic validation of Vague's early hypothesis. The concept of abdominal obesity as a serious health hazard is now more and more widely recognized, and the study of the etiology of abdominal fat accumulation as well as the pathophysiology of the complications resulting from the presence of abdominal obesity are under active investigation.

Visceral Adipose Tissue Accumulation

Although the WHR is a simple measurement to perform, it should be recognized that this variable only provides, at best, a crude estimation of the proportion of abdominal fat.[22] With the development of imaging techniques such as magnetic resonance imaging and computed tomography, it has been possible to measure body fat distribution with a high level of accuracy, especially when distinguishing the amount of subcutaneous abdominal fat from the amount of adipose tissue (AT) located in the abdominal cavity—the so-called

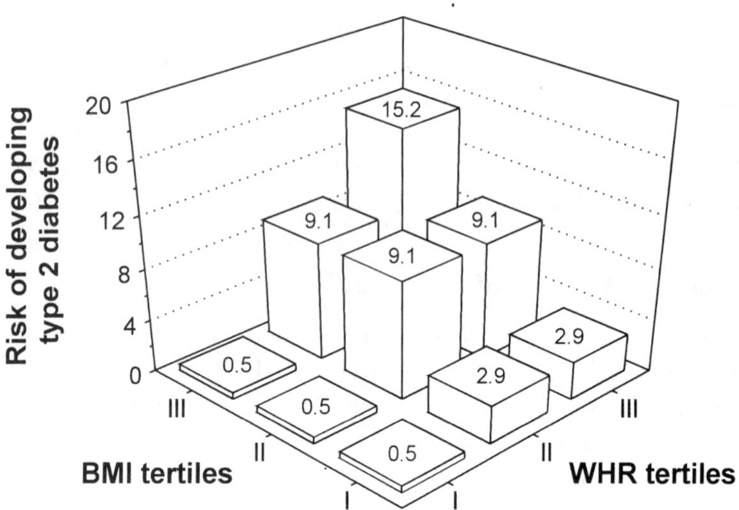

FIGURE 11.1 Risk of developing type 2 diabetes according to total body fatness (BMI) and fat distribution (WHR) in men.

Reproduced with permission from Ohlson et al.[21]

intra-abdominal or visceral AT (Fig. 11.2).[23–27] With this methodology, studies have been conducted to quantify the respective contributions of total body fatness, subcutaneous abdominal fat accumulation, and visceral AT deposition as correlates of the metabolic complications commonly observed among obese patients. When we first examined this issue, we matched obese individuals having the same amount of total body fat but who had either a low or high

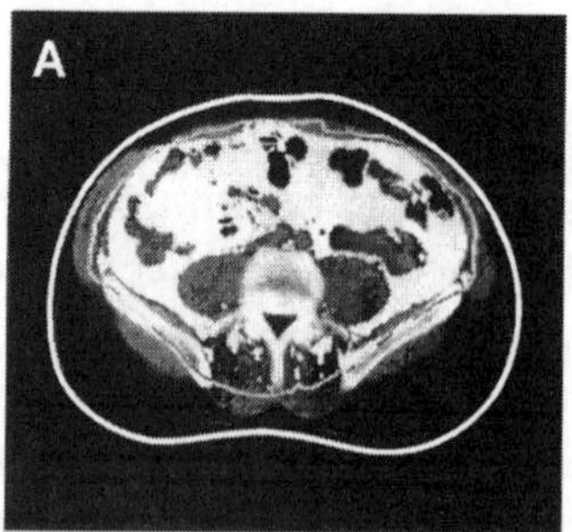

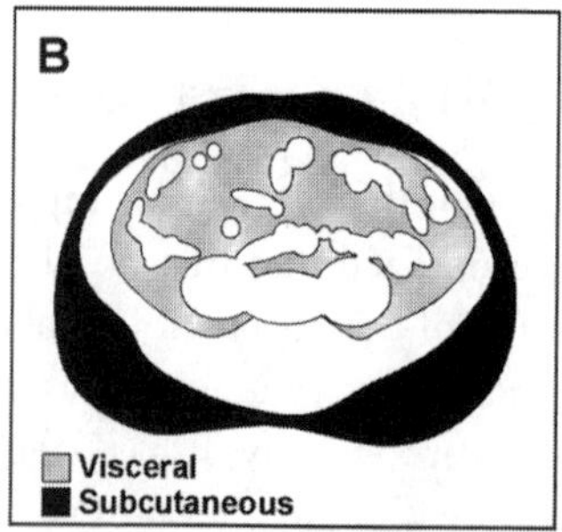

FIGURE 11.2 *A:* Abdominal scan obtained by computed tomography. *B:* Schematic view of abdominal AT accumulation.

accumulation of visceral AT measured by computed tomography[14,28] and found that obesity per se was associated with significant alterations in the metabolic risk factor profile, which included moderate increases in fasting plasma insulin and TG concentrations.[14,28] However, in both men and women, obesity accompanied by a high accumulation of visceral AT was associated with a cluster of metabolic abnormalities (Table 11.1), which included hypertriglyceridemia, hypoalphalipoproteinemia, increased plasma insulin concentrations measured in the fasting state and after a 75-g oral glucose load, and a deterioration in glucose tolerance.[14,28] Thus, visceral obesity is a better correlate of the metabolic complications commonly found in obese patients than excess body weight or body fatness per se. Additional measurements of the plasma lipid-lipoprotein profile revealed that the reduction in plasma HDL cholesterol levels found in viscerally obese patients was largely explained by the preferential reduction in the plasma concentration of cardioprotective HDL_2 cholesterol.[29]

Although excess fatness including an elevated accumulation of subcutaneous adipose tissue has, at least to a certain extent, a deleterious effect on in vivo insulin action and on plasma lipoprotein levels, it appears that obese subjects with the highest accumulation of visceral AT are characterized by the most deteriorated metabolic risk profile. Thus, visceral AT accumulation is an important factor to consider in the evaluation of the risks associated with obesity. We believe that this interpretation reconciles our results with those of

TABLE 11.1 Some Metabolic Abnormalities of Visceral Obesity

- Hypertriglyceridemia
- Low HDL cholesterol concentrations
- Elevated apoB levels
- Small, dense LDL particles
- Hyperinsulinemia
- Insulin resistance
- Glucose intolerance
- Impaired fibrinolysis
- Increased susceptibility to thrombosis
- Endothelial dysfunction
- Inflammatory profile (increased interleukin-6 and C-reactive protein levels)

studies that have suggested that both visceral AT and excess subcutaneous fat (a good marker of total body fat) are significant correlates of an impaired in vivo insulin action.[30]

Effects of Sex and Age on Body Fat Distribution

We are all aware of the well-known sex difference in abdominal fat accumulation—men being more prone to this condition than women before menopause. To examine this phenomenon, we studied the relationship between visceral AT accumulation and total body fatness in both men and premenopausal women.[31] We found that for any level of total body fat, men had on average twice the amount of visceral AT found in premenopausal women.[31] Because visceral AT is a highly significant correlate of the cluster of metabolic complications of obesity,[6,13,14,28,32–41] we also tested whether this greater accumulation of visceral AT found in men compared with premenopausal women could explain the greater susceptibility of men to the related complications. For that purpose, we matched men and women for the same amount of visceral AT. After this procedure, a similar cardiovascular disease (CVD) risk profile was observed in men and women, despite the fact that matched women were characterized by a greater accumulation of subcutaneous fat than men.[42] These results support the view that the low accumulation of visceral AT found in women before menopause helps explain their more favorable CVD risk profile. In addition to sex, age is another important correlate of visceral AT accumulation because there is a selective deposition of visceral AT with increased age in both men and women. Furthermore, the relative estrogen deficiency that occurs at menopause has been suggested to be associated with an acceleration in visceral AT deposition leading to the progressive development of insulin resistance and to a dyslipidemic profile.[43] Interestingly, women on hormone replacement therapy are characterized by a lower relative accumulation of abdominal AT and a more favorable metabolic risk profile than postmenopausal women not on hormone replacement therapy.[44] Additional work in this area is needed to establish to what extent the expanding visceral AT depot observed at menopause is contributing to the deterioration of the CVD risk profile found in postmenopausal women. Furthermore, whether this potentially deleterious accumulation of visceral fat can be prevented by *1*) lifestyle modifications, *2*) proper hormonal replacement therapy, and/or *3*) pharmacotherapy is an unanswered question of great relevance to public health.

Ethnic Group Differences in Body Fat Distribution

Although numerous studies on regional AT distribution have been performed in Caucasians, several studies have shown that body fat distribution differs across ethnic groups.[45] For instance, Mexican-Americans have been shown to have a greater propensity to abdominal fat accumulation than Caucasians.[46] On the other hand, in both men[47] and women,[47–49] Caucasians have been characterized by a greater relative deposition of AT than African-Americans. Other studies have also examined fat patterning in Japanese-Americans,[34,50,51] North American Natives,[52–54] and Asian Indians.[55,56] Thus, the reported race-related differences in body fat distribution suggest that the genetic factors could modulate the magnitude of the interrelationships between adiposity, body fat distribution, and the metabolic risk profile. However, further studies are needed to sort out the respective contributions of cultural and genetic influences to the differences in body fat distribution noted among ethnic groups.

Atherogenic Dyslipidemia of the Viscerally Obese Insulin-Resistant Patient

Visceral obesity is associated with an insulin-resistant hyperinsulinemic state that may lead to glucose intolerance, with this condition potentially evolving to type 2 diabetes in the presence of genetic factors that are presently poorly understood.[7,12,57] In addition, this insulin-resistant hyperinsulinemic condition is associated with a typical dyslipidemic profile that includes hypertriglyceridemia, hyperapolipoprotein B, low HDL cholesterol levels, and an increased proportion of small, dense LDL particles.[6,13,14,39,58–60]

The Québec Cardiovascular Study

Prospective studies have shown that the aforementioned dyslipidemic profile is associated with an increased risk of IHD.[61,62] In a prospective study conducted in Québec City (the Québec Cardiovascular

Study[63]), we had the opportunity to study a sample of 2,103 middle-aged men initially free from IHD and to follow them for incidence of a first IHD event over a period of 5 years. When we first compared the prevalence of various dyslipidemic phenotypes in the 114 men who developed IHD to that of the remaining sample of 1,989 men who remained healthy, ~50% of men who remained free from IHD had a normal lipid profile, whereas less than one-third of the 114 men who developed IHD had a normal lipid profile.[63] Thus, the various dyslipidemic phenotypes were more prevalent among men who developed IHD than among men who remained healthy, and multiple regression analyses revealed that diabetes, apolipoprotein (apo)B, age, smoking, and elevated systolic blood pressure were the best predictors of the risk of IHD in this cohort.[64] Therefore, apoB, not cholesterol or LDL cholesterol, was the best metabolic predictor of IHD risk in this sample of French Canadian men.[64]

A New Metabolic Triad: An Atherogenic Profile Linked to Visceral Obesity

Although only one prospective study has indicated that visceral AT is an independent risk factor for IHD,[65] the metabolic abnormalities found in this condition have been shown to substantially increase the risk of IHD. For instance, we found that the hyperinsulinemic state of visceral obesity was predictive of an increased risk of IHD, especially when it was accompanied by an increased apoB concentration.[66] Visceral obesity also has been associated with an increased proportion of small, dense LDL particles.[67] We measured LDL peak particle diameter in men of the Québec Cardiovascular Study[68] and stratified our subjects on the basis of apoB concentrations (using the 50th percentile of the distribution) and of LDL peak particle diameter to identify subjects with small, dense LDL particles. Among men with normal apoB concentrations, we found that small, dense LDL particles were not associated with an increased risk of IHD.[68] However, men with both small, dense LDL particles and elevated apoB concentrations were characterized by a more than fivefold increase in the risk of IHD, indicating that the concentration of the small, dense LDL particles was a major risk factor for IHD.[68] It should be emphasized that visceral obesity is not only associated with a reduction in LDL peak particle diameter, but also with an increased concentration of LDL particles.[6]

Because abdominal obesity is associated with hyperinsulinemia (resulting from insulin resistance), an increased apoB concentration (reflecting an increased concentration of atherogenic lipoproteins), and small, dense LDL, we were interested to quantify the IHD risk associated with the simultaneous presence of hyperinsulinemia, hyperapolipoprotein B, and small, dense LDL particles. In the sample of middle-aged men of the Québec Cardiovascular Study, we found that the simultaneous presence of hyperinsulinemia, hyperapolipoprotein B, and small, dense LDL particles (a cluster that we refer to as the "atherogenic metabolic triad") was associated with essentially a 20-fold increase in the risk of having a first IHD event over 5 years—this increase in risk being largely unaffected by adjustment for fasting plasma TG, LDL cholesterol, and HDL cholesterol levels (Fig. 11.3).[69] Thus, it

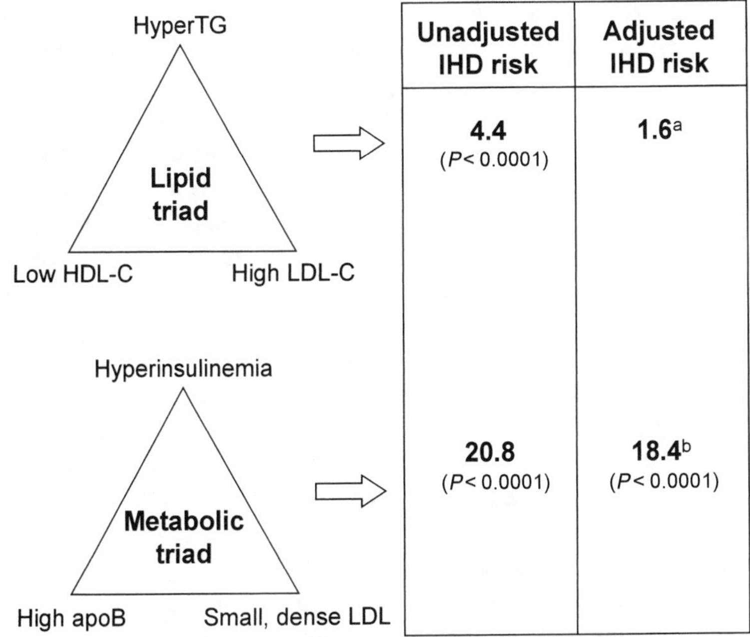

FIGURE 11.3 Five-year relative risk of IHD in men of the Québec Cardiovascular Study. All ratios are adjusted for systolic blood pressure, family history of IHD, and use of medication. [a]Additional adjustment for nontraditional risk factors (metabolic triad). [b]Additional adjustment for traditional risk factors (lipid triad). HDL-C, HDL cholesterol; LDL-C, LDL cholesterol.

Adapted from Lamarche et al.[69]

appears that this new triad of metabolic risk factors found in the insulin-resistant state of visceral obesity substantially increases the risk of IHD. This increased risk is such that this cluster of metabolic alterations may represent one of the most prevalent causes of CHD in affluent societies and may even be more deleterious to cardiovascular health than hypercholesterolemia per se.

Hypertriglyceridemic Waist: A Simple Clinical Phenotype to Screen for the High-Risk Form of Abdominal Obesity

After having recognized the health hazards of the new metabolic triad as it relates to IHD risk, we were interested in the development of a simple screening approach to help general physicians and health care professionals identify these high-risk abdominally obese patients.

In a recent study, we reported that waist circumference was the simplest and best correlate of plasma insulin and apoB levels, whereas another simple parameter, fasting TG concentration, was the best predictor of LDL size. Sensitivity and specificity analyses revealed that, in middle-aged men, the identification of carriers and noncarriers of the metabolic triad (elevated insulin and apoB levels as well as small, dense LDL particles) was best obtained with cutoff points of 90 cm for waist circumference and 2.0 mmol/l for TG (Fig. 11.4). For instance, middle-aged men with a waist circumference <90 cm and fasting TG levels <2.0 mmol/l had a low chance (10%) of being carriers of the triad. However, >80% of men with a waist girth ≥90 cm and TG levels ≥2.0 mmol/l had all features of the metabolic triad.[70] Thus, we believe that we have developed a simple and inexpensive screening test to identify a high-risk form of abdominal obesity. Because there is no prospective data available in women to quantify the IHD risk associated with the metabolic triad, there is an urgent need to validate this approach in women. Finally, it should also be emphasized that there are differences in susceptibility to develop visceral obesity and related complications (diabetes, hypertension, and CHD) among ethnic groups, and our approach should only be considered valid for Caucasian men. Specific cutoffs will likely be obtained, for instance, for our native population as well as for the African-American and South Asian populations.

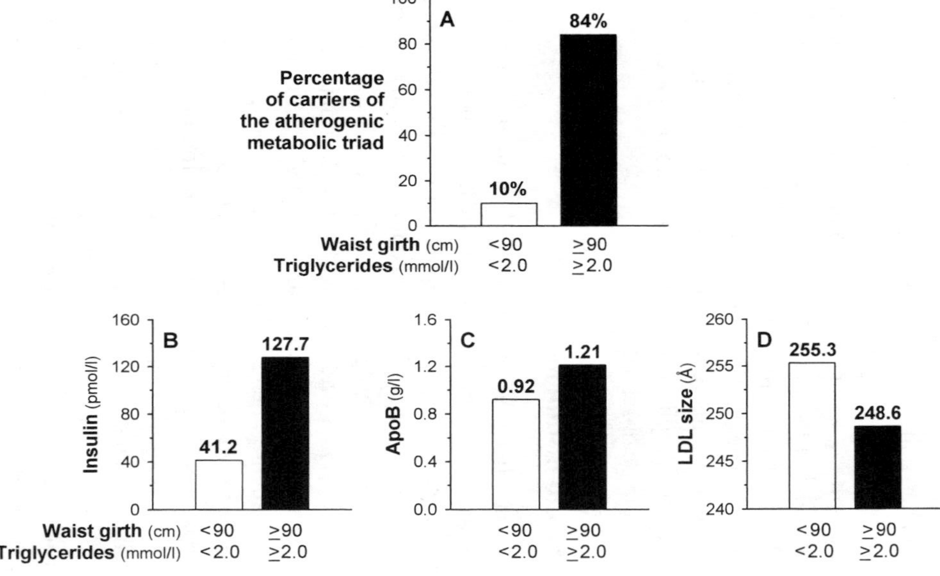

FIGURE 11.4 *A:* Proportion of subjects with the atherogenic metabolic triad (hyperinsulinemia, high apoB, and small, dense LDL particles) in middle-aged men according to waist circumference and fasting plasma TG levels. Fasting plasma insulin (*B*) and apoB (*C*) concentrations as well as LDL peak particle diameter (*D*) in men classified on the basis of waist circumference and fasting plasma TGs are shown.

Adapted from Lemieux et al.[70]

Visceral Obesity and the Plurimetabolic Syndrome: A Causal Relationship?

The etiology of the insulin-resistant state of visceral obesity is not fully understood, although it is known that an impaired insulin action can be found in both obese and nonobese subjects.[71] Studies conducted among insulin-resistant or type 2 diabetic patients have shown that a family history of diabetes alters the relationship of abdominal fat accumulation to indexes of plasma glucose–insulin homeostasis.[72,73] We have reported that among subjects with similar deteriorations in plasma glucose–insulin homeostasis, those with a family history of diabetes had lower levels of abdominal fat than subjects without a family history of diabetes.[73] These results suggest that the presence of genetic susceptibility factors could reduce the threshold of abdominal fat above which metabolic complications predictive of an increased risk of type 2 diabetes could be observed.

Free Fatty Acids and Insulin Resistance

Visceral adipocytes have been shown to display a high lipolytic activity that is poorly inhibited by insulin. This unrepressed hyperlipolytic state could contribute to a greater flux of free fatty acids to the liver through the portal circulation,[12,14,39] a situation that could explain why viscerally obese patients are frequently characterized by liver steatosis and a fatty liver.[74] Interestingly, new evidence suggests that liver fat content is an important determinant of hepatic insulin sensitivity in both nondiabetic and type 2 diabetic patients.[75,76] Thus, high levels of portal free fatty acids contribute to reduce hepatic insulin extraction,[77,78] exacerbating systemic hyperinsulinemia. The increased esterification of these portal fatty acids into TG leads to an increased synthesis of very-low-density lipoproteins (VLDLs) and to a reduced hepatic degradation of apoB, which in turn contributes to an overproduction of apoB-associated lipoproteins by the liver.[6,79] Furthermore, increased hepatic lipid oxidation is associated with impaired glycolysis,[80,81] providing precursors for gluconeogenesis[82] explaining the increased hepatic glucose output, which is a major factor contributing to the glucose intolerance of visceral obesity. In addition, the fat content within muscle is increased in obesity and has been shown to be a strong correlate of insulin resistance.[83–87] Although the mechanisms by which fatty acids accumulate in skeletal muscle are not well known, the metabolic capacity of skeletal muscle of obese individuals appears to be geared toward fat esterification rather than oxidation.[87] Finally, insulin-sensitive glycogen synthase is reduced in skeletal muscle of insulin-resistant obese patients, and this factor could also contribute to the state of insulin resistance assessed in vivo.[88] Thus, in vivo insulin action is altered in subjects with visceral obesity, and compensatory hyperinsulinemia is required to regulate glucose levels in these subjects.

Lipoprotein and Hepatic TG Lipase Activities

Lipoprotein lipase (LPL), the enzyme responsible for the catabolism of TG-rich lipoproteins, also appears to be affected by the insulin-resistant state of visceral obesity. Indeed, its activity has been shown to be reduced in postheparin plasma, whereas the activity of hepatic TG lipase (HTGL) (an enzyme with high affinity for small, TG-rich lipoproteins) is substantially increased in visceral obesity.[29] Thus, these reciprocal changes in LPL and HTGL activities reduce the catabolic rate of large TG-rich lipoproteins and increase the catabolism of HDL particles by HTGL, leading to their increased conversion to HDL_3, which contains smaller HDL particles than HDL_2.[6,14,29,39] Skeletal muscle LPL activity is reduced in insulin-resistant subjects,[89] and in vivo insulin sensitivity is positively correlated with skeletal muscle LPL activity. The hypertriglyceridemia resulting from an increased hepatic VLDL production and a slower clearance of TG-rich lipoproteins due to reduced LPL activity also contributes to an increased transfer of TG from VLDL to LDL and HDL particles in exchange for cholesterol esters from LDL and HDL, ultimately leading to the TG enrichment of LDL and HDL.[29,90] Such TG enrichment is associated with a reduced cholesterol content of HDL, partly explaining the low HDL cholesterol levels in visceral obesity.[90] In addition, a TG-rich LDL particle is an adequate substrate for HTGL generating atherogenic small, dense LDL particles.[39] In this regard, we found marked differences in visceral AT accumulation and in the related dyslipidemic profile between blacks and whites, with whites being more prone to visceral AT accumulation.[47] We also reported that the overall more atherogenic lipoprotein profile found in obese white individuals than in obese black individuals was explained by the greater deposition of visceral AT in whites than in blacks. In accordance with this difference, we observed that the lower HDL cholesterol levels in white subjects with excess visceral AT could be explained by a substantial difference in the ratio of HTGL to LPL activities, with this ratio being higher in white individuals than in black individuals.[47]

Endocrine Disorders

Although it is well established that visceral AT is a strong correlate of metabolic abnormalities, increasing the risk of type 2 diabetes and IHD, such evidence should not be considered the ultimate demonstration of a cause and effect relationship. Indeed, the possibility cannot be excluded that visceral obesity is only a marker of a more primary defect leading to both visceral fat deposition and metabolic complications. For example, Björntorp[91] suggested that visceral obesity may be a marker of a "civilization syndrome" associated with a maladaptive response to stress (Fig. 11.5). Under this model, the in-

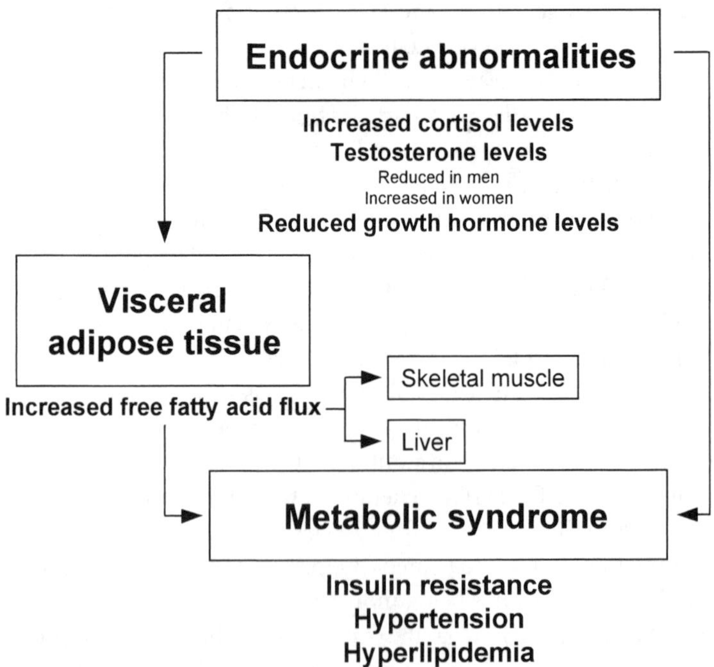

FIGURE 11.5 Relationships between endocrine disorders, excessive visceral adipose tissue accumulation, and the metabolic syndrome.

Adapted from Björntorp.[91]

ability to adequately cope with stress would be associated with an activation of the hypothalamic-pituitary-adrenal axis,[91] which would increase the control of carbohydrate and lipid metabolism by glucocorticoids[92,93] and reduce the production of gonadal steroids.[91] In concordance with this model, women with a high proportion of abdominal fat, as estimated by an elevated WHR, have been characterized by reduced sex hormone–binding globulin (SHBG) and increased free testosterone levels.[15,94,95] Reduced SHBG concentrations have also been associated with increased plasma glucose and insulin levels as well as with hypertriglyceridemia in women.[15,94] Plasma testosterone and SHBG concentrations have also been found to be reduced in viscerally obese individuals.[96,97]

Visceral adipose cells have a greater density of glucocorticoid receptors than subcutaneous adipocytes. This phenomenon helps explain the greater sensitivity of visceral adipocytes to stressor agents.[98,99] Furthermore, the effects of glucocorticoids on skeletal muscle and the liver help generate a state of insulin resistance and the metabolic alterations observed in visceral obesity.[92,93] In addition, glucocorticoids have been reported to stimulate VLDL and apoB production, to reduce the activity of LDL receptors, and to induce in vivo insulin resistance.[92,93]

On the other hand, increased tumor necrosis factor-α (TNF-α) levels have been associated with insulin resistance in rodents.[100] Because adipocytes secrete TNF-α, their contribution to the development of obesity-related insulin resistance and type 2 diabetes in humans deserves to be further investigated, although such studies have not yet been able to demonstrate a physiological link between these metabolic processes.[100] Furthermore, the treatment of normal mice with resistin, a newly discovered signaling molecule secreted by adipose tissue, has been shown to impair glucose tolerance and insulin action.[101] In this regard, the discovery of resistin could be an important breakthrough in the understanding of the development of insulin resistance and type 2 diabetes.

Finally, it has often been suggested that it is difficult to sort out the primary factor responsible for the relationship between abdominal obesity and insulin resistance–hyperinsulinemia. Clinical studies using peroxisome proliferator-activated receptor (PPAR)-γ agonists (insulin sensitizers) have clearly shown that improving insulin action does not lead to weight loss and to a mobilization of visceral AT.[102] On the other hand, losing weight has been shown to improve insulin sensitivity.[103]

Therefore, these observations provide further support that it is abdominal obesity that generates insulin resistance, not insulin resistance that generates abdominal obesity.

Effect of Weight Loss on the Metabolic Risk Profile of Obese Patients

Globally, the literature available on diet-induced weight loss indicates that reductions in body weight and the amount of abdominal fat are associated with significant improvements in the CVD risk profile, which includes decreased blood pressure, increased in vivo insulin action, and improvements in the plasma lipoprotein-lipid profile.[35,104,105] Despite these favorable metabolic effects, it should be pointed out that there is a lack of randomized weight loss trials showing that body weight loss and related metabolic improvements lead to reductions in hard clinical end points, such as decreased morbidity and mortality from CVD. In addition, there is no universal acceptance of the critical amount of weight loss necessary to substantially improve the metabolic risk profile and to significantly decrease morbidity and mortality. Although the notion that a 10% weight loss is generally associated with substantial improvements in the metabolic risk profile is gaining wider acceptance,[35] we need to keep in mind that the magnitude of improvement in the metabolic risk profile associated with a 10% weight loss obviously depends on the patient's initial body weight and on his or her initial metabolic risk profile. For example, a 10% weight loss in a patient with a BMI of 45 kg/m^2 and a body weight of 150 kg would only be associated with a 15-kg weight loss. Thus, the patient's residual body weight (135 kg) may still be associated with a high risk of CVD (although some benefits could be expected from such weight loss). However, a 10% weight loss in a high-risk abdominally obese patient weighing 100 kg may be enough to substantially reduce abdominal fat accumulation and improve his or her metabolic risk profile, especially if this patient is insulin-resistant and characterized by hypertriglyceridemia–low HDL cholesterol atherogenic dyslipidemia (Fig. 11.6).[6] If we refer to abdominally obese patients who may not be very obese, the normalization of body weight and of body fat content may not be necessary to substantially improve insulin sensitivity and reduce CVD risk, although no randomized weight loss trial has confirmed this hypothesis. On the other hand, the loss and normalization

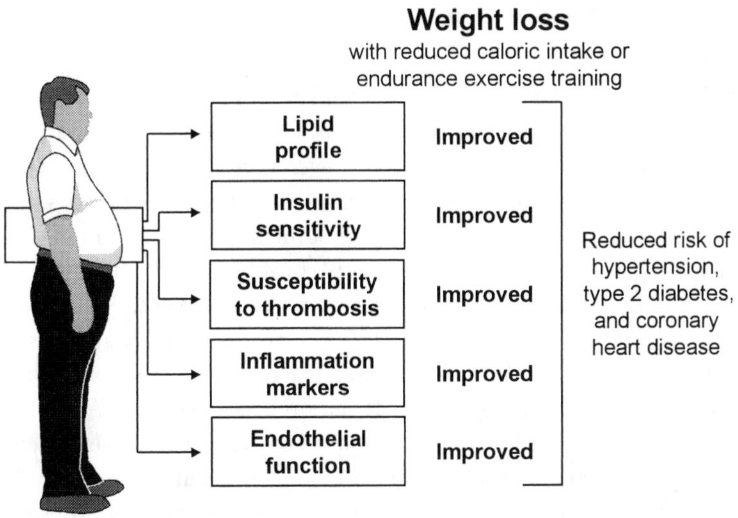

FIGURE 11.6 Summary of the impact of weight loss on the metabolic risk profile.

of the visceral adipose depot is a critically important therapeutic target. Thus, several factors need to be considered when establishing the therapeutic targets in a weight loss program (Table 11.2). For instance, the patient's initial body weight and his or her body fat distribution, family history of complications, and initial metabolic risk profile need to be taken into account.

TABLE 11.2 Risk Assessment of the Obese Patient

- How much fat?
  BMI
- Where is the fat?
  Waist circumference
- What are the traditional risk factors?
  Blood pressure, cholesterol, smoking, and diabetes
- Do I have the insulin resistance syndrome?
  Waist circumference plus TGs, cholesterol/HDL cholesterol
- Genes?
  Family history of hypertension, CHD, and diabetes

Exercise, Physical Activity, and Cardiovascular Health: The "Metabolic Fitness" Concept

As for diet-induced weight loss, it should be emphasized that currently there is no large-scale randomized trial of exercise and its impact on CVD risk in overweight patients. However, there is a large body of evidence indicating that endurance exercise training may generate some weight loss in obese patients as well as some improvements in in vivo insulin action and in the metabolic risk profile. These metabolic improvements would be predictive of a reduced risk of developing type 2 diabetes[106–108] and premature CVD.[105,109] Such observations are consistent with the notion that both physically active[110–112] and fit individuals[113–116] are at reduced risk of CHD and related mortality. Although the identification of the minimal amount of exercise necessary to optimally reduce CHD risk remains a matter of debate, it is generally considered that a physically active lifestyle may favor body weight control and improve the metabolic risk profile (Table 11.3).[105,109,117–122]

Intensity and Duration of Exercise

When the issues of physical activity, exercise, and health are addressed, a critical question is whether an increase in maximal oxygen consumption (VO_{2max}) is necessary to reduce the risk of complications in sedentary obese patients or whether increasing daily energy expenditure per se through a more active lifestyle would reduce CHD risk.[109] Based on the literature indicating that VO_{2max} or the performance on a treadmill test are powerful predictors of CHD and related mortal-

TABLE 11.3 Physical and Metabolic Improvements Associated With Exercise Training and Obesity

Decrease	Increase
Body weight	Muscle mass
Total body fat	HDL cholesterol
Visceral adipose tissue	HDL_2 cholesterol
Triglycerides	
ApoB	
Total/HDL cholesterol ratio	
Insulin	

ity,[113–116] it may be suggested that improving fitness should be an important component of an exercise program designed for poorly fit and sedentary obese patients. However, results from our laboratory and from the published literature suggest that an individual should focus on increasing energy expenditure rather than improving cardiorespiratory fitness to improve the metabolic risk factor profile.[109] It is well established that exercise sessions of at least 20 min of high-intensity aerobic exercise performed three times per week may eventually improve cardiorespiratory fitness over several weeks.[123] However, if the net increase in daily energy expenditure associated with such an exercise regimen is calculated, this change is unlikely to have a substantial effect on energy balance, body weight, and metabolic risk variables.[109] However, an exercise program performed at a lower intensity, such as 50% of VO_{2max} (which would approximately correspond to the exercise intensity associated with a brisk walk), performed over a longer duration (up to 45 min) and on an almost daily basis would likely have a greater impact on daily energy expenditure, body composition, and the metabolic risk profile.[105,109]

Exercise, Body Weight, and Body Fat Distribution

Several exercise training studies have shown that regular endurance exercise may eventually lead to reductions in total body fat and to the mobilization of abdominal AT, leading to improvements in the metabolic risk profile as long as the energy expenditure generated by the exercise program is sufficient.[109,118–120,124–131] Recently, Ross et al.[132] studied the effects of equivalent diet- or exercise-induced weight loss and also quantified the effects of exercise without weight loss on subcutaneous and visceral fat, skeletal muscle, and insulin sensitivity in 52 obese men. Although total body fat decreased in both weight loss groups (diet- vs. exercise-induced), the average reduction was greater in the exercise-induced weight loss group than in the diet-induced weight loss group. Similar reductions in abdominal subcutaneous and visceral fat were observed in the two weight loss groups as well as in the exercise without weight loss group. However, plasma glucose and insulin values (fasting and after an oral glucose challenge) did not change in the treatment groups when compared with control subjects. The authors also reported that the average improvement of in vivo insulin sensitivity measured by the euglycemic-hyperinsulinemic clamp technique was similar in the diet-induced weight loss group and the exercise-induced weight loss group. However, such improvement was significantly greater than that in the control group and in the exercise without weight loss group. These observations led the authors to conclude that weight loss induced by increased daily physical activity without caloric restriction substantially improves insulin sensitivity and that the loss of abdominal fat produced by the exercise training–induced energy deficit is an important correlate of such improvement in in vivo insulin action.[132]

Although apparently discordant results regarding the effect of exercise on the metabolic risk profile can be found in the literature,[124,133–135] it is important to point out that several factors could explain such discrepancies among studies. For instance, variation in subjects' age, initial CVD risk profile, initial body composition, level of abdominal fat, sex, and relevant candidate genes as well as in other undetermined but potentially important genes are all factors that may explain individual differences in the response to a standardized exercise training program. For example, a premenopausal woman with a normal metabolic risk profile is more likely to show trivial changes in her metabolic risk profile in response to exercise training. On the other hand, an abdominally obese insulin-resistant dyslipidemic man is likely to show substantial metabolic improvements in response to the same endurance exercise training program. This notion is often ignored in the interpretation of the literature on exercise training and CHD risk factors.

Metabolic Benefits of Exercise Training

Although it is fairly well accepted that endurance exercise training has a beneficial effect on the CVD risk profile, there is some controversy regarding the exercise prescription that should be recommended to optimally reduce CVD risk. The American College of Sports Medicine[136] stated that the minimal exercise stimulus needed to improve cardiorespiratory fitness may not be sufficient to improve health-related fitness,[122] and it has been recognized that its minimal exercise recommendations should not be considered adequate for overweight or obese patients trying to lose weight to improve their metabolic profile and reduce their risk of complications. An exercise program for the high-risk abdominally obese patient should focus on the improvement of health-related variables rather than on the improvement of exercise tolerance (which is nevertheless an additional legitimate therapeutic target). As discussed above, metabolic variables predictive of diabetes and CHD risk appear to be more substantially altered by the volume of exercise than by its intensity.[105,109] Thus, exercise training programs performed at ~70% VO_{2max} induce favorable changes in both cardiorespiratory fitness and in the CVD risk profile when the net increase in energy expenditure associated with the exercise training program is sufficient.[109,118–120,128,130,131] Generally, such exercise programs induce reductions in plasma TG and apoB-containing lipoproteins and increase plasma HDL cholesterol concentrations, although not all studies have reported such benefits.[118–120,123,128,131,137] Again, it is important to keep in mind that the more deteriorated the initial CVD risk profile, the greater the likelihood of finding significant improvements with regular exercise training.[109] Furthermore, endurance exercise training programs that have not reported substantial changes in the plasma lipoprotein profile may not have had sufficient duration and frequency of sessions to generate metabolic improvements. In this regard, exercise training studies that have induced large increases in energy expenditure were those that reported the most substantial weight losses and related improvements in the metabolic profile predictive of CVD risk.[105,109] For instance, Williams et al.[127] reported that improvements in both VO_{2max} and treadmill duration after training were poor predictors of changes in plasma HDL cholesterol levels. However, they found a highly significant correlation between the increase in plasma HDL concentration and the number of miles ran per week—a finding consistent with the results of Kokkinos et al.[138] Because exercise is also associated with an acute response of metabolic variables (Fig. 11.7), optimal metabolic improvements may be obtained when prolonged exercise is performed on an almost daily basis. In this regard, Rogers et al.[139] showed that a substantial increase in energy expenditure generated by daily prolonged exercise could improve insulin action and reduce plasma insulin levels in a matter of a few days among subjects with an initially deteriorated metabolic profile.[139] Furthermore, two distinct groups have shown that exercise training prevented the incidence of type 2 diabetes over a 6-year period.[140,141] These studies are incidentally discussed in more detail elsewhere in this book (see Chapters 8 and 10). Thus, a moderate-intensity endurance exercise program in

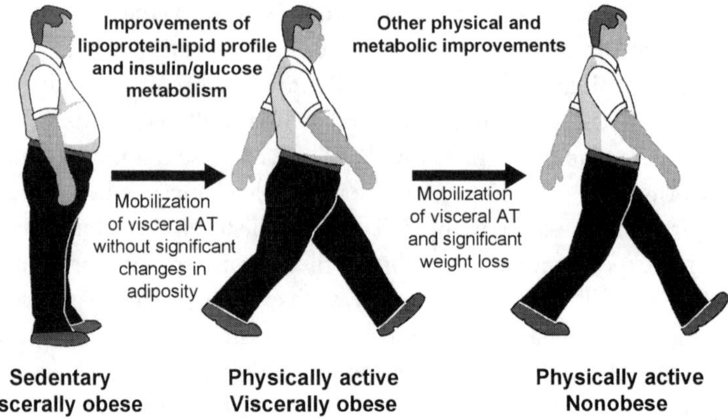

FIGURE 11.7 Combined metabolic benefits of acute and chronic exercise on body fatness and metabolic risk profile.

which subjects exercise for at least 1 h on a daily basis can rapidly improve insulin sensitivity, which leads to an improvement in plasma lipoprotein levels (Fig. 11.8). These studies support the notion that the improvements in the metabolic risk profile resulting from endurance exercise training are more related to the volume of exercise than to its intensity.

Conclusions

Our high-fat, high–refined sugar intake combined with our sedentary lifestyle are contributing factors in the high prevalence of hyperinsulinemia and insulin resistance in our population.[71,105] Because insulin resistance is a significant correlate of a dyslipidemic profile predictive of an increased risk of CHD,[71] it has been proposed that the insulin-resistant dyslipidemic state frequently observed in subjects with visceral obesity may be the most prevalent cause of CHD in North America.[13,40,60,71,142] Consequently, maintaining an adequate level of insulin sensitivity through regular exercise may not only reduce the risk of developing type 2 diabetes, it may also be associated with a more favorable metabolic risk factor profile, thereby reducing the risk of CHD.[105,109] Prolonged endurance exercise, which is associated with an increased oxidation of lipids and mobilization of glycogen stores, has been shown to acutely improve insulin sensitivity, an effect that may

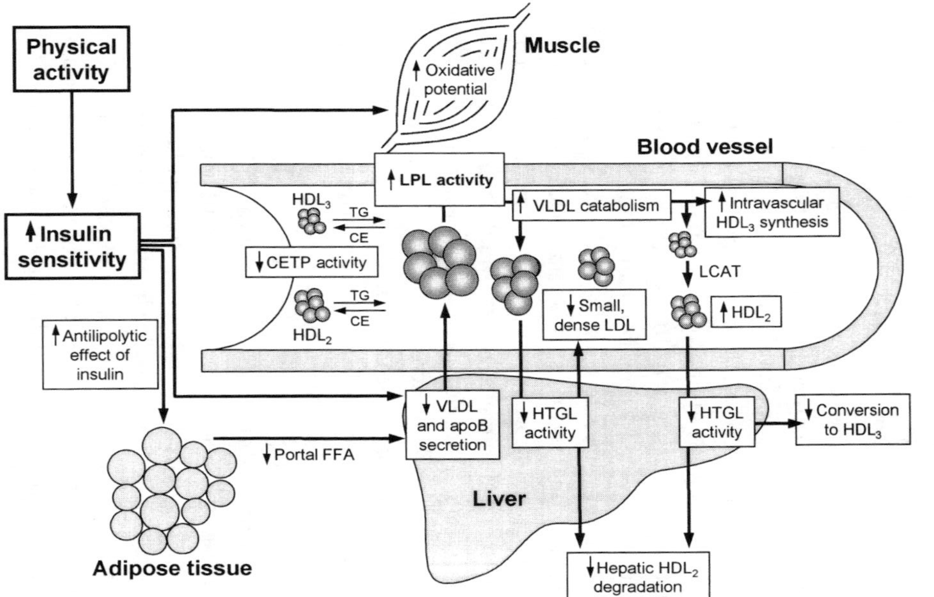

FIGURE 11.8 Effects of endurance exercise training on insulin sensitivity and lipoprotein-lipid metabolism. CE, cholesterol ester; CETP, cholesterol ester transfer protein; FFA, free fatty acid; LCAT, lecithin-cholesterol acyl transferase.

Adapted from Després and Lamarche.[109]

last 48–72 h.[108,143] Thus, rapid improvements in the plasma lipoprotein lipid profile of the sedentary abdominally obese dyslipidemic patient may be obtained through daily improvements in insulin action generated by repeated daily sessions of prolonged exercise. These metabolic adaptations also appear to be dissociated from the improvement in physical fitness because they are related to the degree of weight loss,[144] an indicator of the increased energy expenditure associated with exercise.

Overall, it appears that further increasing the level of physical activity may be associated with an additional reduction in risk because additional improvements in metabolic risk variables have been reported as a function of increasing levels of physical activity among runners.[145,146] However, from a public health standpoint, it should be recognized that the greatest benefit to the population would be to transform our largely sedentary population into moderately active individuals.[134,147,148] Although we do not have evidence from a randomized weight loss exercise trial that such an approach has a favorable impact on morbidity and mortality, it appears warranted to recommend that the level of daily physical activity should be increased in our population. Furthermore, individuals should expect beneficial effects on the CVD risk profile when increasing daily physical activity, although the benefits may vary depending on the subjects' initial characteristics and genetic background. In practical terms, physicians and health professionals should keep in mind that the changes in lifestyle associated with the best compliance are those that are likely to have the greatest long-term impact on cardiovascular health. With the dramatic increase in the prevalence of obesity in our affluent population, it is critical to develop environments in schools, parks, cities, and workplaces that favor a physically active lifestyle. This objective goes far beyond the field of exercise physiology and medicine and will require the involvement and cooperation of a multidisciplinary team as well as greater commitment of our political leaders toward physical activity and health.

Acknowledgments

Results from the authors' laboratory presented in this chapter were obtained with the financial support of the Natural Sciences and Engineering Research Council of Canada, the Canadian Institutes for Health Research of Canada, the Canadian Diabetes Association, and the Heart and Stroke Foundation of Canada.

References

1. Seidell JC: Obesity in Europe: scaling an epidemic. *Int J Obes* 19 (Suppl. 3):S1–S4, 1995
2. Seidell JC, Flegal KM: Assessing obesity: classification and epidemiology. *Br Med Bull* 53:238–52, 1997
3. World Health Organization: *Obesity: Preventing and Managing the Global Epidemic: Report of a WHO Consultation on Obesity.* Geneva, World Health Org., 1998, p. 1–276
4. Barrett-Connor EL: Obesity, atherosclerosis, and coronary artery disease. *Ann Intern Med* 103:1010–19, 1985
5. Bray GA: Complications of obesity. *Ann Intern Med* 103:1052–62, 1985
6. Després JP: Dyslipidaemia and obesity. *Baillieres Clin Endocrinol Metab* 8:629–60, 1994
7. Kissebah AH, Peiris AN: Biology of regional body fat distribution: relationship to non-insulin-dependent diabetes mellitus. *Diabetes Metab Rev* 5:83–109, 1989
8. Kissebah AH, Freedman DS, Peiris AN: Health risks of obesity. *Med Clin North Am* 73:111–38, 1989
9. Manson JE, Willett WC, Stampfer MJ, Colditz GA, Hunter DJ, Hankinson SE, Hennekens CH, Speizer FE: Body weight and mortality among women. *N Engl J Med* 333:677–85, 1995
10. Kissebah AH, Vydelingum N, Murray R, Evans DJ, Hartz AJ, Kalkhoff RK, Adams PW: Relation of body fat distribution to metabolic complications of obesity. *J Clin Endocrinol Metab* 54: 254–60, 1982
11. Björntorp P: Hazards in subgroups of human obesity. *Eur J Clin Invest* 14:239–41, 1984
12. Björntorp P: Abdominal obesity and the development of non-insulin-dependent diabetes mellitus. *Diabetes Metab Rev* 4:615–22, 1988
13. Després JP: Abdominal obesity as important component of insulin-resistance syndrome. *Nutrition* 9:452–59, 1993

14. Després JP, Moorjani S, Lupien PJ, Tremblay A, Nadeau A, Bouchard C: Regional distribution of body fat, plasma lipoproteins, and cardiovascular disease. *Arteriosclerosis* 10:497–511, 1990
15. Kissebah AH, Evans DJ, Peiris A, Wilson CR: Endocrine characteristics in regional obesities: role of sex steroids. In *Metabolic Complications of Human Obesities.* Vague J, Björntorp P, Guy-Grand B, Rebuffé-Scrive M, Vague P, Eds. Amsterdam, Elsevier Science, 1985, p. 115–30
16. Vague J: Sexual differentiation, a factor affecting the forms of obesity (in French). *Presse Médicale* 30:339–40, 1947
17. Vague J: The degree of masculine differentiation of obesities: a factor determining predisposition to diabetes, atherosclerosis, gout and uric-calculous disease. *Am J Clin Nutr* 4:20–34, 1956
18. Krotkiewski M, Björntorp P, Sjöström L, Smith U: Impact of obesity on metabolism in men and women: importance of regional adipose tissue distribution. *J Clin Invest* 72:1150–62, 1983
19. Lapidus L, Bengtsson C, Larsson B, Pennert K, Rybo E, Sjöström L: Distribution of adipose tissue and risk of cardiovascular disease and death: a 12-year follow up of participants in the population study of women in Göthenburg, Sweden. *Br Med J* 289:1257–61, 1984
20. Larsson B, Svardsudd K, Welin L, Wilhelmsen L, Björntorp P, Tibblin G: Abdominal adipose tissue distribution, obesity, and risk of cardiovascular disease and death: 13 year follow up of participants in the study of men born in 1913. *Br Med J* 288:1401–04, 1984
21. Ohlson LO, Larsson B, Svardsudd K, Welin L, Eriksson H, Wilhelmsen L, Björntorp P, Tibblin G: The influence of body fat distribution on the incidence of diabetes mellitus: 13.5 years of follow-up of the participants in the study of men born in 1913. *Diabetes* 34:1055–58, 1985
22. Pouliot MC, Després JP, Lemieux S, Moorjani S, Bouchard C, Tremblay A, Nadeau A, Lupien PJ: Waist circumference and abdominal sagittal diameter: best simple anthropometric indexes of abdominal visceral adipose tissue accumulation and related cardiovascular risk in men and women. *Am J Cardiol* 73:460–68, 1994
23. Borkan GA, Gerzof SG, Robbins AH, Hults DE, Silbert CK, Silbert JE: Assessment of abdominal fat content by computed tomography. *Am J Clin Nutr* 36:172–77, 1982

24. Ferland M, Després JP, Tremblay A, Pinault S, Nadeau A, Moorjani S, Lupien PJ, Thériault G, Bouchard C: Assessment of adipose tissue distribution by computed axial tomography in obese women: association with body density and anthropometric measurements. *Br J Nutr* 61:139–48, 1989
25. Kvist H, Chowdhury B, Grangard U, Tylen U, Sjöström L: Total and visceral adipose-tissue volumes derived from measurements with computed tomography in adult men and women: predictive equations. *Am J Clin Nutr* 48:1351–61, 1988
26. Sjöström L, Kvist H, Cederblad A, Tylen U: Determination of total adipose tissue and body fat in women by computed tomography, 40K, and tritium. *Am J Physiol* 250:E736–45, 1986
27. Tokunaga K, Matsuzawa Y, Ishikawa K, Tarui S: A novel technique for the determination of body fat by computed tomography. *Int J Obes* 7:437–45, 1983
28. Pouliot MC, Després JP, Nadeau A, Moorjani S, Prud'homme D, Lupien PJ, Tremblay A, Bouchard C: Visceral obesity in men: associations with glucose tolerance, plasma insulin, and lipoprotein levels. *Diabetes* 41:826–34, 1992
29. Després JP, Ferland M, Moorjani S, Nadeau A, Tremblay A, Lupien PJ, Thériault G, Bouchard C: Role of hepatic-triglyceride lipase activity in the association between intra-abdominal fat and plasma HDL cholesterol in obese women. *Arteriosclerosis* 9:485–92, 1989
30. Abate N, Garg A, Peshock RM, Stray-Gundersen J, Grundy SM: Relationships of generalized and regional adiposity to insulin sensitivity in men. *J Clin Invest* 96:88–98, 1995
31. Lemieux S, Prud'homme D, Bouchard C, Tremblay A, Després JP: Sex differences in the relation of visceral adipose tissue accumulation to total body fatness. *Am J Clin Nutr* 58:463–67, 1993
32. Després JP, Moorjani S, Ferland M, Tremblay A, Lupien PJ, Nadeau A, Pinault S, Thériault G, Bouchard C: Adipose tissue distribution and plasma lipoprotein levels in obese women: importance of intra-abdominal fat. *Arteriosclerosis* 9:203–10, 1989
33. Després JP, Nadeau A, Tremblay A, Ferland M, Moorjani S, Lupien PJ, Thériault G, Pinault S, Bouchard C: Role of deep abdominal fat in the association between regional adipose tissue distribution and glucose tolerance in obese women. *Diabetes* 38:304–09, 1989

34. Fujioka S, Matsuzawa Y, Tokunaga K, Tarui S: Contribution of intra-abdominal fat accumulation to the impairment of glucose and lipid metabolism in human obesity. *Metabolism* 36:54–59, 1987
35. Fujioka S, Matsuzawa Y, Tokunaga K, Kawamoto T, Kobatake T, Keno Y, Kotani K, Yoshida S, Tarui S: Improvement of glucose and lipid metabolism associated with selective reduction of intra-abdominal visceral fat in premenopausal women with visceral fat obesity. *Int J Obes* 15:853–59, 1991
36. Fujioka S, Matsuzawa Y, Tokunaga K, Keno Y, Kobatake T, Tarui S: Treatment of visceral fat obesity. *Int J Obes* 15 (Suppl. 2): 59–65, 1991
37. Peiris AN, Sothmann MS, Hennes MI, Lee MB, Wilson CR, Gustafson AB, Kissebah AH: Relative contribution of obesity and body fat distribution to alterations in glucose insulin homeostasis: predictive values of selected indices in premenopausal women. *Am J Clin Nutr* 49:758–64, 1989
38. Sparrow D, Borkan GA, Gerzof SG, Wisniewski C, Silbert CK: Relationship of fat distribution to glucose tolerance: results of computed tomography in male participants of the Normative Aging Study. *Diabetes* 35:411–15, 1986
39. Després JP: Obesity and lipid metabolism: relevance of body fat distribution. *Curr Opin Lipidol* 2:5–15, 1991
40. Després JP: Visceral obesity: a component of the insulin resistance-dyslipidemic syndrome. *Can J Cardiol* 10:17B–22B, 1991
41. Després JP: Visceral obesity, insulin resistance, and related dyslipoproteinemias. In *Diabetes.* Rifkin H, Colwell JA, Taylor SI, Eds. Amsterdam, Elsevier Science, 1991, p. 95–99
42. Lemieux S, Després JP, Moorjani S, Nadeau A, Thériault G, Prud'homme D, Tremblay A, Bouchard C, Lupien PJ: Are gender differences in cardiovascular disease risk factors explained by the level of visceral adipose tissue? *Diabetologia* 37:757–64, 1994
43. Tchernof A, Poehlman ET: Effects of the menopause transition on body fatness and body fat distribution. *Obes Res* 6:246–54, 1998
44. Tchernof A, Calles-Escandon J, Sites CK, Poehlman ET: Menopause, central body fatness, and insulin resistance: effects of hormone-replacement therapy. *Coron Artery Dis* 9:503–11, 1998
45. Lemieux S: Genetic susceptibility to visceral obesity and related clinical implications. *Int J Obes Relat Metab Disord* 21:831–38, 1997

46. Haffner SM, Stern MP, Hazuda HP, Pugh J, Patterson JK, Malina R: Upper body and centralized adiposity in Mexican Americans and non-Hispanic whites: relationship to body mass index and other behavioral and demographic variables. *Int J Obes* 10:493–502, 1986
47. Després JP, Couillard C, Gagnon J, Bergeron J, Leon AS, Rao DC, Skinner JS, Wilmore JH, Bouchard C: Race, visceral adipose tissue, plasma lipids and lipoprotein lipase activity in men and women: The HERITAGE Family Study. *Arterioscler Thromb Vasc Biol* 20:1932–38, 2000
48. Conway JM, Chanetsa FF, Wang P: Intraabdominal adipose tissue and anthropometric surrogates in African American women with upper- and lower-body obesity. *Am J Clin Nutr* 66:1345–51, 1997
49. Lovejoy JC, de la Bretonne JA, Klemperer M, Tulley R: Abdominal fat distribution and metabolic risk factors: effects of race. *Metabolism* 45:1119–24, 1996
50. Boyko EJ, Leonetti DL, Bergstrom RW, Newell-Morris L, Fujimoto WY: Visceral adiposity, fasting plasma insulin, and blood pressure in Japanese-Americans. *Diabetes Care* 18:174–81, 1995
51. Yamashita S, Nakamura T, Shimomura I, Nishida M, Yoshida S, Kotani K, Kameda-Takemuara K, Tokunaga K, Matsuzawa Y: Insulin resistance and body fat distribution. *Diabetes Care* 19: 287–91, 1996
52. Risica PM, Ebbesson SO, Schraer CD, Nobmann ED, Caballero BH: Body fat distribution in Alaskan Eskimos of the Bering Straits region: the Alaskan Siberia Project. *Int J Obes Relat Metab Disord* 24:171–79, 2000
53. Gautier JF, Milner MR, Elam E, Chen K, Ravussin E, Pratley RE: Visceral adipose tissue is not increased in Pima Indians compared with equally obese Caucasians and is not related to insulin action or secretion. *Diabetologia* 42:28–34, 1999
54. Katzmarzyk PT, Malina RM: Obesity and relative subcutaneous fat distribution among Canadians of First Nation and European ancestry. *Int J Obes Relat Metab Disord* 22:1127–31, 1998
55. Snehalatha C, Ramachandran A, Satyavani K, Vallabi MY, Viswanathan V: Computed axial tomographic scan measurement of abdominal fat distribution and its correlation with anthropometry and insulin secretion in healthy Asian Indians. *Metabolism* 46:1220–24, 1997

56. Banerji MA, Faridi N, Atluri R, Chaiken RL, Lebovitz HE: Body composition, visceral fat, leptin, and insulin resistance in Asian Indian men. *J Clin Endocrinol Metab* 84:137–44, 1999
57. Lemieux S, Després JP: Metabolic complications of visceral obesity: contribution to the aetiology of type 2 diabetes and implications for prevention and treatment. *Diabete Metab* 20:375–93, 1994
58. Després JP: Lipoprotein metabolism in visceral obesity. *Int J Obes* 15 (Suppl. 2):45–52, 1991
59. Després JP, Marette A: Relation of components of insulin resistance syndrome to coronary disease risk. *Curr Opin Lipidol* 5:274–89, 1994
60. Després JP, Lemieux S, Lamarche B, Prud'homme D, Moorjani S, Brun LD, Gagné C, Lupien PJ: The insulin resistance-dyslipidemic syndrome: contribution of visceral obesity and therapeutic implications. *Int J Obes* 19 (Suppl. 1):S76–86, 1995
61. Assmann G, Schulte H: Relation of high-density lipoprotein cholesterol and triglycerides to incidence of atherosclerotic coronary artery disease (the PROCAM experience): Prospective Cardiovascular Munster Study. *Am J Cardiol* 70:733–37, 1992
62. Manninen V, Tenkanen L, Koskinen P, Huttunen JK, Manttari M, Heinonen OP, Frick MH: Joint effects of serum triglyceride and LDL cholesterol and HDL cholesterol concentrations on coronary heart disease risk in the Helsinki Heart Study: implications for treatment. *Circulation* 85:37–45, 1992
63. Lamarche B, Després JP, Moorjani S, Cantin B, Dagenais GR, Lupien PJ: Prevalence of dyslipidemic phenotypes in ischemic heart disease: prospective results from the Québec Cardiovascular Study. *Am J Cardiol* 75:1189–95, 1995
64. Lamarche B, Moorjani S, Lupien PJ, Cantin B, Bernard PM, Dagenais GR, Després JP: Apolipoprotein A-I and B levels and the risk of ischemic heart disease during a five-year follow-up of men in the Québec Cardiovascular Study. *Circulation* 94:273–78, 1996
65. Fujimoto WY, Bergstrom RW, Boyko EJ, Chen KW, Leonetti DL, Newell-Morris L, Shofer JB, Wahl PW: Visceral adiposity and incident coronary heart disease in Japanese-American men: the 10-year follow-up results of the Seattle Japanese-American Community Diabetes Study. *Diabetes Care* 22:1808–12, 1999

66. Després JP, Lamarche B, Mauriège P, Cantin B, Dagenais GR, Moorjani S, Lupien PJ: Hyperinsulinemia as an independent risk factor for ischemic heart disease. *N Engl J Med* 334:952–57, 1996
67. Tchernof A, Lamarche B, Prud'homme D, Nadeau A, Moorjani S, Labrie F, Lupien PJ, Després JP: The dense LDL phenotype: association with plasma lipoprotein levels, visceral obesity, and hyperinsulinemia in men. *Diabetes Care* 19:629–37, 1996
68. Lamarche B, Tchernof A, Moorjani S, Cantin B, Dagenais GR, Lupien PJ, Després JP: Small, dense low-density lipoprotein particles as a predictor of the risk of ischemic heart disease in men: prospective results from the Québec Cardiovascular Study. *Circulation* 95:69–75, 1997
69. Lamarche B, Tchernof A, Mauriège P, Cantin B, Dagenais GR, Lupien PJ, Després JP: Fasting insulin and apolipoprotein B levels and low-density lipoprotein particle size as risk factors for ischemic heart disease. *J Am Med Assoc* 279:1955–61, 1998
70. Lemieux I, Pascot A, Couillard C, Lamarche B, Tchernof A, Alméras N, Bergeron J, Gaudet D, Tremblay G, Prud'homme D, Nadeau A, Després JP: Hypertriglyceridemic waist: a marker of the atherogenic metabolic triad (hyperinsulinemia; hyperapolipoprotein B; small, dense LDL) in men? *Circulation* 102:179–84, 2000
71. Reaven GM: Banting lecture 1988: Role of insulin resistance in human disease. *Diabetes* 37:1595–1607, 1988
72. Fujimoto WY, Leonetti DL, Newell-Morris L, Shuman WP, Wahl PW: Relationship of absence or presence of a family history of diabetes to body weight and body fat distribution in type 2 diabetes. *Int J Obes* 15:111–20, 1991
73. Lemieux S, Després JP, Nadeau A, Prud'homme D, Tremblay A, Bouchard C: Heterogeneous glycaemic and insulinaemic responses to oral glucose in non-diabetic men: interactions between duration of obesity, body fat distribution and family history of diabetes mellitus. *Diabetologia* 35:653–59, 1992
74. Kral JG, Schaffner F, Pierson RN Jr, Wang J: Body fat topography as an independent predictor of fatty liver. *Metabolism* 42:548–51, 1993
75. Ryysy L, Häkkinen AM, Goto T, Vehkavaara S, Westerbacka J, Halavaara J, Yki-Järvinen H: Liver fat content, insulin absorption and action as determinants of insulin requirements in type 2 diabetes (Abstract). *Diabetologia* 42 (Suppl. 1):A83, 1999

76. Seppälä-Lindroos A, Häkkinen AM, Goto T, Ryysy L, Vehkavaara S, Bergholm R, Halavaara J, Yki-Järvinen H: Liver fat content quantified by proton spectroscopy is a more important determinant of insulin resistance than obesity or visceral fat in nondiabetic subjects (Abstract). *Diabetologia* 43 (Suppl. 1):A58, 2000
77. Hennes MM, Shrago E, Kissebah AH: Receptor and postreceptor effects of free fatty acids (FFA) on hepatocyte insulin dynamics. *Int J Obes* 14:831–41, 1990
78. Svedberg J, Björntorp P, Smith U, Lonnroth P: Free-fatty acid inhibition of insulin binding, degradation, and action in isolated rat hepatocytes. *Diabetes* 39:570–74, 1990
79. Björntorp P: "Portal" adipose tissue as a generator of risk factors for cardiovascular disease and diabetes. *Arteriosclerosis* 10:493–96, 1990
80. Randle PJ, Garland PB, Hales CN, Newsholme EA: The glucose fatty-acid cycle: its role in insulin sensitivity and the metabolic disturbances of diabetes mellitus. *Lancet* i:785–89, 1963
81. Taylor SI, Mukherjee C, Jungas RL: Regulation of pyruvate dehydrogenase in isolated rat liver mitochondria: effects of octanoate, oxidation-reduction state, and adenosine triphosphate to adenosine diphosphate ratio. *J Biol Chem* 250:2028–35, 1975
82. Jahoor F, Klein S, Wolfe R: Mechanism of regulation of glucose production by lipolysis in humans. *Am J Physiol* 262:E353–58, 1992
83. Pan DA, Lillioja S, Kriketos AD, Milner MR, Baur LA, Bogardus C, Jenkins AB, Storlien LH: Skeletal muscle triglyceride levels are inversely related to insulin action. *Diabetes* 46:983–88, 1997
84. Phillips DI, Caddy S, Ilic V, Fielding BA, Frayn KN, Borthwick AC, Taylor R: Intramuscular triglyceride and muscle insulin sensitivity: evidence for a relationship in nondiabetic subjects. *Metabolism* 45:947–50, 1996
85. Simoneau JA, Colberg SR, Thaete FL, Kelley DE: Skeletal muscle glycolytic and oxidative enzyme capacities are determinants of insulin sensitivity and muscle composition in obese women. *FASEB J* 9:273–78, 1995
86. Goodpaster BH, Thaete FL, Simoneau JA, Kelley DE: Subcutaneous abdominal fat and thigh muscle composition predict insulin sensitivity independently of visceral fat. *Diabetes* 46:1579–85, 1997

87. Simoneau JA, Kelley DE: Metabolic aspects of skeletal muscle in obesity. In *Progress in Obesity Research.* Ailhaud G, Guy-Grand B, Eds. London, John Libbey, 1999, p. 411–14
88. Felber JP: From obesity to diabetes: pathophysiological considerations. *Int J Obes* 16:937–52, 1992
89. Pollare T, Vessby B, Lithell H: Lipoprotein lipase activity in skeletal muscle is related to insulin sensitivity. *Arterioscler Thromb* 11:1192–1203, 1991
90. Després JP, Moorjani S, Tremblay A, Ferland M, Lupien PJ, Nadeau A, Bouchard C: Relation of high plasma triglyceride levels associated with obesity and regional adipose tissue distribution to plasma lipoprotein-lipid composition in premenopausal women. *Clin Invest Med* 12:374–80, 1989
91. Björntorp P: Visceral fat accumulation: the missing link between psychosocial factors and cardiovascular disease? *J Intern Med* 230:195–201, 1991
92. Brindley DN: Neuroendocrine regulation and obesity. *Int J Obes* 16 (Suppl. 3):S73–79, 1992
93. Brindley DN, Rolland Y: Possible connections between stress, diabetes, obesity, hypertension and altered lipoprotein metabolism that may result in atherosclerosis. *Clin Sci* 77:453–61, 1989
94. Evans DJ, Hoffmann RG, Kalkhoff RK, Kissebah AH: Relationship of androgenic activity to body fat topography, fat cell morphology, and metabolic aberrations in premenopausal women. *J Clin Endocrinol Metab* 57:304–10, 1983
95. Peiris AN, Mueller RA, Struve MF, Smith GA, Kissebah AH: Relationship of androgenic activity to splanchnic insulin metabolism and peripheral glucose utilization in premenopausal women. *J Clin Endocrinol Metab* 64:162–69, 1987
96. Tchernof A, Després JP, Bélanger A, Dupont A, Prud'homme D, Moorjani S, Lupien PJ, Labrie F: Reduced testosterone and adrenal C19 steroid levels in obese men. *Metabolism* 44:513–19, 1995
97. Seidell JC, Björntorp P, Sjöström L, Kvist H, Sannerstedt R: Visceral fat accumulation in men is positively associated with insulin, glucose, and C-peptide levels, but negatively with testosterone levels. *Metabolism* 39:897–901, 1990
98. Pedersen SB, Jonler M, Richelsen B: Characterization of regional and gender differences in glucocorticoid receptors and lipoprotein

lipase activity in human adipose tissue. *J Clin Endocrinol Metab* 78:1354–59, 1994

99. Rebuffé-Scrive M, Lundholm K, Björntorp P: Glucocorticoid hormone binding to human adipose tissue. *Eur J Clin Invest* 15:267–71, 1985
100. Hotamisligil GS: Molecular mechanisms of insulin resistance and the role of the adipocyte. *Int J Obes Relat Metab Disord* 24 (Suppl. 4):S23–27, 2000
101. Steppan CM, Bailey ST, Bhat S, Brown EJ, Banerjee RR, Wright CM, Patel HR, Ahima RS, Lazar MA: The hormone resistin links obesity to diabetes. *Nature* 409:307–12, 2001
102. Scheen AJ, Lefebvre PJ: Troglitazone: antihyperglycemic activity and potential role in the treatment of type 2 diabetes. *Diabetes Care* 22:1568–77, 1999
103. Goodpaster BH, Kelley DE, Wing RR, Meier A, Thaete FL: Effects of weight loss on regional fat distribution and insulin sensitivity in obesity. *Diabetes* 48:839–47, 1999
104. Leenen R, van der Kooy K, Deurenberg P, Seidell JC, Weststrate JA, Schouten FJ, Hautvast JG: Visceral fat accumulation in obese subjects: relation to energy expenditure and response to weight loss. *Am J Physiol* 263:E913–19, 1992
105. Després JP, Lamarche B: Effects of diet and physical activity on adiposity and body fat distribution: implications for the prevention of cardiovascular disease. *Nutr Res Rev* 6:137–59, 1993
106. Björntorp P: The effects of exercise on plasma insulin. *Int J Sports Med* 2:125–29, 1981
107. Björntorp P, De Jounge K, Sjöström L, Sullivan L: The effect of physical training on insulin production in obesity. *Metabolism* 19:631–38, 1970
108. Consensus Development Conference on Diet and Exercise in Non-Insulin-Dependent Diabetes Mellitus: National Institutes of Health. *Diabetes Care* 10:639–44, 1987
109. Després JP, Lamarche B: Low-intensity endurance exercise training, plasma lipoproteins and the risk of coronary heart disease. *J Intern Med* 236:7–22, 1994
110. Morris JN, Chave SP, Adam C, Sirey C, Epstein L, Sheehan DJ: Vigorous exercise in leisure-time and the incidence of coronary heart-disease. *Lancet* i:333–39, 1973

111. Paffenbarger RS, Hale WE: Work activity and coronary heart mortality. *N Engl J Med* 292:545–50, 1975
112. Paffenbarger RS Jr, Wing AL, Hyde RT: Physical activity as an index of heart attack risk in college alumni. *Am J Epidemiol* 108:161–75, 1978
113. Peters RK, Cady LD Jr, Bischoff DP, Bernstein L, Pike MC: Physical fitness and subsequent myocardial infarction in healthy workers. *J Am Med Assoc* 249:3052–56, 1983
114. Lie H, Mundal R, Erikssen J: Coronary risk factors and incidence of coronary death in relation to physical fitness: seven-year follow-up study of middle-aged and elderly men. *Eur Heart J* 6:147–57, 1985
115. Ekelund LG, Haskell WL, Johnson JL, Whaley FS, Criqui MH, Sheps DS: Physical fitness as a predictor of cardiovascular mortality in asymptomatic North American men: The Lipid Research Clinics Mortality Follow-up Study. *N Engl J Med* 319: 1379–84, 1988
116. Blair SN, Kohl HW, Paffenbarger RS Jr, Clark DG, Cooper KH, Gibbons LW: Physical fitness and all-cause mortality: a prospective study of healthy men and women. *J Am Med Assoc* 262:2395–2401, 1989
117. Bouchard C, Tremblay A, Després JP, Nadeau A, Lupien PJ, Thériault G, Dussault J, Moorjani S, Pinault S, Fournier G: The response to long-term overfeeding in identical twins. *N Engl J Med* 322:1477–82, 1990
118. Haskell WL: Exercise-induced changes in plasma lipids and lipoproteins. *Prev Med* 13:23–36, 1984
119. Haskell WL: The influence of exercise training on plasma lipids and lipoproteins in health and disease. *Acta Med Scand* 711: 25–37, 1986
120. Krauss RM: Exercise, lipoproteins, and coronary artery disease. *Circulation* 79:1143–45, 1989
121. Bouchard C, Després JP, Tremblay A: Exercise and obesity. *Obes Res* 1:40–54, 1993
122. Bouchard C, Shephard RJ, Stephens T: Physical activity, fitness and health: the consensus statement. In *Physical Activity, Fitness and Health: International Proceedings and Consensus Statement.* Bouchard C, Shephard RJ, Stephens T, Eds. Champaign, IL, Human Kinetics, 1994, p. 9–76

123. American College of Sports Medicine Position Stand: The recommended quantity and quality of exercise for developing and maintaining cardiorespiratory and muscular fitness in healthy adults. *Med Sci Sports Exerc* 22:265–74, 1990
124. Katzel LI, Bleecker ER, Colman EG, Rogus EM, Sorkin JD, Goldberg AP: Effects of weight loss vs aerobic exercise training on risk factors for coronary disease in healthy, obese, middle-aged and older men: a randomized controlled trial. *J Am Med Assoc* 274:1915–21, 1995
125. Leon AS, Conrad J, Hunninghake DB, Serfass R: Effects of a vigorous walking program on body composition, and carbohydrate and lipid metabolism of obese young men. *Am J Clin Nutr* 32: 1776–87, 1979
126. Oshida Y, Yamanouchi K, Hayamizu S, Sato Y: Long-term mild jogging increases insulin action despite no influence on body mass index or VO2 max. *J Appl Physiol* 66:2206–10, 1989
127. Williams PT, Wood PD, Haskell WL, Vranizan K: The effects of running mileage and duration on plasma lipoprotein levels. *J Am Med Assoc* 247:2674–79, 1982
128. Wood PD, Haskell WL: The effect of exercise on plasma high density lipoproteins. *Lipids* 14:417–27, 1979
129. Wood PD, Stefanick ML, Dreon DM, Frey-Hewitt B, Garay SC, Williams PT, Superko HR, Fortmann SP, Albers JJ, Vranizan KM, Ellsworth NM, Terry RB, Haskell WL: Changes in plasma lipids and lipoproteins in overweight men during weight loss through dieting as compared with exercise. *N Engl J Med* 319: 1173–79, 1988
130. Wood PD, Stefanick ML: Exercise, fitness and atherosclerosis. In *Exercise, Fitness and Health: A Consensus of Current Knowledge.* Bouchard C, Shephard RJ, Stephens T, Sutton JR, McPherson BD, Eds. Champaign, IL, Human Kinetics, 1988, p. 409–20
131. Wood PD, Williams PT, Haskell WL: Physical activity and high-density lipoproteins. In *Clinical and Metabolic Aspects of High-Density Lipoproteins.* Miller NE, Miller GJ, Eds. Amsterdam, Elsevier Science, 1984, p. 133–65
132. Ross R, Dagnone D, Jones PJ, Smith H, Paddags A, Hudson R, Janssen I: Reduction in obesity and related comorbid conditions after diet-induced weight loss or exercise-induced weight loss

in men: a randomized, controlled trial. *Ann Intern Med* 133: 92–103, 2000

133. Blair SN, Connelly JC: How much physical activity should we do? The case for moderate amounts and intensities of physical activity. *Res Q Exerc Sport* 67:193–205, 1996
134. Blair SN, Kohl HW, Gordon NF, Paffenbarger RS Jr: How much physical activity is good for health? *Med Sci Sports Exerc* 28: 335–49, 1996
135. Whaley MH, Blair SN: Epidemiology of physical activity, physical fitness and coronary heart disease. *J Cardiovasc Risk* 2:289–95, 1995
136. American College of Sports Medicine Position Stand: The recommended quantity and quality of exercise for developing and maintaining cardiorespiratory and muscular fitness, and flexibility in healthy adults. *Med Sci Sports Exerc* 30:975–91, 1998
137. Seals DR, Hagberg JM: The effect of exercise training on human hypertension: a review. *Med Sci Sports Exerc* 16:207–15, 1984
138. Kokkinos PF, Holland JC, Narayan P, Colleran JA, Dotson CO, Papademetriou V: Miles run per week and high-density lipoprotein cholesterol levels in healthy, middle-aged men: a dose-response relationship. *Arch Intern Med* 155:415–20, 1995
139. Rogers MA, Yamamoto C, King DS, Hagberg JM, Ehsani AA, Holloszy JO: Improvement in glucose tolerance after 1 wk of exercise in patients with mild NIDDM. *Diabetes Care* 11:613–18, 1988
140. Pan XR, Li GW, Hu YH, Wang JX, Yang WY, An ZX, Hu ZX, Lin J, Xiao JZ, Cao HB, Liu PA, Jiang XG, Jiang YY, Wang JP, Zheng H, Zhang H, Bennett PH, Howard BV: Effects of diet and exercise in preventing NIDDM in people with impaired glucose tolerance: The Da Qing IGT and Diabetes Study. *Diabetes Care* 20:537–44, 1997
141. Eriksson KF, Lindgärde F: Prevention of type 2 (non-insulin-dependent) diabetes mellitus by diet and physical exercise: the 6-year Malmö feasibility study. *Diabetologia* 34:891–98, 1991
142. Lamarche B, Després JP, Pouliot MC, Moorjani S, Lupien PJ, Thériault G, Tremblay A, Nadeau A, Bouchard C: Is body fat loss a determinant factor in the improvement of carbohydrate and lipid metabolism following aerobic exercise training in obese women? *Metabolism* 41:1249–56, 1992
143. Burnstein R, Polychronakos C, Toews CJ, MacDougall JD, Guyda HJ, Posner BI: Acute reversal of the enhanced insulin action in

trained athletes: association with insulin receptor changes. *Diabetes* 34:756–60, 1985

144. Després JP, Pouliot MC, Moorjani S, Nadeau A, Tremblay A, Lupien PJ, Thériault G, Bouchard C: Loss of abdominal fat and metabolic response to exercise training in obese women. *Am J Physiol* 261:E159–67, 1991
145. Williams PT: High-density lipoprotein cholesterol and other risk factors for coronary heart disease in female runners. *N Engl J Med* 334:1298–1303, 1996
146. Williams PT: Relationships of heart disease risk factors to exercise quantity and intensity. *Arch Intern Med* 158:237–45, 1998
147. Blair SN, Horton E, Leon AS, Lee IM, Drinkwater BL, Dishman RK, Mackey M, Kienholz ML: Physical activity, nutrition, and chronic disease. *Med Sci Sports Exerc* 28:335–49, 1996
148. Wei M, Macera CA, Hornung CA, Blair SN: Changes in lipids associated with change in regular exercise in free-living men. *J Clin Epidemiol* 50:1137–42, 1997

Jean-Pierre Després, PhD, and Charles Couillard, PhD, are from the Québec Heart Institute, Laval Hospital Research Center; the Lipid Research Center, Laval University Medical Research Center; and the Department of Food Sciences and Nutrition, Laval University, Ste-Foy, Québec, Canada. Jean Bergeron, MD, is from the Lipid Research Center, Laval University Medical Research Center, Ste-Foy, Québec, Canada. Benoît Lamarche, PhD, is from the Lipid Research Center, Laval University Medical Research Center, and the Department of Food Sciences and Nutrition, Laval University, Ste-Foy, Québec, Canada.

12

A Target Population for Diabetes Prevention: The Metabolically Obese, Normal-Weight Individual

NEIL RUDERMAN, MD, DPHIL

Highlights

- Epidemiological evidence suggests that regular physical activity may prevent, or at least retard, the development of type 2 diabetes and coronary heart disease.
- This benefit of exercise is likely to be most prominent in individuals predisposed to the insulin resistance syndrome.
- Individuals with this syndrome often have generalized obesity; however, they also may not be obese or even overweight by present standards. The latter have been referred to as metabolically obese, normal-weight (MONW) individuals.
- Exercise may be therapeutically more efficacious in MONW individuals than in patients with established type 2 diabetes and overt obesity.
- People at risk for type 2 diabetes and the insulin resistance syndrome, including MONW individuals, may

be identifiable early by such factors as family history, birth weight, and the presence of gestational diabetes, polycystic ovarian syndrome, and central adiposity.

- Whether lifestyle modification programs of diet and exercise should be targeted specifically at these high-risk individuals or aimed at the general population is a major public health issue.

Exercise Reduces the Risk for Type 2 Diabetes and Coronary Heart Disease

As reviewed elsewhere in this book, both clinical and epidemiological evidence suggest that physical activity prevents, or at least retards, the development of type 2 diabetes and coronary heart disease (see Chapters 8–11). Thus, several studies have shown that the prevalence of type 2 diabetes and heart attack is 30–55% lower in men and women who exercise regularly than in their sedentary counterparts (see Chapter 9). In addition, a decreased progression from impaired glucose tolerance (IGT) to overt diabetes over 5–6 years has been reported in three prospective studies in which exercise, alone or in combination with diet, has been used as an intervention (see Chapters 8 and 10). In one of these studies,[1] major decreases in overall and cardiovascular mortality were observed after 12 years (Table 12.1). Such data prompt

TABLE 12.1 Mortality Rates and Causes of Death in Men With Normal and Impaired Glucose Tolerance and Diabetes in the Malmo Prevention Trial

	NGT	IGT Intervention	IGT Routine	Diabetes
Ischemic heart disease	1.8	3.6	7.3*	14.6*
Total mortality	6.2	6.5	14.0*	22.6*

All data are given as mortality per 1,000 patient-years. Results are for 12 years of follow-up in 6,389, 288, 134, and 144 men in the normal glucose tolerance (NGT), IGT Intervention, IGT Routine, and Diabetes groups, respectively. Intervention in the IGT group consisted of dietary instructions and regular exercise: patients selected for routine therapy and intervention were not randomized. *$P < 0.05$ vs. the NGT group.

Adapted from Eriksson and Lindgarde.[1]

many important questions, including the following: *1*) by what mechanism does exercise exert these effects, and *2*) how can patients who are most likely to benefit from regular exercise be identified?

Hyperinsulinemia and Insulin Resistance

Exercise and diet most likely exert these beneficial effects by diminishing hyperinsulinemia and insulin resistance. Insulin resistance has been defined as a state (of a cell, tissue, organ, or body) in which greater than normal amounts of insulin are required to elicit a quantitatively normal response. In humans, it is generally diagnosed on the basis of high plasma insulin levels, either fasting or during an oral glucose tolerance test, or by a decreased rate of glucose disappearance during a hyperinsulinemic-euglycemic clamp. It has long been associated with central obesity and, in particular, increases in intra-abdominal fat.[2]

Physical activity acutely[3] and chronically[4] (Table 12.2) diminishes insulin resistance and enhances insulin sensitivity in peripheral tissue; indeed, it was for this reason that the utility of exercise in the treatment of IGT[5] and type 2 diabetes was first assessed[6] (see Chapter 1). Hyperinsulinemia and insulin resistance are not only more prevalent in patients with IGT and type 2 diabetes, they are also associated with hypertension, certain dyslipoproteinemias, and premature

TABLE 12.2 Characteristics of Athletic and Sedentary Middle-Aged Swedish Men

	Skiers	Nonathletes
Age (years)	54	55
Weight (kg)	71	75
Body fat (kg)	10*	16
Triglycerides (mg/dl)	80*	109
Cholesterol (mg/dl)	203*	257
Glucose (mg/dl)		
Fasting	73	64
Postglucose (1 h)	79*	108
Insulin (μU/ml)		
Fasting	2*	10
Postglucose (1 h)	34*	95

*$P < 0.05$, significantly different from nonathletes.

Adapted from Bjorntorp et al.[4]

coronary heart disease, all of which are more common in people with type 2 diabetes and IGT[7–9] (see Chapters 3 and 11). They appear to be part of an insulin resistance syndrome, sometimes referred to as syndrome X or the metabolic syndrome,[8] which antedates these disorders and may contribute to their pathogenesis (Fig. 12.1). Thus, hyperinsulinemia and insulin resistance have been observed in off-

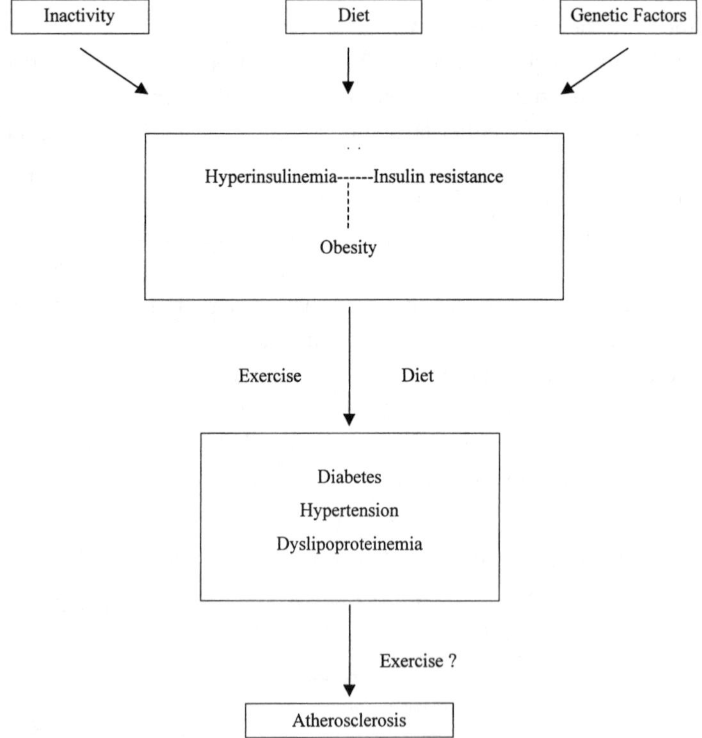

FIGURE 12.1 Exercise and atherosclerosis. According to this scheme, inactivity and diet cause hyperinsulinemia and insulin resistance and increase central fat (obesity) in genetically predisposed individuals. Both exercise and appropriate diet therapy could prevent these abnormalities from occurring or be used to treat them once already established. It is proposed that by doing this, the propensity of genetically predisposed individuals to develop type 2 diabetes, hypertension, certain dyslipoproteinemias, and hemostatic abnormalities is diminished (not shown). The anti-atherogenic action of exercise could be attributable to any or all of these effects. The report that exercise diminishes the severity of coronary heart disease in monkeys fed an atherogenic diet,[37] independent of changes in plasma lipoproteins, glucose, or blood pressure, suggests that exercise has a more direct anti-atherogenic effect. As shown here, it is unclear whether obesity is a cause and/or a consequence of the hyperinsulinemia and insulin resistance.

spring and/or other first-degree relatives of patients with type 2 diabetes,[10,11] hypertension[12] (Table 12.3), and hypertriglyceridemia.[12,13] In addition, they are often present in people who are at increased risk for coronary heart disease, even in the absence of these disorders.[7] It has been estimated by Reaven that 60 million people in the U.S. are insulin resistant.

As shown in Fig. 12.1, current theory holds that the insulin resistance syndrome results from genetic factors (e.g., susceptibility genes), acting in concert with obesity and/or physical inactivity, each of which can have both genetic and environmental determinants (see Chapter 7). In turn, depending on the genetic makeup of the individual, hyperinsulinemia and insulin resistance may lead to type 2 diabetes, hypertension, dyslipoproteinemias, or all three combined.[8] It has been proposed that the high prevalence of hyperinsulinemia and insulin resistance in individuals leading a Western lifestyle accounts for the reported benefits of physical activity in decreasing the incidence of type 2 diabetes and heart attacks.[14] In keeping with this contention, the most marked benefit of exercise in preventing type 2 diabetes in one study was observed in men at high risk because of a family history of diabetes or the presence of obesity.[15]

TABLE 12.3 Metabolic Comparison of Young Men and Women With and Without Hypertensive Parents

	Normotensive Parents	Hypertensive Parents
Age (years)	24	24
n (M/W)	70/8	64/6
BMI (kg/m^2)	22.3	22.4
Fasting plasma insulin (μU/ml)	8.6	9.9*
Serum or plasma triglycerides (mmol/l)	0.83	1.03*
Plasma glucose (mmol/l)	4.7	4.8
Systolic blood pressure (mmHg)	123	127*
Insulin sensitivity ($10^{-4} \times min^{-1}$/μU/ml)	13.2	9.4*

Insulin sensitivity is based on minimal modeling of an intravenous glucose tolerance test performed on 38 individuals with normotensive parents and 41 individuals with one hypertensive parent. *$P < 0.05$ vs. subjects with normotensive parents.

Adapted from Ferrari and Weidmann.[12]

Relation of the Insulin Resistance Syndrome to Obesity: The Metabolically Obese, Normal-Weight Individual

Hyperinsulinemia and insulin resistance accompany adult-onset obesity and most likely account for the close linkage of obesity (defined as a BMI >27 kg/m^2), and particularly central obesity, to type 2 diabetes and other cardiovascular risk factors (see Chapter 11). However, insulin resistance is often present in individuals with these disorders who are not overtly obese or even overweight (BMI >25 kg/m^2).[17–19] Such metabolically obese, normal-weight (MONW) individuals[16] are probably quite common in the general population[17–19] (Table 12.4) and may cluster at the upper end of the normal range of BMI.[20] Some of them may have a predominantly android (central) fat distribution (i.e., central obesity) due to an increase in intra-abdominal fat[2,21,22] that may be evident from measurement of waist circumference or waist-to-hip ratio or which may require more sensitive tests, such as computerized axial tomography or magnetic resonance imaging, for detection. A listing of some of the metabolic and physiological characteristics of young,

TABLE 12.4 Characteristics of Italian Factory Workers With Hyperinsulinemia and Normal Glucose Tolerance

	Hyperinsulinemia	Normal Glucose Tolerance
Age (years)	39	39
BMI (kg/m^2)	24.7	24.7
Glucose (mg/dl)		
Fasting	86	86
Postglucose (1 h)	110*	94
Insulin (μU/ml)		
Fasting	14*	7
Postglucose (1 h)	94*	35
Triglycerides (mmol/l)	1.7*	1.2
Cholesterol (mmol/l)	5.1	4.8
HDL cholesterol (mmol/l)	1.2*	1.4
Blood pressure (mmHg)		95
Systolic	126*	119
Diastolic	85*	78

Results are for 32 subjects (22 men) in each group. *$P < 0.05$, significantly different from the normal glucose tolerance group.

Adapted from Zavaroni et al.[19]

TABLE 12.5 Characteristics of MONW Women

	Control	MONW
n	58	13
Age (years)	28	29
BMI (kg/m^2)	21	22.5
Truncal fat (g)	6.3	8.2
Glucose (mg/dl)		
Fasting	79	79
2-h postload	83	103*
Insulin (pmol/ml)		
Fasting	49	60*
2-h postload	281	481*
VO_{2max} (l/min)	2.3	2.2
PAEE (mJ/day)	4.4	2.7*

MONW women were identified by a decreased glucose disposal rate during a euglycemic-hyperinsulinemic clamp (11 vs. 6.5 mg/kg fat-free mass/min: control vs. MONW). *$P < 0.05$ vs. control women. PAEE, physical activity energy expenditure.

Adapted from Dvorak et al.[26]

MONW women is presented in Table 12.5. As already noted, increases in intra-abdominal fat can be associated with hyperinsulinemia and insulin resistance, even in the absence of an increase in BMI, and these increases predispose an individual to both type 2 diabetes and coronary heart disease.[2,21,22] Based on epidemiological data (Fig. 12.2), it has been hypothesized that many MONW individuals may have been thin when young and that increases in central adiposity during adolescence and adulthood bring them to a normal population mean for body weight.[2,17] Such individuals may also be characterized by the presence of large adipocytes.[23] To a certain extent, such increases in fat cell size and intra-abdominal fat occur in all individuals in Westernized societies and may account for the correlation between weight gain in adult life and the incidence of diabetes and other disorders associated with insulin resistance[2] (Fig. 12.2).

Inactivity as a Cause of Insulin Resistance

Just as physical activity appears to diminish insulin resistance, inactivity appears to have the opposite effect. In this context, a sedentary lifestyle has long been associated with coronary heart disease and diabetes.[2] Likewise, a decreased VO_{2max} has been observed in individ-

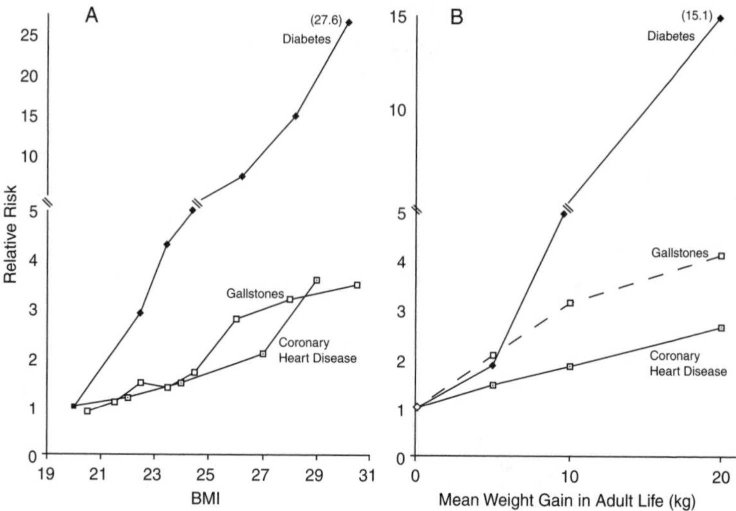

FIGURE 12.2 Relation of BMI (*A*) and weight gain (*B*) since 18 years of age to relative risks for diabetes, coronary heart disease, and gallstones in the Nurses Health Study. Numbers in parentheses are relative risks for diabetes if mean weight gain was >20 kg or BMI was >30 kg/m^2.

Reproduced with permission from Ruderman et al.[2]

uals with type 2 diabetes[24] and in their nonobese, nondiabetic first-degree relatives.[25] The relationship of these findings to insulin resistance and central obesity is presently under study. In MONW women, Dvorak et al.[26] recently demonstrated that a decreased daily energy expenditure due to physical activity can correlate with insulin resistance and increased central adiposity, independent of differences in VO_{2max} (Table 12.5).

Rationale for Use of Exercise Before the Onset of Diabetes

Although exercise can improve glucose tolerance, diminish insulin resistance, and improve coronary risk factors in patients with overt type 2 diabetes, its therapeutic efficacy in this population may sometimes be limited. Most patients with type 2 diabetes are over 40 years of age at the time of diagnosis, they are often obese, and they tend to be resistant to the lifestyle changes required by a lifelong exercise (or diet) program.[27]

Also, many of them (20–40%) have clinically significant ischemic heart disease at the time of diagnosis,[28–30] and a somewhat smaller percentage show evidence of microvascular complications.[30] As stated previously, "these factors do not negate the therapeutic value of exercise in patients with type 2 diabetes; however, they strongly suggest that exercise and other preventive measures (e.g., diet) may be more efficacious if they are instituted earlier in life."[2,14] The recent observation that type 2 diabetes is now appearing with increasing frequency in adolescents, in association with an increase in adiposity,[31] provides further support for this notion. In addition, numerous studies have shown that regular physical activity can diminish hypertension[32] and other coronary risk factors in nondiabetic individuals with hyperinsulinemia and insulin resistance (see Chapter 11).

Target Populations

Genetic markers do not as yet allow us to identify people at risk for developing type 2 diabetes and related disorders, and, as already noted, in the absence of obesity, the task is somewhat difficult. However, it may be possible to do so on the basis of family history, the presence of components of the insulin resistance syndrome (such as hypertriglyceridemia, low HDL cholesterol, or hypertension), and/or the presence of central obesity[2] (see Chapter 11) (Table 12.6). In addition, serial measurements of parameters such as plasma glucose and triglycerides, body weight, and waist size in individuals at high risk because of family history or ethnicity (see below) might prove useful. Groups that are already routinely identified (although not always followed) are women with gestational diabetes (see Chapter 30) and polycystic ovarian syndrome. Yet another group may be men or women who had low birth weights for gestational age. Studies in several English populations have shown a dramatically higher prevalence of both type 2 diabetes and syndrome X in middle-aged individuals who had a low birth weight.[31] Thus, in one population of 64-year-old men whose birth weights were <6.5 lb, 22% had syndrome X, compared with a prevalence of 2% in those with birth weights >9.5 lb. Likewise, in another group of 64-year-old men, the prevalence of diabetes and IGT (40%) was nearly threefold greater in the low–versus high–birth weight group. This effect of birth weight has also been demonstrated in other populations.[2] How a low birth weight relates to subsequent diabetes is unknown. The observation

TABLE 12.6 Predicted Characteristics of Normal-Weight Young Individuals Most Likely to Benefit From Exercise and Diet Therapy

Family history
Type 2 diabetes
Premature atherosclerosis
Hypertriglyceridemia
Low HDL cholesterol
Hypertension
Presence of central obesity
Manifestations of insulin resistance syndrome
Gestational diabetes
Polycystic ovarian syndrome
Low birth weight
Certain ethnic groups
Latinos
Blacks
Japanese-Americans
Native-Americans
Serial increases in at-risk individuals
Body weight
Glucose
Triglycerides
Blood pressure

that people with a low BMI at birth have a somewhat greater BMI than higher birth weight individuals in middle-age suggests that a predisposition to central obesity may be a factor. Finally, certain ethnic groups, such as Native-Americans, Japanese-Americans, Mexican-Americans, Australian aborigines, and African-Americans,[33–35] are more prone to obesity and type 2 diabetes when living a Western lifestyle. Where studied, these groups have shown an excellent response to exercise and diet therapy.[33–35] Presumably, such individuals also go through a state in which insulin resistance develops in the absence of what is commonly diagnosed as obesity.

Exercise Prescription

The principles of exercise and diet prescription described elsewhere in this book (see Chapters 14, 15, 17, and 18) apply to individuals with the insulin resistance syndrome even when they are normoglycemic and not obese or overweight. Many individuals who fit this classification will be young (<40 years of age) and not require an extensive cardiac workup (see Chapter 13). The exception will be patients in whom symptoms or specific risk factors for coronary heart disease, such as dyslipoproteinemia or hypertension, are already present. As in patients with overt diabetes, the exercise and diet prescription should take into account the individual's social and cultural background and specific preferences. This is an especially important consideration in the U.S., where an extremely high prevalence of diabetes is found in African-Americans, Native-Americans, Latinos, Mexican-Americans, and Japanese-Americans (see Chapter 8).

Conclusions

Existing studies strongly suggest that exercise and diet therapy can be used to prevent (or at least retard) the development of type 2 diabetes and other disorders associated with the insulin resistance syndrome. Results from the U.K. Prospective Diabetes Study suggest that diet and exercise do not permanently halt the progression of new-onset diabetes, type 2 diabetes, or its complications.[36] Likewise, although other studies have shown that interventions with exercise or diet can diminish the progression of IGT to overt type 2 diabetes by 50%, nearly 20% of the intervention group still became diabetic after 5 years. Whether even better results can be obtained when interventions are carried out before the onset of IGT is unknown, and the author is unaware of studies to test this possibility. On the other hand, the risk from such a therapeutic approach is low, and the likelihood that it will be beneficial is high. For this reason, and because of the high prevalence of insulin resistance in Western populations, programs of exercise and diet that prevent excess adiposity and increase insulin sensitivity are probably justified. Whether they should target the general population or, more specifically, individuals at high risk for type 2 diabetes and related disorders is a major public health issue (see Chapter 8).

Acknowledgments

This work was supported in part by National Institutes of Health Grant DK-19514. The author thanks Angie Liu and Deanna Chung for typing the manuscript.

References

1. Eriksson KF, Lindgarde F: No excess mortality in men with impaired glucose tolerance in the Malmo Preventive Trial with diet and exercise. *Diabetologia* 41:1010–16, 1998
2. Ruderman N, Chisholm D, Pi-Sunyer X, Schneider S: The metabolically-obese, normal-weight individual revisited. *Diabetes* 47:699–713, 1998
3. Richter EA, Garetto LP, Goodman MN, Ruderman NB: Muscle glucose metabolism following exercise in the rat. *J Clin Invest* 69:785–93, 1982
4. Bjorntorp P, Fahlen M, Grimby G, Gustafson A, Holm J, Renstrom P, Schersten T: Carbohydrate and lipid metabolism in middle-aged, physically well-trained men. *Metabolism* 21:1037–44, 1972
5. Saltin B, Lindgarde F, Houston M: Physical training and glucose tolerance in middle-aged men with chemical diabetes. *Diabetes* 28 (Suppl. 1):30–37, 1979
6. Ruderman NB, Ganda OP, Johansen K: The effect of physical training on glucose tolerance and plasma lipids in maturity-onset diabetes. *Diabetes* 28:89–92, 1979
7. Schneider SH, Vitug A, Ruderman N: Atherosclerosis and physical activity. *Diabetes Metab Rev* 1:513–53, 1986
8. Reaven GM: Role of insulin resistance in human disease. *Diabetes* 37:1595–607, 1988
9. DeFronzo RA, Ferrannini E: Insulin resistance: a multi-faceted syndrome responsible for NIDDM, obesity, hypertension, dyslipidemia and atherosclerotic cardiovascular disease. *Diabetes Care* 14:173–94, 1991
10. Ericksson J, Franssila-Kallunki A, Ekstand A, Groop L: Early metabolic defects in persons at increased risk for non-insulin dependent diabetes mellitus. *N Engl J Med* 6:337–43, 1989
11. Vaag A, Henriksen JE, Beck-Neilson H: Decreased insulin activation of glycogen synthase in skeletal muscles in young non-obese Caucasian relatives of patients with non-insulin dependent diabetes mellitus. *J Clin Invest* 89:782–88, 1992
12. Ferrari P, Weidmann P: Insulin, insulin sensitivity and hypertension. *J Hypertens* 8:491–500, 1990
13. Werbin B, Tamir I, Heidenberg D, Ayalen D, Adler M, Lenton O: Immunoreactive insulin response to oral glucose in offspring of

patients with endogenous hypertriglyceridemia. *Clin Chim Acta* 76:35–40, 1977
14. Ruderman NB, Schneider SH: Diabetes, exercise, and atherosclerosis. *Diabetes Care* 15 (Suppl. 4):1787–93, 1992
15. Helmreich SP, Ragland DR, Leung RW, Paffenbarger RS: Physical activity and reduced occurrence of non-insulin dependent diabetes mellitus. *N Engl J Med* 325:147–52, 1991
16. Manson JE, Nathan DM, Krowlewski AS, Stampfer MJ, Willett WC, Hennekens CH: A prospective study of exercise and the incidence of diabetes among male physicians. *JAMA* 268:63–67, 1992
17. Ruderman NB, Schneider SH, Berchtold P: The metabolically-obese, normal-weight individual. *Am J Clin Nutr* 34:1617–21, 1981
18. Zavaroni I, Bonini L, Fantuzzi M, Dall'Aglio E, Passeri M, Reaven GM: Hyperinsulinemia, obesity and syndrome X. *J Intern Med* 235:51–56, 1994.
19. Zavaroni I, Bonora E, Pagliara M, Dall'Aglio E, Luchetti L, Buonanno G, Bonati PA, Bergonzani M, Gnudi L, Passeri M, Reaven G: Risk factors for coronary artery disease in healthy persons with hyperinsulinemia and normal glucose tolerance. *N Engl J Med* 320:702–06, 1989
20. Chan JM, Rimm EB, Colditz GA, Stampfer MJ, Willett WC: Obesity, fat distribution, and weight gain as risk factors for clinical diabetes in men. *Diabetes Care* 17:961–69, 1994
21. Kissebah AH, Vydelingum N, Murray R, Evans DJ, Hartz AJ, Kalkhoff RK, Adams PW: Relation of body fat distribution to metabolic complications of obesity. *J Clin Endocrinol Metab* 54:254–60, 1980
22. Bjorntrop P: Metabolic implications of body fat distribution. *Diabetes Care* 14:1132–43, 1991
23. Bernstein RS, Grant N, Kipnis DM: Hyperinsulinemia and enlarged adipocytes in patients with endogenous hyperlipoproteinemia without obesity or diabetes mellitus. *Diabetes* 24:207–13, 1975
24. Schneider SH, Amorosa LF, Clemow L, Ruderman NB: Ten year experience with an exercise-based lifestyle modification program in the treatment of diabetes mellitus. *Diabetes Care* 15 (Suppl. 4): 1800–10, 1992
25. Nyholm B, Mehgel A, Nielson S, Skjaerback C, Moller N, Albert KGMM, Schmitz O: Insulin resistance in relatives of NIDDM

patients: the role of physical fitness and muscle metabolism. *Diabetologia* 39:813–22, 1996

26. Dvorak RV, Denirow F, Ades PA, Poehlman ET: Phenotypic characteristics associated with insulin resistance in metabolically obese but normal-weight young women. *Diabetes* 48:2210–14, 1999
27. Skarfors ET, Wegener TA, Lithell H, Selinus I: Physical training as treatment for type 2 (non-insulin-dependent) diabetes in elderly men: a feasibility study over 2 years. *Diabetologia* 30:930–33, 1987
28. Nesto RW, Phillips RT, Kett KG, Hill T, Perper E, Young E, Leland S: Angina and exertional myocardial ischemia in diabetic and non-diabetic patients: assessment by exercise thallium scintigraphy. *Am Intern Med* 107:170–75, 1988
29. Uusitupa M, Siltonen O, Pyorala K, Aro A, Hersio K, Pentilla I, Voutilainen E: The relationship of cardiovascular risk factors to the prevalence of coronary heart disease in recently diagnosed type II (non-insulin-dependent) diabetes. *Diabetologia* 28:653–59, 1985
30. Expert Committee on the Diagnosis and Classification of Diabetes Mellitus: Report of the Expert Committee on the Diagnosis and Classification of Diabetes Mellitus. *Diabetes Care* 20:1183–97, 1997
31. Barker DJP, Hales CN, Fall CHD, Osmond C, Phipps K, Clark PMS: Type 2 (non-insulin-dependent) diabetes mellitus, hypertension and hyperlipidaemia (syndrome X): relation to reduced fetal growth. *Diabetologia* 36:62–67, 1993
32. Krotkiewski M, Mandrovkas K, Sjostrom L, Sullivan L, Wetterquist H, Bjorntorp P: Effects of long-term physical training on body fat, metabolism and blood pressure in obesity. *Metabolism* 28:650–58, 1979
33. Ruderman NB, Apelian AZ, Schneider SH: Exercise in the therapy and prevention of type II diabetes: implications for blacks. *Diabetes Care* 13 (Suppl. 4):1163–68, 1990
34. O'Dea K: Marked improvement in carbohydrate and lipid metabolism in diabetic Australian Aborigines after temporary reversion to traditional lifestyle. *Diabetes* 33:596–603, 1984
35. Heath GW, Leonard BE, Wilson RH, Kendrick JS, Powell KE: Community-based exercise intervention: Zuni Diabetes Project. *Diabetes Care* 10:579–83, 1987

36. UK Prospective Diabetes Study (UKPDS) Group: Intensive blood-glucose control with sulphonylureas and insulin compared to conventional treatment and risk of complications in patients with type 2 diabetes (UKPDS 33). *Lancet* 352:837–53, 1998
37. Kramsch DM, Apsen AJ, Abramowitz BM, Kreimendahl T, Hood W: Reduction of coronary atherosclerosis by moderate conditioning exercise in monkeys on an atherogenic diet. *N Engl J Med* 305:1483–91, 1981

Neil Ruderman, MD, DPhil, is from the Boston University School of Medicine, Boston, MA.

The Treatment Plan

13

Application of the American Diabetes Association's Guidelines for the Evaluation of the Diabetic Patient Before Recommending an Exercise Program

STEPHEN H. SCHNEIDER, MD,
AND DANIEL SHINDLER, MD

Highlights

- There is a high prevalence of asymptomatic coronary artery disease in type 1 and type 2 diabetic patients.
- Patients with significant coronary artery disease have an increased risk of experiencing an acute cardiac event during or immediately after exercise.
- Noninvasive exercise testing before the initiation of an exercise program can be used in appropriate patients to assess cardiovascular risk and to generate specific exercise recommendations.
- The value of exercise testing depends on an assessment of the prior probability of significant coronary artery disease in the asymptomatic patient with diabetes. Low-risk patients may not benefit from formal exercise testing before initiating a modest exercise program.

- Nontraditional risk factors, such as autonomic neuropathy, peripheral vascular disease, proteinuria, and azotemia, are important predictors of cardiovascular risk in the diabetic population.

Increased Cardiac Risk During Exercise

It is well established that both type 1 and type 2 diabetic patients have at least twice the morbidity and mortality related to myocardial infarction as the general population. In addition, many studies indicate that the incidence of asymptomatic coronary artery disease (CAD) or CAD associated with atypical symptoms is higher in the diabetic population.[1–3] A 10% prevalence of occult clinically significant CAD in the typical clinic population with type 2 diabetes without classic symptoms of ischemia is probably a conservative estimate.[4–8] Those patients with diabetes who are free of classic symptoms of CAD are nevertheless at increased risk for having an acute event.[9] Framingham Study data suggest that asymptomatic diabetic patients with multiple risk factors have a >3% per year incidence of cardiac events—about twice that of the general population. The benefits of regular physical activity for these patients are outlined in Chapters 14 and 24, but the presence of asymptomatic or atypical CAD raises important concerns.

One of the most feared risks of initiating an exercise program is that of inducing sudden death secondary to an arrhythmia or an ischemic event. This is most likely to occur when underlying CAD is undiagnosed.[4,10] In a population-based study in Rhode Island, 12 cases of cardiovascular death during jogging were reported over a period of 6 years. The age-adjusted relative risk was 7 when compared with the risk during sedentary activities.[11–13] On the other hand, regular physical activity clearly and substantially reduces the risk of sudden death during or immediately after an individual exercise session. One study reported a relative risk of 107 for an exercise-related ischemic event in sedentary patients. For individuals who exercise one to two times a week, the risk was 19.4, and for those who exercise five or more times a week, the risk was only 2.4.[14,15] Although the absolute as opposed to relative risk of sudden death during or immediately after exercise is quite small, it remains a particular concern for the population with diabetes because of its high incidence of asymptomatic ischemic heart disease.

Evaluation of the Patient With Diabetes Who Wishes to Start an Exercise Program

Formal exercise testing before the initiation of a training program in patients with diabetes can be helpful in a variety of ways. In addition to identifying undiagnosed ischemic heart disease, the pulse and blood pressure response to various levels of exercise intensity can be quantified, the patient's ability to use ratings of perceived exertion can be tested, and more accurate assessments for heart rate recommendations can be made. Nevertheless, it is the concern over the risk of exercise-related sudden death has led to formal recommendations for noninvasive cardiac testing before initiating an exercise program in patients with diabetes and other high-risk groups.[16] Before starting an exercise program of moderate to high intensity, current American Diabetes Association (ADA) recommendations for type 2 diabetes[17] suggest that previously sedentary individuals >35 years of age or sedentary individuals of any age with duration of diabetes >10 years undergo exercise stress testing. In addition, nephropathy, autonomic neuropathy, and peripheral vascular disease indicate the need for exercise testing. The definition of low intensity in the ADA position statement[17] is <60% of maximal heart rate. Recommendations for asymptomatic individuals by the American Heart Association and the American College of Sports Medicine suggest pre-exercise noninvasive testing in the presence of two or more coronary risk factors or in patients >40 years of age with only one risk factor. These recommendations do not specify for what exercise training intensity formal testing is required nor is there a consensus on the nature of the specific exercise test to be done. Such recommendations raise great practical concerns because they could be interpreted to encompass the great majority of patients with type 2 diabetes, and the costs of following these recommendations indiscriminately would probably be prohibitive. For example, if more than 25 million people are expected to have diabetes in the U.S. in 2010 and 20% wanted to engage in exercise programs, then, at a cost of $250 per test, the total cost to society would be more than 1 billion dollars. Whereas this does not include potential but unproven savings from early intervention, the vast majority of positive tests in this population will be false-positives, and the consequences of such a result include the costs and risks of additional unnecessary tests and the psychological and societal costs of being labeled a cardiac patient.

Patient Selection

The cardiac evaluation of the diabetic patient who wishes to start a physical training program should be aimed at assessing the risk for a clinically important exercise-related cardiac event. Information that would be helpful in deciding whether formal exercise testing is necessary and, if so, which type of test would be most useful include the following: *1*) factors that predict a high risk of occult CAD (pretest probability), *2*) the intrinsic limitations of the testing procedure to be used (positive and negative predictive value), *3*) the type and intensity of exercise being planned, *4*) the ability of the individual to successfully complete the test, and *5*) the cost of the procedure.

Pretest Probability

Based on an estimate of the pretest probability of CAD, it is possible to gauge the utility of exercise testing as a screening tool. An important first step is to stratify patients for their risk of sudden death or myocardial infarction by clinical evaluation. The evaluation begins with the history and physical examination and scrutiny of the resting 12-lead electrocardiogram (ECG). A typical history of chest pain or pressure is most helpful, but it is quite possible that a diabetic patient may not provide this in the presence of significant disease. Other symptoms, such as dyspnea on exertion or unexplained gastrointestinal complaints, may also be useful. The presence of prior myocardial infarction or of resting ST segment abnormalities on the 12-lead ECG is useful for predicting the presence of CAD. Documenting the presence of additional traditional cardiac risk factors is also important. Also, because the increment in risk is a continuum, not only the prevalence, but the severity of the risk factors needs to be assessed. For patients with diabetes, an increased risk for more extensive CAD has been clearly associated with the presence of smoking, hyperlipidemia, cardiomegaly, and congestive heart failure. In a multivariate analysis that includes a history of prior myocardial infarction, 12-lead ECG abnormalities, smoking, and hyperlipidemia, diabetes per se had only a modest additional effect on the likelihood of significant CAD.[18] In fact, there are few studies that have attempted to determine the prognostic value of specific noninvasive tests in the diabetic population relative to the general population, and extrapolation from the results of studies done on largely healthy populations could be misleading. In addition, data on minorities are scant. Extensive data in patients with diabetes about the value of revascularization, anti-ischemic treatment, and other preventive therapies in the face of occult CAD are not available.

Nontraditional risk factors for CAD in patients with diabetes are powerful predictors of cardiac risk. Of these, renal disease, peripheral vascular disease,[19,20] cerebrovascular disease,[21] and autonomic neuropathy are particularly important. For example, angiographic studies of asymptomatic patients with diabetes and renal failure have found a roughly 50% incidence of significant CAD.[22–24] Autonomic neuropathy is also an important risk factor for sudden death in this population. In one study, >50% of patients with autonomic neuropathy died in a 5-year follow-up, mostly as a result of sudden death.[25] Some studies reported that >50% of patients with diabetes with no overt clinical evidence of heart disease who were to undergo vascular surgery for peripheral vascular disease had a positive thallium stress test.[26,27]

Type 1 Diabetes

Because there are more patients with type 2 diabetes than with type 1 diabetes, most information about the risks of exercise training has been obtained from type 2 diabetic patients. Although they are at higher risk for coronary heart disease, even in the absence of traditional risk factors, little is known about type 1 diabetic patients. Roughly 50% of patients with type 1 diabetes have clinically evident CAD by age 55. Until additional information is available, anyone with the onset of type 1 diabetes in childhood or adolescence who is over the age of 35 years or who has diabetes for >15 years should be considered a high-risk patient.

Assessing the Value of Exercise Testing

The positive and negative predictive value of various noninvasive tests can be assessed over a range of possibilities. For example, if a routine exercise test has a sensitivity (proportion of patients with CAD who have a positive test) of 90% and a specificity (proportion of patients without CAD who have a negative test) of 90% in the general population, then the negative predictive value (proportion of patients with a negative stress test who do not have CAD) would be 99% for patients with diabetes at low risk of disease (~10%).[4–8] However, the test would have a positive predictive value (proportion of patients with a positive stress test who have CAD) of only 50%. This result is no better than flipping a coin. In one large study of 3,617 hypercholesterolemic men, the predictive value of a positive stress test was only 0.3% at 1 year and 4% at 7.4 years.[28] There are no such large studies specifically in patients with diabetes, but in a small study, 34 asymptomatic diabetic patients were found to have positive stress tests. On angiography, only 12 patients had lesions requiring intervention, and 15 had patent coronary arteries. In a similar study from Japan, only 14 of 36 patients had significant angiographic findings.[29] Studies using cardiac events rather then angiographic findings as end points are probably more pertinent in assessing the clinical value of exercise testing because the relationship between angiographic findings and events is quite complex. Such studies are unfortunately not available for the diabetic population. In general, it appears that a positive exercise test in a patient with diabetes has a poor predictive value.

On the other hand, in a high-risk population, such as patients with renal disease and prevalence of CAD close to 50%, a positive exercise test would have a positive predictive value of 90%. It is generally accepted that stress tests are most useful when the pretest probability of CAD is intermediate (at around 50%).

In summary, a negative exercise test in an asymptomatic patient with a normal pretest ECG and average risk is sufficient to allow participation in an exercise program. It is true that false-negative tests occur in the presence of CAD. However, most of these individuals have single-vessel disease, and it is not clear that they are at an importantly increased risk for a clinically significant exercise-related coronary event. The strong prognostic value of a negative exercise test is not as widely accepted as it should be, and imaging stress tests tend to be overused in patients with normal resting ECGs. A positive test is less useful and may require further screening. A number of factors common in patients with diabetes are known to interfere with the sensitivity and specificity of noninvasive tests. These factors include hypertension, underlying diabetic cardiomyopathy, autonomic neuropathy, and renal insufficiency. The clearest example of a group of patients for whom exercise testing would be most useful are those with a prior coronary event and those with nontraditional risk factors, i.e., autonomic neuropathy, peripheral vascular disease, proteinuria, and azotemia (Table 13.1). The prognostic value of noninvasive exercise testing to assess the risk of the increasingly popular light resistance exercise being recommended for patients with diabetes is almost totally unknown. One suggested protocol can be found in Chapter 14.

TABLE 13.1 Characteristics of Asymptomatic Patients Who Might Benefit From Exercise Testing Before Starting a Physical Training Program

- Prior CAD
- Peripheral vascular disease
- Cerebrovascular disease
- Proteinuria or azotemia
- Documented autonomic neuropathy
- Type 1 diabetes of long duration

Stress Testing Modalities

Once the decision has been made that a patient needs further screening, a number of options are available (Table 13.2). The standard stress test that is used to screen patients for CAD remains the treadmill ECG. The ECG pattern during and after standard exercise testing is interpreted as positive when the ST segment is horizontally depressed ≥1 mm below the baseline. The T-P segment is used as the baseline. The ST depression is measured 80 ms after the J point. The test is considered negative if the ST segment criteria are not met and the patient reaches a heart rate of 85% of the age-predicted maximum. The test is considered nondiagnostic if there are no diagnostic ECG changes but the target heart rate is not reached. Asymptomatic diabetic patients with hypotension during exercise, a positive test at a heart rate of <120 beats/min, exercise capacity <6 min or 5 metabolic equivalents, ST depression in five or more leads, and a >2 mm ST depression in two or more leads are at high risk and should undergo coronary angiography. Patients taking insulin are at a risk for exercise-related hypoglycemia during an exercise test, which could precipitate a vascular event. For this reason, patients who are insulin-dependent should be scheduled for exercise testing early in the

TABLE 13.2 Representative Sensitivity and Specificity of Commonly Used Noninvasive Exercise Tests

Test	Sensitivity (%)	Specificity (%)	Reference
Standard ECG exercise test	68	77	Gibbons et al.[35]
Thallium 201 scintigraphy	83	88	Ritchie et al.[36]
Stress echocardiogram	84	87	Cheitlin et al.[37]

morning. If testing is delayed, patients can often receive their usual dose of long-acting insulin, and an infusion of dextrose (50–75 ml/h) can be maintained until resuming normal diet and activity. Traditional formal exercise testing protocols may be difficult for patients with long-standing diabetes. Complications such as loss of vision and neurological dysfunction can make it difficult, if not impossible, for such individuals to undergo standard exercise protocols. In many cases, the type of exercise used must be improvised. Any exercise using large muscle groups can be substituted as long as it includes those muscle groups likely to be used during the training program. For example, substitution of an arm exercise protocol in a patient unable to walk might more accurately reflect the hemodynamic stress associated with upper-body activity.

Nuclear Stress Imaging

For individuals with abnormal resting ECGs, some imaging modality is needed to supplement the electrocardiographic evaluation. In addition, although asymptomatic diabetic patients with a mildly positive stress test (i.e., 1–1.5 mm ST depression at a moderate to high exercise level) are generally a low-risk group, follow-up perfusion imaging excludes false-positive responses, and if perfusion imaging suggests a fixed defect rather than ischemia, these patients may not require coronary angiography before initiating a supervised exercise rehabilitation program.[5,23,30] The standard nuclear isotope is thallium, but the technetium compound sestamibi has been encroaching on thallium in volume of use. Both modalities require radionuclide imaging at rest as well as at peak stress. This means that the diabetic patient has to be capable of walking a treadmill or pedaling a bicycle. The protocol can be adjusted to the needs of someone who is not physically fit or suffers from peripheral vascular disease. Even if CAD is present, a negative perfusion study is associated with a low annual cardiac event rate in diabetic patients of around 2%.[31] Conversely, large perfusion defects indicate a significant risk of events over the next 1–2 years. Abnormal lung uptake and left ventricular dilation during exercise are also indicators of high-risk patients. The clinical value of perfusion imaging is reinforced by a longitudinal study of 1,271 patients with diabetes undergoing either rest thallium or sestamibi testing.[32] Yearly event rates were 1–2% for individuals with mildly abnormal scans, 3–4% for those with intermediate tests, and >70% for those with severely abnormal scans at baseline.

Bicycle and Treadmill Echocardiography

Echocardiographic stress techniques can be used in place of nuclear techniques in diabetic patients and have their own distinct advantages. Nuclear imaging is preferable when echocardiographic image quality is poor. Conversely, specificity of echocardiography seems better than that of nuclear techniques in patients with left ventricular hypertrophy and left bundle branch block.[33]

The echocardiographic stress test involves exercise with echocardiographic imaging. Specifically, a treadmill stress echocardiogram is performed by having the patient undergo resting echocardiographic imaging to display left ventricular wall motion. The patient then walks a treadmill, and at peak stress, the treadmill is halted and the patient is immediately transferred to a stretcher, with rapid imaging of left ventricular contractility for ~2 min. This test generates a fairly strenuous physical response, and the wall motion abnormalities are in response to fairly significant exercise workloads.

One advantage of exercise echocardiography using either a treadmill or a bicycle is the fact that an intravenous infusion is not required in most cases. Also, the test is shorter than nuclear imaging modalities because the patient does not have to return for a second set of images.

Pharmacological Stress Testing

For patients disabilities or medical status does not permit them to exercise using standardized protocols, there is a subset of nuclear and echocardiographic techniques that may be useful. Specifically, the nuclear techniques involve the injection of a pharmaceutical agent that results in a coronary vessel response. The heart is imaged along with electrocardiographic monitoring and the patient completes the test without having exercised. Some patients with diabetes find this to be the only type of test that they can complete.

Pharmacological stress tests using nuclear techniques to display myocardial perfusion use persantine or adenosine. Both agents have their drawbacks. For pharmacological stress testing with echocardiography, the most popular agent remains dobutamine. Echocardiography shows evidence of myocardial ischemia as regional left ventricular wall motion abnormalities.

Other Tests

Other noninvasive modalities, such as ambulatory ECG monitoring, carotid ultrasound, PET scanning,[34] and determination and quantification of coronary calcification with super-fast CAT scans, have not been shown to have predictive value for exercise-related coronary events, and their role, if any, remains to be determined.

Conclusions

When is an exercise test indicated for the patient with diabetes who wishes to participate in a program of physical training? It is important to remember that exercise testing may be useful for reasons other than the detection of occult ischemic heart disease. Accepted recommendations for routine screening of patients for occult coronary artery disease in high-risk populations (independent of any planned changes in physical activity) can be found in the position statement of the American College of Cardiology and American Heart Association.[35] Indications for exercise testing before initiating an exercise program for diabetic patients are meant as an adjunct to these general recommendations and are not intended to supplant them.

In the U.S., the diabetic population may approach 30 million in the next decade. Formal exercise testing before recommending a training program for asymptomatic patients with diabetes can be a useful tool for determining the type and intensity of exercise and for assessing potential cardiac risks. When recommending exercise training as a therapy for these patients, application of guidelines, such as those of the ADA, will require sound clinical judgment and a pragmatic approach. It is likely that the majority of individuals who limit their planned exercise to brisk walking will be able to safely initiate their program without formal stress testing (Table 13.3). Avoiding unnecessary testing

TABLE 13.3 Characteristics of Asymptomatic Patients Who Might Initiate Mild to Moderate Exercise Without Prior Exercise Testing

- Low or average traditional cardiac risk factors
- Normal resting ECG
- Absence of nontraditional risk factors
- Anticipated activity level not greatly exceeding that of daily living

would result in significant savings in time and money and remove a barrier to initiating exercise training for the population with type 2 diabetes (Fig. 13.1). On the other hand, efforts should be made to carry out appropriate testing in all high-risk asymptomatic patients with diabetes who wish to start a more intensive exercise program and to encourage third-party payers to provide adequate reimbursement.

Suggested Approaches to Applying the ADA Guidelines on Exercise Testing to Patients Encouraged to Start an Exercise Program

- Asymptomatic patients with type 2 diabetes and normal physical examinations and resting ECGs can participate in a modest exercise program, such as walking, without exercise

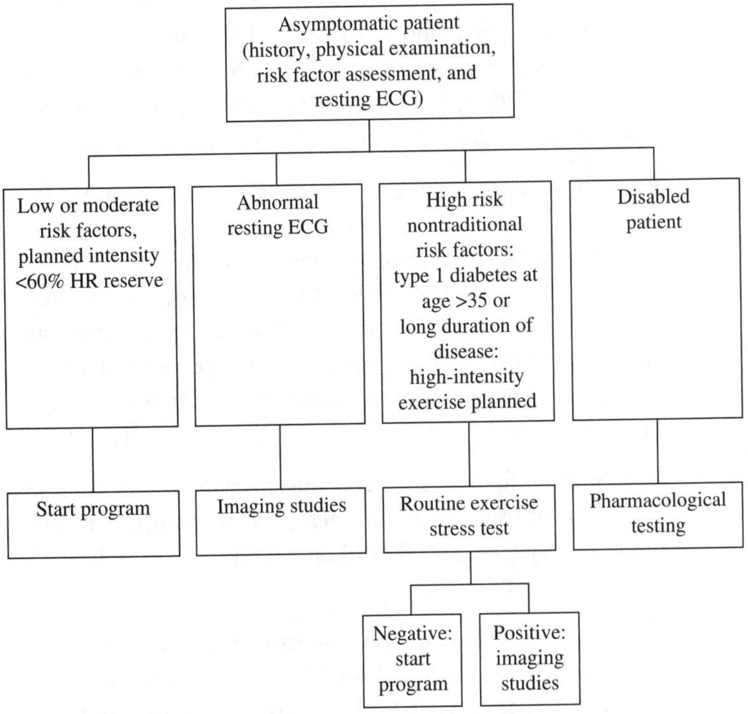

FIGURE 13.1 Pre-exercise evaluation.

stress testing. A modest exercise program is defined as *1*) <60% maximum heart rate (HR), *2*) <40% HR or VO_2 reserve, or *3*) rating of perceived exertion <14 (see Chapter 14). Patients should be carefully instructed on the signs and symptoms of cardiac disease so that any abnormalities can be immediately reported to their physician. Take for example a 50-year-old man with a resting HR of 70 beats/min: HR reserve = 170 beats/min (i.e., estimated maximum HR) – 70 beats/min (i.e., resting HR) = 100 beats/min. Then, 40% of the heart rate reserve would be 0.4 × 100 beats/min = 50 beats/min. Adding this to the resting heart rate leads to the recommendation that there is no need for prior testing if the proposed activity results in an HR of <110 beats/min.

- Previously sedentary asymptomatic patients over the age of 35 years with normal resting ECGs who will be exercising at a moderate to high intensity (>40–50% of HR reserve) should undergo routine exercise stress testing before initiating an exercise program. Abnormal exercise ECGs should be evaluated further. Repeat stress testing with nuclear cardiac imaging or echocardiography may be the next step, but in some cases, coronary angiography may be the proper choice.

- Patients with nontraditional risk factors include those with *1*) proteinuria and/or azotemia; *2*) a history of long duration of poor metabolic control; *3*) evidence of autonomic neuropathy, such as a decreased R-R interval variation on deep respiration (see Chapter 27); and *4*) evidence of peripheral vascular or cerebrovascular disease. These are exceptionally strong risk factors, and noninvasive evaluation is indicated in all such patients.

- Until more information is available, previously sedentary individuals with type 1 diabetes of >15 years' duration or those older than age 35 years should undergo noninvasive baseline exercise evaluation.

- Individuals with baseline ECG abnormalities that preclude the diagnosis of ischemia should be evaluated with a stress test that includes imaging using isotopes or echocardiography before initiating an exercise program.

- Properly performed high-volume resistance exercise induces hemodynamic changes similar to aerobic exercise at moderate intensity. Therefore, in the absence of available data, it seems reasonable to recommend that any individual who will be performing high-volume resistance exercise (as currently recommended by the ADA) should have routine cardiac stress testing using criteria similar to those recommended for moderate-intensity aerobic exercise programs. Validations of protocols to evaluate the risks of resistance exercise are still needed.

References

1. Nesto RW, Phillips RT, Kett KG, Hill T, Perper E, Young E, Leland OS: Angina and exertional myocardial ischemia in diabetic and nondiabetic patients: assessment by exercise thallium scintigraphy. *Ann Intern Med* 108:170–75, 1988
2. Scheidt-Nave C, Barrett-Conner E, Wingard DL: Resting electrocardiographic abnormalities suggestive of asymptomatic ischemic heart disease associated with non insulin-dependent diabetes mellitus in a defined population. *Circulation* 81:899–906, 1990
3. Thompson PD, Klocke FJ, Levine BD, Van Camp SP: Task force 5: coronary artery disease. *Med Sci Sports Exerc* 26:S271–75, 1994
4. Schneider SH, Khachadurian AK, Amorosa LF, Clemow L, Ruderman NB: Ten-year experience with an exercise-based outpatient lifestyle modification program in the treatment of diabetes mellitus. *Diabetes Care* 15 (Suppl. 4):1800–10, 1992
5. Milan Study on Atherosclerosis and Diabetes Group: Prevalence of unrecognized silent myocardial ischemia and its association with atherosclerotic risk factors in insulin-dependent diabetes mellitus. *Am J Cardiol* 79:134–39, 1997
6. Koistinen MJ: Prevalence of asymptomatic myocardial ischemia in diabetic subjects. *Br Med J* 301:92–95, 1990
7. Langer A, Freeman MR, Josse RG, Steiner G, Armstrong PW: Detection of silent myocardial ischemia in diabetes mellitus. *Am J Cardiol* 67:1073–78, 1991
8. Viviani V, Valensi P, Paycha F, Sachs RN, Ramadan A, Tonton-Moderc M, Nitenberg A, Attali JR: The stress test should be the first test performed when assessing silent myocardial ischemia in diabetic subjects. *Diabetes* 47 (Suppl. 1):119A, 1998

9. American Diabetes Association: Consensus development conference on the diagnosis of coronary heart disease in people with diabetes: 10–11 February 1998, Miami, Florida. *Diabetes Care* 21:1551–58, 1998
10. Kohl HW, Gordon NF, Powell KE, Blair SN, Paffenbarger RS: Physical activity, physical fitness and sudden cardiac death. *Epidemiol Rev* 14:37–58, 1992
11. Thompson PD, Funk EJ, Carleton RA, Sturner WQ: Incidence of death during jogging in Rhode Island from 1975 through 1980. *JAMA* 247:2535–38, 1982
12. Estes M: *Sudden Cardiac Death in the Athlete.* Deeb N, Salem PJ, Eds. Armonk, NY, Wang Futura Publishing, 1998
13. Allen WR: *The Athlete and Heart Disease: Diagnosis, Evaluation and Management.* Allen WR, Ed. Philadelphia, Lippincott, 1999
14. Mittleman M, Maclure M, Tofler GH, Sherwood JB, Goldberg RJ, Muller JE: Triggering of acute myocardial infarction by heavy physical exertion: protection against triggering by regular exertion. *N Engl J Med* 329:1677–83, 1993
15. Muller JE, Mittleman MA, Maclure M, Sherwood JB, Tofler GH: Triggering myocardial infarction by sexual activity: low absolute risk and prevention by regular physical exertion. *JAMA* 275: 1405–59, 1996
16. Caracciolo EA, Chaitman BR, Forman SA, Stone PH, Bourassa MG, Sopko G, Geller NL, Conti CR, Nesto RW: Screening for asymptomatic coronary artery disease in diabetes. *Diabetes Care* 22:1393–95, 1999
17. American Diabetes Association: Diabetes mellitus and exercise (Position Statement). *Diabetes Care* 24 (Suppl. 1):S51–55, 2001
18. Pryor DB, Harrell FE, Lee KL, Califf RM, Rosati RA: Estimating the likelihood of significant coronary artery disease. *Am J Med* 75:771–80, 1983
19. Criqui MH, Langer RD, Fronek A, Feigeison HS, Klauber MR, McCann TJ, Browner D: Mortality over 10 years in patients with peripheral arterial disease. *N Engl J Med* 326:381–86, 1992
20. Katzel LI, Sorkin J, Bradham D, Gardner AW: Comorbidities and the entry of patients with peripheral arterial disease into an exercise rehabilitation program. *J Cardiopulm Rehabil* 20:165–71, 2000

21. Giral P, Bruckert E, Dairou F, Boubrit K, Drobinski G, Chapman JM, Beucler I, Turpin G: Usefulness in predicting coronary artery disease by ultrasonic evaluation of the carotid arteries in asymptomatic hypercholesterolemic patients with positive exercise stress tests. *Am J Cardiol* 84:14–17, 1999
22. National Diabetes Data Group: *Diabetes in America.* Washington, DC, U.S. Dept. of Health and Human Services, 1994
23. Janand-Delenne B, Savin B, Habib G, Bory M, Vague P, Lassmann-Vague V: Silent myocardial ischemia in patients with diabetes: who to screen. *Diabetes Care* 22:1396–1400, 1999
24. Savage S, Estacio RO, Jeffers B, Schrier RW: Urinary albumin excretion as a predictor of diabetic retinopathy, neuropathy, and cardiovascular disease in NIDDM. *Diabetes Care* 19:1243–48, 1996
25. Ewing DJ, Campbell IW, Clarke BF: Assessment of cardiovascular effects in diabetic autonomic neuropathy and prognostic implications. *Ann Intern Med* 92:308–11, 1980
26. Lane SE, Lewis SM, Pippin JJ, Kosinski EJ, Campbell D, Nesto RW, Hill T: Predictive value of quantitative dipyridamole-thallium scintigraphy in assessing cardiovascular risk after vascular surgery in diabetes mellitus. *Am J Cardiol* 64:1275–79, 1989
27. Nesto RW, Wattson FS, Kowalchuk GJ, Zarich SW, Hill T, Lewis SM, Lane SE: Silent myocardial ischemia and infarction in diabetics with peripheral vascular disease: assessment by dipyridamole thallium-201 scintigraphy. *Am Heart J* 120:1073–77, 1990
28. Siscovick DS, Ekelund LG, Johnson JL, Truong Y, Adler A: Sensitivity of exercise electrocardiography for acute cardiac events during moderate and strenuous physical activity: the Lipid Research Clinics Prevention Trial. *Arch Int Med* 151:325–30, 1991
29. Naka M, Hiramatsu K, Aizawa T, Momose A, Yoshizawa K, Shigematsu S, Ishihara F, Niwa A, Yamada T: Silent myocardial ischemia in patients with non insulin-dependent diabetes mellitus as judged by treadmill exercise testing and coronary angiography. *Am Heart J* 123:46–53, 1992
30. Vandenberg BF, Rossen JD, Grover-McKay M, Shammas NW, Burns TL, Rezai K: Evaluation of diabetic patients for renal and pancreas transplantation: noninvasive screening for coronary artery disease using radionuclide methods. *Transplantation* 62:1230–35, 1996

31. Bell DS, Yumuk VD: Low incidence of false-positive exercise thallium 201 scintigraphy in a diabetic population. *Diabetes Care* 19:185–86, 1996
32. Katzel LI, Sorkin JD, Goldberg AP: Exercise-induced silent myocardial ischemia and future cardiac events in healthy, sedentary, middle-aged and older men. *J Am Geriatr Soc* 47:923–29, 1999
33. Fleischmann KE, Hunink MG, Kuntz KM, Douglas PS: Exercise echocardiography or exercise SPECT imaging? A meta-analysis of diagnostic test performance. *JAMA* 280:913–20, 1998
34. Kang X, Berman DS, Lewin HC, Cohen I, Friedman JD, Germano G, Hachamovitch R, Shaw LJ: Incremental prognostic value of myocardial perfusion single photon emission computed tomography in patients with diabetes mellitus. *Am Heart J* 138:1025–32, 1999
35. Gibbons RJ, Balady GJ, Beasley JW, Bricker JT, Duvernoy WF, Froelicher VF, Mark DB, Marwick TH, McCallister BD, Thompson PD Jr, Winters WL, Yanowitz FG, Ritchie JL, Gibbons RJ, Cheitlin MD, Eagle KA, Gardner TJ, Garson A Jr, Lewis RP, O'Rourke RA, Ryan TJ: ACC/AHA Guidelines for Exercise Testing: A Report of the American College of Cardiology/American Heart Association Task Force on Practice Guidelines (Committee on Exercise Testing). *J Am Coll Cardiol* 30:260–311, 1997
36. Ritchie JL, Bateman TM, Bonow RO, Crawford MH, Gibbons RJ, Hall RJ, O'Rourke RA, Parisi AF, Verani MS: Guidelines for clinical use of cardiac radionuclide imaging. *J Am Coll Cardiol* 25: 521–47, 1995
37. Cheitlin MD, Alpert JS, Armstrong WF, Aurigemma GP, Beller GA, Bierman FZ, Davidson TW, Davis JL, Douglas PS, Gillam LD: ACC/AHA Guidelines for the Clinical Application of Echocardiography: a report of the American College of Cardiology/American Heart Association Task Force on Practice Guidelines (Committee on Clinical Application of Echocardiography). Developed in collaboration with the American Society of Echocardiography. *Circulation* 95:1686–744, 1997

Stephen H. Schneider, MD, and Daniel Shindler, MD, are from the Robert Wood Johnson Medical School, University of Medicine and Dentistry of New Jersey, New Brunswick, NJ.

14

The Exercise Prescription

NEIL F. GORDON, MD, PhD, MPH

Highlights

- To optimize the likelihood of a safe and effective response, the exercise prescription should take into consideration safety aspects as well as the mode, frequency, duration, intensity, rate of progression, and timing of physical activity.
- The foremost priority in compiling the exercise prescription is to minimize the potential adverse effects of exercise via appropriate screening, program design, monitoring, and patient education.
- Before embarking on an exercise program, all people with diabetes should undergo a complete medical history and physical examination aimed at the identification of macrovascular, microvascular, and neurological complications. A continuing-care plan with follow-up medical evaluations is also necessary.
- An exercise electrocardiogram is recommended for individuals with one or more of the following: *1*) known

or suspected coronary artery disease, *2*) type 1 diabetes of >15 years' duration or type 2 diabetes of >10 years' duration, *3*) age >35 years, *4*) any additional risk factor for coronary artery disease, *5*) microvascular disease (proliferative retinopathy or nephropathy, including microalbuminuria), *6*) peripheral vascular disease, or *7*) autonomic neuropathy. In the absence of an exercise electrocardiogram, light to moderate rather than vigorous exercise should be prescribed for these individuals.

- The type, frequency, duration, and intensity of exercise training should be modulated to achieve an energy expenditure of 700–2,000 calories/week.
- Generally, to accomplish the desired weekly energy expenditure, aerobic exercise should be performed for 20–60 min, 3–5 days/week, at an intensity corresponding to 55–79% of maximum heart rate (intensities between 55 and 65% of maximum heart rate are most applicable to individuals who are unfit).
- Exercise training should begin at a comfortable intensity and gradually progress in accordance with baseline cardiorespiratory fitness level, age, weight, health status, personal preferences, and individual goals.
- Appropriately designed resistance training programs may be safe and effective for select patients.
- Exercise participation should be timed so that it does not coincide with periods of peak insulin absorption.
- Specific steps should be taken to enhance compliance with exercise training.

Exercise prescription is the process whereby a person's physical activity regimen is formulated in a systematic and individualized manner. Recent advances in basic and clinical exercise physiology have facilitated a more precise approach to exercise prescription for healthy people and those with chronic medical conditions. However, the existing body of scientific information is not so extensive as to warrant its application in a highly rigid fashion. In this respect, it must be emphasized that although the principles for exercise prescription outlined in this chapter are based on a solid foundation of scientific knowledge, they should not be construed as being theorems or laws. Rather, the recommended procedures should be viewed as guidelines that may be applied to a given person in a flexible manner. Health professionals who compile exercise prescriptions should recognize that the process is an art as well as a science.[1]

To optimize the likelihood of a safe and effective response, the exercise prescription should take into consideration safety aspects as well as the mode, frequency, duration, intensity, rate of progression, and timing of physical activity. These fundamental components are interrelated and partly dependent on the purposes for which exercise is prescribed in a given person. The purposes will vary depending on the individual's interests, needs, background, and health status. For people with diabetes, the major potential benefits of a physically active lifestyle include increased physical fitness, improved glycemic control, reduced risk for cardiovascular disease, decreased adiposity, and enhanced psychological well-being.[2,3] From a health promotion perspective, the various components of the exercise prescription should therefore be modulated with these purposes in mind. However, the purposes need not carry equal or consistent weight in all people with diabetes. In some instances, for example, in an overweight person with type 2 diabetes, decreased adiposity and improved insulin sensitivity may be the central concerns. In other instances, for example, in a young person with type 1 diabetes, enhancement of physical fitness and psychological well-being may be the primary goal. Thus, the exercise prescription should focus on achieving the potential health-related benefits of exercise while reflecting the specific outcomes that are sought by a particular person with diabetes.

Safety: The Pre-Exercise Evaluation

Exercise is a normal human function that can be undertaken with a high level of safety by most people, including those with diabetes. However, exercise is not without risks, and the recommendation that people with diabetes participate in an exercise program is based on the premise that the benefits outweigh these risks. Therefore, the foremost priority in compiling the exercise prescription is to pay careful attention to minimizing the potential adverse effects of exercise via appropriate screening, program design, monitoring, and patient education (Table 14.1).

As is the case for the general population, the major potential health hazards of exercise for people with diabetes include musculoskeletal in-

TABLE 14.1 Summary of Exercise Recommendations for Patients With Diabetes

Screening

- Search for vascular and neurological complications, including silent ischemia
- Exercise ECG recommended for patients with one or more of the following: *1*) known or suspected CAD, *2*) type 1 diabetes of >15 years' duration or type 2 diabetes of >10 years' duration, *3*) age >35 years, *4*) any additional risk factor for CAD, *5*) microvascular disease, *6*) peripheral vascular disease, or *7*) autonomic neuropathy. In the absence of an exercise ECG, light to moderate rather than vigorous exercise should be prescribed for these patients

Exercise program

- Type: aerobic
- Frequency: three to five times per week
- Duration: 20–60 min of continuous or intermittent exercise (minimum of 10-min bouts)
- Intensity: 55–79% of HR_{max} or 40–74% of VO_2R or HRR
- Energy expenditure: modulate type, frequency, duration, and intensity to attain an energy expenditure of 700–2,000 calories/week
- Timing: time participation so that it does not coincide with peak insulin absorption

Avoiding complications

- Warm up and cool down
- Careful selection of exercise type and intensity
- Patient education
- Proper footwear
- Avoid exercise in extreme heat or cold
- Inspect feet daily and after exercise
- Avoid exercise when metabolic control is poor
- Maintain adequate hydration
- Monitor blood glucose if taking insulin or oral hypoglycemic agents, and follow guidelines to prevent hypoglycemia

Compliance

- Make exercise enjoyable
- Convenient location
- Positive feedback from involved medical personnel and family

Adapted in part from the American Diabetes Association.[2,3]

jury and sudden cardiac death. Other potential adverse effects that apply specifically to people with diabetes are listed in Table 14.2. Health professionals who counsel patients on exercise should be familiar with these adverse effects and how to prevent them.

Specific safety precautions for people with diabetes who participate in exercise are addressed in detail later (see Chapters 4, 13, 15, and 20–34). Depending on the severity of diabetic complications and other coexisting medical conditions, certain patients may need to participate in a medically supervised exercise program. However, before embarking on an exercise program, it is recommended that all people with diabetes undergo a complete medical history (Table 14.3), usually the most important part of the pre-exercise evaluation, and physical examination (Table 14.4) aimed at identifying macrovascular, microvascular, and neurological complications as well as other medical conditions that constitute a contraindication to exercise or require special consideration (Table 14.5).[2] Because diabetes is potentially a progressive chronic disease, a continuing care plan with follow-up medical evaluations is also necessary. Follow-up evaluations may be integrated into the patient's regular office visits, which should be scheduled at least quarterly until treatment goals are achieved and at least semi-annually thereafter. The

TABLE 14.2 Potential Adverse Effects of Exercise in Patients With Diabetes

Cardiovascular
- Cardiac dysfunction and arrhythmias due to ischemic heart disease (often silent)
- Excessive increments in blood pressure during exercise
- Postexercise orthostatic hypotension

Microvascular
- Retinal hemorrhage
- Increased proteinuria
- Acceleration of microvascular lesions

Metabolic
- Worsening of hyperglycemia and ketosis
- Hypoglycemia in patients on insulin or oral hypoglycemic agents

Musculoskeletal and traumatic
- Foot ulcers (especially in presence of neuropathy)
- Orthopedic injury related to neuropathy
- Accelerated degenerative joint disease
- Eye injuries and retinal hemorrhage

Adapted with permission from the American Diabetes Association.[3]

TABLE 14.3 Major Components of the Pre-Exercise Medical History

Individuals should be asked about their past and present medical history. Appropriate components of the medical history may include the following:

- Medical diagnosis: cardiovascular disease including myocardial infarction; percutaneous coronary artery procedures including angioplasty, coronary stent(s), and atherectomy; coronary artery bypass surgery; valvular surgery(s) and valvular dysfunction (e.g., aortic stenosis/mitral valve disease); other cardiac surgeries such as left ventricular aneurysmectomy and cardiac transplantation; pacemaker and/or implantable cardioverter defibrillator; presence of aortic aneurysm; ablation procedures for arrhythmias; symptoms of ischemic coronary syndrome (angina pectoris); peripheral vascular disease; hypertension; obesity; pulmonary disease including asthma, emphysema, and bronchitis; cerebrovascular disease including stroke and transient ischemic attacks; anemia and other blood dyscrasias (e.g., lupus erythematosis); phlebitis, deep vein thrombosis, or emboli; cancer; pregnancy; osteoporosis; musculoskeletal disorders; emotional disorders; eating disorders; other chronic complications associated with diabetes (eye, renal, and neurological)
- Previous physical examination findings: murmurs, clicks, gallop rhythms, other abnormal heart sounds, and other unusual cardiac and vascular findings; abnormal pulmonary findings (e.g., wheezes, rales, or crackles); abnormal blood lipids and lipoproteins or other significant laboratory abnormalities (e.g., microalbuminuria); high blood pressure; edema
- History of symptoms: discomfort (pressure, tingling, pain, heaviness, burning, tightness, squeezing, or numbness) in the chest, jaw, neck, back, or arms; lightheadedness, dizziness, or fainting; temporary loss of visual acuity or speech, transient unilateral numbness or weakness; shortness of breath; rapid heart beats or palpitations, especially if associated with physical activity, eating a large meal, emotional upset, or exposure to cold (or any combination of these activities); frequency, severity, and cause of acute diabetic complications, such as ketoacidosis and hypoglycemia; other symptoms (and treatment) of chronic complications associated with diabetes (eye, heart, kidney, nerve, peripheral vascular, and cerebral vascular)
- Recent illness, hospitalization, new medical diagnoses, or surgical procedures
- Orthopedic problems including arthritis, joint swelling, or any condition that would make ambulation or use of certain exercise modalities difficult
- Medication use; drug allergies; current treatment of diabetes including medications, diet, and results of glucose monitoring
- Other habits including caffeine, alcohol, tobacco, or recreational (illicit) drug use
- Exercise history: information on readiness for change and habitual level of activity; type of exercise, frequency, duration, and intensity
- Work history with emphasis on current or expected physical demands, noting upper- and lower-extremity requirements
- Family history of cardiac, pulmonary, or metabolic disease; stroke; or sudden death

Adapted with permission from the American College of Sports Medicine[1] and the American Diabetes Association.[4]

TABLE 14.4 Major Components of the Pre-Exercise Physical Examination, Including Laboratory Testing

The physical examination should be thorough. Appropriate components of the physical examination may include the following:

- Body weight; in many instances, determination of BMI, waist-to-hip ratio, waist girth, and/or body composition (percent body fat) is desirable
- Apical pulse rate and rhythm
- Resting blood pressure, seated, supine, and standing
- Auscultation of the lungs with specific attention to uniformity of breath sounds in all areas (absence of rales, wheezes, and other breathing sounds)
- Palpation of the cardiac apical impulse (point of maximal impulse)
- Auscultation of the heart with specific attention to murmurs, gallops, clicks, and rubs
- Palpation and auscultation of carotid, abdominal, and femoral arteries
- Evaluation of the abdomen for bowel sounds, masses, visceromegaly, and tenderness
- Palpation and inspection of lower extremities for edema and presence of arterial pulses
- Foot examination
- Ophthalmoscopic examination
- Absence or presence of tendon xanthoma and skin xanthelasma
- Follow-up examination related to orthopedic or other medical conditions that would limit exercise participation
- Tests of neurological function, including reflexes and cognition (as indicated)
- Inspection of the skin, especially of the lower extremities
- Laboratory tests (if not recently performed and clinically indicated), including fasting blood glucose, glycosylated hemoglobin, fasting serum lipids and lipoproteins, serum creatinine, urinalysis, testing for microalbuminuria, thyroid function tests, resting ECG, exercise ECG, pulmonary studies, and review of results of previous pertinent tests (e.g., coronary angiography, echocardiographic studies, nuclear medicine studies)

Adapted with permission from the American College of Sports Medicine[1] and the American Diabetes Association.[4]

precise frequency and nature of follow-up physician visits, of course, will also depend on other factors, such as changes in the treatment regimen and the presence of complications or other medical conditions.[4]

From a pre-exercise evaluation perspective, it must be emphasized that the most serious complication of exercise participation is sudden cardiac death. Although habitual physical activity is associated with an overall reduction in the risk of sudden cardiac death in the general adult population and the chances of sustaining a fatal cardiac event during exercise training are extremely small, it is well established that exercise can precipitate sudden cardiac death.[5–7] Moreover, several studies have now shown that in adults, the transiently increased risk of

TABLE 14.5 Contraindications to Exercise Participation

Absolute contraindications

- Recent significant change in the resting ECG that has not been adequately investigated and managed
- Unstable angina pectoris
- Uncontrolled cardiac arrhythmias causing symptoms or hemodynamic compromise
- Uncontrolled symptomatic heart failure
- Severe symptomatic aortic stenosis
- Suspected or known dissecting aneurysm
- Acute myocarditis or pericarditis
- Acute thrombophlebitis or intracardiac thrombi
- Acute pulmonary embolus or pulmonary infarction
- Untreated high-risk proliferative retinopathy
- Recent significant retinal hemorrhage
- Acute or inadequately controlled renal failure
- Acute infections

Relative contraindications

- Fasting blood glucose >300 mg/dl or >250 mg/dl with urinary ketone bodies
- Uncontrolled hypertension with resting systolic blood pressure >200 mmHg or diastolic blood pressure >110 mmHg
- Severe autonomic neuropathy with exertional hypotension
- Moderate stenotic valvular heart disease
- Hypertrophic cardiomyopathy and other forms of outflow tract obstruction
- Tachyarrhythmias or bradyarrhythmias
- High-degree atrioventricular block
- Ventricular aneurysm
- Electrolyte abnormalities (e.g., hypokalemia, hypomagnesemia)
- Uncontrolled metabolic disease (e.g., thyrotoxicosis, myxedema)
- Chronic infectious disease (e.g., hepatitis, AIDS)
- Neuromuscular, musculoskeletal, or rheumatoid disorders that are exacerbated by exercise
- Complicated pregnancy

Adapted with permission from the American College of Sports Medicine[1] and Gordon NF: *Diabetes: Your Complete Exercise Guide.* Champaign, IL, Human Kinetics, 1993.

cardiac arrest that occurs during exercise results primarily from the presence of preexisting coronary artery disease (CAD).[8,9] In view of this, and because diabetes increases the risk for CAD by about threefold in men and possibly even more in women and is associated with a high prevalence of silent ischemia,[3] it is recommended that individuals with diabetes perform a graded exercise test with electrocardiogram (ECG) monitoring as part of a medical evaluation before beginning an exercise program if any one or more of the following are present: *1*) known or suspected CAD, *2*) type 1 diabetes of >15 years' duration or type 2 diabetes of >10 years' duration, *3*) age >35 years, *4*) any additional risk factor for CAD, *5*) microvascular disease (proliferative retinopathy or nephropathy, including microalbuminuria), *6*) peripheral vascular disease, or *7*) autonomic neuropathy. Graded exercise testing in these individuals should be conducted in accordance with traditional guidelines that are outlined in detail elsewhere.[1]

From a practical standpoint, it is recognized that it may not be possible, for a variety of reasons, for many of these individuals with diabetes to perform an exercise test before beginning an exercise program. For patients for whom an exercise ECG is recommended but not performed, light to moderate rather than vigorous exercise should be prescribed (for more details, see INTENSITY).

Fitness Versus Health Benefits of Exercise: Implications for Exercise Prescription

Much is known about the physiological adaptations that result from regular exercise. In particular, the exercise stimuli that are needed to improve maximum oxygen uptake—the most widely accepted index of cardiorespiratory fitness—have been well documented. Based on existing research in this area, guidelines for the quality and quantity of exercise required to promote cardiorespiratory fitness have been formulated.[10] Because cardiorespiratory fitness and health are frequently considered synonymous, such guidelines are often extrapolated to the prescription of exercise for the purpose of disease prevention and rehabilitation.[11] In reality, however, changes in clinical status and health do not necessarily parallel increases in maximum oxygen uptake. Interestingly, recent epidemiological studies strongly suggest that regular participation in light to moderate–intensity physical activities, which are unlikely to exert an optimal effect on maximum oxygen uptake, may be beneficial for the prevention of several diseases, including CAD, hypertension, and type 2 diabetes.[5,12,13] Furthermore, these studies suggest that strenuous exercise may not offer substantially more benefit from a health standpoint. Similarly, moderate levels of cardiorespiratory fitness, which probably are attainable by most adults without resorting to particularly strenuous exercise, have been shown to be partially protective against premature mortality.[14] In addition, longitudinal training studies indicate that exercising at intensities that do not have an optimal effect on maximum oxygen uptake may produce equally favorable changes in CAD risk factors, including serum lipids and lipoproteins, blood pressure, and adiposity.[12,15] Unlike improvements in maximum oxygen uptake, which are closely coupled with the volume and intensity of exercise training, the effectiveness of exercise in the possible prevention of CAD appears to depend primarily on the total energy expenditure.[16] Thus, provided the frequency and duration are modulated appropriately, even physical activity performed at an intensity below the critical threshold above which significant improvements in maximum oxygen uptake occur may be beneficial.[11]

How can such knowledge be used to help promote physical activity participation among people with diabetes? Many individuals dislike strenuous exercise. Therefore, one approach is to reassure these individuals that they will derive important health benefits from less strenuous exercise training, place no emphasis on the intensity component of their exercise prescription (with the exception of ensuring that they do not exercise at too high an intensity), and focus on attainment of the desired level of energy expenditure.[11] A potential disadvantage to this approach is that the efficacy of such low-intensity exercise in enhancing insulin sensitivity is unknown at present. Another disadvantage is that although any increase in physical activity may increase a sedentary person's maximum oxygen uptake, clinically relevant changes would be unlikely to result. Because important goals of exercise training for people with diabetes include enhancement of insulin sensitivity and physical fitness, a somewhat modified version of this approach may be preferable. Rather than completely ignoring the intensity component, a middle ground may be reached. This can be accomplished by encouraging people to achieve the desired energy expenditure level while exercising at intensities of their choice that are above the minimal threshold needed to significantly increase maximum oxygen uptake but below that which may elicit undesirable physiological responses or clinical consequences (such as hypoglycemia, hyperglycemia, ketosis, myocardial ischemia, arrhythmia, exacerbation of proliferative retinopathy, and orthopedic injury).[11]

Mode of Exercise

A key goal of the exercise prescription is caloric energy expenditure.[1,16] To accomplish this, activities that use large muscle groups, that can be maintained for a prolonged period, and that are rhythmic and aerobic in nature are preferred. Typical examples include walking, jogging, swimming, cycling, cross-country skiing, rowing, dancing, skating, rope skipping, stair climbing, and various endurance game activities. For a given level of energy expenditure, the health-related benefits of exercise appear to be independent of the mode of aerobic activity. Therefore, provided no contraindications exist, the types of aerobic exercise a patient performs are a matter of personal preference.

Aerobic activities that require running and jumping are considered high-impact types of exercise. Generally, in beginning as well as long-term exercisers, these activities are associated with a higher incidence of musculoskeletal injuries than low-impact and non–weight-bearing activities.[1] This increased risk for musculoskeletal injury is particularly evident in the elderly. Such activities are also more likely to traumatize the feet in patients with peripheral neuropathy and precipitate vitreous hemorrhage or traction retinal detachment in patients with active diabetic retinopathy.[2,3] Thus, these factors must be considered when the exercise modality is prescribed.

When precise control of exercise intensity is needed, as in the early stages of an exercise program for patients with diabetic complications, preferred activities are those that can be readily maintained at a constant intensity and for which interindividual variability in energy expenditure is relatively low.[1] Such activities include walking and stationary cycling.

Although aerobic exercise is of primary importance, a persuasive body of scientific evidence indicates that resistance training sufficient to develop and maintain strength should also be an integral component of an adult physical activity program. Based on existing research, both the American College of Sports Medicine (ACSM) and the American Association of Cardiovascular and Pulmonary Rehabilitation have added resistance training guidelines to their exercise recommendations for healthy adults and low-risk cardiac patients.[10,17] Recent studies suggest that appropriately designed resistance training programs may be safe and effective for patients with diabetes who do not have contraindications to such exercise[18,19] (see Chapter 16).

Frequency, Intensity, Duration, Rate of Progression, and Timing of Exercise

According to the American Heart Association, leisure-time activity for minimum physical conditioning and health benefits should burn at least 700 calories/week.[16] They further recommend that individuals be encouraged to engage in activities requiring up to 2,000 calories/week for maximum health benefits.[16] There is little convincing evidence of substantially greater health benefit at more than 2,000 calories/week.[16]

In addition to the mode of exercise, weekly energy expenditure during training depends on the frequency, intensity, and duration of physical activity. Therefore, these factors should be modulated in accordance with the patient's clinical status and personal preferences to achieve the desired weekly energy expenditure.

Frequency

The frequency at which exercise should be performed depends in part on the duration and intensity of each exercise session. Existing research indicates that a frequency of <2 days/week generally does not evoke a meaningful change in maximum oxygen uptake.[10] In contrast, the magnitude of improvement in maximum oxygen uptake tends to plateau when the frequency of training is increased above 3 days/week, with little additional benefit with training >5 days/week.[10] Available evidence further suggests that the duration of glycemic improvement after the last bout of exercise in patients with diabetes is >12 but <72 h.[20] In view of the above, it is recommended that aerobic exercise be performed on at least 3 nonconsecutive days each week and ideally on 5 days/week. Patients on insulin who experience difficulty in balancing their daily insulin and caloric needs may find it preferable to exercise daily. Similarly, obese patients may need to exercise more frequently (that is, 6–7 days/week) to optimize weight loss.

Multiple shorter bouts of exercise spread throughout the day may produce improvements in exercise capacity similar to a single longer session.[21] Although more comprehensive scientific inquiry is needed, note that multiple short bouts of exercise closely resemble the physical activity that typically has been measured in epidemiological studies.[22] In these studies, the accumulation of energy expenditure has been found to be inversely related to the risk for CAD and the development of type 2 diabetes. Therefore, while additional confirmatory data are needed, it is thought that if the total daily energy expenditure is the same, comparable health benefits should accrue with multiple versus single bouts of exercise. For multiple bouts of exercise, a minimum of 10 min/bout is recommended by the ACSM.[10]

Intensity

The prescription of the appropriate exercise intensity is the most difficult problem in designing exercise programs. According to the ACSM, the minimum training intensity threshold for improvement in maximum oxygen uptake is between 55 and 65% of the maximum heart rate (HR_{max}).[10] The minimal threshold for improving maximum oxygen uptake is greatly affected by the individual's initial level of fitness. The person who has a low level of fitness can achieve a significant training effect with a training heart rate as low as 55–65% of HR_{max}, whereas individuals with higher fitness levels require a higher training stimulus. A training heart rate of 55–65% of HR_{max} corresponds to 40–50% of maximum oxygen uptake reserve (VO_2R) or HR_{max} reserve (HRR) and a rating of perceived exertion (RPE) of 12 on the Borg 6–20 scale (Table 14.6). It should be noted that the ACSM now relates HR_{max} and HRR to a percentage of VO_2R rather than to a percentage of VO_{2max} ($VO_2R = VO_{2max} - \text{resting } VO_2$).

The ACSM recommends an intensity of exercise for healthy adults corresponding to between 55 and 90% of HR_{max} or to between 40 and 85% of HRR or VO_2R. However, higher-intensity exercise is associated with greater cardiovascular risk, greater chance for musculoskeletal injury, and lower compliance to training than lower-intensity exercise. Therefore, programs emphasizing low to moderate–intensity exercise may be preferable for most people with diabetes. If the complications of diabetes permit, it is recommended that exercise generally be prescribed at an intensity corresponding to 55–79% of HR_{max}, 40–74% of VO_2R or HRR, or an RPE of 12–15 (intensities

TABLE 14.6 Classification of Intensity of Exercise Based on 20–60 min of Aerobic Exercise Training

HR_{max} (%)	VO_2R or HRR (%)	RPE	Intensity
<35	<20	<10	Very light
35–54	20–39	10–11	Light
55–69	40–59	12–13	Moderate
70–89	60–84	14–16	Hard
≥90	≥85	17–19	Very hard
100	100	20	Maximal

Adapted with permission from the American College of Sports Medicine.[10]

between 55 and 65% of HR_{max}, between 40 and 50% of VO_2R or HRR, or eliciting an RPE of 12 are most appropriate for individuals who are unfit). For patients for whom an exercise ECG is recommended but not performed, it may be prudent not to exceed an exercise intensity corresponding to 69% of HR_{max}, 59% of VO_2R or HRR, or an RPE of 13.

As indicated above, various techniques can be used to prescribe and monitor exercise intensity. These include heart rate, VO_2, and RPE.[1] Patients usually find the concept of heart rate and RPE easier to understand than the concept of VO_2, and these two methods are generally preferred.[23] Generally for people with diabetic complications, both heart rate and RPE should be used. Although the use of heart rate as an estimate of exercise intensity is the recommended approach, for those without diabetic complications or coexisting medical conditions that may be worsened by exercise, RPE may be used on its own.

The heart rate method of exercise prescription is based on the linear relationship that exists between heart rate and exercise intensity. Ideally, target heart rates should be prescribed using the individual's HR_{max} determined during graded exercise testing. This is particularly important for patients with cardiovascular complications or autonomic neuropathy or those receiving medications, such as β-blockers, that may alter the heart rate response to exercise. When the true HR_{max} is unknown, it can be estimated by the equation $HR_{max} = 220 -$ the patient's age (provided the person does not have autonomic neuropathy or any other medical condition known to alter HR_{max} and is not taking a medication that alters HR_{max}).

The two most commonly used ways of prescribing target heart rates are the percent HR_{max} method and the percent HRR method.[1,10,23] The percent HR_{max} method simply involves multiplying HR_{max} by 0.55 and 0.79, respectively, to determine the lower and upper limits of the target heart rate range. The percent HRR method differs from this in that the individual's true resting heart rate (HR_{rest}), determined before rising in the morning, is also taken into consideration, as follows:

$$\text{Lower limit} = 0.4\,(HR_{max} - HR_{rest}) + HR_{rest}$$

$$\text{Upper limit} = 0.74\,(HR_{max} - HR_{rest}) + HR_{rest}$$

The use of RPE has become a valid method of monitoring and prescribing exercise intensity. It is generally regarded as an adjunct to heart rate monitoring, but it can be used in place of heart rate in patients in whom a precise knowledge of heart rate is not clinically indicated. It should be kept in mind, however, that ~10% of participants tend to select unrealistic RPE scores. In these individuals, the RPE method for exercise prescription is inappropriate. The commonly used Borg 6–20 scale is shown in Table 14.7.

Irrespective of the precise manner of exercise intensity prescription, importance should be placed on an adequate warm-up and cooldown. Patients should warm up with low-intensity aerobic exercise for at least 5 min. The most practical way to accomplish this is to perform the prescribed aerobic activity at a lower intensity. Ideally, the aerobic warm-up should raise the heart rate to within at least 20 beats/min of the lower limit of the prescribed target heart rate range. On completion of the aerobic phase of the exercise session, it is also important to keep exercising at a reduced intensity for at least 5 min before stopping completely. This cooldown helps ensure the gradual return of heart rate and blood pressure to near-resting levels and reduces the potential for postexercise hypotension together

TABLE 14.7 Borg 6–20 Perceived Exertion Scale

RPE	Verbal Description of RPE
6	
7	Very, very light
8	
9	Very light
10	
11	Fairly light
12	
13	Somewhat hard
14	
15	Hard
16	
17	Very hard
18	
19	Very, very hard
20	

From Borg GA: Psychophysical bases of perceived exertion. *Med Sci Sports Exerc* 14:377–87, 1982.

with its adverse clinical sequelae. The importance of an adequate aerobic warm-up and cooldown is emphasized by the observation in one study that of 61 cardiac complications during the exercise training of CAD patients, 44 occurred at the beginning or end of an exercise session.[24] To help prevent musculoskeletal injuries, stretching exercises may also be included in the warm-up and/or cooldown. However, patients must do these stretches without holding their breath because that can result in increases in systolic blood pressure due to a Valsalva effect. For patients with microvascular or coronary disease, such increases in systolic blood pressure are potentially detrimental.[3]

Duration

The appropriate duration of each exercise session is inversely related to the intensity at which the exercise is performed. Thus, lower-intensity physical activity should be conducted over a longer period of time than higher-intensity exercise. When performed 3–5 days/week at 55–79% of HR_{max}, exercise sessions will typically need to last 20–60 min to achieve the desired weekly energy expenditure. Shorter exercise sessions will need to be performed several times during the day. Longer exercise sessions may result in a higher incidence of musculoskeletal injury and difficulty with compliance.

Rate of Progression

The rate of progression in the exercise training program depends on several factors. These include baseline cardiorespiratory fitness level, age, weight, health status, personal preferences, and individual goals. It is usually best initially to alter the duration of exercise rather than the intensity of effort. Generally, exercise training should begin at a comfortable intensity that is well within the individual's current capacity. Exercise sessions initially should be no more than 10–15 min in duration and should be gradually increased in accordance with the individual's capabilities. Once a desired duration is reached, exercise intensity may likewise be gradually increased. To prevent musculoskeletal injury and untoward physiological responses, beginning exercisers should be advised to progress gradually and be cautioned against attempting to perform too much exercise too soon.[1]

Timing of Exercise

Ideally, exercise training should be performed at the time of day that is most convenient for the participant. However, because exercise can potentiate the effects of insulin, hypoglycemia during or after exercise is a definite risk for individuals receiving treatment with insulin (and, to a lesser degree, oral hypoglycemic agents). It is important when prescribing exercise to time participation so that it does not coincide with periods of peak insulin absorption (details of hypoglycemia prevention are presented in Chapter 20). Initially, to enhance blood glucose control, it may be preferable for patients on insulin to exercise at a similar time each day. However, this is not absolutely necessary, especially once the patient gains adequate experience with hypoglycemia prevention.

Compliance

Research on adherence to exercise training reveals that 50% of participants drop out within 1 year.[1] Specific steps can be taken to enhance exercise compliance. These are discussed in detail elsewhere[1,3] and include *1*) ensuring that the person has reasonable expectations at the start of the program, *2*) having the new participant make a firm commitment to adhere to the program via a written contract, *3*) starting the exercise program at a comfortable level and progressing gradually, *4*) choosing enjoyable activities that can be performed at a convenient time and location, *5*) setting realistic goals to ensure gradual progression of exercise training, *6*) reviewing the person's performance on a regular basis and giving him or her feedback about progress, *7*) reinforcing positive changes in behavior via appropriate rewards, *8*) using stimulus control strategies (e.g., writing exercise time in appointment books, setting watch alarms for exercise time, laying out clothes the night before) and cognitive strategies (e.g., having participants systematically consider the pros and cons of exercise), *9*) optimizing social support from friends and relatives, and *10*) training in relapse prevention.

The Role of Physicians and Other Health Care Professionals in the Exercise Prescription

Physicians have both the opportunity and responsibility to promote regular exercise to their patients with diabetes. If the physician does not have the time or does not feel knowledgeable enough to personally prescribe and supervise an exercise program, he or she may delegate the task to other appropriately qualified members of the health care team. In this respect, the services of nurses, exercise physiologists, physical therapists, and other health care professionals may be extremely useful. However, the physician must set the agenda because staff members under a physician's supervision cannot deliver preventive and rehabilitative services, such as the exercise prescription, unless the physician defines the services as medically appropriate.[5]

References

1. American College of Sports Medicine: *Guidelines for Exercise Testing and Prescription.* Philadelphia, Lippincott Williams and Wilkins, 2000
2. American Diabetes Association: Diabetes mellitus and exercise (Position Statement). *Diabetes Care* 23 (Suppl. 1):S50–54, 2000
3. American Diabetes Association: Exercise and NIDDM (Technical Review). *Diabetes Care* 16 (Suppl. 2):54–58, 1993
4. American Diabetes Association: Standards of medical care for patients with diabetes mellitus (Position Statement). *Diabetes Care* 23 (Suppl. 1):S32–42, 2000
5. Fletcher GF, Balady G, Blair SN, Blumenthal J, Caspersen C, Chaitman B, Epstein S, Sivarajan Froelicher ES, Froelicher VF, Pina IL, Pollock ML: Benefits and recommendations for physical activity programs for all Americans (Statement on Exercise). *Circulation* 94:857–62, 1996
6. Thompson PD, Funk EJ, Carleton RA, Sturner WQ: Incidence of death during jogging in Rhode Island from 1975 through 1980. *JAMA* 247:2535–38, 1982
7. Siscovick DS, Weiss NS, Fletcher RH, Lasky T: The incidence of primary cardiac arrest during vigorous exercise. *N Engl J Med* 311:874–77, 1984
8. Kohl HW, Gordon NF, Powell KE, Blair SN, Paffenbarger RS: Physical activity, physical fitness and sudden cardiac death. *Epidemiol Rev* 14:37–58, 1992
9. Thompson PD, Klocke FJ, Levine BD, Van Camp SP: Task force 5: coronary artery disease. *Med Sci Sports Exerc* 26:S271–75, 1994

10. American College of Sports Medicine: The recommended quantity and quality of exercise for developing and maintaining cardiorespiratory and muscular fitness and flexibility in healthy adults (Position Stand). *Med Sci Sports Exerc* 30:975–91, 1998
11. Gordon NF, Kohl HW, Blair SN: Lifestyle exercise: a new strategy to promote physical activity for adults. *J Cardiopulm Rehab* 13:161–63, 1993
12. American College of Sports Medicine: Physical activity, physical fitness, and hypertension (Position Stand). *Med Sci Sports Exerc* 25:i–x, 1993
13. Helmrich SP, Ragland DR, Leung RW, Paffenbarger RS: Physical activity and reduced occurrence of non-insulin-dependent diabetes mellitus. *N Engl J Med* 325:147–52, 1991
14. Blair SN, Kohl HW III, Paffenbarger RS Jr, Clark DG, Cooper KH, Gibbons LW: Physical fitness and all-cause mortality: a prospective study of healthy men and women. *JAMA* 262:2395–401, 1989
15. Duncan JJ, Gordon NF, Scott CB: Women walking for health and fitness: how much is enough? *JAMA* 266:3295–99, 1991
16. Fletcher GF, Balady G, Froelicher VF, Hartley LH, Haskell WL, Pollock ML: A statement for health professionals from the American Heart Association Exercise Standards. *Circulation* 91:580–612, 1995
17. American Association of Cardiovascular and Pulmonary Rehabilitation: *Guidelines for Cardiac Rehabilitation and Secondary Prevention Programs.* Champaign, IL, Human Kinetics, 1999
18. Miller WJ, Sherman WM, Ivy JL: Effect of strength training on glucose tolerance and post-glucose insulin response. *Med Sci Sports Exerc* 16:539–43, 1984
19. Durak EP, Jovanovic-Peterson L, Peterson CM: Randomized crossover study of effect of resistance training on glycemic control, muscular strength, and cholesterol in type I diabetic men. *Diabetes Care* 13:1039–43, 1990
20. Vranic M, Wasserman D: Exercise, fitness, and diabetes. In *Exercise, Fitness, and Health.* Bouchard C, Shephard RJ, Stephens T, Sutton J, McPherson B, Eds. Champaign, IL, Human Kinetics, 1990, p. 467–90
21. De Busk RF, Stenestrand U, Sheehan M, Haskell WL: Training effects of long versus short bouts of exercise in healthy subjects. *Am J Cardiol* 65:1010–13, 1990

22. De Busk RF, Haskell WL: Do multiple short bouts of exercise really produce the same benefits as single long bouts? (Letter) *Am J Cardiol* 67:326, 1991
23. Campaigne BN, Lampman RM: *Exercise in the Clinical Management of Diabetes.* Champaign, IL, Human Kinetics, 1994
24. Haskell WL: Cardiovascular complications during exercise training of cardiac patients. *Circulation* 57:920–24, 1978

Neil F. Gordon, MD, PhD, MPH, is from the Center for Heart Disease Prevention, Savannah, GA.

15

Initiation and Maintenance of Exercise in Patients With Diabetes

DAVID G. MARRERO, PHD

Highlights

- It is important that the health care provider give specific recommendations concerning types of exercise and its frequency, intensity, and duration. Moreover, this prescription should account for the patient's personal health status and situation.
- An effective exercise program should include activities that result in expending a minimum cumulative total of 1,000 kcal/week in aerobic activity. To improve muscular strength and endurance as well as body composition, a well-rounded resistance training program should also be incorporated.
- To develop and maintain cardiorespiratory endurance as well as desirable caloric expenditure, individuals with diabetes should exercise at least 3 nonconsecutive days and up to 5 days each week.
- The duration of physical activity for individuals with diabetes is directly related to the caloric expenditure

needs and inversely related to the intensity. For patients who have not exercised before, each session should last 10–15 min. It is recommended that physical activity be increased to at least 30 min per session to achieve the recommended energy expenditure.

- To account for the necessary energy expenditure, 30 min of activity can be divided into three 10-min sessions in a single day. When weight loss is a primary goal, intensity needs to be low to moderate and duration needs to be incrementally increased to ~60 min.
- There are potential risks associated with exercise for the person with diabetes and some limitations for those who have preexisting diabetic complications. These include hypoglycemic reactions resulting from exercise and the risk of exacerbating specific diabetic complications and provoking musculoskeletal injuries.
- To help motivate the person to do regular exercise, the program must be viewed as desirable and intrinsically reinforcing. The activities recommended must be perceived as realistic and feasible. Strategies for avoiding the potential negative consequences of exercise, particularly those associated with diabetes, must be taught.
- The reasonableness of an activity selected by the patient should be determined by reviewing the Ease of Access and Ease of Performance indexes. These are self-assessments of how realistic the activity is for a patient given his or her lifestyle and health status.
- There are several factors that can help individuals with diabetes maintain an exercise program. These include using appropriate training and equipment to avoid injury, progressing slowly in exercise intensity and duration, setting realistic training goals, learning to identify and treat hypoglycemia, setting a training schedule in advance and sticking to it, using a training

partner, encouraging self-rewards, identifying alternative exercise activities to reduce boredom, and understanding the difference between failure and backsliding.

"*Exercise in the days before insulin we regarded as useful, but by no means did we appreciate it as vital in the care of diabetes. . . . We should return to it to help us in the treatment of all of our cases. . . .*" (Joslin et al., *Treatment of Diabetes Mellitus*, 1959)

Over 40 years of research has proven Joslin's observation prophetic: regular exercise has many benefits for individuals with type 1 or type 2 diabetes. Exercise has been shown to help individuals with diabetes reduce their need for insulin and/or oral hypoglycemic agents, lose weight, improve glycemic control, and reduce the risk for cardiovascular disease and other diabetic complications. In spite of these benefits, however, many patients with diabetes do not incorporate regular exercise as an integral part of their therapy. Moreover, even when exercise is prescribed, poor adherence to exercise programs is frequently observed.[1,2]

There are several reasons why exercise is not optimally used in diabetes treatment. Health care providers often are unsure what constitutes an appropriate exercise regimen for their patients with diabetes. Their uncertainty is heightened by the possibility of acute diabetes-related problems associated with exercise, such as hypoglycemia, and the potential for some forms of exercise to exacerbate existing complications. Equally problematic, many individuals with diabetes, notably those with type 2, are simply not inclined to implement an exercise regimen. The high rates of obesity and histories of low levels of physical activity often observed in this patient population contribute to this tendency.

In spite of these problems, exercise can effectively be incorporated into the therapy plan. Indeed, health care professionals are in a unique and influential position to motivate their nonactive patients to begin and maintain an effective and safe long-term exercise program. In this chapter, several suggestions are offered on how best to accomplish this goal, with emphasis on factors that should be addressed to maximize patient motivation and willingness to maintain a long-term exercise program.

Recommended Physical Activity Program for People With Type 2 Diabetes

To initially get an inactive person to exercise, it is important that the health care provider give specific recommendations for a program in terms of the types of exercise and its frequency, intensity, and duration. Moreover, this prescription should account for the patient's personal health status and situation. As a referent point, individuals with diabetes who have no significant complications or limitations should combine physical activities designed to build and maintain cardiorespiratory fitness and muscular strength and endurance. In this context, it is recommended that an effective program should include activities that result in expending a minimum cumulative total of 1,000 kcal/week in aerobic activity.[3–5] To improve muscular strength and endurance as well as body composition, a well-rounded resistance training program should also be incorporated. For both modes of exercise, it is essential that the appropriate frequency, intensity, and duration of each physical activity be selected.

Frequency

To develop and maintain cardiorespiratory endurance as well as desirable caloric expenditure, individuals with diabetes should exercise at least 3 nonconsecutive days and up to 5 days each week.[5] Recently, the U.S. Surgeon General[6] recommended that physical activity should be performed most, if not all, days of the week to produce favorable health-related benefits such as weight loss, blood pressure reduction, and favorable lipid and lipoprotein changes. Because the acute effect of a single exercise session on blood glucose levels lasts <72 h,[7,8] it is important that individuals with diabetes engage in regular physical activity to lower blood glucose. Individuals taking insulin may find it easier to balance caloric needs with insulin dosage by engaging in daily physical activity. Moreover, obese individuals may need to engage in daily physical activity to maximize caloric expenditure for effective weight management.[5]

Intensity

For most individuals with diabetes, particularly type 2, low to moderate–intensity physical activity is recommended to achieve cardiorespiratory and metabolic improvements. Low to moderate intensity is defined as 40–65% of the individual's maximum oxygen uptake (VO_{2max}). This is sufficient to both lower blood glucose and increase insulin sensitivity. There is also evidence that favorable metabolic changes also occur with higher-intensity exercise (e.g., 70–90% of VO_{2max}).[9–12] It is important to note that low-intensity exercise may not meet the recommended minimum threshold of exercise intensity (i.e., ≥50% of VO_{2max}) for improving cardiorespiratory endurance.[5] However, this limitation should be balanced against the reduced risk of acute stress associated with physical activity for this population. Specifically, lower-intensity activity affords a more comfortable level of exertion and enhances the likelihood of adherence while lessening the likelihood of musculoskeletal injury and foot trauma, particularly when weight-bearing activity is recommended.[12]

To ensure safety, it is important to monitor the intensity level of physical activity in individuals with diabetes. This may require the use of heart rate monitors. Although a percentage of heart rate reserve (50–85%) or maximal heart rate (60–90%) is commonly used to identify exercise intensity for nondiabetic individuals, those with type 2 diabetes may develop autonomic neuropathy, which affects the heart rate response to exercise. Consequently, using heart rate as the only means to monitor intensity may be unsuitable for some with type 2 diabetes. A more appropriate adjunct to gauge the intensity of physical activity may be to use a rating of perceived exertion (RPE)[4,5] (see Chapter 27).

Duration

The duration of physical activity for individuals with diabetes is directly related to the caloric expenditure needs and inversely related to the intensity. For patients who have not exercised before, each session should last 10–15 min.[4,5] It is recommended that physical activity be increased to at least 30 min per session to achieve the recommended energy expenditure.[4] However, 30 min of activity can be divided into three 10-min sessions in a single day to account for the necessary energy expenditure. When weight loss is a primary goal, the intensity needs to be low to moderate (50% VO_{2max}), and the duration needs to be incrementally increased to ~60 min.[13,14]

Increasing the Level of Exercise Over Time

The pace at which a person with diabetes increases his or her rate of physical activity depends on age, functional ability, health status, and, most importantly, goals and motivation.[4,5,15] As a rule, initial increases should focus on the frequency and duration of physical activity rather than intensity. This helps to maintain an activity level that can be performed without undue discomfort, thereby increasing the likelihood that the activity will be repeated and sustained.[5,13,15,16] Initially, it is recommended that individuals with diabetes engage in physical activity at a comfortable level (RPE of 10–12) for about 10–15 min at a very low intensity at least three times per week but preferably five times per week.[14,17,18] Duration should be gradually increased to accommodate the person's functional capacity and clinical status. Given that older age and obesity are common elements of type 2 diabetes, a longer period of time may be necessary for the older and/or obese person to achieve a desired level of physical activity.[14,17] After the desired duration of activity is achieved, any increase in intensity should be small and approached with caution to minimize the risk of undue fatigue, musculoskeletal injuries, and/or relapse.

Risks and Complications of Exercise

There are potential risks associated with exercise for the person with diabetes and some limitations for those who have preexisting diabetic complications.[19,20] These include hypoglycemic reactions resulting from exercise and the risk of exacerbating specific diabetic complications and provoking musculoskeletal injuries. The issues surrounding these concerns are discussed in detail elsewhere in this book (see Chapters 1 and 2). In any case, before commencing exercise, all individuals with diabetes, particularly those with type 2, should have a physical examination to ensure that a safe and effective individualized activity program is developed. Emphasis should be placed on assessing if macro- and/or microvascular complications are present. For those with type 2 diabetes ≥35 years of age, it is recommended that a stress test be conducted to assess cardiovascular and respiratory systems.[15] Moreover, the stress test electrocardiography will identify target heart rate limits within which the person with or without autonomic neuropathy can safely exercise. Additionally, physical exertion may induce a recognizable hypertensive response in some with diabetes.[21] Exercise-induced hypertension can be identified during a stress test and avert abnormal blood pressure excursions during normal physical activity by identifying appropriate physical activities (e.g., intensity or selection of activity) (see Chapters 13 and 14).

Increasing Motivation to Exercise

In spite of the benefits of exercise for diabetes health status, little is known about factors likely to affect exercise adoption and maintenance. Two theoretical models are useful for understanding these factors: the transtheoretical model (i.e., "stages of change" theory)[22] and self-efficacy theory.[23] The transtheoretical model postulates that individuals are at different cognitive stages with regard to their readiness to adopt and maintain a particular behavior such as exercise, ranging from precontemplation and contemplation to preparation, action, and maintenance. The implication of this stage-based model is that interventions designed to encourage adoption of an exercise regimen must be responsive to the current stage of readiness in which the individual is and focus effort on moving the individual through the stages.

The self-efficacy theory postulates that adoption of exercise is a function of a person's judgment concerning his or her ability to do exercise in relation to the probable benefits and costs associated with the activity.[24,25] In this context, research has demonstrated that individuals with previous exercise experience and, particularly, previous success have substantially higher exercise efficacy expectations.[26–29] In addition, physical status may be of equal importance to developing exercise efficacy expectations among older adults, who are more likely to have type 2 diabetes and also suffer from more physical limitations generally associated with age.[26]

Outcome expectations are viewed as an important element of models of health behavior and may contribute significantly to a person's motivation to adopt a particular behavior. A person's confidence that he or she will adopt a behavior is influenced in part by the extent to which that person believes rewards are associated with that behavior.[23] Thus, outcome expectations will have important implications for the form of information and education delivered by health care providers.[27–29] This is supported by research that found having a physician discuss physical activity was a strong predictor of exercise adoption among African-American women.[30]

Factors Influencing the Contemplation Stage

Several factors should be addressed to help motivate the person in the contemplation stage to initiate an exercise program.[31] First, the program must be viewed by the person as desirable and intrinsically reinforcing. Second, the activities recommended must be perceived as realistic and feasible. Third, strategies for avoiding the potential negative consequences of exercise, particularly those associated with diabetes, must be taught.

The failure of individuals with diabetes to engage in regular exercise is due, in part, to their outcome expectations. Many are not familiar with the benefits of exercise on their diabetes. Even when the benefits are known, health care professionals often describe exercise to their patients using a negative reinforcement paradigm, i.e., exercise is done to avoid the onset of punishment in the form of complications, not as an intrinsically enjoyable activity with health benefits. Often, attempts at exercise have resulted in physical discomfort, injury, or hypoglycemia, thus demonstrating that the costs outweigh the potential long-term benefits.

To help increase a better outcome expectation, the rationale for the prescription of exercise should include discussion of its social, psychological, and general health benefits in all people and in individuals with diabetes in particular. Social benefits include participation of family members and friends and involvement in organized, community-based activities. Psychological benefits include reduction in stress, anxiety, and depression and increased feelings of well-being. Health benefits include the factors discussed above: improvements in glucose regulation, weight control, lipid profiles, hypertension, and increased work capacity.

To help address efficacy expectations, several key points should be emphasized:

- To benefit diabetes control, exercise needs to be part of a lifelong management program that starts gradually and works up to a higher intensity.

- To sustain an exercise program, select one that reflects the individual's goals, desires, and availability of appropriate support.
- Teach the patient how to perform the activity so that discomfort, injury, and problems with diabetes are avoided.
- Assure patients that they don't have to figure out how to set up an exercise program alone. There are several health care professionals who can help them accomplish these goals.

Factors Influencing the Action Stage

An important component to increasing exercise adoption is providing patients with specific exercise prescriptions. Frequently, the recommendation to exercise is a generic prescription with no specific instructions about what to do or how to do it. As a result, most individuals with diabetes do not have a clear idea about what type of exercise will work best for their particular situation. Moreover, they are not given much guidance concerning how to adjust their diabetes regimen to exercise safely. As a result, they often choose activities without any reflection as to their suitability or safety. Discussing patients' answers to two simple questions can help them to more critically consider factors that can contribute to or inhibit their selection of an exercise method they are likely to enjoy. These questions are as follows:

What are your personal goals for exercise? Finding out the patient's goal for exercising helps identify a method that will help him or her achieve those goals. Their goals may not reflect what the clinician feels is most important but may result in achieving the same end point.

What types of physical activity do you like or think you would like to do? This question is designed to help guide patients in selecting an activity they are motivated to do. If they do not have preferences, ask them to indicate their preference between the following options: *1*) long or short duration, *2*) high versus low intensity, *3*) exercising by themselves or with others, *4*) exercising at home or at a facility, *5*) exercising indoors versus outdoors, and *6*) a competitive or cooperative sport.

Their responses to these types of preference trade-offs will help them to consider more critically what is truly reinforcing to them. It will also help the health care provider in supplying suggestions as to the suitability of a given activity and how patients may best adapt their diabetes regimen to its demands.

It is equally important to counsel patients as to what types of exercise will have the optimum impact on their diabetes. In general, for individuals with type 2 diabetes, physical activities that afford greater control of intensity, have little interindividual variability in energy expenditure, are easily maintained, and require little skill are recommended.[4,5,9] Combined with personal interests and goals, the mode of physical activity is an important aid in motivating the person with diabetes to begin physical activity and to sustain a life-long physical activity habit. The mode of physical activity dictates that the level of energy expended and/or improvement in cardiorespiratory endurance be directly influenced by the amount of muscle mass used over the time of activity, as well as the rhythmic and aerobic nature of the activity. For those with type 2 diabetes, it is important to identify a mode of physical activity that can safely and effectively maximize caloric expenditure. Walking is the most commonly performed exercise for those with type 2 diabetes and is the most convenient low-impact mode of physical activity. However, because of complications or coexisting conditions such as peripheral neuropathy or degenerative arthritis, those with type 2 diabetes may require alternative modes of physical activity that are non–weight-bearing (e.g., stationary cycling, swimming, or aquatic activities) or may alternate between weight-bearing and non–weight-bearing activities.[4,5]

It is also useful to discuss resistance training with the patient because it has the potential to improve muscular strength and endurance, enhance flexibility, improve body composition, and decrease risk factors for cardiovascular disease.[32–37] Data on the use of resistance training in individuals with type 2 diabetes are limited,[34,36] but available results appear to be consistent with the findings in nondiabetic subjects: improvements in glucose tolerance and insulin sensitivity,[38,39] prevention of muscle mass loss,[40–42] and reduction in intra-abdominal obesity.[42]

It is recommended that, whenever possible, resistance training of at least 2 days per week be included as part of a well-rounded exercise program for individuals with type 2 diabetes (see Chapter 16). A minimum of eight to ten exercises involving the major muscle groups should be performed with a minimum of one set of 10–15 repetitions to near fatigue. Increased intensity of exercise, additional sets, or combinations of volume and intensity may produce greater benefits and may be appropriate for certain individuals. All individuals with type 2 diabetes should be carefully screened before beginning this type of training and should receive proper supervision and monitoring. Caution should be used in cases of advanced retinal and cardiovascular complications (see Chapter 23). Modifications such as lowering the intensity of lifting, preventing exercise to the point of exhaustion, and eliminating the amount of sustained gripping or isometric contractions should be considered in these patients. More detailed information for developing a resistance exercise training plan for people with diabetes is available elsewhere in this book (see Chapter 16).

Determining Whether a Specific Activity Is Right for the Patient: the Ease of Access and Ease of Performance Indexes

Once the patient has narrowed down the possibilities, or even selected a specific exercise method, the reasonableness of the activity given his or her personal situation should be considered by reviewing the Ease of Access and Ease of Performance indexes. These are self-assessments of how realistic the activity is given the patient's lifestyle.[31]

Ease of Access Index

The Ease of Access index addresses the question "how easily can I engage in my activity of choice where I live?" Many people have a tendency to begin an exercise program only to find that participation on a regular basis is simply too difficult for a variety of reasons that were either ignored, rationalized, or simply not considered before the program was begun. To determine their Ease of Access index for a given activity, ask patients to consider the following questions:

- ***Does the activity require special facilities, and are these facilities available?***
- ***Does it require special equipment, and is this equipment available and affordable?***
- ***Does it require special training or instruction, and is this instruction readily available, at convenient times, easy to get to, and affordable?***
- ***Does it involve others, and will you always be able to find partners when you want or need to play?***
- ***Is it seasonal, and what will you do other times of the year?***

Ease of Performance Index

If the exercise activity of interest has an acceptable Ease of Access index, encourage evaluation in terms of ease of performance. The Ease of Performance index has the patient consider the question, "how suitable is a specific purpose of activity given my physical attributes and lifestyle?" By its nature, this type of assessment is more difficult and requires that the patients be honest with themselves. It also requires greater input from the health care professional. To determine the Ease of Performance index, have patients consider the following questions:

- ***Does the activity suit your physical attributes?*** Patients are most likely to stick to an activity or sport for which they are physically suited and maximize the probability of having positive experiences.
- ***Do you have physical limitations?*** Before diabetic patients begin any exercise, they need to be aware of physical limitations that may affect their ability to engage in the activity. These include poor physical conditioning and preexisting chronic conditions. As noted above, it is a good idea that all individuals with diabetes undergo a medical examination to determine whether they have any musculoskeletal/orthopedic problems that rule out or limit various exercise activities. Similarly, any existing comorbidities should be identified and considered in the exercise prescription. There are excellent reviews of exercising with diabetic complications (see Chapters 22–27),[3,17,20] so an extensive discussion is not offered here. Table 15.1 provides a brief overview of risks, recommendations, and precautions that are associated with three of the more common complications of diabetes: neuropathy, reti-nopathy, and nephropathy. In addition to the physical examination, a graded exercise test before beginning an exercise program is also recommended. The exercise test is not only intended to identify contraindications to exercise; equally important, by establishing work capacity limits, it can greatly facilitate the exercise prescription.
- ***Can you realistically integrate the activity into your lifestyle?*** This is a critical issue to address. For many, the greatest barrier to beginning an exercise program is finding the time to do it.

TABLE 15.1. Exercising With Diabetic Complications: Risks, Recommendations, and Precautions

			Neuropathy	
	Retinopathy	Nephropathy	Autonomic	Peripheral
Risks	■ Elevations in blood pressure ■ Possible retina detachment from jarring of head	■ Marked changes in hemodynamics ■ Marked elevations in blood pressure ■ Presence of retinopathy likely	■ Hypoglycemia ■ Abnormal blood pressure response ■ Abnormal heart rate response ■ Impaired sympathetic/parasympathetic nerves ■ Abnormal thermoregulation (prone to dehydration)	■ Superficial pain ■ Impaired balance/reflexes ■ Numbness/weakness in hands ■ Decreased proprioception ■ Weakness/atrophy of thigh muscles (when severe)
Recommendations	■ Use heart rate and RPE based on blood pressure response (which should not exceed 170 mmHg systolic; >200 increases damage to retina) ■ Use low-impact activities ■ Use submaximal exercise testing ■ If possible, monitor blood pressure during exercise ■ Consider stationary cycling, walking, swimming, and low-intensity rowing	■ Include dynamic, weight-bearing, low-impact activity ■ Use submaximal isometric or light weight lifting when blood pressure is controlled and left ventricular functioning is normal ■ Develop specific programs for hemodialysis patients	■ Use submaximal exercise testing ■ Use RPE to gauge exercise intensity ■ Use water activities, stationary cycling, or both	■ Use RPE to monitor exercise intensity ■ Use non–weight-bearing activities ■ Use activities to improve balance

(*continued*)

TABLE 15.1. (*Continued*)

	Retinopathy	Nephropathy	Neuropathy	
			Autonomic	Peripheral
Precautions	■ Avoid Valsalva maneuvers ■ Avoid heavy weight lifting, breath-holding stretches, high-intensity exercise, and strenuous upper arm exercise ■ Exercise is contraindicated if recent photo-occulation treatment or surgery has occurred	■ Avoid lifting heavy weight, intense aerobic activities, and Valsalva maneuvers ■ Use cushioned shoes (gel/air) ■ Maintain hydration	■ Avoid high-intensity activity ■ Avoid rapid changes in body position ■ Avoid extremes of temperature	■ Examine feet frequently ■ Use proper footwear ■ Perform gentle, pain-free stretching

All too often, the good intention of going to the gym every day is derailed by competing demands. Therefore, when selecting a method of exercise, it is useful to have the patient consider, "will this fit into my existing schedule or will I have to make special adjustments?" It is useful to point out to patients that they are more likely to maintain a program that smoothly meshes with their basic routine.

- ***Can you afford it?*** Many forms of exercise activity require a small, possibly one-time investment. Others require a bigger fee, and others require ongoing fees. This last category has surprised many when they begin to add up the cost of exercise when reviewing their home budget.
- ***Do you have a good support network?*** Any activity is easier to engage in if the patient has the support and encouragement of family and friends. In this regard, patients are more likely to maintain a program if they can involve others in whatever way best suits their needs.

How the above questions are discussed can be facilitated by having patients fill out a brief activity profile to help them think about these issues. The health care provider can review their answers and discuss with them their options. An example of an activity profile is included in Fig. 15.1.

1. My typical day includes:

   ___ hours of sleep
   ___ hours of low activity (driving, reading, watching television, etc.)
   ___ hours of moderate activity (walking, gardening, housework, etc.)
   ___ hours of vigorous activity (aerobic exercise, heavy labor, competitive sports)

2. The physical activities I enjoy most are:

3. The physical activities I would like to learn are:

4. I see the following as obstacles to exercising (check all that apply):

___Time	___Fear of hypoglycemia	___Skills/coordination
___Age	___Boredom	___Energy
___Money	___Family support	___Lack of facilities
___Arthritis	___Pain during or after exercise	

FIGURE 15.1 Activity profile.

Factors Influencing the Maintenance Stage

There are several factors that can help individuals with diabetes to maintain an exercise program. These include the following:

- ***Use appropriate training and equipment to avoid injury.*** The quickest way for patients to destroy motivation to exercise is to injure themselves early in their program. The smart athlete reduces or avoids downtime by training to avoid injuries (see Chapter 28). This involves proper stretching and warming up before exercise. It also means using proper equipment, especially footwear. Also, encourage patients to seek out lessons from a qualified instructor if they are not sure how to properly perform an exercise.
- ***Progress slowly in exercise intensity and duration.*** The new exerciser needs to be cautioned to avoid the temptation of doing too much too fast. This will help to avoid stopping the program because of soreness or injury.
- ***Set realistic training goals.*** Patients are more likely to keep up their motivation to exercise if they set specific goals for themselves and work to accomplish them. It is important that the goals they select are precisely defined and realistically attainable. It is also important that the goals be defined by exercise behavior (e.g., walking for 30 min three times per week) rather than defined by an outcome of exercise behavior (e.g., losing 20 lb). Many individuals will have a tendency to set a big goal, e.g., "I want to walk for an hour every day." They then attempt this for 2 months only to discover that they have only walked 35 min four times per week. This less-than-desired outcome is not likely to reinforce exercising, resulting in poor motivation to continue. Moreover, we tend to be our own worst critics, focusing on what we did not rather than what we did achieve. A more realistic approach is to set a series of smaller, stepwise goals for which patients can observe success and progress.
- ***Learn to identify and treat hypoglycemia.*** It is important that individuals with diabetes treated with insulin and some oral agents (e.g., sulfonylureas) (see Chapter 20) understand that the increased utilization of glucose during exercise can

result in hypoglycemia both during the activity and for several hours after its completion. A serious exercise-induced hypoglycemic episode can have a devastating effect on motivation to exercise. Patients need to be instructed to always carry some form of a quick carbohydrate during exercise sessions to treat hypoglycemia. This will help them reduce the number of times exercise results in a punishing experience.

- ***Set a training schedule in advance and stick to it.*** Long-term habits are developed through practice. Moreover, a regular schedule makes diabetes regimen adjustments easier to establish, thereby improving glycemic control.
- ***Use a training partner.*** A training partner can help encourage and motivate an individual to maintain a training schedule. In addition, the partner may be of assistance in the event of a hypoglycemic episode.
- ***Encourage self-rewards.*** An effective strategy is to suggest to patients that they select rewards that they give to themselves when achieving a specific goal. For example, a patient might decide to purchase athletic equipment or clothing when a certain number of consecutive workouts have been reached. Such a reward also helps to perpetuate the goal of maintaining regular physical activity. Patients may want to increase the size of the reward as they reach successive goals. This helps create a more positive reinforcement paradigm that can aid in increasing motivation to stay with the exercise program.
- ***Identify alternative exercise activities to reduce boredom.*** Individuals who become bored with a single activity should be encouraged to select alternative activities that will help them remain active. The goal is to do some form of physical activity.
- ***Understand the difference between failure and backsliding.*** For some individuals, any deviation from a schedule or not meeting expectations is viewed as failure. It is important to help such individuals understand and accept off-days as part of any long-term exercise program. When off-days do occur, the concept of a backslide (i.e., a temporary state) should be reinforced, and a return to the regular schedule should be encouraged.

In summary, helping patients with diabetes incorporate exercise into their daily routine is a significant challenge. This chapter provides some guidelines that hopefully will help health care providers in this process. Finally, it is important to remember that it is the norm rather than the exception to experience periodic frustration with lack of success in adopting and maintaining an effective exercise program. When this occurs, it is important to team up with the patient by asking how the problem(s) may best be resolved. Not only will this help patients get back on track, it will enhance the doctor-patient relationship in general.

References

1. Herman WH: Leisure-time physical activity patterns in the U.S. diabetic population. *Diabetes Care* 18:27–33, 1995
2. McNabb WL, Quinn MT, Rosing L: Weight loss programs for inner-city black women with non-insulin-dependent diabetes mellitus: PATHWAYS. *J Am Diet Assoc* 93:75–77, 1993
3. American Diabetes Association: Diabetes mellitus and exercise (Position Statement). *Diabetes Care* 22 (Suppl. 1):S49–53, 1999
4. Fletcher GF, Blair SN, Blumenthal J, Caspersen C, Chaitman B, Epstein S: Statement on exercise: benefits and recommendations for physical activity programs for all Americans. *Circulation* 86: 340–44, 1992
5. American College of Sports Medicine: *Guidelines to Exercise Testing and Exercise Prescription.* 5th ed. Philadelphia, Williams & Wilkins, 1995
6. U.S. Department of Health and Human Services: *Physical Activity and Health: a Report of the Surgeon General.* Atlanta, GA, U.S. Department of Health and Human Services, Centers for Disease Control and Prevention, National Center for Chronic Disease Prevention and Health Promotion, 1996
7. Schneider SH, Amorosa LF, Khachadurian AK, Ruderman NB: Studies on the mechanism of improved glucose control during regular exercise in type 2 (non-insulin-dependent) diabetes. *Diabetologia* 26:355–60, 1984
8. Schneider SH: Long-term exercise programs. In *The Health Professional's Guide to Diabetes and Exercise.* Ruderman N, Devlin JT, Eds. Alexandria, VA, American Diabetes Association, 1995, p. 123–32

9. Vranic M, Wasserman D: Exercise, fitness, and diabetes. In *Exercise, Fitness, and Health.* Bouchard C, Shephard RJ, Stephens T, Sutton J, MacPherson B, Eds. Champaign, IL, Human Kinetics, 1990, p. 467–90
10. Bogardus C, Ravussin E, Robbins DC, Wolfe RR, Horton ES, Sims EAH: Effects of physical training and diet therapy on carbohydrate metabolism in patients with glucose intolerance and non-insulin-dependent diabetes mellitus. *Diabetes* 33: 311–18, 1984
11. Krotkiewski M, Lonnroth P, Mandroukas K, Wroblewski Z, Rebuffe-Scrive M, Holm G, Smith U, Bjorntorp P: The effects of physical training on insulin secretion and effectiveness and on glucose metabolism in obesity and type 2 (non-insulin-dependent) diabetes mellitus. *Diabetologia* 28:881–90, 1985
12. American Diabetes Association: Diabetes mellitus and exercise (Position Statement). *Diabetes Care* 14 (Suppl. 1): S51–55, 2001
13. Wing RR: Exercise and weight control. In *The Health Professional's Guide to Diabetes and Exercise.* Ruderman N, Devlin JT, Eds. Alexandria, VA, American Diabetes Association, 1995, p. 109–14
14. Wing RR, Epstein LH, Paternostro-Bayles M, Kriska A, Norwalk MP, Gooding W: Exercise in a behavioural weight control programme for obese patients with type 2 (non-insulin-dependent) diabetes. *Diabetologia* 31:902–09, 1988
15. Albright AL: *Exercise Management for Persons With Chronic Diseases and Disabilities.* Champaign, IL, Human Kinetics, 1997, p. 94–98
16. Gordon N: The exercise prescription. In *The Health Professional's Guide to Diabetes and Exercise.* Ruderman N, Devlin JT, Eds. Alexandria, VA, American Diabetes Association, 1995, p. 69–82
17. Zierath A Jr, Wallberg-Henricksson H: Exercise training in obese diabetic patients: special considerations. *Sports Med* 14: 171–89, 1992
18. Wallberg-Henricksson H: Exercise and diabetes mellitus. In *Exercise and Sport Science Reviews.* Vol. 22. Holloszy JO, Ed. Philadelphia, Williams and Wilkins, 1992, p. 339–68
19. American Diabetes Association: *Medical Management of Type 2 Diabetes.* 4th ed. Alexandria, VA, American Diabetes Association, 1998

20. American Diabetes Association: *The Health Professional's Guide to Diabetes and Exercise.* Ruderman N, Devlin JT, Eds. Alexandria, VA, American Diabetes Association, 1995
21. Blake GA, Levin SR, Koyal SN: Exercise induced hypertension in normotensive patients with NIDDM. *Diabetes Care* 13:799–801, 1990
22. Prohaska TR, Glasser M: Older adult health behavior change in response to symptom experiences. *Advances Med Soc* 4:141–61, 1994
23. Ajzen I, Fishbein M: *Understanding Attitudes and Predicting Social Behavior.* Englewood Cliffs, NJ, Prentice-Hall, 1980
24. Bandura A: Self-efficacy mechanism in psychobiologic functioning. In *Self-Efficacy: Thought Control and Action.* Schwarzer R, Ed. Washington, DC, Hemisphere Publishing, 1992
25. Strecher VJ, McEvoy B, Becker MH, Rosenstock IM: The role of self-efficacy in achieving health behavior change. *Health Educ Q* 13:73–91, 1986
26. Clark DO, Patrick DL, Grembowski D, Durham M: Socioeconomic status and exercise self-efficacy in late life. *J Behav Med* 18:355–76, 1995
27. McAuley E, Lox C, Duncan TE: Long-term maintenance of exercise, self-efficacy, and physiological change in older adults. *J Gerontol* 48:218–24, 1993
28. McAuley E: Self-efficacy and the maintenance of exercise participation in older adults. *J Behav Med* 16:103–12, 1993
29. Strecher VJ, Seijts GH, Kok GJ, Latham GP, Glasgow R, DeVellis B, Meertens RM, Bulger DW: Goal setting as a strategy for health behavior change. *Health Educ Q* 22:190–200, 1995
30. Macera CA, Croft JB, Brown DR, Ferguson JE, Lane MJ: Predictors of adopting leisure-time physical activity among a biracial community cohort. *Am J Epidemiol* 142:629–35, 1995
31. Marrero DG, Sizemore JM: Motivating patients with diabetes to exercise. In *Practical Psychology for Diabetes Physicians: How to Deal With Key Behavioral Issues Faced by Health Care Teams.* Anderson BJ, Rubin RR, Eds. Alexandria, VA, American Diabetes Association, 1996, p. 73–81
32. Stone MH, Fleck SJ, Triplett NT, Kraemer WJ: Health- and performance-related potential of resistance training. *Sports Med* 11:210–31, 1991

33. Soukup JT, Kovaleski JE: A review of the effects of resistance training for individuals with diabetes mellitus. *Diabetes Educ* 19:307–12, 1993
34. Smutok MA, Kokkinos PF, Farmer C, Dawson P, Shulman R, DeVane-Bell J, Patterson J, Charabogos C, Goldberg AP, Hurley BF: Aerobic versus strength training for risk factor intervention in middle-aged men at high risk for coronary heart disease. *Metabolism* 42:177–84, 1993
35. Eriksson JS, Taimela K, Eriksson S, Parvianen J, Peltonen J, Kujala U: Resistance training in the treatment of non-insulin-dependent diabetes mellitus. *Int J Sports Med* 18:242–46, 1997
36. Hurley BF, Seals DR, Ehsani AA, Carter LJ, Dalsky GP, Hagberg JM, Holloszy JO: Effects of high-intensity strength training on cardiovascular function. *Med Sci Sports Exerc* 16:483–88, 1984
37. Miller WJ, Sherman WM, Ivy JL: Effect of strength training on glucose tolerance and post-glucose insulin response. *Med Sci Sports Exerc* 16:539–43, 1984
38. Ryan AS, Pratley RE, Goldberg AP, Elahi D: Resistive training increases insulin action in postmenopausal women. *J Gerontol A Biol Sci Med Sci* 51:M199–205, 1996
39. Ballor DL, Harvey-Berino JR, Ades PA, Cryan J, Calles-Escandon J: Contrasting effects of resistance and aerobic training on body composition and metabolism after diet-induced weight loss. *Metabolism* 45:179–83, 1996
40. Bryner RW, Ullrich IH, Sauers J, Donley D, Hornsby G, Kolar M, Yeater R: Effects of resistance vs. aerobic training with an 800 calorie liquid diet on lean body mass and resting metabolic rate. *J Am Col Nutr* 18:115–21, 1999
41. Geliebter A, Maher MM, Gerace L, Gutin B, Heymsfield SB, Hashim SA: Effects of strength or aerobic training on body composition, resting metabolic rate, and peak oxygen composition in obese dieting subjects. *Am J Clin Nutr* 66:557–63, 1997
42. Treuth MS, Hunter GR, Kekes-Szabo T, Weinsier RL, Goran MI, Berland L: Reduction in intra-abdominal adipose tissue after strength training in older women. *J Appl Physiol* 78:1425–31, 1995

David G. Marrero, PhD, is from the Indiana University School of Medicine, Indianapolis, IN.

16

Resistance Training

W. GUYTON HORNSBY, JR., PhD, CDE,
AND ROBERT D. CHETLIN, MS, CSCS

Highlights

- Properly designed resistance training programs may provide important benefits for patients with diabetes.
- Patients should be carefully screened before beginning resistance training and should receive proper supervision and monitoring.
- Intense resistive exercise often produces an acute hyperglycemic effect. Patients on insulin or oral hypoglycemic agents may develop hypoglycemia in the hours after resistance training.
- Proper technique should be taught for all of the exercises used in the program. Patients should be instructed to perform lifting movements through a full range of motion while breathing freely and rhythmically.
- Exercise prescriptions for resistance training must be developed on an individual basis after consideration of

the patient's goals and limitations, as well as selection of the appropriate modality, choice of exercise, and the intensity, volume, and frequency of training.

Resistance training refers to forms of exercise that use muscular strength to move a weight or work against a resistive load. Resistance training may provide substantial benefits to patients with diabetes. As with any form of exercise, benefits must outweigh risks. Resistance training has previously been regarded as unsafe for many patients with cardiovascular disease or for those with microvascular or neurological complications. With thorough pre-exercise screening, proper supervision and monitoring, and appropriate attention to modifications of the training regimen, resistance training may allow many patients to safely improve muscular strength and endurance, enhance flexibility, improve insulin sensitivity and glucose tolerance, enhance body composition, and decrease risk factors for cardiovascular disease.[1–4]

Cardiovascular and Metabolic Effects

Chronic resistance training has been associated with a number of favorable metabolic and cardiovascular effects in nondiabetic study groups. Improvements in oral glucose tolerance and insulin sensitivity, similar to those produced by aerobic training, have been reported after resistance training.[5] Miller et al.[6] demonstrated lower fasting plasma insulin after resistance training that was correlated with increased lean body mass. Ullrich et al.[7] found that resistance training improved plasma lipids and enhanced cardiovascular function. Furthermore, favorable reductions in intra-abdominal obesity have been associated with moderately intense resistance training.[8]

Circuit-type resistance training has increased insulin sensitivity in subjects with impaired glucose tolerance.[9] Improvements in glycemic control have been reported in subjects with type 1 diabetes when resistance training is combined with aerobic exercise[10] and when resistance training is used exclusively.[11] Several recent studies demonstrated beneficial effects of resistance training in subjects with type 2 diabetes, including improvements in HbA_{1c}, insulin sensitivity, and lipoprotein profiles. These studies used either moderate-intensity, high-volume training[12] or circuit-type resistance training.[13–15] The American College of Sports Medicine recommends that resistance training be included in the exercise prescription for patients with type 2 diabetes whenever possible.[16]

Little is known about the acute effects of resistance exercise in diabetes. An informal survey of members of the Diabetes Exercise and Sports Association suggests that resistance exercise is often associated with hyperglycemia during and shortly after acute training sessions. This anecdotal evidence is consistent with findings of hyperglycemic responses to intense (>80% VO_{2max}) aerobic exercise in subjects with type 1[17] and type 2 diabetes.[18] Glucoregulation with intense exercise has been reviewed by Marliss et al.[19] Short-term increases in blood glucose with resistance exercise are frequently followed by hypoglycemia, which may appear many hours after the exercise has ended. This postexercise hypoglycemia is likely due to restoration of muscle glycogen.[20]

Acute resistance exercise has been associated with extreme elevations in both systolic and diastolic blood pressure in healthy subjects performing high-intensity exhaustive exercise.[21] Increased arterial pressure and heart rate increase the work of the heart and myocardial requirements for oxygen. Holding your breath during maximal tension exercise may cause reductions in venous return and can lead to inadequate blood flow to the heart and brain. Increases in blood pressure are most pronounced during Valsalva maneuvers with sustained isometric contractions. There is a fear that inappropriate hemodynamic responses may place an excessive burden on patients with diabetes. Caution should be observed in patients with advanced retinal and cardiovascular complications (see Chapters 23 and 24).

Safety

The safety of resistance training has been well documented in geriatric patients[22] (see Chapter 32) as well as in patients with cardiac disease[23] and diabetes.[11] Attention to modifications in training, such as lowering the intensity of lifting, eliminating exercising to the point of exhaustion, and limiting the amount of sustained gripping or isometric contractions, may be useful in reducing exercise-induced blood pressure elevations. Patients should be instructed to perform lifting movements while breathing freely and rhythmically, without holding their breath. Exhalation should occur during the lifting phase of the movement, and inhalation should be done while lowering the weight. If patients are unable to perform this breathing pattern, telling them to "breathe regularly and do not hold your breath" is usually adequate to help them avoid the Valsalva maneuver.

Whereas intense resistance exercises are expected to produce a short-term hyperglycemic effect, it is important to instruct patients that responses can vary. Hypoglycemic responses after resistance exercise have been reported[11] and should always be considered a possible consequence. Any patient on insulin or an oral hypoglycemic agent should be advised to monitor blood glucose before, during, and after exercise and should be instructed to take appropriate action in response to undesirable glycemic effects.

To reduce the risk of injury, proper technique should be learned for each exercise. Whenever possible, exercises should be done through a full range of motion. Adequate warm-up and cooldown periods should always be performed. A 5- to 10-min general warm-up period consisting of light aerobic activity and stretching should be done before resistance training. If moderate or intense lifting is to be performed, this should be preceded by low-resistance movements. Light aerobic activity and stretching should be done for 5–10 min in the cooldown period.

All patients should have a thorough medical examination before beginning a resistive training program to detect the presence of macrovascular, microvascular, or neurological complications, as well as to determine any orthopedic limitations. The evaluation should include a symptom-limited graded exercise test with electrocardiographic and blood pressure monitoring for all patients with known or suspected coronary artery disease and all people who have had type 1 diabetes >15 years, who have type 1 diabetes and are >30 years of age, or who have type 2 diabetes and are >35 years of age. Heart rate, blood pressure, and rating of perceived exertion should be determined during lifting movements.

Types of Resistance Training

Modalities for resistance training include calisthenic activities using body weight for resistance; various types of springs, rubber bands, or elastic tubing; free weights, such as barbells or dumbbells; and weight machines that provide resistance by pulleys, chains, hydraulic cylinders, or electromagnets. The resistance that is applied may be described as *1*) constant, if the load remains the same throughout the exercise, or *2*) variable, if the resistance is altered during the exercise by special pulleys or cams. Muscular contractions are classified as *1*) isometric or static, with force being applied without movement; *2*) isotonic or dynamic, with force being applied to produce movement; or *3*) isokinetic, with variable force being applied to move a resistance at a constant speed.

The Resistive Exercise Prescription

Once patients have been properly screened, various techniques can be used to establish initial resistance training loads. One of the safest methods is to begin with the lightest weight that can be set for each exercise and monitor patient responses for six to ten repetitions. Heart rate and blood pressure should be within individual limits established by exercise testing, and the rating of perceived exertion should be no greater than 13 (somewhat hard). If the patient tolerates this weight well, he or she can increase repetitions to 10–15 and then 15–20 every 1–2 weeks. After patients are comfortable with the movements and have demonstrated good technique, the number of sets can be increased to two to three, and heavier weight can be added. Typically, 2–5 lb for upper-body exercises and 5–10 lb for lower-body exercises will be appropriate.

Alternatively, the maximal weight lifted in one full range of motion (the one repetition maximum [1 RM]) or the maximal weight that can be lifted for 10 (10 RM) or 15 (15 RM) repetitions can be determined, and initial training loads can be set as percentages of these values. Generally, resistive loads are classified as light (40–60% 1 RM), moderate (60–80% 1 RM), or heavy (80–100% 1 RM). Although 1 RM testing is the standard for determining initial loads in most research studies, the previously described technique of starting with the lightest weight is more practical in clinical settings. This method puts less initial stress on patients, allows for better patient orientation, and may allow for a more accurate exercise prescription.

Circuit-type training may be a good option for patients who should be limited to light resistive loads. This type of program involves alternating between upper- and lower-body exercises with short rest periods (<30 s) between sets. Loads are typically prescribed at 40–60% of 1 RM, and 10–15 repetitions are performed in one or more circuits of 8–12 different exercises. This type of training has been found to be effective in improving insulin sensitivity in subjects with impaired glucose tolerance[9] and improving glycemic control in patients with type 2 diabetes.[14,15] Although improvements in maximal oxygen consumption have not been demonstrated with circuit-type training in patients with type 2 diabetes, improvements of 4–8% have been reported in healthy men and women training for periods of 8–20 weeks.[24] The extent to which a program of circuit-type resistance exercise can improve cardiorespiratory fitness is likely due to the duration and/or volume of training.

The volume of resistance training depends on the number of complete movements or repetitions that are performed for a given exercise. Repetitions are typically performed in groups or sets, depending on the intensity of training and the goals of the program. Rest between sets should be adequate to allow successful completion of the next set. For low-intensity training, rest periods are as brief as 15 s to 1 min. Moderate-intensity training usually requires 1–2 min of rest, and high-intensity exercise may require 2–5 min for adequate recovery.

Exercises should be selected for each major muscle group including *1*) the hip and legs (gluteal, quadriceps, and hamstring group), *2*) the chest (pectoral group), *3*) the shoulders (deltoid and trapezius groups), *4*) the back (latissimus dorsi, rhomboid, and teres and erector spinae groups), *5*) the arms (biceps, triceps, and wrist flexor and extensor groups), and *6*) the abdominal muscle groups. For each muscle group, at least 48 h recovery should be allowed between training sessions. Two resistance training sessions per week appear to be the minimum number required to produce positive physiological effects. Concepts involved in prescribing resistance training have been described by Fleck and Kraemer.[25,26]

The National Strength and Conditioning Association

The National Strength and Conditioning Association certifies exercise professionals who demonstrate fundamental competencies to plan and supervise resistance training programs. This organization may be helpful in providing physicians and health care professionals with a list of Certified Strength and Conditioning Specialists who can work with the health care team to instruct patients on proper exercise technique and training and can be reached at the following: National Strength and Conditioning Association, 1955 N. Union Blvd., Colorado Springs, CO 80909. Tel: 800-815-6826.

References

1. Poehlman ET, Gardner AW, Ades PA, Katzman-Rooks SM, Montgomery SM, Atlas OK, Ballor DL, Tyzbir RS: Resting metabolism and cardiovascular disease risk in resistance-trained and aerobically trained males. *Metabolism* 41:1351–60, 1992
2. Smutok MA, Reece C, Kokkinos PF, Farmer CM, Dawson P, Shulman R, DeVane-Bell J, Patterson J, Charabogos C, Goldberg AP, Hurley BF: Aerobic versus strength training for risk factor intervention in middle-aged men at high risk for coronary heart disease. *Metabolism* 42:177–84, 1993
3. Soukup JT, Kovaleski JE: A review of the effects of resistance training for individuals with diabetes mellitus. *Diabetes Educ* 19:307–12, 1993
4. Stone MH, Fleck SJ, Triplett NT, Kraemer WJ: Health- and performance-related potential of resistance training. *Sports Med* 11:210–31, 1991
5. Hurley BF, Seals DR, Ehsani AA, Carter L-J, Dalsky GP, Hagberg JM, Holloszy JO: Effects of high-intensity strength training on cardiovascular function. *Med Sci Sports Exerc* 16:483–88, 1984
6. Miller WJ, Sherman WM, Ivy JL: Effect of strength training on glucose tolerance and post-glucose insulin response. *Med Sci Sports Exerc* 16:539–43, 1984
7. Ullrich IH, Reid CM, Yeater RA: Increased HDL-cholesterol levels with a weight lifting program. *Southern Med J* 80:328–31, 1987
8. Treuth MS, Hunter GR, Kekes-Szabo T: Reduction in intra-abdominal adipose tissue after strength training in older women. *J Appl Physiol* 78:1425–31, 1995
9. Eriksson J, Tuominen J, Valle T, Sundberg S, Sovijarvi A, Lindholm H, Tuomilehto J, Koivisto V: Aerobic endurance exercise or circuit-type resistance training for individuals with impaired glucose tolerance? *Horm Metab Res* 30:37–41, 1998
10. Peterson CM, Jones RL, DuPuis A, Levine BS, Bernstein R, O'Shea ML: Feasibility of improved blood glucose control in patients with insulin-dependent diabetes mellitus. *Diabetes Care* 2:329–35, 1979

11. Durak EP, Jovanovic-Peterson L, Peterson CM: Randomized crossover study of effect of resistance training on glycemic control, muscular strength, and cholesterol in type I diabetic men. *Diabetes Care* 13:1039–43, 1990
12. Ishii T, Yamakita T, Sato T, Tanaka S, Fujii S: Resistance training improves insulin sensitivity in NIDDM subjects without altering maximal oxygen uptake. *Diabetes Care* 21:1353–55, 1998
13. Dunstan DW, Puddey IB, Beilin LJ, Burke V, Morton AR, Stanton KG: Effects of short-term circuit weight training program on glycaemic control in NIDDM. *Diabetes Res Clin Pract* 40: 53–61, 1998
14. Eriksson J, Taimela S, Eriksson K, Parviainen S, Peltonen J, Kujala U: Resistance training in the treatment of non-insulin-dependent diabetes mellitus. *Int J Sports Med* 18:242–46, 1997
15. Honkola A, Forsen T, Eriksson J: Resistance training improves the metabolic profile in individuals with type 2 diabetes. *Acta Diabetol* 34:245–48, 1997
16. Albright A, Franz M, Hornsby G, Kriska A, Marrero D, Ullrich I, Verity L: ACSM position stand on exercise and type 2 diabetes. *Med Sci Sports Exerc* 32:1345–60, 2000
17. Mitchell TH, Abraham G, Schiffrin A, Leiter LA, Marliss EB: Hyperglycemia following intense exercise in insulin-dependent diabetic subjects during continuous subcutaneous insulin infusion. *Diabetes Care* 11:311–17, 1988
18. Kjaer M, Hollenbeck CB, Frey-Hewitt B, Galbo H, Haskell W, Reaven GM: Glucoregulation and hormonal responses to maximal exercise in non-insulin-dependent diabetes. *J Appl Physiol* 68:2067–74, 1990
19. Marliss EB, Purdon C, Miles PDG, Halter JB, Sigal RJ, Vranic M: Glucoregulation during and after intense exercise in control and diabetic subjects. In *Diabetes Mellitus and Exercise.* Devlin JT, Horton ES, Vranic M, Eds. London, Smith-Gordon, 1992, p. 173–90
20. Ivy JL: Resynthesis of muscle glycogen after exercise. In *Diabetes Mellitus and Exercise.* Devlin JT, Horton ES, Vranic M, Eds. London, Smith-Gordon, 1992, p. 153–64
21. MacDougall JD, Tuxen D, Sale DG, Moroz JR, Sutton JR: Arterial blood pressure response to heavy resistance exercise. *J Appl Physiol* 58:785–90, 1985

22. Fiatarone MA, Marks EC, Ryan ND, Meredith CN, Lipsitz LA, Evans WJ: High-intensity strength training in nonagenarians. *JAMA* 263:3029–34, 1990
23. Ghilarducci LE, Holly RG, Amsterdam EA: Effects of high resistance training in coronary artery disease. *Am J Cardiol* 64:866–70, 1989
24. Fleck S, Kraemer W: Resistance training systems. In *Designing Resistance Training Programs.* 2nd ed. Champaign, IL, Human Kinetics, 1997, p. 121
25. Fleck SJ, Kraemer WJ: Resistance training: basic principles (part 1 of 4). *Physician and Sportsmedicine* 16 (no. 3):160–71, 1988
26. Fleck SJ, Kraemer WJ: Resistance training: exercise prescription (part 4 of 4). *Physician and Sportsmedicine* 16 (no. 6):69–81, 1988

Suggested Reading

Baechle TR, Earle RW, Eds: *Essentials of Strength Training and Conditioning.* 2nd ed. Champaign, IL, Human Kinetics, 2000

W. Guyton Hornsby, Jr., PhD, CDE, and Robert D. Chetlin, MS, CSCS, are from the West Virginia University School of Medicine, Morgantown, WV.

17

Nutrition, Physical Activity, and Diabetes

MARION J. FRANZ, MS, RD, CDE

Highlights

- In individuals with diabetes, many factors influence the glycemic response to physical activities, making it impossible to give precise nutrition (and insulin) guidelines that will apply to everyone with diabetes. Furthermore, few studies have been done examining the need for carbohydrate, fluids, and calories for exercise in individuals with diabetes. Therefore, recommendations are usually extrapolated from studies on exercisers without diabetes. To meet individual needs, frequent blood glucose monitoring is important to modify general guidelines to ingest carbohydrate after (or before) exercise and to reduce insulin doses before (and/or after) exercise.
- Carbohydrate intake before, during, and after exercise can be important for the exerciser with diabetes.
- A higher carbohydrate intake (~60% of daily calories) on a fairly consistent basis during training with

adequate blood glucose control is necessary to maintain maximal muscle and liver glycogen stores.

- Eating a meal containing carbohydrate 3–4 h before activities or consuming a carbohydrate feeding within the hour before exercise can improve performance. During moderate-intensity exercise, glucose uptake is increased by 8–13 g/h, and this is the basis for the recommendation to add 15 g carbohydrate for every 30–60 min of activity (depending on the intensity) over and above the normal routine. Blood glucose levels at the time of exercise and the time of day that exercise is performed will determine if carbohydrate is needed or not needed and if the carbohydrate should be eaten before or after exercise.

- During exercise, blood glucose levels decline gradually. Ingesting a carbohydrate feeding during prolonged exercise can improve performance by maintaining the availability and oxidation of blood glucose. For the exerciser with diabetes whose blood glucose levels may drop sooner and lower, ingesting carbohydrate after 40–60 min of exercise is important and may also assist in preventing hypoglycemia. Drinks containing ≤8% carbohydrate empty from the stomach as quickly as water and have the advantage of providing both needed fluids and carbohydrate.

- Consuming carbohydrate immediately after exercise optimizes repletion of muscle and liver glycogen stores. This takes on added importance for the exerciser with diabetes, who is also at increased risk for late-onset hypoglycemia.

- Fluids are important for all exercisers. For the first 60–90 min, water is the preferred beverage, after which fluids containing ≤8% carbohydrate are recommended. For the exerciser with diabetes, fluids with carbohydrate should be ingested after ~40–60 min. This can also help prevent hypoglycemia.

- An adequate caloric intake should be planned for the person with diabetes who participates in regular exercise. A nutrition assessment of usual food intake followed by monitoring of weight, growth (if pertinent), and appetite (hunger) is the best way to judge adequacy of caloric intake.

Adequate and appropriate nutrition is important for any person engaging in physical activity or fitness programs. For the person with diabetes, however, it takes on added importance. Not only can adequate nutrition help with physical performance, but nutrition also plays a pivotal role in the regulation of blood glucose levels before, during, and after physical activities.

In individuals with diabetes, factors that influence the glycemic response to physical activities, and therefore nutrition recommendations for exercise, include timing, intensity, duration, and type of activity; the individual's fitness level and nutritional state (glycogen stores); and relation to prior food intake and the macronutrient content of that food. Other considerations include the type of diabetes, state of metabolic control, blood glucose values at the start of exercise, and the type and timing of insulin injections or oral medications.

Despite the increase in glucose uptake by muscles during moderate-intensity exercise, glucose levels change little in individuals without diabetes. Hepatic glycogenolysis and gluconeogenesis closely match the increase in glucose uptake. Muscular work causes a fall in plasma insulin and a rise in counterregulatory hormones—glucagon being the primary counterregulatory hormone at the start of exercise.[1,2] This balance is the major determinant of hepatic glucose production, underscoring the need for insulin adjustments in addition to adequate carbohydrate intake during training for people with diabetes.

Acute responses to exercise that affect nutritional intake include both hypoglycemia and hyperglycemia. Hypoglycemia is reported to be most common after exercise, especially after exercise of long duration, after strenuous activity or play, or after sporadic exercise.[3] Thus, depending on the time of day exercise is performed, adding carbohydrate (and reducing insulin doses) may be more important after exercise than before. However, hypoglycemia can occur during exercise as well. The blood glucose level before exercise only reflects the value at that time, and it is unknown if this is a stable blood glucose level or a blood glucose level that is dropping. If blood glucose levels are dropping before exercise, adding exercise can contribute to hypoglycemia.[4] Furthermore, hypoglycemia on the day before exercise is reported to increase the risk of hypoglycemia on the day of exercise.[5] After ~90 min of exercise, the increase in endogenous glucose production may be absent as a result of hypoglycemia the day prior. This is due to a reduced neuroendocrine response in both insulin and counterregulatory hormones.

Hyperglycemia can also result from exercise. This may occur because an individual is exercising at what for him or her is a high intensity, causing a greater than normal increase in counterregulatory hormones. As a result, hepatic glucose release exceeds the rise in glucose utilization. The elevated glucose levels may also extend into the postexercise state.[6,7] Hyperglycemia can also result from insulin deficiency, which causes a decreased ability of cells to take up glucose and an increase in hepatic glucose production.[8] The latter cause is not as likely to occur as the first.

All of the above contribute to the difficulty in giving precise nutrition (and insulin) guidelines that will apply to everyone with diabetes. Frequent glucose monitoring before, during, and after exercise helps individuals identify their response to physical activities. To meet their individual needs, they must modify general guidelines to ingest carbohydrate after (or before) exercise and to reduce insulin doses before (and/or after) exercise.

Fatigue that causes anyone (with or without diabetes) to stop exercising can result from deficiencies of oxygen, fluid, or fuel. These shortages can occur separately or in combination. The ability to take in and process an adequate supply of oxygen is related to physical training, whereas fluid and fuel status and use are primarily related to nutrition. Dehydration leads progressively to fatigue, heat cramps, heat exhaustion, and heat stroke. However, for exercise to continue, muscles must also have a source of fuel. Although all athletes will eventually need fuel replacements to continue exercising, individuals with diabetes may need replenishment of fuel, especially carbohydrates, sooner than other athletes.[9] Fluid and carbohydrate ingestion are immediate concerns related to physical activities; however, adequate calories must also be ingested to meet the energy requirements of the exerciser.

Few studies examining the need for carbohydrate, fluids, and calories for exercise have been done on individuals with diabetes. Therefore, recommendations are usually extrapolated from studies done on exercisers without diabetes. However, it has been suggested that exercisers with diabetes use glucose and lipid fuel sources differently than nondiabetic individuals during moderate, but not intense, exercise. In individuals with type 1 diabetes, glucose uptake into muscles was reported to be less and fat oxidation greater during moderate-intensity exercise.[10] Until more studies are reported on subjects with diabetes, we are left with general nutrition guidelines to enable patients with diabetes to exercise safely and to the best of their ability.

Carbohydrate

An adequate carbohydrate intake on a fairly consistent basis is necessary to maintain maximal muscle and liver glycogen stores in all endurance athletes.[11] Chronic low intake of carbohydrate leads to a progressive depletion of glycogen stores. If liver and muscle glycogen is not replenished on a daily basis, chronic fatigue results.

For the athlete with diabetes, blood glucose control is also essential. Therefore, coordination of insulin doses with carbohydrate intake is essential to ensure both glucose control and desirable muscle and liver glycogen stores.

Carbohydrate for Daily Training

For individuals without diabetes who train ≤1 h per day, carbohydrate intake of 5–6 g/kg body wt/day is needed on a regular basis to replenish muscle glycogen stores. For most individuals, this means the carbohydrate content will be ~60% of the daily calories. For individuals training ≥2 h/day, 8 g carbohydrate/kg body wt/day may be needed.[11] Because average intake is generally 4–5 g of carbohydrate/kg body wt/day (~45% of calories), increasing carbohydrate requires effort and concentration on the part of the exerciser. Although research has not been conducted in exercisers with diabetes, there is no apparent reason why individuals with diabetes in good metabolic control would be different.

Carbohydrate Feedings Before Exercise

On days of athletic events, meals eaten 3 or 4 h before activity or carbohydrate feedings 1–4 h before activity have been shown to improve performance.[12,13] For a morning event, athletes can eat 1 h before exercise. This can enhance performance compared with exercising in a fasting state. Exercising or competing in the early morning after an overnight fast may cause liver and muscle glycogen to be low at the start of exercise and may contribute to fatigue and poor performance. For events later in the day, a small meal may be eaten 3–4 h before the event. The meal should contain mostly carbohydrate and some protein but a minimal amount of fat. The menu could include pasta or potatoes, bread, fruit, skim milk, and lean meat (fish or poultry without skin). Three to four cups of fluid should be included with the meal.

For the athlete with diabetes, additional carbohydrate may be needed ~20 min before an event. Nathan et al.[14] reported that a simple snack of 15 g carbohydrate, 15–30 min before or after exercise of short duration (<45 min), can prevent postexercise hypoglycemia. Furthermore, sugars (simple) or starches (complex carbohydrates) work equally well.[15] Carbohydrate foods (such as crackers, muffins, yogurt, or soups), rather than sugary sweets, are good choices. Other nutritious snacks include crackers, fig bars, oatmeal-raisin cookies, dried fruit, bread sticks, and granola bars. Fruit juices and fruits such as apples, peaches, plums, and pears not only have natural sugars, vitamins, and minerals, but also are 85% water.[16]

Guidelines for increasing carbohydrate intake and decreasing insulin doses should be based on blood glucose levels before and after exercise, how close to scheduled meals and snacks exercise will occur, and how often the person exercises. The more regular the exercise, the more the body adapts. As a result, not as much extra carbohydrate is required. If exercise is done on a regular basis, the snacks should be part of the usual meal plan, and usual insulin doses can be adjusted. Self-monitoring of blood glucose can provide valuable information to document and maximize the benefits of nutrition. This will give the athlete with diabetes the information needed to modify food choices and portions and to adjust insulin for best results for both performance and blood glucose control.

Several studies[17,18] have reported that people with type 1 diabetes tend to overeat rather than undereat with exercise, possibly because of concern and an overcautious approach to preventing hypoglycemia or because of a belief that exercise will alleviate the high blood glucose levels caused by overeating.

Moderate-intensity exercise (50–60% VO_{2max}) is reported to increase muscle glucose uptake and utilization by 2–3 mg/kg body wt/min above usual daily requirements.[4] When exercising, a 70-kg person would need an added 140–210 mg glucose for every minute of moderate-intensity exercise or an added 8.4–12.6 g for every hour. During very high-intensity exercise (80–100% VO_{2max}), glucose uptake may increase by 5–6 mg/kg body wt/min above usual needs. As a result, 350–420 mg glucose is used every minute. Despite this increased rate of glucose use for very high-intensity exercise, the demand on glucose stores and the risk of hypoglycemia is less because exercise of this intensity cannot be sustained for long intervals.[4] This increase in glucose uptake is the basis for the recommendation to add one carbohydrate choice (15 g) for every 30–60 min of activity (depending on the intensity) over and above normal routine.

Therefore, it may be prudent for exercisers with diabetes to eat a carbohydrate snack before or after a short period (~1 h) of moderate-intensity exercise; 15 g carbohydrate (60 kcal) may be enough to prevent hypoglycemia while not adding excessive calories. The time of day that exercise is performed will also determine if carbohydrate is or is not needed and if the carbohydrate should be ingested before or after exercise. For example, Soo et al.[15] reported that 45 min of moderate-intensity exercise before the morning insulin injection resulted in a small or absent fall in plasma glucose, and, therefore, the exerciser with type 1 diabetes should consider reducing or omitting carbohydrate after monitoring the response to early-morning exercise. After completion of the exercise session, the morning insulin dose can be given and the usual breakfast eaten. On the other hand, exercise in the late afternoon may require 15–30 g carbohydrate before exercise to prevent hypoglycemia. For exercise at this time of day, it may not be as easy to adjust insulin doses and it has usually been several hours since food was eaten. For exercise during the evening or after dinner, if needed, the extra carbohydrate should be added to the bedtime snack to prevent overnight hypoglycemia.

Reduction in the dose of insulin before exercise (and possibly after) may also be required. Several guidelines are available for decreasing insulin. A 30–50% reduction of the short-acting insulin has been reported to decrease the risk of hypoglycemia.[19] Another method is to decrease the insulin acting during the time of exercise by 10% of the total daily insulin dose.[16]

Carbohydrate loading is a technique used to increase glycogen stores by athletes doing events of long duration.[20] Individuals with diabetes who carbohydrate-load must monitor blood glucose levels carefully and adjust insulin doses appropriately, both to preserve glucose control and to accomplish the goals of the carbohydrate-loading process.

Carbohydrate Intake During Exercise

All exercisers, with or without diabetes, need carbohydrate during events that last longer than 60–90 min. The rate of glucose use by contracting muscles peaks at 90–180 min, after which it declines in parallel with a gradual fall in blood glucose levels.[21] Ingesting carbohydrate during prolonged moderate- to high-intensity exercise can improve performance by maintaining the availability and oxidation of blood glucose late in exercise,[22,23] but it does not conserve glycogen stores.[24]

Exercisers without diabetes given a carbohydrate feeding of 1 g/kg at 20 min and 0.25 g/kg every 20 min thereafter maintained their blood glucose levels better and exercised longer than exercisers receiving no carbohydrate.[25] For the exerciser with diabetes, whose blood glucose levels may drop sooner, faster, and to lower levels, carbohydrate feedings during exercise take on added importance. In general, during events of long duration, a minimum of 30–60 g carbohydrate should be consumed every hour, preferably distributed at 15- to 30-min intervals. Along with carbohydrate feedings, appropriate adjustments in insulin doses are needed. This allows hepatic glycogenolysis to proceed, thus decreasing the risk of hypoglycemia and lessening the need for supplemental food to manage exercise.

Solid or liquid forms of carbohydrate work equally well.[26] Each form has its advantages: liquids provide fluid for hydration, whereas solids may prevent hunger. For exercise lasting longer than 60–90 min, a liquid carbohydrate has the advantage of also providing fluids.[27] Rapid gastric emptying allows fluids into the plasma and glucose into cells as quickly as possible. Gastric emptying is affected by temperature, volume, osmolarity, and sugar content of the solution. As volume increases, so does the rate of gastric emptying. The higher the sugar content, the slower the rate of emptying. Fluids consumed should be cooled, if possible, to increase gastric emptying, although the effect of temperature on gastric emptying is less than the volume and sugar content effect.[28]

Solutions containing ≤8% carbohydrate empty from the stomach as quickly as plain water. Drinks with a concentration of carbohydrate or sugars >10% can cause osmotic problems and lead to gastrointestinal upset, such as cramps, nausea, diarrhea, or bloating.[29] Fruit juice and most regular soft drinks contain about 12% carbohydrate and need to be diluted with an equal amount of water (½ cup juice, ½ cup water = 15 g carbohydrate). For the exerciser with diabetes, diluted fruit juice or fluid replacement beverages can provide both needed fluids and a source of carbohydrate (Table 17.1).

Carbohydrate Intake After Exercise

Carbohydrate intake before and during events increases performance ability, but of equal importance is carbohydrate ingestion after exercise. Carbohydrate should be consumed as soon as possible after exercise of long duration to replenish glycogen stores. To optimize repletion of muscle glycogen after exhaustive exercise, 1.5 g carbohydrate/kg body wt should be consumed within 30 min after exercise, and a second 1.5 g carbohydrate/kg body wt should be consumed 1–2 h later.[30] This is a time when high-carbohydrate bars or feedings may be most useful. In individuals without diabetes, when muscle glycogen is depleted, a carbohydrate-rich diet will restore glycogen to its pre-exercise levels within 24 h.[31]

For the athlete with diabetes, replacing carbohydrate after exercise is important to prevent late-onset hypoglycemia. Monitoring blood glucose levels at 1- to 2-h intervals allows individuals to assess their response to exercise and to make necessary adjustments in insulin and food intake.

Fluids

Exercisers without diabetes should not forget the importance of ingesting fluids. During exercise, water should be consumed on a set

TABLE 17.1 Nutritive Analysis of Sports Drinks

	Portion	Carbohydrate (g)	Carbohydrate Concentration (%)	Sodium (mg)	Potassium (mg)	Calories
Sports drinks						
AllSport (PepsiCo, Inc.)	8 fl oz	20	8	55–80	50	70
CeraSport (Cera Products, LLC)	8 fl oz	16	7	102	37	76
Cytomax (CytoSport, Inc.)	8 fl oz	15	6	70	77	80
Gatorade Thirst Quencher (The Gatorade Company)	8 fl oz	14	6	110	30	50
Met-Rx ORS (Met-Rx, Inc.)	8 fl oz	19	8	125	40	75
Metabolol Endurance (Champion Nutrition)	8 fl oz	16	7	140	200	133
Powerade (The Coca-Cola Company)	8 fl oz	19	8	53	33	72
PowerBar Perform (PowerBar, Inc.)	8 fl oz	16	7	110	35	60
Pro-Hydrator (InterNutria, Inc.)	8 fl oz	0	0	2.5	4.5	0
Revenge (Champion Nutrition)	8 fl oz	10	4	48	80	50
Ultima (Ultima Replenisher)	8 fl oz	4	2	8	16	16
Non-sports drinks						
Coca-Cola (The Coca-Cola Company)	8 fl oz	27	11	35	0	100
Mountain Dew (PepsiCo, Inc.)	8 fl oz	31	13	50	0	110
Orange Juice	8 fl oz	27	11	7	446	112

schedule. Because the thirst mechanism is blunted with exercise, it is essential for athletes and trainers to monitor and meet fluid needs. Athletes should note weight changes from fluid losses during exercise and drink 2 cups of water for every pound lost.

For exercise sessions of up to ~60–90 min (for exercisers with diabetes, 40–60 min), plain water is usually the best replacement beverage. For exercise lasting longer, water and extra carbohydrate may be needed. Fruit juices (diluted with water) and fluid replacement beverages are good sources of fluids and carbohydrate.

After competition or training, athletes should continue to drink water periodically until weight has been regained. Lost fluids need to be fully replaced at the time the fluid deficit occurs. If rehydration is delayed, the body's altered fluid compartments may not be restored until well into the next day.

Energy Needs

People participating in regular physical activity programs usually have higher energy needs than sedentary individuals. Total daily caloric requirements for individuals engaged in physical training programs vary and may range from 2,000 kcal (e.g., for a gymnast) to ≥6,000 kcal (e.g., for a football player or body builder).[32] The lower caloric density of the recommended high-carbohydrate/low-fat diet often makes it difficult to provide sufficient food to meet high-energy requirements. High-carbohydrate food choices in a pattern of more frequent eating, with planned snacks, are often necessary. Nutritional beverages (liquid meal supplements) or energy bars may be helpful for the athlete wanting to gain weight or maintain a high weight because they provide a high-carbohydrate snack in a ready-to-consume concentrated form (Table 17.2).

Men may require up to 50 kcal/kg body wt or more during periods of regular heavy physical activity. This is in contrast to 40 kcal/kg body wt for more moderate physical activity and 30 kcal/kg body wt for very light physical activity. Women may require 44 kcal/kg body wt for regular heavy physical activity compared with 37 kcal/kg body wt for more moderate activity and 30 kcal/kg body wt for very light physical activity.[33] However, there is considerable person-to-person variation in caloric needs. In general, these values, along with the in-

TABLE 17.2 Nutritive Analysis of Sport, Energy, Breakfast, and Candy Bars

	Serving Size	Carbohydrate [g (% kcal)]	Protein (g)	Fat [g (% kcal)]	Calories	Other Ingredients
Sport and energy bars						
Balance Bar (chocolate-banana)	1.76 oz	22 (44)	14	6 (27)	200	25 vit/min
Clif Bar (peanut butter)	2.4 oz	45 (72)	10	4 (14)	250	15 vit/min
Clif Luna (chocolate pecan pie)	1.69 oz	24 (53)	10	5 (25)	180	22 vit/min, soy protein
CHOICEdm (fudge brownie)	1.23 oz	19 (54)	6	4.5 (13)	140	23 vit/min, resistant starch
Extreme Ripped Force (triple shot mocha)	1.6 oz	33 (78)	3	3 (17)	160	Caffeine, ma huang, quercetin
Met-Rx Bar (fudge brownie)	3.53 oz	48 (60)	27	2.5 (7)	320	26 vit/min, L-glutamine
Met-Rx Source One Food (chocolate-peanut)	2.2 oz	30 (63)	15	3 (14)	190	26 vit/min, sugar alcohol
PowerBar (chocolate)	2.25 oz	42 (75)	10	10 (8)	225	20 vit/min
PowerBar Essential (chocolate)	1.87 oz	28 (62)	10	4 (20)	180	21 vit/min
PowerBar Harvest (chocolate)	2.3 oz	45 (75)	7	4 (15)	240	19 vit/min
PowerBar Protein Plus (chocolate fudge)	3.0 oz	15 (21)	32	8 (25)	290	21 vit/min
PR Bar Ironman	2.0 oz	24 (2)	17	7 (27)	230	Yes*
ProGram 16 (peanut butter)	2.3 oz	34 (54)	16	5 (18)	250	5 vit/min
Slim-Fast Meal On-the-Go	1.97 oz	36 (65)	8	5 (20)	220	22 vit/min

Tiger Protein Bar (chocolate)	1.2 oz	18 (50)	7	5 (31)	145	16 vit/min
Tiger Sport Bar (mocha)	2.3 oz	43 (75)	10	2 (8)	230	19 vit/min
Tiger Milk Bar (milk chocolate)	1.2 oz	24 (74)	4	2.5 (17)	130	5 vit/min
TwinLab Ironman (chocolate)	2.0 oz	25 (43)	16	7 (27)	230	21 vit/min
Breakfast and candy bars						
Hershey's Milk Chocolate Bar	1.55 oz	25 (43)	3	13 (51)	230	No†
Kellogg's Nutri-Grain Cereal Bar (blueberry)	1.3 oz	27 (77)	2	3 (19)	140	12 vit/min
Nature Valley Granola Bar (peanut butter)	1.5 oz	29 (64)	5	6 (30)	180	No
Milky Way Bar	2.05 oz	41 (61)	2	10 (33)	270	No
Snickers Bar	2.07 oz	280 (50)	4	14 (45)	280	No
Liquid meal supplements						
Boost (Mead Johnson)	8 fl oz	41 (68)	10	4 (9)	240	Yes
CHOICEdm (Mead Johnson)	8 fl oz	25 (40)	15	12 (43)	250	Yes
Ensure (Ross Labs)	8 fl oz	34 (54)	9	9 (32)	250	Yes
Resource Diabetic (Sandoz Nutrition)	8 fl oz	23 (37)	15	11 (40)	250	Yes
Sustacal (Mead Johnson)	8 fl oz	33 (55)	9	9 (33)	240	Yes

*Yes indicates that the product contains added vitamins/minerals or added multivitamin/minerals; †No indicates that the product does not contain added vitamins/minerals. vit/min, vitamins/minerals.

TABLE 17.3 Approximate Calorie Requirements for Different Activity Levels

Activity Level	Men (kcal/kg body wt)	Women (kcal/kg body wt)
Heavy	50	44
Moderate	40	37
Light	30	30

dividual's weight, growth (if pertinent), and hunger, can be used to evaluate adequacy of caloric intake (Tables 17.3 and 17.4).

Without sufficient energy intake, both fat stores and body proteins are used to fuel daily activities. As a consequence, circulating levels of protein by-products increase as lean tissue is degraded, and water and electrolytes are lost in the excretion of these by-products. Because active people do not want to lose muscle mass, matching individual intake with energy expenditure is critical.

For exercisers with diabetes, the best way to determine caloric needs is to begin with a detailed nutrition history. Compare current intake with estimated caloric needs and develop a meal plan based on the nutrition assessment. Weight and appetite should be monitored and used to evaluate caloric adequacy.

TABLE 17.4 Examples of Estimated Daily Nutrient Needs for Typical Athletes

Weight	Calories	Carbohydrate	Protein
70-kg man	50 kcal/kg 3,500 kcal	8 g/kg 560 g (64%)	1.2 g/kg 84 g (10%)
		6 g/kg 420 g (48%)	
55-kg woman	44 kcal/kg 2,420 kcal	8 g/kg 440 g (73%)	1.2 g/kg 66 g (11%)
		6 g/kg 330 g (55%)	

Summary

Although guidelines can help all exercisers get started, individuals with diabetes vary in their response to training and physical stress. Adjustments that work for one person may not work for another. Both awareness of the signals the body provides and blood glucose monitoring data allow the person with diabetes to become an expert at interpreting this information and to exercise safely.

References

1. Wasserman DH, Lacy DB, Goldstein RS, William PE, Cherrington AD: Exercise-induced fall in insulin and hepatic carbohydrate during exercise. *Am J Physiol* 256:E500–08, 1989
2. Wasserman DH, Spalding JS, Lacy DBB, Colburn CA, Goldstein RE, Cherrington AD: Glucagon is a primary controller of the increments in hepatic glycogenolysis and gluconeogenesis during exercise. *Am J Physiol* 257:E108–17, 1989
3. MacDonald MJ: Postexercise late-onset hypoglycemia in insulin-dependent diabetic patients. *Diabetes Care* 10:584–88, 1987
4. Wasserman DH, Zinman B: Exercise in individuals with IDDM (Technical Review). *Diabetes Care* 17:924–37, 1994
5. Davis SN, Galassetti P, Wasserman DH, Tate D: Effects of antecedent hypoglycemia on subsequent counterregulatory responses to exercise. *Diabetes* 49:73–81, 2000
6. Mitchell TH, Abraham G, Schriffrin A, Leiter LA, Marliss EF: Hyperglycemia after intense exercise in IDDM subjects during continuous insulin infusion. *Diabetes Care* 11:311–17, 1988
7. Purdon C, Brousson M, Nyveen L, Miles PDG, Halter JB, Vranic M, Marliss EB: The role of insulin and catecholamines in the glucoregulatory response to exercise during intense exercise and early recovery in insulin-dependent diabetic and control subjects. *J Clin Endocrinol Metab* 76:566–73, 1993
8. Berger M, Berchtold P, Cuppers HJ, Drost H, Kley HK, Muller WA, Wiegelmann W, Zimmerman-Telschow H, Gries FA, Kruskemper HL, Zimmerman H: Metabolic and hormonal effects of muscular exercise in juvenile type diabetics. *Diabetologia* 13: 355–65, 1977
9. Franz MJ: Fuel metabolism, exercise and nutritional needs in type 1 diabetes. *Can J Diabetes Care* 22:59–63, 1998

10. Raguso CA, Coggan AR, Gastaldelli A, Sidossis LS, Bastry EJ, Wolfe RR: Lipid and carbohydrate metabolism in IDDM during moderate and intense exercise. *Diabetes* 44:1066–74, 1995
11. Sherman WM, Doyle JA, Lamb DR, Strauss RH: Dietary carbohydrate, muscle glycogen, and exercise performance during 7 d of training. *Am J Clin Nutr* 57:27–31, 1993
12. Neuffer PD, Costill DL, Flyn MG, Kirwan JP, Mitchell JB, Houmard J: Improvements in exercise performance: effects of carbohydrate feeding and diet. *J Appl Physiol* 62:983–88, 1987
13. Wright DA, Sherman WM, Dernbach AR: Carbohydrate feedings before, during, or in combination improve cycling endurance performance. *J Appl Physiol* 71:1082–88, 1991
14. Nathan DN, Madnek S, Delahanty L: Programming pre-exercise snacks to prevent post-exercise hypoglycemia in intensively treated insulin-dependent diabetics. *Ann Intern Med* 4:483–86, 1985
15. Soo K, Furler SM, Samaras K, Jenkins AB, Campbell LV, Chisholm DJ: Glycemic responses to exercise in IDDM after simple and complex carbohydrate supplementation. *Diabetes Care* 19:575–79, 1996
16. Franz MJ: Nutrition: can it give athletes with diabetes a boost? *Diabetes Educ* 17:163–72, 1991
17. Zinman B, Zunuga-Guajardo S, Kelly D: Comparison of the acute and long-term effects of exercise on glucose control in type I diabetics. *Diabetes Care* 7:515–19, 1984
18. Wallberg-Henriksson H, Gunnarsson R, Henriksson J, DeFronzo R, Felig P, Ostman J, Wahren J: Increased peripheral insulin sensitivity and muscle mitochondrial enzymes but unchanged blood glucose control in type I diabetes after physical training. *Diabetes* 11:311–17, 1982
19. Schiffrin A, Parikh S: Accommodating planned exercise in type I diabetic patients on intensive treatment. *Diabetes Care* 8:337–43, 1985
20. Sherman WM, Costill DL, Fink WJ, Miller JM: The effect of exercise and diet manipulation on muscle glycogen and its subsequent use during performance. *Int J Sports Med* 2:114–18, 1981
21. Wahren J, Felig P, Hagenfeldt L: Physical exercise and fuel homeostasis in diabetes metabolism. *Diabetologia* 14:213–22, 1978
22. Coggan AR, Coyle EF: Carbohydrate ingestion during prolonged exercise: effects on metabolism and performance. *Exerc Sport Sci Rev* 19:1–40, 1991

23. Coggan AR, Swanson SC: Nutritional manipulation before and during endurance exercise: effects on performance. *Med Sci Sports Exerc* 24:S331–35, 1992
24. Coyle EF, Coggan AR, Hemmert MK, Ivy JL: Muscle glycogen utilization during prolonged strenuous exercise when fed carbohydrate. *J Appl Physiol* 61:165–72, 1986
25. Coyle EF, Hagberg JM, Hurley BF, Martin WH, Ehsani AA, Holloszy JO: Carbohydrate feeding during prolonged strenuous exercise can delay fatigue. *J Appl Physiol* 55:230–35, 1983
26. Mason WL, McConell G, Hargreaves M: Carbohydrate ingestion during exercise: liquid vs. solid feedings. *Med Sci Sports Exerc* 25:966–69, 1993
27. Coyle EF, Montain SJ: Benefits of fluid replacement with carbohydrate during exercise. *Med Sci Sports Exerc* 24:S324–30, 1992
28. Lamb DR, Brodowicz GR: Optimal use of fluids of varying formulations to minimize exercise-induced disturbances in homeostasis. *Sports Med* 3:247–74, 1986
29. Wagenmakers AJM, Brouns F, Saris WHM, Halliday D: Oxidation rates of orally ingested carbohydrates during prolonged exercise in men. *J Appl Physiol* 75:2774–80, 1993
30. Ivy JL, Katz SL, Cutler CL, Sherman WM, Coyle EF: Muscle glycogen synthesis after exercise: effect of time of carbohydrate ingestion. *J Appl Physiol* 64:1480–85, 1988
31. Zachwieja J, Costill DL, Pascoe DD, Robergs RA, Fink WJ: Influence of muscle glycogen depletion on the rate of resynthesis. *Med Sci Sports Exerc* 23:44–48, 1991
32. Position of the American Dietetic Association and the Canadian Dietetic Association: Nutrition for physical fitness and athletic performance for adults. *J Am Diet Assoc* 93:691–96, 1993
33. National Research Council: *Recommended Dietary Allowances.* 10th ed. Washington, DC, National Academy Press, 1989

Marion J. Franz, MS, RD, CDE, is from Nutrition Concepts by Franz, Inc., Minneapolis, MN.

18

Nutritional Strategies to Optimize Athletic Performance

W. MICHAEL SHERMAN, PHD,
KEVIN A. JACOBS, PHD, AND
CYNTHIA FERRARA, PHD

Highlights

- The primary substrate that is oxidized during moderate-intensity exercise (60–75% VO_{2max} lasting 90–120 min) is carbohydrate.
- The body's stores of carbohydrate are limited; thus, it is important to consume adequate dietary carbohydrate during all phases of endurance training and performance.
- Endurance athletes should concentrate on consuming 8–10 g carbohydrate/kg body wt/day, at least 1.2 g protein/kg body wt/day, and the balance of energy from fat.
- Recreational athletes, however, should concentrate on consuming a healthy diet that contains <30% of total energy from fat, at least 0.8 g protein/kg body wt/day, and the balance of energy from carbohydrate.

- Both endurance and recreational athletes should consume fluids during exercise to match the fluid lost from sweating.

Fuel Use During Endurance Exercise

The bodily fuel reserves, protein, fat, and carbohydrate, are metabolized to provide the energy necessary for muscular contraction during endurance exercise. Protein metabolism may make a small contribution to energy expenditure but only when bodily carbohydrate stores are low or when the exercise is of long duration. Fat and carbohydrate are the primary substrates that are metabolized to produce energy for muscle contraction. The duration, intensity, and mode of exercise as well as the nutritional state influence the relative proportion of fat and carbohydrate that are metabolized to provide the energy required for muscle contraction during endurance exercise.

Does the Availability of Fat Limit Endurance Performance?

During low-intensity long-duration exercise such as walking, the primary fuel that is metabolized to produce energy for muscle contraction is fat. Fat circulates in the blood as a fatty acid–albumin complex, or fat is stored in muscle or adipose tissues as triglyceride. After 40 min of exercise at 30% VO_{2max} (walking), fat contributes 40% of the total energy expenditure, whereas after 240 min of exercise at this walking intensity, fat contributes 70% of the total energy expenditure.[1] However, because the body's fat stores are so large, the depletion of bodily fat stores has not been identified as a factor that limits performance (i.e., depletion of bodily fat stores or available fat energy almost never occurs and thus does not contribute to fatigue during endurance exercise).

Does the Availability of Protein Limit Endurance Performance?

Metabolism of protein during exercise may provide a relatively small proportion of the total energy expenditure, depending on nutritional status and the duration of exercise. During exercise at 60% VO_{2max} for longer than 1 h, protein oxidation may contribute up to 5% of the total energy expenditure.[2] If muscle glycogen stores are low, the contribution of protein oxidation may increase to 10–15% of the total energy expenditure.[3] These findings indicate that metabolism of protein contributes an increasing proportion of the energy expenditure as the duration of exercise increases and the bodily carbohydrate stores decrease. However, there is no association between the onset of fatigue and a low content of muscle protein or the rate of protein breakdown during endurance exercise. This seems reasonable because the body protects this critical tissue to preserve the essential elements for muscle contraction and bodily structure. Therefore, it is unlikely that protein oxidation is a limiting factor during prolonged exercise (i.e., depletion of bodily protein reserves or available protein energy almost never occurs and thus does not contribute to fatigue during endurance exercise).

Does the Availability of Carbohydrate Limit Endurance Performance?

During moderate-intensity exercise, a large proportion of the energy for muscle contraction is provided by the metabolism of the body's carbohydrate stores.[4] Moderate-intensity exercise is between 60 and 75%VO_{2max}: within this range of exercise intensities, it would be slightly to extremely difficult to carry on a normal conversation during the exercise session. The bodily stores of carbohydrate include muscle and liver glycogen and blood glucose. Because bodily carbohydrate stores are limited, a significant reduction in or depletion of the bodily carbohydrate stores can limit the ability of the muscle to continue producing force at the required rate (i.e., a lowering of the muscle glycogen or blood glucose concentrations or muscle glycogen depletion causes fatigue during endurance exercise).

Stored carbohydrate energy in a 70-kg person is ~2,000 kcal.[5] This carbohydrate energy is found in muscle (79%) and liver (14%) as glycogen and in the blood (7%) as glucose.[6] These carbohydrate stores can sustain moderate-intensity exercise for only about 120 min if carbohydrates are the only fuels metabolized to produce energy for muscular contraction during endurance exercise.

The rate of muscle glycogen degradation increases with increasing exercise intensity.[7] At exercise intensities between 60 and 85% VO_{2max}, fatigue appears to be related to a low muscle glycogen concentration. Furthermore, the pre-exercise muscle glycogen concentration is directly proportional to the endurance time to fatigue.[8,9] For exercise at <60% VO_{2max}, fatigue likely occurs as a result of boredom, dehydration, hyperthermia, or orthopedic injury. For exercise at >90% VO_{2max}, fatigue is related to a variety of factors, including decreased muscle pH, potassium efflux, and a failure of processes responsible for muscle fiber excitation.

Blood glucose is also metabolized to provide energy for muscle contraction. Low blood glucose concentration (i.e., hypoglycemia) during exercise may impair endurance performance.[10,11] These blood glucose responses can occur during moderate-intensity exercise that lasts for longer than 90–120 min. Therefore, it is extremely important to maintain a blood glucose concentration in the normal range during prolonged moderate-intensity endurance exercise.

The blood glucose concentration during exercise is dependent on the rate of muscle glucose uptake and the rate of glucose released from the splanchnic areas.[1] The liver degrades glycogen to glucose and releases the glucose into the blood to maintain the blood glucose concentration. In a 70-kg person exercising at 75% VO_{2max}, the blood glucose concentration remains at ~90 mg/dl for 90–120 min. The blood glucose concentration is maintained because the rate of splanchnic glucose release equals the rate of glucose uptake by the contracting muscles. If exercise continues at a moderate intensity for longer than 90–120 min, glucose uptake by the contracting muscle remains constant, but splanchnic glucose release declines because of the depletion of liver glycogen.[12] Formation of glucose by glucose precursors (gluconeogenesis) cannot completely compensate for the decreased splanchnic glucose release that is due to liver glycogen depletion, and, consequently, the blood glucose concentration declines.[1,11,12]

In conclusion, carbohydrate, fat, and protein may be metabolized and contribute by varying degrees to the total energy expenditure during prolonged moderate-intensity exercise. The major energy sources for exercise at intensities appropriate for improving cardiovascular endurance (between 60 and 75% VO_{2max}) are the bodily carbohydrate stores (e.g., muscle and liver glycogen and blood glucose).[4] When exercise is undertaken at these intensities for longer than 90–120 min, a reduction of these carbohydrate reserves can limit exercise performance (e.g., a lowering or depletion of muscle and liver glycogen and/or blood glucose causes fatigue).

Nutritional Strategies to Optimize Body Carbohydrate Stores

Normally active, untrained individuals have an energy expenditure between 2,000 and 2,500 kcal/day, whereas an athlete undertaking strenuous, prolonged exercise training may have an energy expenditure that is 1.5–3 times higher.[13,14] The typical American diet contains 40–45% of the total energy from carbohydrate, 40% of the total energy from fat, and 10–15% of the total energy from protein. The recommended amounts of these nutrients in the diet for active people should probably be based on body weight.[14] Thus, physically active people should consume at least 5–6 g carbohydrate/kg body wt/day, 0.8 g protein/kg body wt/day, and no more than 30% of the total calories from fat. Those with diabetes must evaluate the effect of any dietary manipulation on glycemic control.

The endurance athlete should choose foods during training that will maintain bodily carbohydrate stores to optimize training and performance capabilities. Because carbohydrates are the primary source of fuel for exercising muscle, the carbohydrate intake must be carefully monitored.

Athletes undertaking intense daily exercise should consume additional energy equal to the energy expenditure of exercise to maintain a constant body weight. The percent of energy consumed as fat should not exceed 30% of the total energy intake in most people. Additionally, the endurance athlete should probably increase protein intake to 1.2 g/kg body wt/day, with the balance of energy intake derived primarily from dietary carbohydrate. Based on these recommendations, an endurance athlete may consume as much as 8–10 g carbohydrate/kg body wt/day.[15] This high carbohydrate intake should maintain or increase glycogen stores in the muscle and liver. It is possible that some athletes participating in strength or endurance activities, or those athletes subjecting their muscles to recurring muscle trauma or sudden increases in training load, may require a slightly higher protein intake.[2] However, it is likely that the increased protein requirement for these conditions will be adequately met by the increased food intake to meet the energy expenditure associated with exercise.

Nutritional Strategies for the Endurance Athlete

For the endurance athlete, nutritional strategies to optimize carbohydrate stores in muscle and liver are essential to optimize training and performance capabilities. These nutritional strategies should be used in every phase of the endurance athlete's training regimen, including daily training, the week before a competition, the hours before a competition, during a competition, and the 4–6 and 24 h after a competition or training. The applications of these recommendations to the endurance and recreational athlete are summarized in Table 18.1.

Nutritional Strategies During Daily Heavy Training

Intense daily training will acutely reduce the bodily stores of carbohydrate. If inadequate dietary carbohydrate is consumed on a daily basis, there may be a suboptimal level of bodily carbohydrate that may impair daily training capabilities. Consuming 10 g carbohydrate/kg body wt/day during twice-daily intense rowing training for 28 days produced higher muscle glycogen and significantly better training/performance responses than consuming 5 g carbohydrate/kg body wt/day.[16] Thus, adequate dietary carbohydrate intake on a daily basis has the potential to facilitate a more "optimal" training adaptation.

Nutritional Strategies the Week Before an Important Event

Because of the direct relationship between a low muscle glycogen concentration and fatigue, it has been hypothesized that starting exercise with a supra-elevated muscle glycogen concentration (supercompensation) may extend, in time, the point at which fatigue occurs during endurance exercise.

An accepted glycogen supercompensation regimen reported by Sherman et al.[17] incorporates dietary manipulation with a tapering of the duration of exercise during the 6 days before an important endurance competition. Exercise is undertaken during these days at a

TABLE 18.1 Synopsis of Nutritional Strategies and Phases of Training/Competition for Endurance and Recreational Athletes

Phase of Training	Endurance Athlete	Recreational Athlete
During daily training	Consume <0.4 g fat/kg body wt/day; 0.8–1.2 g protein/kg body wt/day; 8–10 g CHO/kg body wt/day	Consume <30% total daily energy from fat, 10–12% total daily energy from protein, and balance of energy from CHO
Week before event (CHO loading; note cautions in text for type 1 diabetes)	Do 90, 40, 40, 20, 20, and 0 min of exercise at moderate intensity; consume 5 g CHO/kg body wt/day during first 3 days followed by 8–10 g CHO/kg body wt/day during second 3 days	Probably not applicable
Hours before event (see cautions in text for those who might be sensitive to an early lowering of blood glucose)	Consume 4–5 g liquid CHO/kg body wt 3–4 h before event, or consume 1–2 g liquid CHO/kg body wt 1 h before event, or solids may be used as tolerated; test individual responsiveness to recommendation	Exercise need not be undertaken on an empty stomach, although the work-enhancing effect of a pre-exercise CHO meal for the recreational athlete is doubtful
During the event	Consume fluids at a rate equal to sweat loss, or at minimum, consume 250 ml every 20 min during exercise; do not wait until thirst develops to begin consuming fluids; desirable fluids are CHO/electrolyte beverages (6–10% wt/vol); consume at a rate to provide 40–65 g CHO/h. If CHO consumption is delayed, consume 200 g of liquid CHO before completing 2 h of exercise and then consume 40–65 g CHO/h	Consume fluids at a rate equal to sweat loss, or at minimum, consume 250 ml every 20 min during exercise to produce moderate to heavy sweating; do not wait until thirst develops to begin consuming fluids; fluids may be CHO/electrolyte beverages, water, or other fluids according to individual preference
4–6 h after event	Consume 0.7–3.0 g CHO/kg body wt immediately after and every 2 h thereafter for 4 h; if tolerated, consume 0.4 g CHO/kg body wt every 15 min after exercise for 4 h	Probably not applicable

(continued)

TABLE 18.1 (*Continued*)

Phase of Training	Endurance Athlete	Recreational Athlete
24 h after event	Consume 8–10 g CHO/kg body wt/day; mixed CHO foods can be consumed; high–glycemic index foods probably promote glycogen synthesis	See daily training recommendation

Individual tolerances to these recommendations may vary. Before individuals with diabetes undertake these nutritional strategies, they should consult a physician or diabetes educator about appropriate activity level. CHO, carbohydrate.

moderate intensity for 90, 40, 40, 20, 20, and 0 min, respectively. During the first 3 days, the diet should contain 5 g carbohydrate/kg body wt/day, and during the next 3 days, the diet should contain 8–10 g carbohydrate/kg body wt/day. The protein intake should be 0.8–1.2 g/kg body wt/day over the 6-day period. This regimen increases muscle glycogen to more than 210 mmol/kg wet wt: 1.6-fold above the "normal" glycogen concentration of 130 mmol/kg wet wt that is found in trained athletes consuming a diet containing 5 g carbohydrate/kg body wt/day.[17]

It should be emphasized that muscle glycogen supercompensation may only benefit long-duration (>90 min) exercise that is limited by carbohydrate availability.[17–19] In addition, the mechanism for the ergogenic effect of muscle glycogen supercompensation is not well understood and has recently been suggested to be due to a placebo effect.[20]

The supercompensation or carbohydrate-loading regimen must be used with caution in people with diabetes. Specifically, among type 1 diabetic individuals, careful manipulation of the insulin regimen and doses guided by frequent blood glucose monitoring will be needed to maintain glucose control while achieving the goals of the regimen.

Nutritional Strategies During the Hours Before Competition

Many endurance athletes train or compete after an overnight fast. An overnight fast will reduce the liver glycogen concentration, and this may produce a premature lowering of the blood glucose concentration and premature fatigue during endurance exercise. Thus, endurance athletes should consider consuming a pre-exercise carbohydrate meal during the hours before training and/or competition in endurance events.

Moderately trained cyclists who consumed 312 g carbohydrate 4 h before 95 min of exercise showed a 15% improvement in performance compared with placebo.[21] Wright et al.[22] reported an 18% increase in total work and a 36-min increase in endurance time to exhaustion in well-trained cyclists who consumed 5 g liquid carbohydrate/kg body wt compared with a placebo solution 3 h before exercise. Additionally, consuming either 1.1 or 2.2 g liquid carbohydrate/kg body wt 1 h before endurance exercise produced a significant 12% increase in cycling time trial performance in moderately trained cyclists.[23] Pre-exercise carbohydrate feedings do not affect muscle glycogen use during exercise[24] and likely improve exercise performance by sparing liver glycogen for use later in exercise.[25]

If blood insulin is elevated at the start of exercise as a result of a pre-exercise carbohydrate feeding, there may be an initial lowering of the blood glucose concentration by as much as 18 mg/dl during the first 15–20 min of exercise.[26] Thus, pre-exercise carbohydrate feedings may cause fatigue in those individuals who may be sensitive to this lowering of blood glucose. Therefore, the athlete should evaluate adoption of this strategy to improve endurance performance in advance and not for the first time during an important competition.

Nutritional Strategies During Competition

During endurance exercise, it is imperative to maintain the body's fluid balance and available carbohydrate energy. The body's heat content increases during exercise. The body attempts to minimize the increase in body temperature primarily by sweating. As sweat evaporates, heat is lost from the body. The heat that is dissipated by sweating is especially critical for minimizing the increase in body temperature during exercise in a warm or hot environment.

Sweating reduces the amount of fluid in the body. The loss of body water and electrolytes during exercise may lead to heat cramps, heat exhaustion, and even heat stroke, which can cause death. When sweating occurs during exercise, the primary objective is to consume as much water as is lost. The sweat rate may range from 0.75 to 1.0 l/h; thus, at least 250 ml fluid should be consumed every 20 min during exercise.[14,27] Because the sensation of thirst occurs after there is already a significant body fluid deficit, the consumption of fluid should begin within the first 20 min of exercise.

Carbohydrate consumption during moderate-intensity exercise lasting longer than 90–120 min will delay the onset of fatigue during endurance exercise. Endurance time until exhaustion may be extended by as much as 60 min with carbohydrate feeding during exercise.[10,11,22,28] The preservation of exercise tolerance is attributed largely to the maintenance of a high rate of carbohydrate oxidation during the later stages of exercise that is facilitated by maintaining the availability of blood glucose.[10,11,28,29] Blood glucose availability is maintained by the sparing of liver glycogen stores with carbohydrate supplementation during exercise.[30,31] Based on many studies of carbohydrate feedings during endurance exercise, it appears that the endurance athlete should ingest 40–65 g carbohydrate/h, consumed as a 6–10% (wt/vol) solution.[14,29,32]

Under certain circumstances, it may not be practical or possible to consume carbohydrate in liquids during the early stages of an endurance event. However, for carbohydrate ingestion to positively affect endurance performance under this circumstance, the carbohydrates must be consumed before the blood glucose concentration begins to decline.[10] If carbohydrate consumption must be delayed during endurance exercise, 200 g liquid carbohydrate should be consumed before completing 2 h of moderate-intensity exercise. Thereafter, carbohydrate should be consumed at a rate to provide 40–65 g carbohydrate/h.[28]

Carbohydrate feedings during variable intensity exercise also improve performance; however, the mechanism for the enhanced performance appears to be the result of a slowing of the degradation of muscle glycogen.[33]

Nutritional Strategies During the 4–6 h After Training or Competition

The rate of glycogen synthesis is linear during the first 6 h after exercise. When muscle glycogen has been depleted, muscle glycogen synthesis occurs at a maximum rate of 6 mmol/kg wet wt/h if 0.7–3.0 g carbohydrate/kg body wt is consumed immediately after exercise and at 2-h intervals thereafter for 4–6 h.[34,35] However, if carbohydrate ingestion is delayed for 2 h after stopping exercise, the rate of muscle glycogen synthesis will be 50% slower (i.e., only 3 mmol/kg wet wt/h).[36] It may be possible to double the rate of muscle glycogen synthesis (10–12 mmol/kg wet wt/h) after exercise by ingesting small amounts of carbohydrate (0.4 g carbohydrate/kg body wt) at 15-min intervals for 4 h after endurance exercise.[37] In addition, consumption of glucose polymers may promote more rapid muscle glycogen resynthesis than sucrose.[38] Ingestion of carbohydrates immediately after glycogen-depleting exercise may be especially important if multiple glycogen-depleting sports events are to be undertaken in a given day.[32]

The ingestion of both carbohydrate and protein results in greater increases in insulin concentration than carbohydrate ingestion alone.[39] This raises the possibility that carbohydrate-protein coingestion may promote greater glucose uptake and muscle glycogen resynthesis.[39,40] The majority of evidence, however, suggests no additional benefit of carbohydrate-protein coingestion compared with carbohydrate ingestion alone in promoting muscle glycogen resynthesis.[41–44]

Nutritional Strategies During the 24 h After Training or Competition

Muscle glycogen synthesis during the 24–48 h after exercise is largely dependent on the amount of carbohydrate ingested. Muscle glycogen can be replenished in 24 h if >525 g carbohydrate or 8 g carbohydrate/kg body wt/day is consumed.[45] One study suggested that consuming complex carbohydrate produced greater muscle glycogen storage during the second 24-h period after exercise; however, this study has not been replicated.[45] More recently, it was demonstrated that a high–glycemic index carbohydrate diet (10 g/kg body wt/day) results in more muscle glycogen storage than consuming a low–glycemic index carbohydrate diet.[46] Exercise that significantly depletes muscle glycogen also often impairs muscle function. Whereas most studies focus on the ideal methods to "normalize" muscle glycogen, few studies have determined if muscle function is also normal when a "normal" muscle glycogen concentration has been achieved.

Nutritional Strategies for Recreational Athletes

Because most recreational athletes will not undertake exercise lasting longer than 90–120 min at a moderate intensity for more than 3 or 4 days/week, it is unlikely that these athletes will benefit from the nutritional strategies outlined above. Most likely, adequate body carbohydrate stores will be maintained by consuming a "healthy" diet that matches caloric expenditure and maintains body weight. Thus, most recreational athletes should consume a diet that contains <30% of total energy from fat, roughly 10–12% of energy as protein, and the balance of energy from carbohydrate. Probably the most significant threat to the endurance capabilities of the recreational athlete is the negative consequence of dehydration due to sweating. Thus, the primary emphasis for the recreational athlete should be to consume fluids at a rate that is equal to the loss of body water from sweating. Normal body weight should be attained between exercise sessions that produce significant sweating to eliminate the consequences of chronic dehydration. Because thirst is increased after significant sweating has already occurred, fluid consumption should begin before the onset of the sensation of thirst during exercise.

Alternative Nutritional Strategies

Several nutritional supplements are now available to athletes of all levels. A majority of the purported performance-enhancing effects of these supplements have no scientific backing. The ability of creatine to improve high-intensity exercise performance has received a great deal of scientific attention. Although the evidence is far from conclusive, creatine may enhance the ability to perform repeated bouts of short-duration (<30 s) high-intensity exercise.[47] Creatine supplementation does not improve endurance performance. Other popular nutritional supplements include carnitine, branched-chain amino acids, and medium-chain triglycerides. However, none of these supplements have been shown to improve exercise performance.[47] Caution should be exerted because the long-term effects of these nutritional supplements are not clear, and they have not been evaluated for use in diabetic individuals.

References

1. Ahlborg G, Felig P, Hagenfeldt L, Hendler R, Wahren J: Substrate turnover during prolonged exercise in man: splanchnic and leg metabolism of glucose, free fatty acids, and amino acids. *J Clin Invest* 53:1080–90, 1974

2. Lemon PWR, Yarasheski KE, Dolony DG: The importance of protein for athletes. *Sports Med* 1:474–84, 1984
3. Lemon PWR, Mullin JP: Effect of initial muscle glycogen levels on protein catabolism during exercise. *J Appl Physiol* 48:624–29, 1980
4. Romijn JA, Coyle EF, Sidossis LS, Gastaldelli A, Horowitz JF, Endert E, Wolfe RR: Regulation of endogenous fat and carbohydrate metabolism in relation to exercise intensity and duration. *Am J Physiol* 265:E380–91, 1993
5. Goodman MN: Amino acid and protein metabolism. In *Exercise, Nutrition, and Energy Metabolism.* 1st ed. Horton ES, Terjung RL, Eds. New York, Macmillan, 1988, p. 89–99
6. Cahill GF, Aoki TT, Rossini AA: Metabolism in obesity and anorexia nervosa. *Nutr Brain* 3:1–70, 1979
7. Saltin B, Karlsson J: Muscle glycogen utilization during work of different intensities. In *Muscle Metabolism During Exercise.* Pernow B, Saltin B, Eds. New York, Plenum, 1971, p. 289–300
8. Bergstrom J, Hermansen L, Hultman E, Saltin B: Diet, muscle glycogen, and physical performance. *Acta Physiol Scand* 71:140–50, 1967
9. Hermansen L, Hultman E, Saltin B: Muscle glycogen during prolonged severe exercise. *Acta Physiol Scand* 71:129–39, 1967
10. Coggan AR, Coyle EF: Reversal of fatigue during prolonged exercise by carbohydrate infusion or ingestion. *J Appl Physiol* 63:2388–95, 1987
11. Coyle EF, Coggan AR, Hemmert MK, Ivy JL: Muscle glycogen utilization during prolonged strenuous exercise when fed carbohydrate. *J Appl Physiol* 61:165–72, 1986
12. Ahlborg G, Felig P: Lactate and glucose exchange across the forearm, legs, and splanchnic bed during and after prolonged leg exercise. *J Clin Invest* 69:45–54, 1982
13. Brotherhood JR: Nutrition and sports performance. *Sports Med* 1:350–89, 1984
14. Sherman WM, Lamb DR: Nutrition and prolonged exercise. In *Perspectives in Exercise Science and Sports Medicine: Prolonged Exercise.* Vol. 1. Lamb DR, Murray R, Eds. Indianapolis, IN, Benchmark, 1988, p. 213–80
15. Sherman WM, Wimer GS: Insufficient dietary carbohydrate: does it impair athletic performance? *Int J Sports Nutr* 1:28–44, 1991

16. Simonsen JC, Sherman WM, Lamb DR, Dernbach AR, Doyle JA, Strauss R: Dietary carbohydrate, muscle glycogen, and power output during rowing training. *J Appl Physiol* 70:1500–05, 1990
17. Sherman WM, Costill DL, Fink WJ, Miller JM: The effect of exercise and diet manipulation on muscle glycogen and its subsequent use during performance. *Int J Sports Med* 2:114–18, 1981
18. Hawley JA, Palmer GS, Noakes TD: Effects of 3 days of carbohydrate supplementation on muscle glycogen content and utilisation during 1-h cycling performance. *Eur J Appl Physiol* 75:407–12, 1997
19. Madsen K, Pedersen PK, Rose P, Richter EA: Carbohydrate supercompensation and muscle glycogen utilization during exhaustive running in highly trained athletes. *Eur J Appl Physiol* 61:467–72, 1990
20. Burke LM, Hawley JA, Schabort EJ, Gibson ASC, Mujika I, Noakes TD: Carbohydrate loading failed to improve 100-km cycling performance in a placebo-controlled trial. *J Appl Physiol* 88:1284–90, 2000
21. Sherman WM, Brodowicz G, Wright DA, Allen WK, Simonsen J, Dernbach A: Effects of 4 h preexercise carbohydrate feedings on cycling performance. *Med Sci Sports Exerc* 21:598–604, 1989
22. Wright DA, Sherman WM, Dernbach AR: Carbohydrate feedings before, during, or in combination improve cycling endurance performance. *J Appl Physiol* 71:1082–88, 1991
23. Sherman WM, Peden MC, Wright DA: Carbohydrate feedings 1 h before exercise improves cycling performance. *Am J Clin Nutr* 54:866–70, 1991
24. Febbraio MA, Stewart KL: CHO feeding before prolonged exercise: effect of glycemic index on muscle glycogenolysis and exercise performance. *J Appl Physiol* 81:1115–20, 1996
25. Marmy-Conus N, Fabris S, Proietto J, Hargreaves M: Preexercise glucose ingestion and glucose kinetics during exercise. *J Appl Physiol* 81:853–57, 1996
26. Costill DL, Coyle EF, Dalsky G, Evans W, Fink W, Hoopes D: Effects of elevated plasma FFA and insulin on glycogen usage during exercise. *J Appl Physiol* 43:695–99, 1977
27. American College of Sports Medicine: Position stand on exercise and fluid replacement. *Med Sci Sports Exerc* 28:i–vii, 1996
28. Coggan AR, Coyle EF: Metabolism and performance following carbohydrate ingestion late in exercise. *Med Sci Sports Exerc* 21:59–65, 1989

29. Coggan AR, Swanson SC: Nutritional manipulations before and during endurance exercise: effects on performance. *Med Sci Sports Exerc* 24:S331–35, 1992
30. Bosch AN, Dennis SC, Noakes TD: Influence of carbohydrate ingestion on fuel substrate turnover and oxidation during prolonged exercise. *J Appl Physiol* 76:2364–72, 1994
31. McConell G, Fabris S, Proietto J, Hargreaves M: Effect of carbohydrate ingestion on glucose kinetics during exercise. *J Appl Physiol* 77:1537–41, 1994
32. Coyle EF: Timing and method of increased carbohydrate intake to cope with heavy training, competition, and recovery. *J Sports Sci* 9:29–52, 1993
33. Yaspelkis BB III, Patterson JG, Anderla PA, Ding Z, Ivy JL: Carbohydrate supplementation spares muscle glycogen during variable intensity exercise. *J Appl Physiol* 75:1477–85, 1993
34. Blom PCS, Hostmark AT, Vaage O, Kardel KR, Maehlum S: Effect of different post-exercise sugar diets on the rate of muscle glycogen synthesis. *Med Sci Sports Exerc* 19:491–96, 1987
35. Ivy JL, Lee MC, Brozinick JT, Reed MJ: Muscle glycogen storage after different amounts of carbohydrate ingestion. *J Appl Physiol* 65:2018–23, 1988
36. Ivy JL, Katz AL, Cutler CL, Sherman WM, Coyle EF: Muscle glycogen synthesis after exercise: effect of time of carbohydrate ingestion. *J Appl Physiol* 64:1480–85, 1988
37. Doyle JA, Sherman WM, Strauss RL: Effects of eccentric and concentric exercise on muscle glycogen replenishment. *J Appl Physiol* 74:1848–55, 1993
38. Bowtell JL, Gelly K, Jackman ML, Patel A, Simeoni M, Rennie MJ: Effect of different carbohydrate drinks on whole body carbohydrate storage after exhaustive exercise. *J Appl Physiol* 88:1529–36, 2000
39. Zawadzki KM, Yaspelkis BB, Ivy JL: Carbohydrate-protein complex increases the rate of muscle glycogen storage after exercise. *J Appl Physiol* 72:1854–59, 1992
40. Van Loon LJC, Saris WHM, Kruijshoop M, Wagenmakers AJM: Maximizing postexercise muscle glycogen resynthesis: carbohydrate supplementation and the application of amino acid or protein hydrolysate mixtures. *Am J Clin Nutr* 72:106–11, 2000
41. Carrithers JA, Williamson DL, Gallagher PM, Godard MP, Schulze KE, Trappe SW: Effects of postexercise carbohydrate-protein feedings on muscle glycogen restoration. *J Appl Physiol* 88:1976–82, 2000

42. Roy BD, Tarnopolsky MA: Influence of differing macronutrient intakes on muscle glycogen resynthesis after resistance exercise. *J Appl Physiol* 84:890–96, 1998
43. Tarnopolsky MA, Bosman M, MacDonald JR, Vandeputte D, Martin J, Roy BD: Postexercise protein-carbohydrate supplements increase muscle glycogen in men and women. *J Appl Physiol* 83:1877–83, 1997
44. Van Hall G, Shirreffs SM, Calbet JAL: Muscle glycogen resynthesis during recovery from cycle exercise: no effect of additional protein ingestion. *J Appl Physiol* 88:1631–36, 2000
45. Costill DL, Sherman WM, Fink WJ, Maresh C, Whitten M, Miller JM: The role of dietary carbohydrates in muscle glycogen resynthesis after strenuous running. *Am J Clin Nutr* 34:1831–36, 1981
46. Burke LM, Collier GR, Hargreaves M: Muscle glycogen storage after prolonged exercise: effect of the glycemic index of carbohydrate feedings. *J Appl Physiol* 75:1019–23, 1993
47. Wagenmakers AJM: Nutritional supplements: effects on exercise performance and metabolism. In *Perspectives in Exercise Science and Sports Medicine: The Metabolic Basis of Performance in Exercise and Sport.* Vol. 12. Lamb DR, Murray R, Eds. Carmel, IN, Cooper, 1999, p. 207–59

W. Michael Sherman, PhD, is from the Ohio State University, Columbus, OH. Kevin A. Jacobs, PhD, is from the University of California at Berkeley, Berkeley, CA. Cynthia Ferrara, PhD, is from the University of Maryland, College Park, MD. While work was being completed for this chapter, Drs. Jacobs and Ferrara were with the Ohio State University.

19

Exercise and Weight Control

RENA R. WING, PHD

Highlights

- Weight loss is important in the treatment and prevention of type 2 diabetes.
- The combination of diet, exercise, and behavior modification is the most effective approach to weight control.
- Exercise may also help prevent weight gain in type 1 diabetic individuals on intensive therapy.
- Current dietary interventions focus on reducing calories and dietary fat; periods of very-low-calorie intake or portion-controlled meals may also be helpful.
- Low-intensity, long-duration exercise is recommended for weight loss.
- A combination of lifestyle exercise and programmed exercise is recommended.
- To increase activity level, it is helpful to divide exercise into multiple short sessions.

- Approaches that teach patients to rearrange their environment to support healthy eating and exercise behaviors are important for long-term maintenance of behavior change.

The majority of patients with type 2 diabetes are overweight. For these individuals, weight loss is an important component of treatment. Lowering body weight can improve glycemic control, reduce insulin resistance, and improve coronary heart disease risk factors. Modest weight losses of 7–14 kg are often sufficient to improve glycemic control and cardiovascular risk factors in patients with type 2 diabetes.

The combination of diet plus exercise may also be important in the prevention of diabetes. Both weight loss and exercise have been shown to be independently related to the risk of developing type 2 diabetes. Changes in weight and exercise behaviors can reduce insulin resistance and visceral abdominal fat and thereby help prevent or delay the development of diabetes.

Exercise as an Adjunct to Diet for Weight Loss and Maintenance

The most successful approach to long-term weight control involves the combination of diet, exercise, and behavior modification. University-based research programs using such combinations of diet, exercise, and behavior modification typically produce weight losses of 9–13.6 kg at the end of a 20-week program. Approximately 60% of this weight loss is maintained over a year of follow-up.[1]

Exercise is an important aspect of weight control intervention because the energy expenditure associated with regular activity has the potential to create a state of negative energy balance. Exercise may also minimize the loss of lean body mass and the decrease in resting energy expenditure that accompanies weight loss[2] and may maximize the cardiovascular benefits.[3]

Recently, the National Heart, Lung and Blood Institute Expert Panel on the Identification, Evaluation, and Treatment of Overweight and Obesity in Adults reviewed the literature on diet and exercise.[4]

A similar review was also conducted by Wing.[5] Both reviews concluded that exercise alone (without a dietary intervention component) produces only modest weight losses (~2 kg). This is because most overweight individuals increase their exercise only modestly, leading to small energy deficits. Moreover, the increase in physical activity may be compensated for by increases in caloric intake and changes in activity patterns after exercise.

Exercise is more effective when used as a component of a weight loss intervention, in combination with caloric restriction, rather than as the sole treatment modality. The combination of diet plus exercise has been shown to improve weight loss compared with diet alone. Across 15 studies comparing diet only to diet plus exercise for short-term weight loss, 12 showed a greater weight loss with diet plus exercise.[4] However, it should be noted that the difference was often small (averaging only 2 kg) and often not statistically significant. The benefits of diet plus exercise, relative to diet alone, are more apparent in studies using moderate caloric restriction rather than very-low-calorie diets (VLCDs) because the severity of caloric restriction of VLCDs may overshadow the potential benefits of exercise.

The combination of diet plus exercise also appears more effective for maintenance of weight loss rather than for initial weight loss. The Expert Panel[4] identified three studies of the long-term effect of diet only versus diet plus exercise; all three favored the combination. In a meta-analysis of the long-term effects of diet only versus diet plus exercise, Miller et al.[6] found that at the 1-year follow-up, patients in the diet only group had maintained a weight loss of 6.6 kg, whereas the diet plus exercise group had maintained a weight loss of 8.6 kg. Wing[5] identified six studies comparing diet and diet plus exercise with follow-up periods of ≥1 year. All six studies indicated larger weight losses with diet plus exercise, but the differences were statistically significant in only two of the six. Thus, these studies consistently suggest that long-term weight losses may be improved by using a combination of diet plus exercise.

Randomized trials may underestimate the long-term benefits of exercise because some participants in the diet only conditions may increase their physical activity over time, whereas some in the diet plus exercise conditions may decrease their activity. Stronger evidence suggesting the benefits of exercise for long-term weight loss is seen in correlational analyses.[7] Consistently, those individuals who report the best long-term weight loss report that they have continued to be physically active. Whether the exercise promotes weight loss maintenance per se or is a marker for a constellation of behaviors related to weight-controlling behaviors is unclear from such correlational studies.

Data from the National Weight Control Registry also highlight the importance of exercise for long-term maintenance of weight loss.[8] In this registry of now over 3,000 individuals who have lost at least 13.6 kg (mean 28 kg) and kept it off for at least 1 year (mean 6 years), exercise appears to be a key maintenance strategy. Participants in the registry report that they maintain their weight loss by continuing to eat a low-calorie, low-fat diet and performing high levels of physical activity. These participants report expending ~2,800 kcal/week in physical activity and typically accomplish this through a combination of walking and light-, medium-, or high-intensity sport activities.

Exercise as a Way to Prevent Weight Gain in Patients on Intensive Insulin Therapy

Several recent studies have suggested that weight gain is a potential negative effect of intensified insulin therapy in subjects with type 1 diabetes.[9] Moreover, the effect of intensive insulin treatment on body weight is related to the degree of improvement in glycemic control. Thus, patients who are initially in poorest control, and apparently wasting a large number of calories in glycosuria, experience the greatest weight gain with intensive therapy. Efforts to prevent weight gain in these individuals have not been systematically investigated, but it would appear that the combination of increased exercise and moderate caloric restriction would again be most successful in these individuals, as in other overweight individuals.

Developing an Effective Weight Loss Program

Given that the combination of diet, exercise, and behavior modification is most effective for long-term weight loss, each of these components will be briefly discussed below.

Modifying Dietary Intake to Promote Weight Loss

The dietary component of behavioral weight loss programs focuses on both decreasing overall caloric intake and lowering the amount of dietary fat. Traditionally, most behavioral weight loss programs have used a diet of 1,200–1,500 kcal/day. Subjects are taught to self-monitor the foods they consume and to calculate the calories in those foods. A great deal of flexibility is provided to subjects in selecting the foods to consume as long as they stay within their calorie goal. Exchange system diets have also been used in many treatment programs to produce weight loss and ensure a balanced dietary intake.

Recently, behavioral treatment programs have placed more emphasis on lowering dietary fat intake. Subjects are given dietary fat goals in the range of 20–30% of calories from fat. Focusing on lowering dietary fat and reducing overall caloric intake appears more effective for weight loss than focusing on caloric restriction alone.[1]

VLCDs, defined as diets of <800 kcal/day, have also been used in the treatment of overweight patients in general and overweight individuals with type 2 diabetes in particular.[10] VLCDs appear safe when used with carefully selected patients and appropriate medical management. Moreover, they are extremely effective in producing initial weight losses and improving glycemic control. Unfortunately, however, techniques are not yet available to help patients maintain these weight losses; consequently, when studied at the 1-year follow-up, subjects treated with behavior modification and a VLCD maintained weight losses comparable to those treated with behavior modification and a more moderate 1,000–1,500 kcal/day regimen. Intermittent use of VLCDs (1 day each week or 1 week each month) may also improve initial weight loss and glycemic control.[11]

Several recent studies have suggested that structured meal plans (which tell patients exactly what they should eat for each meal) and portion-controlled diets (where liquid meal replacement or prepared foods are used for several meals each day) are helpful to participants, especially in the early weeks of weight control interventions.[1,12]

Modifying Physical Activity Patterns to Promote Weight Loss and Maintenance

The physical activity component of weight loss programs is designed to increase overall calorie expenditure. Consequently, the types of activities emphasized are those of low intensity (50% of maximum) and long duration (1 h/session), such as walking, bicycling, or swimming. Subjects are encouraged to exercise frequently (initially five times per week) because frequent exercise has been shown to be most effective for weight loss. No additional benefits in terms of weight loss are seen with high-intensity exercise.[2] Moreover, high-intensity exercise may increase the risk of injuries and attrition. Walking is recommended for the typical overweight patient with type 2 diabetes (60 years of age and 200 lb). Participants are encouraged to start exercise slowly, walking about one-half a mile for 5 days a week. The distance is gradually increased until participants reach a goal of 2 miles per day for 5 days a week (or ~1,000 kcal/week).

Recently, several studies have suggested that weight loss maintainers may actually do far higher levels of physical activity, reporting levels of 2,000–3,000 kcal/week, rather than the typically recommended level of 1,000 kcal/week.[8,13] Further studies to validate these self-report data and to compare prescriptions of 1,000 versus 2,500 kcal/week are needed to determine the most appropriate dose of exercise to recommend for weight loss maintenance.

The major issue in developing an exercise program for overweight patients with type 2 diabetes is the problem of long-term adherence. As noted in other chapters in this book (see Chapters 6 and 13–15), few people are willing to maintain exercise habits long term, and clearly, long-term exercise habits are required to produce long-term weight control. To increase long-term adherence to exercise, the following suggestions are offered:

- **Encourage lifestyle exercise in addition to programmed exercise.** A distinction can be made between increasing daily physical activity (e.g., using stairs instead of elevators and parking farther from your destination) versus programmed exercise (setting aside a time each day for the purpose of exercise). Most behavioral weight loss programs encourage both types of exercise to produce the greatest overall change in caloric expenditure.

- **Supervised exercise may help patients begin exercise, but home-based exercise may be beneficial in the long term.** Providing supervised exercise at the start of a weight loss program has been shown to improve weight loss and maintenance.[14] This supervised exercise may entail simply leading a group of overweight patients on a walk. The group format and the support of the leader may be helpful in maximizing the initial reinforcement value of exercise. However, for long-term maintenance, the home-based formats appear more effective.[15] Perhaps over time, the increased flexibility that is found in a home-based program becomes crucial for maintenance of the behavior change.

- **Break exercise into small sessions.** The number one barrier to physical activity is lack of time. Therefore, it may be easier for patients to find several 10-min time periods in their day for exercise rather than to find a 30- to 40-min block of time. Jakicic et al.[16,17] have shown that encouraging patients to exercise in multiple short sessions promotes initial adherence to exercise and may be beneficial for weight loss. Moreover, improvements in cardiovascular fitness appear equivalent with short- and long-session exercise regimens.
- **Home exercise equipment.** To date, there has been only one study investigating the benefit of providing home exercise equipment to overweight patients.[17] This study suggested that participants in a behavioral weight loss program who were given a treadmill for their home use had better long-term adherence to exercise and better long-term weight losses than participants who were given the same exercise goals but not given the equipment.
- **Focus on decreasing sedentary activity as well as increasing physical activity.** The number of hours of television viewing has been shown to be correlated with the prevalence of obesity. Based on this finding, several researchers have developed clinical programs and school-based interventions that focus on decreasing the time spent on sedentary activities, such as television viewing or computer games. These programs have shown that decreasing sedentary activity can promote weight loss or prevent weight gain in children.[18] Such approaches have not yet been studied in overweight adults.

Behavior Modification

The third component of an effective weight loss program is behavior modification. Behavior modification techniques are designed to help patients change their behavior by changing the cues and reinforcers in their environment. Behavioral strategies are usually taught to patients during a series of 16–24 weekly group sessions. Key behavioral strategies include the following:

- **Self-monitoring.** Participants are instructed to record both the foods they consume and the physical activity they perform. By determining the caloric value of each, patients learn to identify problem foods and patterns in their eating and exercise habits. These records provide helpful feedback to patients on their behavior changes. For example, they can see gradual increases in the number of calories expended through exercise each week. These records can also be used by the therapist to identify behaviors that require further attention.
- **Stimulus control.** Participants are taught to increase cues for appropriate behaviors and decrease cues for inappropriate behaviors. Specifically, in the area of exercise, patients may be encouraged to leave out their exercise shoes to remind them to take a walk and/or to move the television (a cue for inappropriate behavior) to a more distant location.
- **Goal setting and reinforcement.** Participants are encouraged to set short-term, realistic goals (e.g., walking 2 miles per day 5 days this week) and to reinforce themselves when they achieve these goals. Reinforcers can be simple things such as buying a special magazine, or patients can put aside $1.00 for each mile walked until sufficient money is accrued for a larger reward.
- **Continued contact.** One of the key components of a behavioral treatment program is the contact between the patient, the therapist, and the other individuals in the treatment group. Recent studies have shown that continued contact over extended periods of time (biweekly for 18 months) can help overweight patients maintain their weight loss over time.[19] Even phone contacts have been shown to be helpful in maintaining exercise behaviors long term.[20]
- **Social support.** Natural sources of social support (friends and family) and experimentally created social support (sup-

port from peers in a weight loss program; team competitions) have both been shown to be helpful for maintenance of behavior changes and improved long-term weight loss.[21]

References

1. Wing RR: Behavioral approaches to the treatment of obesity. In *Handbook of Obesity*. Bray G, Bouchard C, James P, Eds. New York, Marcel Dekker, p. 855–73, 1998
2. Bouchard C, Depres J, Tremblay A: Exercise and obesity. *Obes Res* 1:133–47, 1993
3. Wood P, Stefanick M, Williams P, Haskell W: The effects on plasma lipoproteins of a prudent weight-reducing diet, with or without exercise, in overweight men and women. *N Engl J Med* 325:461–66, 1991
4. National Heart, Lung and Blood Institute Obesity Education Initiative Expert Panel on the Identification, Evaluation, and Treatment of Overweight and Obesity in Adults: Clinical guidelines on the identification, evaluation, and treatment of overweight and obesity in adults: the evidence report. *Obes Res* 6:51S–210S, 1998
5. Wing R: Physical activity in the treatment of the adulthood overweight and obesity: current evidence and research issues. *Med Sci Sports Exerc* 31:S547–52, 1999
6. Miller WC, Koceja DM, Hamilton EJ: A meta-analysis of the past 25 years of weight loss research using diet, exercise or diet plus exercise intervention. *Int J Obes* 21:941–47, 1997
7. Pronk NP, Wing RR: Physical activity and long-term maintenance of weight loss. *Obes Res* 2:587–99, 1994
8. Klem ML, Wing RR, McGuire MT, Seagle HM, Hill JO: A descriptive study of individuals successful at long-term maintenance of substantial weight loss. *Am J Clin Nutr* 66:239–46, 1997
9. Carlson MG, Campbell PJ: Intensive insulin therapy and weight gain in IDDM. *Diabetes* 42:1700–07, 1993
10. National Task Force on the Prevention and Treatment of Obesity: Very low-calorie diets. *JAMA* 270:967–74, 1993
11. Williams KV, Mullen ML, Kelley DE, Wing RR: The effect of short periods of caloric restriction on weight loss and glycemic control in type 2 diabetes. *Diabetes Care* 21:2–8, 1998

12. Wing RR: Strategies for changing eating and exercise behavior. In *Present Knowledge in Nutrition.* 8th ed. Bowman B, Russell R, Eds. Washington, DC, ILSI Press, 2001, p. 650–61
13. Jeffery RW, Wing RR, Thorson C, Burton LC: Use of personal trainers and financial incentives to increase exercise in a behavioral weight-loss program. *J Consult Clin Psychol* 66:777–83, 1998
14. Craighead LW, Blum MD: Supervised exercise in behavioral treatment for moderate obesity. *Behav Ther* 20:49–59, 1989
15. Perri MG, Martin AD, Leermakers EA, Sears SF, Notelovitz M: Effects of group- versus home-based exercise in the treatment of obesity. *J Consult Clin Psychol* 65:278–85, 1997
16. Jakicic JM, Wing RR, Butler BA, Robertson RJ: Prescribing exercise in multiple short bouts versus one continuous bout: effects on adherence, cardiorespiratory fitness, and weight loss in overweight women. *Int J Obes* 19:893–901, 1995
17. Jakicic J, Wing R, Winters C: Effects of intermittent exercise and use of home exercise equipment on adherence, weight loss, and fitness in overweight women. *JAMA* 282:1554–60, 1999
18. Epstein LH, Valoski AM, Vara LS, McCurley J, Wisniewski L, Kalarchian MA, Klein KR, Shrager LR: Effects of decreasing sedentary behavior and increasing activity on weight change in obese children. *Health Psychol* 14:109–15, 1995
19. Perri MG, McAdoo WG, Spevak PA, Newlin DB: Effect of a multicomponent maintenance program on long-term weight loss. *J Consult Clin Psychol* 52:480–81, 1984
20. King AC, Frey-Hewitt B, Dreon DM, Wood PD: The effects of minimal intervention strategies on long-term outcomes in men. *Arch Intern Med* 149:2741–46, 1989
21. Wing RR, Jeffery RW: Benefits of recruiting participants with friends and increasing social support for weight loss maintenance. *J Consult Clin Psychol* 67:132–38, 1999

Rena R. Wing, PhD, is from Brown University, Providence, RI.

20

Adjustment of Insulin and Oral Agent Therapy

MICHAEL BERGER, MD

Highlights

- Hypoglycemia in patients with insulin-treated diabetes may occur both during and after exercise.
- Rational strategies for its prevention are based on adjustments of insulin therapy.
- Specific insulin adjustments need to be individualized for a given patient based on his or her experience and the intensity and duration of exercise.
- To make adjustments in insulin dosage, the patient must have a sound knowledge of basic principles and must monitor his or her blood glucose frequently.
- Exercise-induced hypoglycemia usually cannot be avoided by changing the insulin injection site.
- Patients on intensive insulin therapy should, in general, be able to participate in sports without an excessively high risk of exercise-induced hypoglycemia.

- During and after long-term exercise, type 2 diabetic patients on sulfonylurea therapy may require a dose reduction of the insulin secretagogue and/or additional carbohydrate intake to prevent hypoglycemia.

Patients with diabetes frequently need to adjust their insulin therapy to prevent hypoglycemia. Reasons for this adjustment include *1*) the dramatic changes in insulin sensitivity that occur in muscle during and after exercise; *2*) the fact that the stimulation of hepatic glucose production, which is essential for maintaining normal blood glucose levels during exercise, is blocked or partially inhibited by the hyperinsulinemia that results from exogenous insulin substitution;[1] and *3*) the physiological decrease of circulating insulin levels (due to decreased β-cell secretion) at the beginning of physical exercise, which is instrumental in allowing an increase in hepatic glucose production, may not take place in patients on insulin treatment. All of these events contribute to the risk of exercise-induced hypoglycemia in insulin-treated diabetic patients.

Hypoglycemia induced by exercise has been recognized as a threat to people with diabetes ever since insulin treatment became available. Unfortunately, it has prevented some young diabetic patients from participating in sports and games for decades. Usually, this lack of participation is because of their own or their teachers' and parents' fear of exercise-induced hypoglycemia and their inability to prevent it. Even today, a high percentage of reported episodes of severe hypoglycemia in children and adolescents occur as a result of exercise.[2,3] This highlights the lack of understanding of all concerned of the means to prevent exercise-induced hypoglycemia, especially by appropriate adjustments of insulin therapy.

Exercise-induced hypoglycemia was described with admirable clarity by R.D. Lawrence in 1926[4] as a phenomenon whereby physical activity acts as a potentiator of the hypoglycemic action of insulin. Based on a single experiment with one diabetic patient, combined with his clinical experience with two others, Lawrence developed his decisive recommendations to prevent exercise-induced hypoglycemia almost 70 years ago. He stated that before vigorous or prolonged exercise, the insulin dose may have to be reduced substantially, often by as much as 50%. Lawrence also pointed out that a patient's insulin dosage after physical activity may also need to be reduced to avoid postexercise episodes of hypoglycemia. According to his experience, these basic recommendations could easily be included in an appropriate educational program: "Patients should and do easily learn to reduce their insulin before unaccustomed exercise or activity. Even after exercise . . . it is usually advisable to reduce the next dose of insulin." It remains unexplained why such sophisticated guidance based on solid clinical research and experience has failed to make its way into routine clinical practice for so long.

Adjustment of Insulin Therapy Before and After Exercise

Any rational strategy to prevent exercise-induced hypoglycemia in insulin-treated patients must be based on an adjustment of insulin therapy. By reducing the iatrogenic hyperinsulinemia at appropriate times,[5] such adjustments are intended to mimic the fall of serum insulin levels early during exercise and to allow for increased insulin sensitivity during and after physical activity. If adjusting insulin therapy is impossible or unnecessary (e.g., in case physical exercise was not anticipated or was of a duration of <30 min), supplemental carbohydrates before and during exercise may be used to counterbalance the iatrogenic hyperinsulinemia (see Chapter 17).

In almost all instances when physical exercise of moderate or higher intensity exceeds 30 min, planned adjustments in insulin therapy are required to ensure optimal performance and to minimize the risk of hypoglycemia. In practice, physicians need to calculate the percentage by which patients should reduce their dosages of short-acting and prolonged insulin preparations or insulin infusion rates at times before, during, and after physical activity. Numerous investigators have directed their attention to this question, and an impressive number of publications have attempted to work out precise and practical recommendations and guidelines. Some of them are described in the following sections.

Altering the Insulin Injection Site

After reports in the 1970s of a paradoxical increase of serum insulin levels in patients exercising shortly after insulin injection, attempts were made to avoid exercise-induced hypoglycemia by changing the site of the insulin injection to parts of the body that were not involved or were substantially less involved in planned physical activity.[6] Thus, it was widely suggested that patients inject their insulin dose into the abdomen or the arm instead of the leg if they were about to jog or ride their bicycles. However, with the possible exception of vigorous exercise initiated within the first 30 min after an injection of regular insulin, this recommendation turned out to be quite useless and, in fact, potentially dangerous: exercise-induced hypoglycemia cannot be avoided by simply changing the insulin injection site.[7]

If the plasma insulin level is high for any reason, hypoglycemia is likely to occur. For this reason, the intramuscular application of insulin should be meticulously avoided because contractions will accelerate the absorption of insulin into the circulation from the musculature.[8] Also, the ambient temperature of the injection site needs to be taken into account because a hot environment may profoundly accelerate insulin absorption kinetics during exercise.[9]

Decreasing Insulin Dosages

In principle, diabetologists and their patients have returned to the basic recommendations of Lawrence[4] in an effort to develop strategies for preventing exercise-induced hypoglycemia. In practice, variables such as type of exercise, mode of insulin therapy, clinical characteristics, and condition of the patient have made the formulation of precise, effective, and safe rules difficult.[10] Nevertheless, a number of basic principles for the prevention of exercise-induced hypoglycemia have been worked out.

In anticipation of a long period of exercise (e.g., hiking, bicycle touring, long distance running, or cross-country skiing) that begins during the morning hours, the prebreakfast insulin dosage will have to be reduced by >50%. On a day of marathon running, insulin dosages may have to be reduced by >80%. A postexercise reduction of insulin dosages is often necessary after prolonged endurance exercise, even on the following day. The amount by which the insulin dose is decreased in these circumstances will also depend on the type of insulin treatment used by the patient. Thus, in patients predominantly treated with long-acting insulin preparations, it may even be necessary to withhold insulin on the morning of a day when prolonged and intense exercise is planned. In type 1 diabetic patients on more modern types of insulin treatment, i.e., intensified insulin therapy (at least 50% of daily insulin requirements administered as regular insulin), a withdrawal of insulin for an entire day of extraordinary physical activity will not be possible without risk of potentially harmful degrees of hyperglycemia.

The longer the physical activity and the better the patient is physically trained and adapted to exercise, the more drastic the insulin dosage reduction needs to be. Shorter-term, exhaustive, and stressful forms of exercise (such as certain highly competitive sports) may lead to transient phases of hyperglycemia, especially in less well-trained individuals. If not adequately informed, these patients may be surprised and disturbed by postexercise hyperglycemia and may wrongly decide to inject extra insulin in this situation. The biological effect of such an extra injection of insulin will often coincide with the postexercise increase in insulin sensitivity, and an episode of potentially severe hypoglycemia can result.

Several authors have tried to link the risk of exercise-induced hypoglycemia to the time of day when the exercise is performed. Obviously, the risk of hypoglycemia is particularly low if patients with type 1 diabetes exercise before their morning insulin injection. In this situation, strenuous exercise might very well precipitate substantial hyperglycemia because of potential hypoinsulinemia at this time of the day.

Not unexpectedly, the risk of nocturnal hypoglycemia is particularly high when exercise is performed in the evening hours. To prevent this, a reduction of the predinner insulin dosages by ≥50% may be required. Some physicians are hesitant to have their patients exercise in the evening hours because of the risk of nocturnal hypoglycemia. However, a great number of our patients can only exercise in the evening, at least on workdays; hence, appropriate adjustments for evening exercise need to be worked out for and with these individuals.

The time span between the onset of exercise and the previous insulin injection, the type of insulin preparation used, and the strategy for insulin substitution are all important considerations for fine-tuning the adjustment of insulin dosage to maintain normoglycemia during and after exercise. Patients also will have to take into account their preferences with regard to the consumption of extra carbohydrates when deciding what insulin dosage adjustments they have to make. For examples of adjustments of insulin dosage to avoid insulin-induced hypoglycemia, see Table 20.1.

TABLE 20.1 Examples of Insulin Adjustments for Two Patients on Intensive Insulin Therapy

	Insulin Units (Regular/NPH)				SMBG (mg/dl)				
Day	Morning Regular/ NPH	Prelunch Regular	Predinner Regular	Bedtime NPH	Morning	Prelunch	Predinner	Bedtime	Remarks
M	6/10	6	6	8	110	90	130	140	
T	6/10	6	3	6	130	100	120	100	Tennis*
W	6/10	6	8	8	110	120	100	120	Dinner party
F	8/14	4	6	8	120	110	100	140	
S	4/6	0	3	4	130	100	90	130	Hiking†
Su	6/10	4	6	8	90	130	120	130	

*Tennis for 2 h at 7:30 P.M. †Hiking all day on the flat.

The recently available, rapidly absorbed (peak at 30–60 min), short-acting (~4 h) insulin analog insulin lispro has been used increasingly to diminish postprandial hyperglycemia. Depending on the temporal relationship between administration and carbohydrate intake, postprandial exercise recommendations for the reduction of preprandial insulin dosages may have to be somewhat adapted to the different time course of action when using insulin lispro.[11]

For type 1 diabetic patients treated predominantly with long-acting insulin preparations (conventional insulin therapy), adjustments of insulin therapy in anticipation of exercise can prove difficult. In particular, insulin preparations with longer half-lives, by causing sustained hyperinsulinemia, can interfere with glycemic control during and after intense, prolonged exercise. Accordingly, diabetic athletes in the U.S. opted for intensified insulin therapy emphasizing shorter-acting insulins to ensure optimal and safe performance long before this form of treatment became generally accepted. Because intensified insulin therapy is gradually becoming the standard treatment for type 1 diabetic patients, comments on potential adjustments of other insulin substitution strategies can be restricted.

For patients with type 1 or type 2 diabetes on conventional (twice-daily) therapy (e.g., twice-daily NPH + regular), the duration and intensity of physical exercise may need to be limited to keep performance and safety at optimal levels because possibilities for adjusting insulin dosages to reflect the changing insulin requirements during and after exercise are limited by variable kinetics of intermediate- and long-acting insulin preparations. Table 20.2 gives some examples of insulin

TABLE 20.2 Examples of Insulin Adjustments for a Patient on Conventional Insulin Therapy

	Insulin Units (30% Regular/70% NPH)		SMBG (mg/dl)			
Day	**Morning**	**Predinner**	**Morning**	**Prelunch**	**Predinner**	**Remarks**
T	32	16	140		130	
W	28	14	130	100	90	Gardening*
Th	32	16	120	120	140	

*Exercise is mild-intensity gardening between 9:00 A.M. and noon.

dose adjustments in connection with exercise for patients on conventional insulin regimens.

Even more complex and unpredictable is the situation for patients with type 2 diabetes on combination therapies (e.g., NPH or ultralente insulin in the evening and a sulfonylurea drug in the morning). If such a patient plans to exercise in the morning, the use of two different hypoglycemic principles with independent mechanisms of action and varying half-lives makes it next to impossible to recommend a rational and effective adjustment of insulin/sulfonylurea dosages to mimic a near-physiological insulinemia. Because these therapeutic regimens seem to be restricted to elderly patients for whom only mild-intensity exercise is appropriate, a reduction (or omission) of the morning sulfonylurea dose, along with some extra carbohydrates, may suffice to counter the increased peripheral glucose use resulting from physical activities. For patients who want to enjoy physical exercise of prolonged duration and a high degree of intensity, who want to exercise irregularly according to changing daily schedules and preferences, or who are competitive athletes and need intensive physical training, it must be concluded that the necessary adjustments of insulin dosages can only be made in the framework of intensified insulin therapy.

Adjustment of Oral Therapy

In patients with type 2 diabetes, Minuk et al.[12] observed a failure of plasma insulin levels to exhibit a normal physiological decline during exercise. However, this finding has remained unconfirmed. In any case, exercise-induced hypoglycemia in diet-treated type 2 diabetic patients has not been observed.[13] With the increasing insulin sensitivity that occurs during or after physical exercise, it may be possible to reduce the dosage of any oral antidiabetic agent (such as is done with insulin treatment). Since the publication of the United Kingdom Prospective Diabetes Study,[14,15] the treatment of type 2 diabetic patients without clinically apparent coronary artery disease with glibenclamide and—for obese patients—with metformin monotherapy can be considered effective and safe according to the principles of evidence-based medicine. However, exercise-induced hypoglycemia has been reported in sulfonylurea-treated patients, although data on incidence rates are not available.

In young healthy subjects treated with glibenclamide, it was shown that exercise-induced hypoglycemia during sulfonylurea treatment could develop via an inability to suppress stimulated insulin secretion during physical activity.[16] However, in overweight, moderately hyperglycemic type 2 diabetic patients, exercise was shown to attenuate the glibenclamide-induced increase in serum insulin levels. Despite this, exercise had a substantial hypoglycemic effect in these glibenclamide-treated patients.[17] Recently, Larsen et al.[18] published a somewhat more systematic study of the interactions between exercise and glibenclamide in postabsorptive individuals with type 2 diabetes. They concluded that in these physically active patients, factors such as medication, extent of exercise, and intake of carbohydrates should be mutually adjusted—in much the same way as they are in insulin-treated diabetic patients. Because most of these studies were carried out after an overnight fast, their clinical relevance with regard to the risk of exercise-induced hypoglycemia in a more typical situation may be limited.

Overall, these reports suggest that during and after long-term exercise in type 2 diabetic patients on sulfonylurea therapy, the prevention of hypoglycemia may require a dose reduction of the insulin secretagogue and/or additional carbohydrate intake. As long as regular carbohydrate intake is maintained, the risk of exercise-induced hypoglycemia during sulfonylurea treatment in type 2 diabetic patients appears to be remote.

Because of their particular modes of action, metformin and other classes of oral antidiabetic agents, such as acarbose or glitazones, are not expected to precipitate exercise-induced hypoglycemia, whereas an exercise-induced increase in lactate levels may be further increased during metformin treatment.

Conclusions

Patients need to adjust their insulin therapy on the basis of personal experiences to avoid exercise-induced hypoglycemia. This adjustment requires a sound knowledge of basic principles and frequent self-monitoring of blood glucose (SMBG). SMBG remains the patient's primary yardstick for managing his or her glycemia and effectively and safely participating in sports and games.

A structured treatment and teaching program that includes instruction on how to deal with exercise-induced hypoglycemia has proven very useful. After 3 years, intensified insulin therapy in an unselected group of ~700 consecutive type 1 diabetic patients resulted in a fall in HbA_{1c} levels to a mean of 7.6% (after 6 years, 7.9%) and a significant decrease in the incidence of severe hypoglycemia to 0.13 cases per patient per year (after 6 years, 0.18).[19,20] In patients with severe hypoglycemia, exercise played only a minor role as a precipitating factor.

This study suggests that patients on intensified insulin therapy should, in general, be able to participate in sports without an excessively high risk of exercise-induced hypoglycemia, provided they have participated in an adequate treatment and teaching program. The educational program may need to include a discussion of hypoglycemia risks because of such factors as hypoglycemia unawareness, nephropathy, early pregnancy, or other factors specific to the individual patient. Suggested general guidelines for patients are given in Table 20.3.

In addition to building up a personal body of experience and growing self-confidence, diabetic patients who are active and ambitious in sports have learned much from each other. The Diabetes Exercise and Sports Association (DESA) is a unique and effective example of a self-help group of diabetic patients experienced and successful in sports and athleticism (see RESOURCES at the end of the book).[21] Among its members are numerous diabetic individuals of international reputation, including several Olympic Gold Medal winners. Within this group, a wealth of personal experiences, ideas, and hints that could never have been provided by the medical profession or by

TABLE 20.3 General Guidelines to Avoid Exercise-Induced Hypoglycemia in Insulin-Treated Patients

- Measure blood glucose before, (during), and after exercise.
- Unplanned exercise should be preceded by extra carbohydrates, e.g., 20–30 g/30 min of exercise; insulin may have to be decreased after exercise.
- If exercise is planned, insulin dosages must be decreased before and after exercise, according to the exercise intensity and duration as well as the personal experience of the patient; insulin dosage reductions may amount to 50–90% of daily insulin requirements.
- During exercise, easily absorbable carbohydrates may have to be consumed.
- After exercise, an extra carbohydrate-rich snack may be necessary.
- Diabetic patients interested in sports need a specific education program for self-treatment; they should contact the DESA.

diabetes educators are exchanged. It is not surprising that almost all of the members of DESA are on intensified insulin therapies. Wherever possible, a member of the DESA (which has chapters in many countries) should be asked to participate in the specific education and counseling of patients who want to begin exercise or competitive sports or who want to continue their careers as amateur or professional athletes despite having developed diabetes.

References

1. Zinman B, Murray FT, Vranic M, McClean PA, Albisser AM, Leibel BS, Marliss EB: Glucoregulation during moderate exercise in insulin-treated diabetics. *J Clin Endocrinol Metab* 45:641–52, 1977
2. McDonald MJ: Post-exercise late-onset hypoglycemia in insulin-dependent diabetic patients. *Diabetes Care* 10:584–88, 1987
3. Bergada I, Suissa S, Dufrense J, Schiffrin A: Severe hypoglycemia in children. *Diabetes Care* 12:239–44, 1989
4. Lawrence RD: The effect of exercise on insulin action in diabetes. *Br Med J* 1:648–50, 1926
5. Zinman B, Vranic M, Albisser AM, Leibel BS, Marliss EB: The role of insulin in the metabolic response to exercise in diabetic man. *Diabetes* 28 (Suppl. 1):76–81, 1979
6. Koivisto VA, Felig P: Effects of leg exercise on insulin absorption in diabetic patients. *N Engl J Med* 298:77–83, 1978
7. Kemmer FW, Berchtold P, Berger M, Starke A, Cüppers HJ, Gries FA, Zimmermann H: Exercise-induced fall of blood glucose in insulin-treated diabetics unrelated to alteration of insulin mobilization. *Diabetes* 28:1131–37, 1979
8. Frid A, Östman J, Linde B: Hypoglycemia risk during exercise after intramuscular injection of insulin in the thigh in IDDM. *Diabetes Care* 13:473–77, 1990
9. Rönnemaa T, Koivisto VA: Combined effect of exercise and ambient temperature on insulin absorption and postprandial glycemia in type I diabetic patients. *Diabetes Care* 11:769–73, 1988
10. Kemmer FW: Prevention of hypoglycemia during exercise in type I diabetes. *Diabetes Care* 15 (Suppl. 4):1732–35, 1992
11. Tuominen JA, Karonen SL, Melamies L, Bolli G, Koivisto VA: Exercise-induced hypoglycemia in IDDM patients treated with a short-acting insulin analogue. *Diabetologia* 38:106–111, 1995

12. Minuk HL, Vranic M, Marliss EB, Hanna AK, Albisser AM, Zinman B: The glucoregulatory response to exercise in obese non-insulin dependent diabetes. *Am J Physiol* 240:E458–64, 1981
13. Vranic M, Rodgers C, Davidson JK, Marliss E: Exercise and stress in diabetes mellitus. In *Clinical Diabetes Mellitus: A Problem Oriented Approach.* 3rd ed. Davidson JK, Ed. New York, Thieme, 2000, p. 267–328
14. UKPDS 33: Intensive blood glucose control with sulfonylureas or insulin compared with conventional treatment and risk of complications in patients with type 2 diabetes. *Lancet* 352:837–53, 1998
15. UKPDS 34: Effect of intensive blood glucose control with metformin on complications in overweight patients with type 2 diabetes. *Lancet* 352:854–65, 1998
16. Kemmer FW, Tacken M, Berger M: Mechanism of exercise-induced hypoglycemia during sulfonylurea treatment. *Diabetes* 36:1178–82, 1987
17. Gudat U, Bungert S, Kemmer F, Heinemann L: The blood glucose lowering effects of exercise and glibenclamide in patients with type 2 diabetes mellitus. *Diabet Med* 15:194–98, 1998
18. Larsen JJ, Fleming D, Madsbad S, Vibe-Petersen J, Galbo H: Interaction of sulfonylureas and exercise on glucose homeostasis in type 2 diabetic patients. *Diabetes Care* 22:1647–54, 1999
19. Jörgens V, Grüsser M, Bott U, Mühlhauser I, Berger DM: Effective and safe translation of intensified insulin therapy to general internal medicine departments. *Diabetologia* 36:99–105, 1993
20. Bott S, Bott U, Berger M, Mühlhauser I: Intensified insulin therapy and the risk of severe hypoglycaemia. *Diabetologia* 40:926–32, 1997
21. Thurm U, Harper P: I'm running on insulin. *Diabetes Care* 15 (Suppl. 4):1811–13, 1992

Michael Berger, MD, is from Heinrich-Heine University Düsseldorf, Düsseldorf, Germany.

21

Insulin Pump Therapy With Continuous Subcutaneous Insulin Infusion and Exercise in Patients With Type 1 Diabetes

BERNARD ZINMAN, MDCM, FRCPC, FACP

Highlights

- Insulin pump therapy with continuous subcutaneous insulin infusion is commonly used to implement intensive diabetes management in patients with type 1 diabetes.
- Insulin pump therapy provides great flexibility for adjusting both meal doses and basal insulin requirements for exercise.
- For certain activities, patients can remove their pumps for short periods (<1 h) without any consequences. Pump removal for a longer period requires subcutaneous administration of a bolus of insulin to cover the insulin pump disconnect time.
- Skill in using insulin pump therapy to modify the infusion rate for particular activities is achieved through frequent self-monitoring of blood glucose and patient experience.

Insulin pump therapy has become a common means of implementing intensive diabetes management. In the U.S., more than 100,000 patients with type 1 diabetes are currently using insulin infusion pumps. It is now well established that the most effective insulin to use with pumps is insulin lispro, a rapid-acting meal insulin analogue.[1] The use of lispro allows for rapid translation of changes in the insulin infusion rate to circulating insulin levels and, thus, biological action. This is particularly important in a number of contexts including the following: adjusting premeal boluses of insulin to changing carbohydrate content of a meal, the modification of the basal rate of insulin infusion to compensate for changing basal requirements as illustrated by the dawn phenomenon, and, most relevant to this discussion, the change in insulin replacement necessitated by exercise. Insulin infusion pumps provide unique flexibility in being able to adjust insulin replacement for both postprandial or postabsorptive exercise.

Meal Dose Adjustments

Because most patients are using insulin lispro in their pumps, adjustment of premeal boluses is required when exercise is being performed at the peak time of action of the insulin lispro—namely, within 1–3 h after the injection. Under these circumstances, the usual insulin dose should be reduced by 50%.[2,3] As an example, a patient who has determined that he or she needs 10 units of insulin for a particular meal, based on the premeal glucose level and the carbohydrate content of that meal, may want to reduce the premeal bolus to 5 units if 45 min of tennis is planned 2 h after the insulin injection. With strenuous short-term exercise of 10 or 15 min, no adjustment in insulin may be required. Indeed, it has been shown that with short periods of strenuous exercise, hyperglycemia may occur.[4] It is of course essential that the patient measures his or her response to a particular insulin dose adjustment for a given activity and then modifies the adjustment algorithm accordingly.

Basal Insulin Modification

The modification in the basal insulin infusion rate is most easily made when patients are exercising before breakfast or 4–6 h after the last meal bolus. The precise changes will be determined by the duration and intensity of the exercise and monitoring of the patient's response to it. When done properly, this can result in excellent glycemic control with little risk of hypoglycemia or hyperglycemia. A useful starting point is to decrease the basal insulin infusion to half of the usual rate. As an example, if someone is on 1 unit/h, then an insulin infusion rate of 0.5 units/h could be tried for a planned jog lasting 1.5 h. Again, the same principle applies—namely, monitoring the response to a particular adjustment in insulin replacement will serve as an important guide to future adjustments in therapy. When the exercise is complete, the original basal rate can be resumed. However, subsequent meal boluses may also have to be adjusted because the exercise period will increase muscle insulin sensitivity. In addition, muscle glycogen repletion would be accelerated with an increased risk of hypoglycemia.[5]

Under some circumstances, the basal rate of insulin infusion may have to be suspended entirely. If this suspension is required, the pump user must be careful to ensure that the catheter is not blocked as a consequence of the lack of flow in the infusion set.

Removing the Pump

For certain activities, patients may prefer to remove their pumps because of excessive contact, movement, or sweating. Generally speaking, if the pump is removed for periods of <1 h, no insulin replacement is required. However, if the pump is removed for periods of 1–4 h, the patient should administer an insulin bolus with the pump before it is disconnected. Clearly, the quantity of the bolus replacement dose has to be modified to avoid hypoglycemia. Again, a good starting point is to reduce the total amount of insulin that would have been infused over that period by 50% and administer that as a bolus injection.

Specific Athletic Activities

Water Sports

The Desitronic pump is waterproof, and the MiniMed pump can be protected from the water by a waterproof case. Thus, the pump can be worn during water activities. Alternatively, the insulin pump can be removed for up to 1 h during water activities without any problems. This would be particularly desirable for vigorous water sports such as surfing, diving, or water polo.

Contact Sports

Although most sports can be safely enjoyed while wearing the insulin pump, there are some contact sports in which extra protection for the pump may be required (e.g., basketball, football, and hockey). Pump users have used a sports guard case and have also learned to wear the pump in a position where it is protected (e.g., the small of the back). In addition, protective padding can be used.

Skiing, Skating, and Winter Sports

It is important to appreciate that insulin can easily freeze when exposed to cold temperatures and that the pump user must protect the pump and tubing during winter sports. Obviously, appropriate clothing and wearing the pump under the inner layer of clothing next to the body provides the best protection from exposure to extremes of cold. Interestingly, patients participating in winter sports appear to use glucose more rapidly, and greater adjustments of both basal and bolus doses may be required as well as more frequent monitoring of glucose.

In summary, the insulin infusion pump provides the most flexibility in insulin dose adjustment and allows an individual to effectively manage insulin treatment in relation to nutrient intake and exercise. Skill in using the insulin pump and experience in determining particular glycemic responses to an exercise event are key elements of achieving successful metabolic control. The flexibility provided by insulin infusion pumps allows individuals to fully benefit from the enjoyments and therapeutic advantages of a healthy, physically active lifestyle.

References

1. Zinman B, Tildesley H, Chiasson JL, Tsui E, Strack T: Insulin lispro in CSII. *Diabetes* 46:440–43, 1997
2. Sonnenberg GE, Kemmer FW, Berger M: Exercise in type 1 (insulin-dependent) diabetic patients treated with continuous subcutaneous insulin infusion. *Diabetologia* 33:696–703, 1990

3. Schiffrin A, Parikh S: Accommodating planned exercise in type 1 diabetic patients on intensive treatment. *Diabetes Care* 8:337–43, 1985
4. Mitchell TH, Abraham G, Schiffrin A, Leiter LA, Marliss EB: Hyperglycemia after intense exercise in IDDM subjects during continuous subcutaneous insulin infusion. *Diabetes Care* 11:311–17, 1988
5. MacDonald MJ: Postexercise late-onset hypoglycemia in insulin-dependent diabetic patients. *Diabetes Care* 10:584–88, 1987

Bernard Zinman, MDCM, FRCPC, FACP, is from Mount Sinai Hospital and the University of Toronto, Toronto, Ontario, Canada.

Exercise in Patients With Diabetic Complications

22

The Diabetic Foot

MARVIN E. LEVIN, MD

Highlights

- Exercise programs play an important role in the management of diabetes.
- Most exercise programs involving the lower extremity are weight-bearing.
- Many people with diabetes have peripheral arterial disease (PAD) and peripheral neuropathy (PN), which can limit such activities.
- The diabetic patient with PN and loss of protective sensation should not engage in repetitive weight-bearing exercises, such as prolonged walking, treadmill, or jogging. Such activity in these patients may result in blistering, ulceration, infection, and amputation. Patients with previous plantar foot ulceration may have a recurrence.
- Patients with insensate feet can engage in non–weight-bearing exercises, such as swimming, bicycling, chair exercises, and arm exercises.

- Exercise programs for patients with PAD and PN should be prescribed by a physician and closely supervised.

Today, there is great enthusiasm for exercise for weight loss and cardiovascular conditioning. The diabetic individual gets an extra benefit because exercise improves glucose tolerance.[1] There is also evidence that brisk walking can reduce the incidence of type 2 diabetes.[2] In fact, the American Diabetes Association uses walking, a weight-bearing exercise, as a fundraiser in America's Walk for Diabetes.

Patients with diabetes frequently have peripheral arterial disease (PAD) and peripheral neuropathy (PN). These complications can limit weight-bearing exercise. Therefore, evaluation of PAD and PN should be carried out before prescribing a program of weight-bearing exercises.

Peripheral Arterial Disease

Evaluation of PAD is based on signs and symptoms (Table 22.1)[3] and on noninvasive vascular laboratory findings.[4] Intermittent claudica-

TABLE 22.1 Signs and Symptoms of PAD

- Intermittent claudication
- Cold feet
- Nocturnal pain
- Rest pain
- Nocturnal and rest pain relieved with leg dependency
- Absent pulses
- Blanching on elevation
- Delayed venous filling after elevation
- Dependent rubor
- Atrophy of subcutaneous fatty tissue
- Shiny appearance of skin
- Loss of hair on foot and toes
- Thickened nails, often with fungal infection
- Gangrene
- Miscellaneous
  - Blue toe syndrome
  - Acute vascular occlusion

tion is one of the most common symptoms of PAD. Charcot[5] was the first to describe a case of intermittent claudication in humans in 1858. The word claudication comes from the Latin meaning "to limp," but patients with claudication do not limp. They stop to rest. Cramping or an aching sensation characterizes pain associated with intermittent claudication, most often in the calf. The pain occurs with walking. It is relieved in a few minutes when the individual stops to rest without the need to sit down. The ischemic pain of intermittent claudication must always be differentiated from nonischemic pain called pseudo-claudication (Table 22.2). Patients with pseudoclaudication do not experience rapid relief with cessation of walking. Pain due to these conditions may last 15–20 min, and patients usually must sit down or change position.[6]

Patients with ischemic claudication are limited in the amount of walking exercise they can do. It should be kept in mind that individuals with diabetes might have significant PAD but no symptoms of intermittent claudication because PN has prevented the sensation of ischemic pain[7] or may be related to the distal distribution of peripheral vascular disease.[8] The basic treatment for intermittent claudication is nonsmoking and a supervised exercise program, provided that the patient does not have PN with loss of protective sensation. This treatment should be carried out under the direction of a physician, and a clearly defined program should be established. If patients are instructed simply to do a walking exercise, treatment may be incomplete and unsuccessful.

A walking program for intermittent claudication may improve not only collateral circulation but also muscle metabolism. Hiatt et al.[9] showed that exercise increases the formation of acylcarnitine from carnitine and acyl-CoA. This substance can produce pain. In Hiatt's

TABLE 22.2 Nonischemic Causes of Pain With Walking (Pseudoclaudication)

- Arthritis
- Muscle pain
- Radicular pain
- Spinal cord compression
- Thrombophlebitis
- Anemia
- Myxedema

series, those who were in a walking exercise program had less formation of acylcarnitine and less pain. In this group of patients, the decrease in pain was not associated with an increase in blood flow.

Rest pain and night pain, not due to neuropathy, are indicative of severe PAD. The presence of rest pain and night pain precludes a walking exercise program. These patients require vascular consultation and probable vascular surgery.

The presence of a dorsalis pedis and posterior tibial pulse does not rule out ischemic changes in the forefoot. Because exercise puts added strain on the forefoot and toes, careful evaluation of the blood flow to these areas should be made. If there is any question about this during physical examination, toe pressures as well as Doppler pressures at the ankle should be carried out.

The vascular laboratory findings can be very helpful in the evaluation of PAD. In most instances, a simple handheld Doppler can provide significant information regarding peripheral vascular status. An ankle-brachial index of ≤0.9 confirms the presence of PAD. Intermittent claudication usually begins when the ankle-brachial index is ≤0.75. However, there is a wide range of values before a patient actually detects ischemic claudication. In the patient with diabetes, the Doppler may give an erroneously high value because of calcification in the vessels, which decreases the compressibility. In the final analysis, a good history relating to ischemic symptoms as well as the experienced hand and eye can give an accurate evaluation of PAD. A complete vascular evaluation requires a workup in the vascular laboratory.

Peripheral Neuropathy

PN causing loss of protective sensation is the most important contraindication to weight-bearing exercise. It is therefore important to document the presence of PN, especially the loss of protective sensation. This is best carried out by using the Semmes-Weinstein monofilament (Fig. 22.1), which is a simple and inexpensive test. It can be performed by the patient at home.[10,11] The monofilament is pressed against the skin of the foot until it buckles. If the patient cannot detect pressure when the 5.07 monofilament, which applies 10 g of linear strength, is applied, protective sensation has been lost, and the patient has a high-risk foot. These patients should not engage in

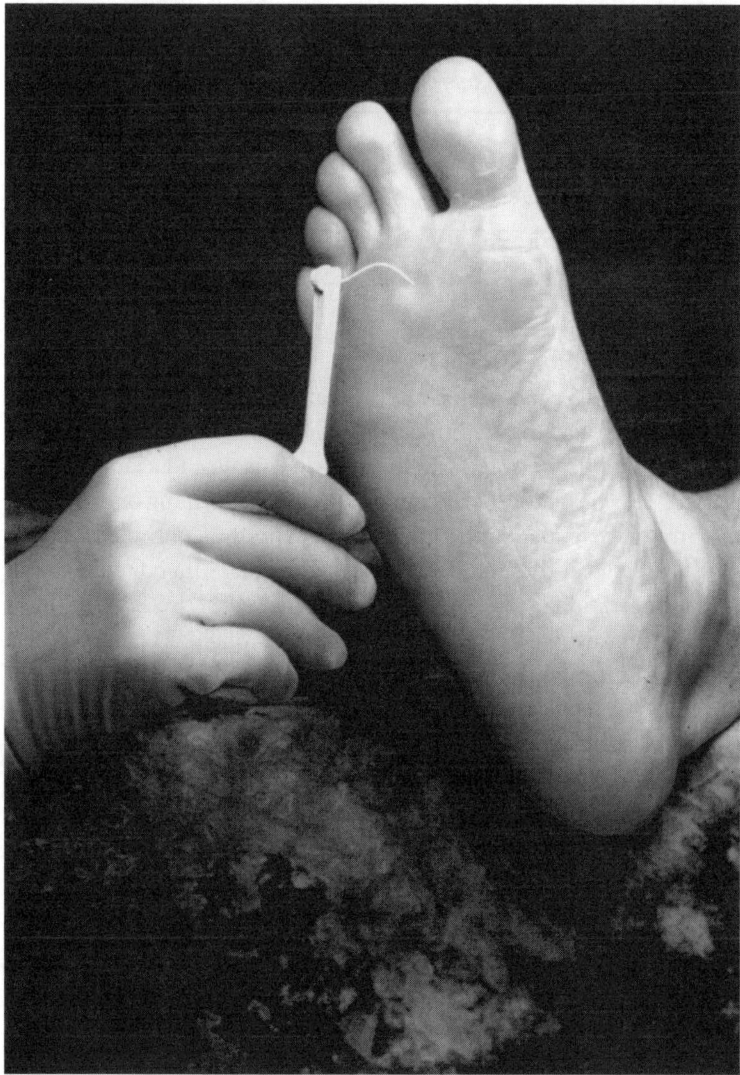

FIGURE 22.1 A 5.07 Semmes-Weinstein monofilament being applied to the plantar surface of the foot. Inability to feel the buckled monofilament indicates a loss of protective sensation.

TABLE 22.3 Contraindicated Exercises for Diabetic Patients With Loss of Protective Sensation

- Treadmill
- Prolonged walking
- Jogging
- Step exercises

weight-bearing exercise (Table 22.3). The areas to be tested are noted in Fig. 22.2.

PN with motor nerve involvement and interosseous muscle atrophy can result in foot deformities—particularly cocked-up or claw toes. This can lead to ulceration at the top and/or tip of the toes unless special in-depth footwear with a protective insole and a large toe box is used. This muscle imbalance can also cause a thinning or shifting of the protective fat pad under the metatarsal heads. Continued walking or exercising on these unprotected, deformed vulnerable areas can lead to ulceration.

Bunions, which are not in areas of direct weight bearing, can be a contraindication to lower-extremity exercise, especially if the patient has PN.

A third type of foot deformity is the Charcot foot. In the acute stage, it is characterized by a red, swollen foot, and the patient must be non–weight-bearing. This is best accomplished by a contact cast. Weight-bearing exercise is contraindicated. If the Charcot foot progresses to a deformed foot, a specially molded shoe is required, and again, weight-bearing exercise is contraindicated.

Diabetic Foot Ulcers

Diabetic plantar foot ulcers result from repetitive stress on insensitive feet that have increased plantar pressure. The presence of a diabetic foot ulcer is an absolute contraindication to any weight-bearing exercise. Diabetic patients with PN have increased pressure; those with ulceration tend to have the highest pressures. Plantar pressures are increased for three reasons: foot deformity, callous buildup, and limited joint mobility with a decrease in flexibility of the foot because of glycosylation of tendons and ligaments. Foot conditions limiting weight-bearing exercises are listed in Table 22.4.

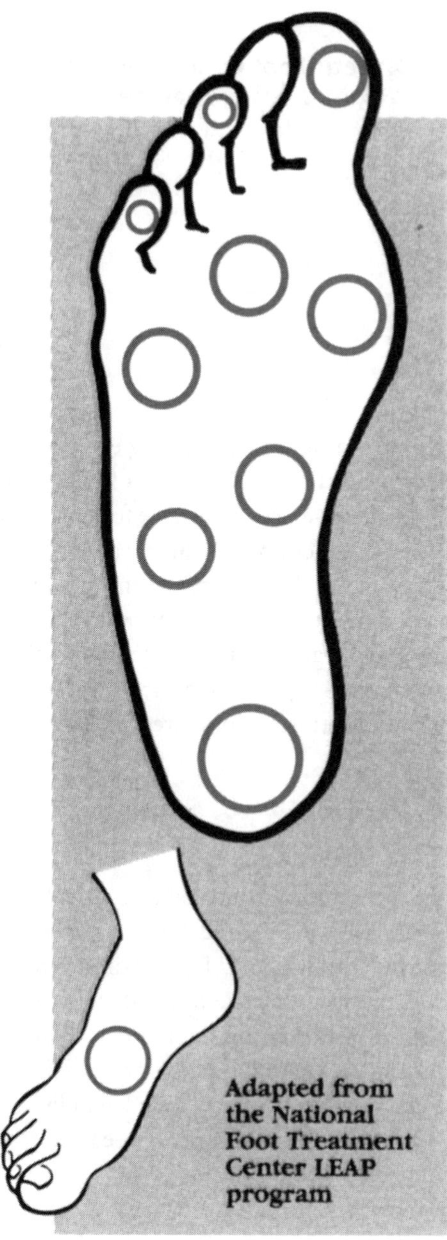

FIGURE 22.2 Areas of application of the Semmes-Weinsten monofilament to test for loss of protective sensation.

Reprinted with permission from Curative Health Services.

TABLE 22.4 Diabetic Foot Conditions Limiting Weight-Bearing Exercise

- Insensate foot
- Foot deformities
    - Cocked-up toes
    - Charcot foot
- Foot ulcer
- Previous foot ulcer

Relieving Foot Pressures

For the patient performing weight-bearing exercise, decreasing foot pressure provides protection against callus buildup and ulceration. A variety of approaches are used to relieve foot pressures. Simply removing the callus will reduce pressure in that area by close to 30%. The use of running or walking shoes decreases the rate of callus buildup[12] because the cushioning that is usually found in this type of shoe decreases pressure. Cavanagh and Ulbrecht[13] found that a cushioned shoe could reduce barefoot pressure by 45%. Special athletic hosiery can also reduce plantar pressure compared with going barefoot.[14]

Contraindicated Exercise in People With Diabetes and PN

Exercises that are contraindicated in diabetic patients with loss of protective sensation are listed in Table 22.3. Figure 22.3 shows the areas of maximum pressures with walking. The maximum pressure is on the forefoot, particularly the metatarsal head, at 20 lb/inch^2. When comparing this with the pressure of riding a stationary bicycle at 20 miles/h, with minimal resistance, we find that the pressure is only 11 lb/inch^2 (Fig. 22.4). Step exercises are contraindicated in individuals with an insensate foot. The repetitive stress and pressure from this type of exercise can result in blisters and ulceration.

Exercises for People With Diabetes and PN

Exercises recommended for patients with PN and loss of sensation are listed in Table 22.5. Swimming is an excellent exercise, but certain pre-

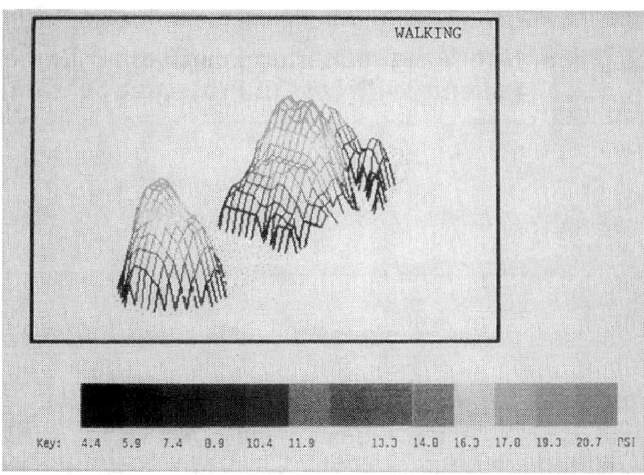

FIGURE 22.3 Foot pressure when walking in ordinary shoes is 20 lb/inch^2 on the forefoot and toes.

cautions must be taken. Diabetic patients who go swimming where there is a hot sandy beach or hot cement around a swimming pool must be cautioned to wear protective footwear to prevent severe burns to insensate feet. Swimming pools frequently have rough cement bottoms. Abrasion of the skin of the feet can occur. Unless the bottom of the pool is tiled, the patient should wear protective footwear in the pool.

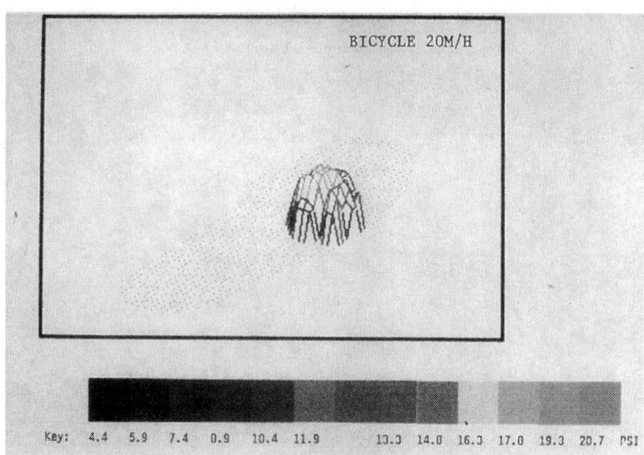

FIGURE 22.4 Pressure on the forefoot while riding a stationary bicycle with minimal resistance is 11 lb/inch^2.

TABLE 22.5 Non–Weight-Bearing Exercises for Diabetic Patients With Loss of Protective Sensation

- Swimming
- Bicycling
- Rowing
- Chair exercises
- Arm exercises

Long exposure to the water can lead to maceration of the skin, making it more susceptible to trauma. Chair exercises, shown in Fig. 22.5, can also involve lifting the legs more vigorously. Arm exercises, shown in Fig. 22.6, may be helpful.

Exercise and Amputation Level

Amputation is a common occurrence in individuals with diabetes. Exercise for the amputee represents a major problem. Velocity in walking is significantly impaired. Pinzur[15] has shown that a normal walk-

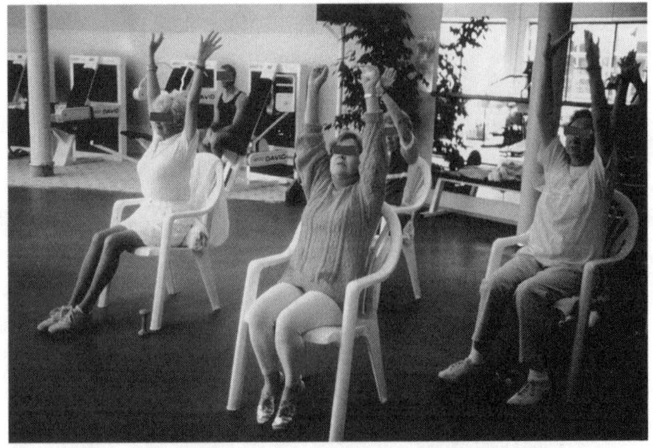

FIGURE 22.5 Chair exercises.

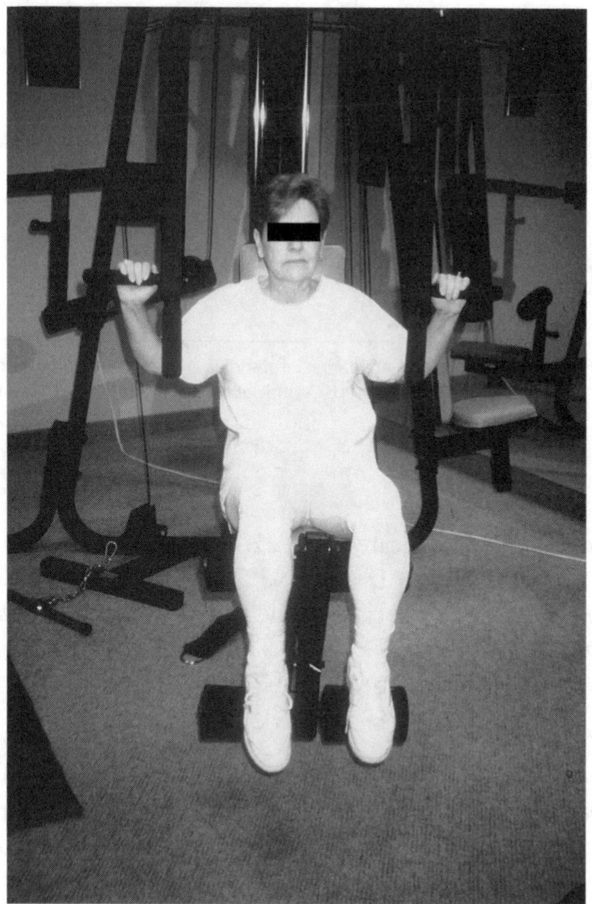

FIGURE 22.6 Arm exercises.

ing speed is 50 m/min or ~2 miles/h, but in a below-the-knee amputee, it is reduced to 40 m/min or ~1.6 miles/h.

A nonamputee's maximum walking speed is 80 m/min. A below-the-knee amputee's maximum walking speed is reduced to 55 m/min.[5] The energy cost of ambulating is also markedly increased (Table 22.6).[16,17] Therefore, walking exercises in the diabetic amputee are extremely limited. In addition, prolonged walking may subject the patient to trauma and ulceration of the stump.

TABLE 22.6 Energy Cost of Ambulation

Subjects	Optimal Speed (m/min)	Energy Cost	
		($ml\ O_2 \cdot min^{-1} \cdot kg^{-1}$)	($ml\ O_2 \cdot m^{-1} \cdot kg^{-1}$)
Normal	82	13.0	0.16
Syme	54	11.5	0.21
Below-the-knee	45	11.7	0.26
Above-the-knee	36	12.6	0.35
Crutches (normal subjects)	40	13.7	0.25

Adapted from Steinberg FU: Rehabilitation of the diabetic amputee and neuropathic disabilities. In *The Diabetic Foot*. 4th ed. Levin ME, O'Neal LW, Eds. St. Louis, MO, Mosby, 1988, p. 310–32.

Foot Care

The instructions for foot care (Table 22.7) are especially important for diabetic patients with PAD and PN.[18] Those patients with diabetes doing weight-bearing exercises should pay particular attention to the instructions.

Summary

Exercise is an important modality in the management of diabetes. However, because of complications of PAD and PN, with the development of the insensate foot, foot deformities, and increased foot pressure, weight-bearing exercises should be curtailed in these patients. The presence of an active foot ulcer is an absolute contraindication for weight-bearing exercise. Patients who have a previously healed ulcer must take special precautions when exercising because recurrence of the ulcer can be accelerated with weight-bearing exercise. Scar tissue is vulnerable to the sheer forces of walking. Patients with PAD, PN, and insensate feet can perform a variety of exercises, such as swimming, bicycling, rowing, chair exercises, and upper-body exercises.

Patients with diabetes, and especially those with PAD and PN, should have specific detailed instructions in foot care and in techniques for decreasing foot pressure before beginning an exercise program. Physical therapists and the personnel in exercise centers should discuss with the referring physician the type of exercise program the diabetic patient can undertake.

TABLE 22.7 Patient Instructions for the Care of the Diabetic Foot

- Do not smoke.
- Inspect feet daily for blisters, cuts, and scratches. The use of a mirror can aid in seeing the bottom of the feet. Always check between the toes.
- Wash feet daily. Dry carefully, especially between the toes.
- Avoid extremes of temperatures. Test water with hand or elbow before bathing.
- If feet feel cold at night, wear socks. Do not apply hot water bottles or heating pads. Do not soak feet in hot water.
- Do not walk on hot surfaces, such as sandy beaches or the cement around swimming pools.
- Do not walk barefoot.
- Do not use chemical agents for the removal of corns and calluses. Do not use corn plasters. Do not use strong antiseptic solutions on your feet.
- Do not use adhesive tape on your feet.
- Inspect the insides of shoes daily for foreign objects, nail points, torn lining, and rough areas.
- If vision is impaired, have a family member inspect your feet daily, trim nails, and buff down calluses.
- Do not soak feet.
- For dry feet, use a thin coat of a lubricating oil, such as baby oil. Apply this after bathing and drying the feet. Do not put the oil or cream between the toes. Consult your physician for detailed instructions.
- Wear properly fitting stockings. Do not wear mended stockings. Avoid stockings with seams. Change stockings daily.
- Do not wear garters.
- Shoes should be comfortable at the time of purchase. Do not depend on them to stretch out. Shoes should be made of leather. Running shoes may be worn after checking with your physician.
- Do not wear shoes without stockings.
- Do not wear sandals with thongs between the toes.
- Take special precautions in wintertime. Wear wool socks and protective footgear, such as fleece-lined boots.
- Cut toenails straight across.
- Do not cut corns and calluses. Follow instructions from your physician or podiatrist.
- See your physician regularly and be sure that your feet are examined at each visit.
- Notify your physician or podiatrist immediately if you develop a blister or sore on your foot.
- Be sure to inform your podiatrist that you have diabetes.

Adapted from Levin.[18]

References

1. American Diabetes Association: Diabetes mellitus and exercise (Position Statement). *Diabetes Care* 22 (Suppl. 1):S49–53, 1999
2. Wunsch H: Risk of type 2 diabetes reduced by regular brisk walking. *JAMA* 282:1433–39, 1999
3. Young JR: Clinical clues to peripheral vascular disease. In *Peripheral Vascular Diseases.* 2nd ed. Young JR, Olin JW, Bartholomew JR, Eds. St. Louis, MO, Mosby, 1996, p. 3–17
4. Strandness DE Jr: Noninvasive vascular laboratory and vascular imaging. In *Peripheral Vascular Diseases.* 2nd ed. Young JR, Olin JW, Bartholomew JR, Eds. Mosby, St. Louis, MO, 1996, p. 33–64
5. Charcot JM: Sur la claudication intermittente, observee dans un cas d'obliteration complete de l'une des arteres iliaque primitive [On the intermittent claudication observed in a case of complete obliteration in one of the primary iliac arteries]. *Compt Rendu Soc Biol* 10:225, 1858
6. Levin ME, Sicard GA, Rubin BG: Peripheral vascular disease in the diabetic patient. In *Ellenberg & Rifkin's Diabetes Mellitus.* 5th ed. Porte D Jr, Sherwin RS, Eds. Stamford, CT, Appleton & Lange, 1997, p. 1127–58
7. Coffman JD: Intermittent claudication. In *Textbook of Vascular Medicine.* lst ed. Tooke JE, Low GDO, Eds. London, Arnold, 1996, p. 207–20
8. The International Working Group on the Diabetic Foot: Peripheral vascular disease. In *International Consensus on the Diabetic Foot.* Amsterdam, International Working Group on the Diabetic Foot, 1999, p. 33–41
9. Hiatt WR, Regensteiner JG, Hargarten ME, Wolfel EE, Brass EP: Benefit of exercise conditioning for patients with peripheral arterial disease. *Circulation* 81:602–09, 1990
10. Levin ME: Diabetes and peripheral neuropathy (Editorial). *Diabetes Care* 21:1, 1998
11. Birke JA, Rolfsen RJ: Evaluation of a self-administered sensory testing tool to identify patients at risk of diabetes-related foot problems. *Diabetes Care* 21:23–25, 1998
12. Soulier SM: The use of running shoes in the prevention of plantar diabetic ulcers. *J Am Podiatr Med Assoc* 76:395–400, 1986

13. Cavanagh PR, Ulbrecht JS: Biomechanics of the foot in diabetes mellitus. In *The Diabetic Foot.* 5th ed. Levin ME, O'Neal LW, Bowker JH, Eds. St. Louis, MO, Mosby, 1993, p. 199–232
14. Murray HJ, Veves A, Young MJ, Richie DH, Boulton AJM, American Group for the Study of Experimental Hosiery in the Diabetic Foot: Role of experimental socks in the care of the high-risk diabetic foot: a multicenter patient evaluation study. *Diabetes Care* 16:1190–92, 1993
15. Pinzur MS: Amputation level selection in the diabetic foot. *Clin Orthop Relat Res* 296:68–70, 1993
16. Fisher SV, Gullickson G: Energy cost of ambulation in health and disability: a literature review. *Arch Phys Med Rehabil* 59:124–33, 1978
17. Waters RL, Perry J, Antonelli D, Hislop H: Energy cost of walking of amputees: the influence of level of amputation (Abstract). *J Bone Jt Surg* 58A:42–46, 1978
18. Levin ME: Pathogenesis and general management of foot lesions in the diabetic patient. In *Levin and O'Neal's The Diabetic Foot.* 6th ed. Bowker JH, Pfeifer MA, Eds. Philadelphia, W.B. Saunders, 2001, p. 219–60

Marvin E. Levin, MD, is from the Washington School of Medicine, St. Louis, MO.

23

Retinopathy

LLOYD P. AIELLO, MD, PHD, JUN WONG, MD,
JERRY D. CAVALLERANO, OD, PHD,
SVEN-ERIK BURSELL, PHD, AND
LLOYD M. AIELLO, MD

Highlights

- Regularly performed exercise is useful in controlling the diabetic condition.
- In general, exercise and physical exertion have no negative impact on the risk of vision loss in cases of diabetic macular edema and nonproliferative diabetic retinopathy.
- In cases of severe nonproliferative diabetic retinopathy and proliferative diabetic retinopathy, especially when vitreous hemorrhage and/or fibrous retinal traction is present, some types of exercise and physical exertion may be contraindicated because of a risk of traction retinal detachment or vitreous hemorrhage.
- It is advisable to determine accurately the level of diabetic retinopathy before suggesting an exercise program for patients with diabetes.

Nearly 100 years ago, Dr. Elliott P. Joslin identified diet, exercise, and proper medical management as the cornerstones of appropriate diabetes care. Despite the subsequent discovery of insulin and innumerable advances in the understanding and treatment of diabetes, these cornerstones remain fundamental to this day. Nevertheless, the appropriate role of exercise in diabetes management is not fully appreciated.

One area of ongoing concern involves possible adverse effects of exercise and physical exertion on the microvascular complications of diabetes in general and diabetic retinopathy in particular. Physical exercise could have potentially detrimental effects on diabetic retinopathy and vision, either by raising systolic blood pressure through exertion, with possible subsequent vitreous hemorrhage mechanically inducing retinal hemorrhage or detachment, or by decreasing already compromised circulating oxygen levels. Conversely, exercise can have positive effects through its action on hormone levels, HDL concentrations, and retinal microcirculatory changes, or by optimization of blood glucose levels.

Despite such conflicting theoretical effects, clinicians and researchers generally agree that appropriate, individually tailored exercise regimens are beneficial in the management of diabetes and in reducing complications of the disease.

Ocular Physiology

Diabetic retinopathy is the most sight-threatening ocular complication of diabetes. The retina is a highly vascularized, light-sensitive tissue that transforms light focused through the refractive media of the eye into neural messages that the brain interprets as vision.

The retina is composed of rod cells, cone cells, and a variety of neural cells that receive, process, and transmit neural signals to the occipital lobe of the brain in response to the light image focused on the retina. Within the retina are numerous arteries and veins that provide the blood supply for the retinal tissue.

Retinal Abnormalities in Diabetes

Diabetes can damage the retinal vessels, impairing the blood's circulation through the retina and causing leakage of blood and blood products into the retina. The retinal vessels undergo ultrastructural damage, such as pericyte or mural cell degeneration and retinal blood flow autoregulatory impairment. These changes result from complex hormonal and biochemical alterations mediated by metabolic abnormalities associated with elevated blood glucose levels. These processes can alter vessel contractility and permeability and other physiological functions. Changes in vessel permeability may lead to diabetic macular edema. In diabetic macular edema, fluid collects in the macula, which is the area of the retina responsible for our most acute vision. Changes in retinal blood flow or nutrient delivery to the retina may result in relative retinal hypoxia that, in the most severe stages, may ultimately lead to new vessel growth and diabetic retinopathy.

Diabetic retinopathy is broadly classified as nonproliferative diabetic retinopathy (NPDR) and proliferative diabetic retinopathy (PDR). Diabetic macular edema can be present with either NPDR or PDR and must always be considered in addition to the level of retinopathy (Table 23.1). NPDR can be further classified as mild, moderate, severe, or very severe, based on the degree of retinal changes (Table 23.2). Each level poses a risk of progression to PDR. Accurate diagnosis of a patient's retinopathy level is critical because the risk of progression to PDR and high-risk PDR varies depending on the specific NPDR level. It is the level of retinopathy that determines appropriate examination schedules and therapeutic regimens (Table 23.3).

Retinopathy marked by new vessel growth on the optic nerve head (neovascularization at the disk [NVD]), by new vessel growth elsewhere in the retina (neovascularization elsewhere [NVE]), or by proliferation of fibrous tissue on the retina is classified as PDR. In the pro-

TABLE 23.1 Clinically Significant Macular Edema

- Retinal thickening at or within 500 μm (⅓ disc diameter) from the center of the macula or
- Hard exudates at or within 500 μm from the center of the macula with thickening of the adjacent retina or
- A zone or zones of retinal thickening ≥1 disc area in size, any portion of which is ≤1 disc diameter from the center of the macula

Clinically significant diabetic macular edema may be present with any level of retinopathy. Specific evaluation for diabetic macular edema requires careful evaluation by a qualified examiner generally using fundus biomicroscopy through dilated pupils on at least an annual basis.

TABLE 23.2 Levels of Diabetic Retinopathy

Mild NPDR
- At least one microaneurysm
- Characteristics not met for more severe diabetic retinopathy

Moderate NPDR
- H/Ma of a moderate degree (i.e., greater than or equal to standard photograph 2A*) and/or
- Soft exudates (cotton wool spots), venous beading, or IRMAs definitely present
- Characteristics not met for more severe diabetic retinopathy

Severe NPDR
- One of the following:
  - H/Ma greater than or equal to standard photograph 2A in four retinal quadrants
  - Venous beading in two retinal quadrants greater than or equal to standard photograph 6B
  - IRMAs in one retinal quadrant greater than or equal to standard photograph 8A
- Characteristics not met for more severe diabetic retinopathy

Very severe NPDR
- Two or more lesions of severe NPDR
- No frank neovascularization

Early PDR
- New vessels definitely present
- Characteristics not met for more severe diabetic retinopathy

High-risk PDR
- One or more of the following:
  - NVD ≥¼–⅓ disc area (i.e., NVD greater than or equal to standard photograph 10A)
  - Any NVD plus vitreous or preretinal hemorrhage
  - NVE on the retina ≥½ disc area plus vitreous or preretinal hemorrhage

PDR is composed of NVD or NVE, preretinal or vitreous hemorrhage, and fibrous tissue proliferation. Specific grading of level of retinopathy requires careful retinal evaluation by a qualified examiner through dilated pupils on at least an annual basis. H/Ma, hemorrhages and/or microaneurysms; IRMA, intraretinal microvascular abnormality. *Standard photographs refer to the Modified Airlie House Classification of Diabetic Retinopathy (see Early Treatment Diabetic Retinopathy Study [ETDRS] report #12).

liferative stage of diabetic retinopathy, new blood vessels form on the surface of the retina, presumably in an attempt to deliver more oxygenated blood to areas of the retina that experience relative hypoxia. These fragile new vessels do not relieve the relative hypoxia and can leak or burst, causing vitreous hemorrhage. Physical exertion, especially Valsalva-type maneuvers, and elevated systolic blood pressure may put added stress on these weakened vessel walls, possibly increasing the risk of vitreous hemorrhage. Furthermore, these vessels are usually accompanied by glial tissue, which may contract and cause traction on the

TABLE 23.3 Eye Examination Schedule

	Recommended First Examination	Routine Minimal Follow-up
Type 1 diabetes	Within 3–5 years after onset once patient is ≥10 years of age	Yearly
Type 2 diabetes	At time of diagnosis of diabetes	Yearly
Diabetes and pregnancy	■ Before conception for counseling ■ Early in first trimester	■ Usually each trimester ■ More frequently as indicated ■ 3–6 months postpartum

Abnormal findings require more frequent follow-up examinations.

retina and subsequent retinal detachment. Physical straining can potentiate this traction, increasing the risk of retinal detachment.

The 5-year risk of severe vision loss (best corrected vision of 5/200 or worse) for eyes with high-risk PDR may be as high as 60%. This risk can be reduced to <4% over 5 years by proper and timely laser photocoagulation. The 3-year risk of moderate vision loss (e.g., a loss of vision from 20/20 to 20/40 or from 20/50 to 20/100) for eyes with macular edema is 25–30%. This risk can be reduced 50% by timely and appropriate laser photocoagulation. Regular eye evaluations are crucial for determining the level of retinopathy, the need for laser photocoagulation, and the impact, if any, of retinopathy on a choice of exercise program (Tables 23.3 and 23.4).

Retinal and Ocular Considerations During Exercise

Type 1 Diabetes

The American Diabetes Association's Position Statement on exercise in type 1 diabetes reiterated that "exercise programs have not been exclusively shown to improve glycemic control."[1] However, it was recommended that individuals with type 1 diabetes be encouraged to participate in exercise to improve cardiovascular and psychological well-being and to promote social interaction in a recreational environment. An individually tailored approach to exercise was recommended, and potential risks of physical exercise in type 1 diabetes were highlighted.

These risks included hypoglycemia, hyperglycemia, ketosis, cardiac ischemia, and exacerbation of complications of proliferative retinopathy.

Several studies have investigated the relationship of exercise to the development of PDR.[2–6] In people diagnosed with diabetes before 30 years of age, of whom most are expected to have type 1 diabetes, there is a suggestion that higher levels of physical activity may result in a reduced risk of PDR in women.[2] Women evaluated in this cross-sectional epidemiological study who either participated in team sports in high school or college or considered their level of activity to be strenuous were less likely to have PDR than women who did not participate in team sports or considered themselves not to be physically active.[2] No such relationship, however, was found in male participants in the study. It has been postulated that the positive effect of exercise in preventing PDR in women may be the result of hormonal influences.

Other studies, however, did not identify any positive effects of exercise in preventing PDR in men or women.[3–6] Moreover, a recent report by the same authors who earlier noted a PDR risk reduction in women who had higher levels of physical activity did not notice any sex-associated differences in retinopathy progression with physical activity.[6] The authors attributed the contrast in the results to the differing nature of the cohort study. The earlier evaluation was a cross-sectional survey[2] and therefore may be subjected to self-selection bias, whereas the more recent report was evaluated prospectively and more objectively.[6] It is important to note that none of the studies observed a deleterious effect of exercise on the development of PDR.

Although the beneficial effects of exercise for people with diabetes are generally accepted, one area of controversy surrounds the effects of exercise on growth hormone (GH). Potentially adverse effects of GH on diabetic retinopathy have been suggested by studies involving diabetic individuals with pituitary ablation and dwarfism.[7,8] In addition, plasma levels of GH rose in individuals who had severe diabetic retinopathy but did not rise significantly for those who exhibited no diabetic retinopathy, suggesting that GH might contribute to the development of diabetic retinopathy.[9,10] Because it is postulated that GH secretion increases in people with diabetes[9,11] under conditions such as muscular exercise, the theoretical potential adverse effects of exercise on diabetic retinopathy have been raised. However, most clinicians and researchers agree that the beneficial effects of an appropriate exercise regimen for people with diabetes outweigh any theoretical detriment. Indeed, a recent large-scale prospective epidemiological study on patients with type 1 diabetes did not report retinopathy worsening with moderate exercise.[6]

Type 2 Diabetes

The National Institutes of Health (NIH), in its consensus paper on diet and exercise in type 2 diabetes, considers the cornerstone of therapy for type 2 diabetes to be a "style of life centered around diet and supplemented, if needed, by insulin or oral agents."[12] A recent prospective study on 198 subjects with type 2 diabetes who attended a diabetic clinic in Thailand suggested that "inadequate exercise" might be related to the development of retinopathy.[13] Exercise is recognized as an auxiliary means to facilitate caloric loss, assist in glucose regulation, and reverse insulin resistance at insulin target tissues, such as the liver, skeletal muscle, and adipose tissue. The NIH consensus panel also recognized potential complications of exercise in patients with type 2 diabetes, including cardiac disease, bone and soft tissue injuries, and eye disease (particularly PDR). The ocular risks include retinal detachment and vitreous hemorrhage, especially during exercise "that requires straining and breath holding (such as weight lifting)."[12]

General Considerations

In general, exercise and physical activity have not been shown to accelerate diabetic retinopathy. There is some indication that physical exercise has a positive effect on reducing the risk of diabetic complications by either direct or indirect mechanisms. In both type 1 and type 2 diabetes, aerobic exercises improve or maintain cardiovascular function, increase levels of HDL, aid in weight control, increase insulin sensitivity, and reduce risk factors for vascular disease.[14–19] Studies of people with diabetic retinopathy have shown that cardiovascular training with moderate levels of exercise results in significant improvements in cardiovascular health.[14]

For patients who have active PDR, strenuous activity may precipitate vitreous hemorrhage or traction retinal detachment.[20,21] One retrospective study[22] involving 72 diabetic patients presenting with 95 episodes of vitreous hemorrhage showed that 80 of the hemorrhages (84%) were associated with exercise no more strenuous than walking.

It is our philosophy that people with PDR should avoid anaerobic exercise and exercise that involves straining, jarring, or Valsalva-type maneuvers. This would include exercises such as high-impact aerobics, jogging, boxing, volleyball, or heavy weight training. There is concern that the loss of circulatory autoregulation in the ophthalmic circulation in individuals with PDR may allow the retinal arteriole perfusion pressure to exceed the hemorrhagic threshold in the abnormal retinal vessels during exercise-induced blood pressure rise. The rise in systolic blood pressure that accompanies strenuous exercise can increase pressure on damaged retinal capillaries and neovascular tufts, resulting in intraretinal, preretinal, and/or vitreous hemorrhage. However, the exact threshold for hemorrhage from the abnormal new vessels in PDR is unknown. In the long term, before the onset of PDR, physical activity and exercise may reduce the risk of PDR and diabetic macular edema indirectly through beneficial effects on blood pressure and HDL, both of which are associated with worsening retinopathy.[23,24]

Special Precautions

Table 23.4 summarizes exercise activities that may be appropriate based on the level of retinopathy. These guidelines reflect the approach to exercise taken at the Beetham Eye Institute and, as such, are suggestions rather than explicit medical directives. In all cases, decisions are based on the patient's individual needs, condition, and physician recommendation.

We suggest that people with PDR avoid exercise regimens that result in systolic blood pressure >170 mmHg.[25] Note, however, that this recommendation is arbitrary and based on other studies.[11] Limiting the blood pressure increase to only 170 mmHg may have little, if any, exercise benefit. One study suggests that the blood pressure increase be limited to <50 mmHg above resting levels or to a maximum systolic blood pressure of 200 mmHg for those patients having residual vision and to 240 mmHg for those patients having no residual light perception.[14] The suggestions recommended in this study, however, are also arbitrary because it was determined that no adverse ophthalmologic events could be directly related to the exercise program over the 2-year duration of the study. Thus, it appears that the blood pressure restrictions given above should be taken as conservative estimates. We do suggest, however, that concurrent monitoring of blood pressure and

TABLE 23.4 Considerations for Activity Limitation in Diabetic Retinopathy

Level of Diabetic Retinopathy	Acceptable Activities	Discouraged Activities	Ocular and Activity Reevaluation
No Diabetic Retinopathy	Dictated by medical status	Dictated by medical status	12 months
Mild NPDR	Dictated by medical status	Dictated by medical status	6–12 months
Moderate NPDR	Dictated by medical status	Activities that dramatically elevate blood pressure: ■ Power lifting ■ Heavy Valsalva maneuvers	4–6 months
Severe and very severe NPDR	Dictated by medical status	Limit systolic blood pressure, Valsalva maneuvers, and active jarring: ■ Boxing ■ Heavy competitive sports	2–4 months (may require laser surgery)
PDR	Low-impact, cardiovascular conditioning: ■ Swimming (not diving) ■ Walking ■ Low-impact aerobics ■ Stationary cycling ■ Endurance exercises	Strenuous activity, Valsalva maneuvers, pounding, or jarring: ■ Weight lifting ■ Jogging ■ High-impact aerobics ■ Racquet sports ■ Strenuous trumpet playing	1–2 months (may require laser surgery)

level of retinopathy is necessary once a person has advanced beyond mild to moderate levels of NPDR.

It has also been demonstrated that people with severe diabetic retinopathy and type 1 diabetes have impaired cardiovascular response to exercise, which is reflected in decreased heart rate, decreased left ventricular ejection fraction, and decreased muscle blood flow.[26] In addition, a prior study[27] demonstrated abnormalities in the autonomic regulation of the ophthalmic circulation during exercise. Similarly, patients with type 2 diabetes without coronary artery disease but with evidence of microvascular disease, including retinopathy, were found to have reduced exercise capacity.[28] These considerations, taken together with suggestions regarding blood pressure elevations, should have an impact on the choice of exercise and the potential therapeutic benefit derived for patients with severe diabetic retinopathy.

Other general restrictions for patients with PDR include avoiding activities that lower the head below waist level, Valsalva-type maneuvers that result in increased blood pressure, and near-maximal isometric contractions.[15,20,21] Similarly, weight lifting with high resistance and low repetitions and exercises that force a person to hold his or her breath should be avoided. Vigorous bouncing, including jogging, high-impact aerobics, and contact sports, is contraindicated because of the risk of retinal tears, retinal detachment, or vitreous hemorrhage in eyes with retinal neovascularization, fibrous tissue proliferation, or retinal traction.[15] Strenuous upper-extremity exercises, such as rowing and arm cycle ergometry, likewise are contraindicated.[15]

Beneficial low-risk exercises include endurance exercise, stationary cycling, low-intensity machine rowing, swimming, and walking. Even patients who have lost vision should attempt to maintain some level of regular physical exercise.[29] With appropriate hemodynamic and glucose monitoring, patients with diabetic retinopathy and autonomic neuropathy may exercise safely.[27,30,31)]

Conclusions

In most cases, exercise is an important component of diabetes care. A person's exercise regimen should be carefully crafted and monitored by his or her health care team, including an exercise physiologist, nutritionist, internist, and eye doctor experienced in the management of diabetic eye disease. Currently, diabetic retinopathy cannot be prevented, but careful evaluation, follow-up, and timely and appropriate laser photocoagulation can reduce the 5-year risk of severe visual loss from PDR to <4% and cut the risk of moderate vision loss from diabetic macular edema by ≥50%. Because even serious retinopathy frequently causes no visual symptoms, especially in the most treatable stages, regular eye examinations are indicated to establish the level of retinopathy. These regular examinations must be obtained at least yearly and will provide the clinical information that determines an appropriate exercise program for people with diabetes.

References

1. American Diabetes Association: Diabetes mellitus and exercise (Position Statement). *Diabetes Care* 18 (Suppl. 1):28, 1995
2. Cruickshanks KJ, Klein R, Moss SE, Klein BEK: Physical activity and proliferative diabetic retinopathy in people diagnosed with diabetes before age 30 yr. *Diabetes Care* 15:1267–72, 1992
3. LaPorte RE, Dorman JS, Tajima N, Cruickshanks KJ, Orchard TJ, Cavender DE, Becker DJ, Drash AL: Pittsburgh Insulin-Dependent Diabetes Mellitus and Mortality Study: physical activity and diabetic complications. *Pediatrics* 78:1027–33, 1986
4. Kriska AM, LaPorte RE, Patrick SL, Kuller LH, Orchard TJ: The association of physical activity and diabetic complications in individuals with insulin-dependent diabetes mellitus: The Epidemiology of Diabetes Complications Study VII. *J Clin Epidemiol* 44:1207–14, 1991
5. Orchard TJ, Dorman JS, Maser RE, Becker DJ, Ellis D, LaPorte RE, Kuller LH, Wolfson SK Jr, Drash AL: Factors associated with avoidance of severe complications after 25 yr of IDDM: Pittsburgh Epidemiology of Diabetes Complications Study I. *Diabetes Care* 13:741–47, 1990
6. Cruickshanks KJ, Moss SE, Klein R, Klein BEK: Physical activity and risk of progression of retinopathy or the development of proliferative diabetic retinopathy. *Ophthalmology* 102:1177–82, 1995
7. Kohner EM, Joplin GF, Blach RK, Cheng H, Fraser TR: Pituitary ablation in the treatment of diabetic retinopathy (a randomized trial). *Trans Ophthalmol Soc* 92:79–90, 1972
8. Merimee TJ: A follow-up study of vascular disease in growth-hormone-deficient dwarfs with diabetes. *N Engl J Med* 298: 1217–22, 1978
9. Passa P, Gauville C, Canivet J: Influence of muscular exercise on plasma level of growth hormone in diabetics with and without retinopathy. *Lancet* 342:72–74, 1994
10. Alzaid AA, Dinneen SF, Melton LJ, Rizza RA: The role of growth hormone in the development of diabetic retinopathy. *Diabetes Care* 17:531–34, 1994
11. Hansen AP: Abnormal serum growth hormone response to exercise in maturity-onset diabetics. *Diabetes* 22:619–28, 1973

12. National Institutes of Health: Consensus development conference on diet and exercise in non-insulin-dependent diabetes mellitus. *Diabetes Care* 10:639–44, 1987
13. Rasmidatta S, Khunsuk-Mengrai K, Warunyuwong C: Risk factors of diabetic retinopathy in non-insulin dependent diabetes mellitus. *J Med Assoc Thai* 81:169–74, 1998
14. Bernbaum M, Albert S, Cohen JD, Drimmer A: Cardiovascular conditioning in individuals with diabetic retinopathy. *Diabetes Care* 12:740–42, 1989
15. Graham C, Lasko-McCarthey P: Exercise options for people with diabetic complications. *Diabetes Educator* 16:212–20, 1990
16. Vranic M, Berger M: Exercise and diabetes. *Diabetes* 28:147–63, 1979
17. Delio D: Aerobic exercise programs and the management of diabetes. *Pract Diabetol* 4:12–20, 1985
18. Franz MJ: Exercise and diabetes: fuel metabolism, benefits, risks and guidelines. *Clin Diabetes* 6:58–70, 1988
19. Horton ES: Role and management of exercise in diabetes mellitus. *Diabetes Care* 11:201–11, 1988
20. Sharuk GS, Stockman ME, Krolewski AS, Aiello LM, Rand LI: Patient activity and the risk of vitreous hemorrhage in eyes with proliferative diabetic retinopathy (Abstract). *Invest Ophthalmol* 27 (Suppl.):5, 1986
21. Sharuk GS, Stockman ME, Krolewski AS, Aiello LM, Rand LI: Patient activity and the risk of vitreous hemorrhage in eyes with proliferative diabetic retinopathy (Abstract). *Invest Ophthalmol* 28 (Suppl.):246, 1987
22. Anderson B Jr: Activity and diabetic vitreous hemorrhages. *Ophthalmology* 87:173–75, 1980
23. Klein R, Klein BEK, Moss SE, Davis MD, DeMets DL: Is blood pressure a predictor of the incidence or progression of diabetic retinopathy? *Arch Intern Med* 149:2427–32, 1989
24. Klein BEK, Moss SE, Klein R, Surawicz TS: The Wisconsin Epidemiologic Study of Diabetic Retinopathy. XIII. Relationship of serum cholesterol to retinopathy and hard exudate. *Ophthalmology* 98:1261–65, 1991
25. Greenlee G: Exercise options for patients with retinopathy and peripheral vascular disease. *Pract Diabetol* 6:9–11, 1987
26. Margonato A, Gerundini P, Vicedomini G, Gilardi M, Pozza G, Fazio F: Abnormal cardiovascular response to exercise in young

asymptomatic diabetic patients with retinopathy. *Am Heart J* 112:554–60, 1986

27. Albert SG, Gomez CR, Russell S, Chaitman BR, Bernbaum M, Kong BA: Cerebral and ophthalmic artery hemodynamic responses in diabetes mellitus. *Diabetes Care* 16:476–82, 1993
28. Estacio RO, Regensteiner JG, Wolfel EE, Jeffers B, Dickenson M, Schrier RW: The association between diabetic complications and exercise capacity in NIDDM patients. *Diabetes Care* 21:291–95, 1998
29. Bernbaum M, Albert SG, Brusca SR, Drimmer A, Duckro P, Cohen JD, Trindade MC, Silverberg AB: A model clinical program for patients with diabetes and vision impairment. *Diabetes Educ* 15:325–30, 1989
30. Bernbaum M, Albert SG, Cohen JD: Exercise training in individuals with diabetic retinopathy and blindness. *Arch Phys Med Rehabil* 70:605–11, 1989
31. Bernbaum M, Albert SG, Brusca SR, Drimmer A, Duckro P: Promoting diabetes self-management and independence in the visually impaired: a model clinical program. *Diabetes Educ* 14: 51–54, 1988

Lloyd P. Aiello, MD, PhD, Jun Wong, MD, Jerry D. Cavallerano, OD, PhD, Sven-Erik Bursell, PhD, and Lloyd M. Aiello, MD, are from the Beetham Eye Institute, Joslin Diabetes Center, and the Department of Ophthalmology, Harvard Medical School, Boston, MA.

24

Cardiovascular Complications

SERGIO WAXMAN, MD, AND
RICHARD W. NESTO, MD

Highlights

- Atherosclerotic heart disease and hypertension are common in patients with diabetes and are major causes of morbidity and mortality.
- Silent myocardial ischemia is more common in the patient with diabetes and may be associated with autonomic dysfunction.
- Autonomic neuropathy is associated with an increased mortality from myocardial infarction and sudden death and may be a marker for clinically unrecognized cardiac disease.
- Exercise may decrease cardiovascular risk in patients with diabetes.
- Before starting an individualized exercise program, the patient with diabetes should undergo a thorough history and physical examination to detect any signs of cardiovascular disease. A graded exercise test is

necessary if the patient is at high risk for underlying cardiovascular disease.

- Exercise of moderate intensity is usually recommended for individuals with stable coronary artery disease and/or hypertension.
- Patients with a recent cardiac event should be stratified according to risk for exercise and should follow a cardiac rehabilitation program.

Cardiovascular Disease and Diabetes

Diabetes constitutes a major risk factor for the development of cardiovascular disease; indeed, its effect greatly exceeds that of many standard risk factors for atherosclerosis, particularly in women and young adults.[1–4] Data from the Framingham Heart Study have demonstrated that cardiovascular mortality is more than doubled in men and more than quadrupled in women who have diabetes compared with their nondiabetic counterparts.[5] The relative risk of myocardial infarction is 50% greater in diabetic men and 150% greater in diabetic women. Myocardial infarction accounts for as many as 30% of all deaths in patients with type 1 diabetes.[6] Coronary atherosclerosis is more extensive, as well as more prevalent, in diabetic individuals than in nondiabetic individuals.[7] Silent myocardial ischemia is also more common in patients with diabetes.[8,9] Asymptomatic coronary artery disease has been reported in up to 10% of type 1 diabetic patients[10,11] and 8–30% of type 2 diabetic patients.[10–12] The prevalence increases when other risk factors for atherosclerosis are present, such as age, hypertension, smoking, and hypercholesterolemia. Both silent ischemia and asymptomatic coronary artery disease may be associated with autonomic dysfunction[13] and appear to be more prevalent in individuals on insulin therapy who have retinopathy.[14] During exercise, the anginal perceptual threshold is prolonged compared with that of nondiabetic individuals, possibly because of the presence of autonomic neuropathy.[15,16]

In addition to atherosclerosis, hypertension is more common and, alone or in combination with coronary artery disease, is a major cause of morbidity and mortality in people with diabetes.[1] The most common type of hypertension in patients with type 2 diabetes is essential hypertension, which may be related to obesity, central adiposity, and insulin resistance (the latter possibly due to increased sympathetic activity[17,18] and sodium retention in the kidney[19]). In type 1 diabetes, diabetic nephropathy and renal artery stenosis due to an increased prevalence of generalized atherosclerosis[20] are also common causes of hypertension.

Cardiac disease may also be present in patients with diabetes in the absence of coronary artery disease. Diabetic cardiomyopathy is associated with abnormalities of systolic and diastolic left ventricular function.[21] Pathological findings in diabetic cardiomyopathy include myocardial enlargement, hypertrophy, and fibrosis, as well as an increase in basement membrane thickening.[22,23] Even in the absence of clinical signs of cardiac impairment, left ventricular function may be impaired in diabetic patients during exercise by mechanisms that are not completely understood but that may involve the presence of microangiopathy or autonomic dysfunction[24–27] or inadequate systemic venous return with limitation in left ventricular filling.[27]

Autonomic neuropathy is frequently present in patients with diabetes[28] (see Chapter 27). It is associated with increased mortality from myocardial infarction and sudden death, and it may be a marker for clinically unrecognized cardiac disease. Alterations in autonomic regulation may lead to ischemia by a number of mechanisms that include the following: *1*) increasing myocardial oxygen demand because of higher resting heart rates, *2*) reducing myocardial blood flow by increasing coronary vascular tone at sites of coronary stenosis, *3*) reducing coronary perfusion pressure during orthostatic hypotension, and *4*) eliminating early warning signs of ischemia.[29]

Cardiovascular Physiology: Benefits of Exercise for Decreasing Cardiovascular Risk

Exercise decreases cardiovascular risk in the general population,[30–33] and its effects are likely to be equally beneficial in the diabetic patient (see Chapters 9 and 12). The potential mechanisms for the decrease in cardiovascular risk associated with exercise are shown in Table 24.1. Exercise is associated with changes in insulin sensitivity and lipid metabolism, events that are likely to have long-term effects on the development of cardiovascular complications. In people at high risk for developing type 2 diabetes, exercise may prevent the onset of diabetes[34] and may affect the course of atherosclerosis-related disease. In patients

TABLE 24.1 Changes Associated With Exercise That May Decrease Cardiovascular Risk

- Decreased blood pressure
- Increased HDL cholesterol level
- Decreased triglyceride level
- Reduced weight
- Increased fibrinolysis in response to thrombotic stimuli
- Increased insulin sensitivity
- Reduced susceptibility to serious ventricular arrhythmias
- Associated behavioral changes (smoking cessation, diet, stress reduction)
- Psychological effects (decreased depression and anxiety)

with type 2 diabetes, the insulin resistance syndrome appears to be an important risk factor for premature coronary disease.[35] These patients tend to have a low level of aerobic fitness, which is associated with many cardiovascular risk factors. Exercise and treatment of risk factors are linked to decreases in plasma insulin levels and improvements in insulin sensitivity, which may be associated with a decrease in cardiovascular risk. However, although exercise can improve lipoprotein profile, reduce blood pressure, and improve overall cardiovascular fitness in patients with established type 2 diabetes, its effect on improving glycemic control is more variable.[35]

Aerobic exercise benefits patients with coronary artery disease by modulating physiological changes that enable the patient to achieve a higher functional state. In previously sedentary individuals, maximal oxygen uptake may increase by 15–25% over baseline after a few months of regular aerobic exercise performed at 60–80% of maximum aerobic capacity for 20–60 min 3–5 days/week.[36] This level of exercise benefits the cardiovascular system by decreasing heart rate at rest and during submaximal exercise, increasing stroke volume at rest and with submaximal and maximal exercise, and increasing maximal cardiac output.[37–39] These changes result in reduced myocardial oxygen demand during submaximal exercise and allow the patient with coronary artery disease to perform a higher workload despite impaired coronary flow reserve. This, in turn, increases the amount of work that can be done at the anginal or ischemic threshold.[40]

In contrast to aerobic physical activity, isometric exercise produces an acute pressor response that is related to the size of muscle mass and the degree of muscular tension exerted. This imposes a greater pressure than volume overload on the left ventricle in relation to the body's ability to supply oxygen. The marked rise in blood pressure is related to an increase in cardiac output with little or no decrease in total peripheral resistance. Because the response to activation of a small muscle group is similar to the response to a large muscle group, the cardiovascular response to this form of exercise is difficult to grade. Although physicians have been hesitant to prescribe isometric exercise for their patients, some studies suggest that regimens incorporating moderate levels of resistance and high repetitions may be safe for patients with coronary artery disease,[41] may favorably alter cardiovascular risk factors such as HDL cholesterol, and may improve insulin sensitivity.[42–44] Use of isometric exercise in elderly individuals (see Chapter 32) as well as in others with diabetes is described in Chapter 16.

Exercise after myocardial infarction has been associated with decreased mortality,[45] a benefit that may be related to a significant reduction in sudden death. Performance of exercise at regular intervals has also been noted to decrease the risk of myocardial infarction.[46] Sedentary individuals experience a higher relative risk of myocardial infarction after an episode of heavy exertion compared with individuals who exercise five or more times per week.[46]

Despite these benefits, exercise may have risks and be contraindicated in certain patients with diabetes. Some risks, however, can be minimized if patients and physicians have a comprehensive knowledge of the medical condition, physical limitations, and safe and appropriate exercises.

Special Problems in Patients With Diabetes

Coronary Artery Disease

The exercise prescription for the patient with diabetes and coronary artery disease differs little from that for the nondiabetic patient and is influenced to a great extent by the presence of other complications of diabetes.

The ischemic response to exercise, ischemic threshold, and the propensity to arrhythmias during exercise should be evaluated. In many cases, left ventricular systolic function at rest and its response to exercise should also be assessed. This information can be used to modify an exercise prescription dependent on the overall risk for subsequent cardiac events, which is based on the presence of ischemia, left ventricular function, and/or arrhythmias.

Exercise of moderate intensity is usually recommended for patients with known coronary artery disease in the absence of ischemia or significant arrhythmias.[47] This level of exercise can be targeted to 60–80% of the maximum heart rate corresponding to 50–74% of the maximum oxygen consumption.[48] In patients with angina, exercise training increases functional capacity at the anginal threshold. For these patients, the target heart rate during aerobic exercise should be set at no less than 10 beats below the ischemic threshold.[49] Sublingual nitroglycerin before exercise may allow patients with low anginal thresholds to achieve higher levels of exercise. In patients without angina, targeting a specific level of activity may be more complicated; in these patients, the ischemic threshold should be determined by exercise electrocardiographic monitoring. Particular attention should be paid to these patients because a lack of angina in the setting of ischemia can be due to autonomic neuropathy (which may also be an indicator of more severe coronary disease), left ventricular dysfunction, and a poor overall cardiovascular prognosis.

Isometric exercise, as discussed earlier, may be beneficial for patients with coronary artery disease—in particular, those with normal or near-normal left ventricular function. Programs that include 8–12 repetitions of loads corresponding to 40–50% of maximum strength appear safe for these patients.[50]

Hypertension

Exercise reduces blood pressure by 5–10 mmHg in some patients with essential hypertension,[51,52] and its effects are usually noted within 10 weeks of training.[53] Although the mechanism for the antihypertensive effects of exercise is unknown, possible explanations may include the attenuation of sympathetic nervous system activity with subsequent reduction in peripheral vascular resistance[44] and improved insulin sensitivity with a reduction in circulating insulin.[54] The latter may decrease sodium reabsorption by the renal tubules.[55]

Before starting an exercise program, the hypertensive patient requires adequate blood pressure control because exercise causes acute increases in systolic pressure, and this increase may be exaggerated in the diabetic patient.[56] The blood pressure response to exercise should be monitored initially, and adjustments in therapy should be made accordingly. Exercise should be performed with a frequency of at least four times per week, with each session lasting between 30 and 60 min. Exercise of moderate intensity is generally recommended for the individual with hypertension.[47] This level of exercise can be targeted to 60–80% of the maximum heart rate, which corresponds to 50–74% of the maximum oxygen consumption.[48] High-intensity and isometric exercises should be minimized because they can cause a significant pressor response.

Autonomic Neuropathy

The presence of autonomic neuropathy may be a marker for severe but clinically unrecognized cardiac disease. Therefore, exercise for these patients should be prescribed with extreme caution (see Chapter 27).

Parasympathetic function is usually impaired before sympathetic function. This is characteristically manifested as a higher basal heart rate; although, during exercise, the heart rate and blood pressure responses tend to be blunted.[57,58] Such abnormalities in the regulation of heart rate and peripheral vascular resistance result in decreased cardiac output with exertion and may account for a reduced exercise capacity. In addition, left ventricular systolic and diastolic function at rest and during exercise may be abnormal, even in the absence of coronary artery disease as a result of diabetic cardiomyopathy. The effects of exercise on the cardiovascular system in diabetic patients with autonomic neuropathy are unknown, although low levels of exercise may be beneficial and safe for some of these patients. Periodic evaluations should be made in the diabetic patient with autonomic neuropathy to detect signs of cardiovascular disease.

Orthostatic hypotension may be present in some patients with autonomic dysfunction, and patients should be screened for it before an exercise regimen is prescribed. The evaluation should be done at rest, and if orthostatic hypotension is present in the absence of symptoms, long warm-up and cooldown periods of low-intensity exercise are recommended before and after each training session. The patient should be educated to recognize early signs of neurocirculatory collapse and report any symptoms to his or her regular physician.

Screening and Evaluation of the Diabetic Patient During Exercise

Before starting an individualized exercise program (see Chapter 13) of more than mild intensity, individuals with diabetes should undergo a thorough interview and physical examination to detect signs and symptoms of cardiovascular disease. The justification for screening is based on the high prevalence of coronary artery disease in this population, although no studies are available to demonstrate a decrease in morbidity or mortality from this approach.[59] Screening seems especially justified as part of the evaluation before renal transplantation or major noncardiac or vascular surgery, where definable periods of excess cardiac risk are identified. A positive outcome of screening would be the discovery of three-vessel or high-risk coronary artery disease, particularly in the presence of left ventricular dysfunction in an asymptomatic patient. Surgical revascularization can prolong life in this otherwise undetected case. According to American Diabetes Association and American College of Cardiology Guidelines,[60] a graded exercise test is also necessary if a patient with diabetes is at high risk for underlying cardiovascular disease, based on the following criteria:

- Age >35 years
- Type 2 diabetes of >10 years' duration
- Type 1 diabetes of >15 years' duration
- Any additional risk factor for coronary artery disease
- Presence of microvascular disease (retinopathy and nephropathy, including proteinuria)
- Peripheral vascular disease
- Autonomic neuropathy

The exercise stress test should be performed in such patients for evaluation of ischemia, arrhythmias, abnormal hypertensive response to exercise, and abnormal orthostatic response during or after exercise. It also provides information regarding initial levels of working capacity, specific precautions that may need to be taken, and heart rates used to prescribe activities. Radionuclide or echocardiographic imaging should accompany ST segment monitoring in patients with resting ST segment abnormalities due to *1*) a prior coronary event, *2*) left ventricular hypertrophy with repolarization abnormalities, *3*) left bundle branch block, *4*) digoxin use, or *5*) electrolyte disturbances affecting repolarization (i.e., diuretics). Another group of patients benefiting from stress imaging includes women because exercise testing with ST segment monitoring results in a higher false-positive rate.

Patients with known coronary artery disease require a supervised evaluation to determine *1*) exercise duration experienced to the onset of ischemia, *2*) heart rate and blood pressure at the onset of ischemia, and *3*) the presence or absence of atrial or ventricular arrhythmias during exercise. Many diabetic individuals may experience an anginal equivalent such as nausea, shortness of breath, profound dyspnea, or undue fatigue on the exercise test.

Although a routine exercise treadmill test is considered the first line of screening, it may not be the most accurate or cost-effective means of evaluation. A number of studies have shown that a positive noninvasive test in patients with diabetes carries a low positive predictive value for significant coronary artery disease on angiography. Of those patients with positive noninvasive tests, either by ST segment changes suggestive of ischemia or perfusion imaging defects, about one-third will have significant lesions (>50% luminal narrowing) on angiography.[10–12] A number of factors specific to the patient with diabetes can affect the sensitivity, specificity, and implications of noninvasive diagnostic tests for coronary artery disease. Hypertension, prevalent in patients with diabetes, can result in greater left ventricular mass[61,62] and produce abnormal ST segment responses and false-positive radionuclide defects during exercise. Diabetic cardiomyopathy can cause segmental wall motion abnormalities or thallium defects mimicking ischemia.[63] Autonomic neuropathy may blunt the chronotropic response to exercise and dissociate the relation between cardiac and external work. Renal insufficiency may be associated with elevated resting levels of adenosine, which may limit maximal coronary flow reserve induced by persantine and decrease sensitivity of stress perfusion thallium or echo imaging.[64] Autonomic neuropathy[65] and endothelial dysfunction[66] may interfere with coronary vasodilatory capacity. Microvascular angina[67,68] and diffuse atherosclerosis may account for abnormalities in exercise testing while failing to demonstrate significant epicardial lesions on coronary angiography. Although these factors are prevalent in patients with diabetes and affect the results of screening tests, it is unlikely that angiography is a practical method for detecting early atherosclerosis and should be reserved only for select individuals at greatest risk for cardiac events.

The exercise stress test should be done near the time of day that the patient would normally exercise to both determine safety and assess the need to modify the exercise prescription. It should also be performed while the patient is taking his or her usual anti-anginal or antihypertensive medications. β-Blockers and calcium-channel blockers may attenuate the heart rate and blood pressure responses to exercise, lessening diagnostic accuracy, and may need to be held the morning of the test. Vasodilator medications, such as calcium-channel blockers and angiotensin-converting enzyme inhibitors, may be associated with postexercise hypotension. In these patients, prolonged cooldown periods may be required. Patients on chronic diuretic therapy may have low serum potassium levels and an increased potential for arrhythmias during exercise. Serum potassium levels should be monitored periodically in these patients.

Cardiac Rehabilitation

Patients with exercise-induced ischemia, heart failure, or a recent cardiac event, such as myocardial infarction, coronary angioplasty, or bypass surgery, should participate in a cardiac rehabilitation program. The risk of cardiac rehabilitation is very low, with one major cardiovascular complication (cardiac arrest or myocardial infarction) per 81,101 patient-hours and one fatality per 783,972 patient-hours.[69] The prevalence of these complications is related to the degree of left ventricular dysfunction and the severity of heart disease. Initial physical activity should be monitored by a professional to record symptoms, heart rate, blood pressure, and rating of perceived exertion. When tolerance and safety are documented, the individual can perform that activity without supervision.

The exercise test is an important part of the rehabilitative process. It provides reassurance to the patient, risk stratification, and information about exercise capacity that is important in determining a safe level of exercise. A symptom-limited exercise test is usually performed 4–8 weeks after hospital discharge, and if no further studies are indicated, a regular conditioning program can be initiated. Low-risk patients (Table 24.2) can participate in a home exercise program. Dura-

TABLE 24.2 Classification of Risk Related to Vigorous Exercise in Patients With Coronary Artery Disease

Low risk (but slightly greater than that for apparently healthy individuals)

Known CAD and the following clinical characteristics:

- New York Heart Association class 1 or 2
- Exercise capacity >6 METs
- No evidence of heart failure
- Free of ischemia or angina at rest or on the exercise test at ≤6 METs
- Appropriate rise in systolic blood pressure during exercise
- No sequential ectopic ventricular contractions
- Ability to satisfactorily self-monitor intensity of activity

Moderate to high risk

Known CAD and any of the following clinical characteristics:

- History of two or more myocardial infarctions
- New York Heart Association class 3 or 4
- Exercise capacity <6 METs
- Ischemic horizontal or downsloping ST depression of ≥4 mm or angina during exercise
- Fall in systolic blood pressure with exercise
- Presence of a life-threatening medical problem
- History of a primary cardiac arrest
- Ventricular tachycardia at a workload of ≥6 METs

Known coronary artery disease (CAD) is defined as history of myocardial infarction, coronary bypass surgery, angioplasty, angina pectoria, abnormal exercise test, or an abnormal coronary angiogram. MET, metabolic equivalent.

Adapted from the American Heart Association.[47]

tion and intensity should be low initially and gradually increased in the absence of symptoms. Because ischemia is frequently asymptomatic in the patient with diabetes, an objective assessment of ischemia should be done periodically as the level of exercise increases. An exercise test is used for this purpose. Patients at moderate to high risk for cardiac complications during exercise (Table 24.2) should participate in a medically supervised program. For a more detailed review on cardiac rehabilitation, see the American Heart Association's Exercise Standards.[47]

The Cardiologist's Role in Prescribing Exercise for Patients With Diabetes

Formulating an exercise prescription for the patient with diabetes should be a multidisciplinary effort involving all members of the health care team and the patient. The cardiologist, as part of the team, should *1*) act as a consultant, providing information on the benefits, potential risks, and appropriateness of exercise for each particular patient; *2*) work in conjunction with the team to screen the patient and formulate an individualized exercise program; *3*) educate the health care team and patient to be aware of and recognize signs, symptoms, and clinical conditions that are associated with coronary artery disease; *4*) institute and promote adherence to treatments proven to reduce cardiac risk, such as lowering of blood pressure and cholesterol; and *5*) monitor the patient's progress.

References

1. Garcia MJ, McNamara PM, Gordon T, Kannel WB: Morbidity and mortality in diabetics in the Framingham population. *Diabetes* 23:105–11, 1974
2. Barrett-Connor E, Orchard TJ: Diabetes and heart disease. In *Diabetes in America.* Harris MJ, Hamman RF, Eds. Bethesda, MD, National Institutes of Health, National Diabetes Data Group, 1985 (NIH publ. no. 85-1468)
3. Barrett-Connor E, Wingard DL: Sex differential in ischemic heart disease mortality in diabetics: a prospective population-based study. *Am J Epidemiol* 118:489–96, 1983
4. Jarrett RJ, McCartney P, Keen H: The Bedford survey: ten-year mortality rates in newly diagnosed diabetics, borderline diabetics and normoglycaemic controls and risk indices for coronary heart disease in borderline diabetics. *Diabetologia* 22:79–84, 1982
5. Kannel W, McGee D: Diabetes and cardiovascular disease: the Framingham Study. *JAMA* 241:2035–38, 1979
6. Barrett-Connor E, Orchard T: Insulin-dependent diabetes mellitus and ischemic heart disease. *Diabetes Care* 8:65–70, 1985
7. Robertson W, Strong J: Atherosclerosis in persons with hypertension and diabetes mellitus. *Lab Invest* 18:538–51, 1968
8. Zarich S, Waxman S, Freeman R, Mittleman M, Hegarty P, Nesto RW: Effect of autonomic nervous system dysfunction on the circadian pattern of myocardial ischemia in diabetes mellitus. *J Am Coll Cardiol* 24:956–62, 1994
9. Nesto RW, Phillips RT, Kett KG, Hill T, Perper E, Young E, Leland OS Jr: Angina and exertional myocardial ischemia in dia-

betic and nondiabetic patients: assessment by exercise thallium scintigraphy. *Ann Intern Med* 108:170–75, 1988

10. Janand-Delenne B, Sabin B, Habib G, Bory M, Vague P, Lassman-Vague V: Silent myocardial ischemia in patients with diabetes: who to screen. *Diabetes Care* 22:1396–1400, 1999
11. Milan Study on Atherosclerosis and Diabetes (MiSAD) Group: Prevalence of unrecognized silent myocardial ischemia and its association with atherosclerotic risk factors in non-insulin dependent diabetes mellitus. *Am J Cardiol* 79:134–39, 1997
12. Koistinen MJ: Prevalence of asymptomatic myocardial ischemia in diabetic subjects. *BMJ* 301:92–95, 1990
13. Langer A, Freeman RM, Josse RG, Steiner G, Armstrong PW: Detection of silent myocardial ischemia in diabetes mellitus. *Am J Cardiol* 67:1073–78, 1991
14. Naka M, Hiramatsu K, Aizawa T, Momose A, Yoshizawa K, Shigematsu S, Ishihara F, Niwa A, Yamada T: Silent myocardial ischemia in patients with non-insulin-dependent diabetes mellitus as judged by treadmill exercise testing and coronary angiography. *Am Heart J* 123:46–53, 1992
15. Umachandran V, Ranjadayalan K, Ambepityia G, Marchant B, Kopelman PG, Timmis AD: The perception of angina in diabetes: relation to somatic pain threshold and autonomic function. *Am Heart J* 121:1649–54, 1991
16. Ambepityia G, Kopelman PG, Ingram D, Swash M, Mills PG, Timmis AD: Exertional myocardial ischemia in diabetes: a quantitative analysis of anginal perceptual threshold and the influence of autonomic function. *J Am Coll Cardiol* 15:72–77, 1990
17. Rowe JW, Young JB, Minaker KL, Stevens AL, Pallota J, Landsberg L: Effect of insulin and glucose infusions on sympathetic nervous system activity in normal men. *Diabetes* 30:219–25, 1981
18. Goldstein DS: Plasma catecholamines and essential hypertension: an analytic review. *Hypertension* 5:86–99, 1983
19. DeFronzo RA: The effect of insulin on renal sodium metabolism. *Diabetologia* 21:165–71, 1981
20. The Working Group on Hypertension in Diabetes: Statement on hypertension in diabetes mellitus: final report. *Arch Intern Med* 147:830–42, 1987
21. Zarich S, Nesto R: Diabetic cardiomyopathy. *Am Heart J* 118: 1000–12, 1989

22. Rubler S, Dlugash J, Yuceoglu YZ, Kumral T, Branwood AW, Grisham A: New type of cardiomyopathy associated with diabetic glomerulosclerosis. *Am J Cardiol* 30:595–602, 1972
23. Fein F: Diabetic cardiomyopathy. *Diabetes Care* 13:1169–79, 1990
24. Vered Z, Battler A, Segal P, Liberman D, Yerushalmi Y, Berezin M, Neufeld HN: Exercise induced left ventricular dysfunction in young men with asymptomatic diabetes mellitus (diabetic cardiomyopathy). *Am J Cardiol* 54:633–37, 1984
25. Mustonen JN, Uusitupa MI, Tahvanainen K, Talwar S, Laasko M, Lansimies E, Kuikka JT, Pyorala K: Impaired left ventricular systolic function during exercise in middle-aged insulin-dependent and non-insulin-dependent diabetic subjects without clinically evident cardiovascular disease. *Am J Cardiol* 62:1273–79, 1988
26. Takahashi N, Iwasaka T, Sugiura T, Hasegawa T, Tarumi N, Matsutani M, Onoyama H, Inada M: Left ventricular dysfunction during dynamic exercise in non-insulin-dependent diabetic patients with retinopathy. *Cardiology* 78:23–30, 1991
27. Borow KM, Jaspan JB, Williams KA, Neumann A, Wolinski-Walley P, Lang R: Myocardial mechanics in young adult patients with diabetes mellitus: effects of altered load, inotropic state and dynamic exercise. *J Am Coll Cardiol* 15:1508–17, 1990
28. Nesto RW: Diabetes and heart disease. In *World Book of Diabetes in Practice.* Vol. 3. Krall LP, Ed. Elsevier, 1988
29. Jacoby RM, Nesto RW: Acute myocardial infarction in the diabetic patient: pathophysiology, clinical course and prognosis. *J Am Coll Cardiol* 20:736–44, 1992
30. Paffenbarger RS, Hyde RT, Wing AL, Hsieh C: Physical activity, all-cause mortality, and longevity of college alumni. *N Engl J Med* 314:605–13, 1986
31. Leon AS, Connett J, Jacobs DR, Rauramaa R: Leisure-time physical activity levels and risk of coronary artery disease and death: the Multiple Risk Factor Intervention Trial. *JAMA* 258:2388–95, 1987
32. Powell KE, Thompson PD, Caspersen CJ, Kendrick JS: Physical activity and the incidence of coronary heart disease. *Annu Rev Public Health* 8:253–87, 1987
33. Blair SN, Kohl HW III, Paffenbarger RS Jr, Clark DG, Cooper KH, Gibbons IW: Physical fitness and all-cause mortality: a prospective study of healthy men and women. *JAMA* 262:2395–401, 1989

34. Helmrich SP, Ragland DR, Leung RW, Paffenbarger RS Jr: Physical activity and reduced occurrence of non-insulin-dependent diabetes mellitus. *N Engl J Med* 325:147–52, 1991
35. American Diabetes Association: Diabetes mellitus and exercise (Position Statement). *Diabetes Care* 24 (Suppl. 1):551–55, 2001
36. American College of Sports Medicine: The recommended quantity and quality of exercise for developing and maintaining cardiorespiratory and muscular fitness in healthy adults. *Med Sci Sports Exerc* 22:265–74, 1990
37. Blomquist CG: Cardiovascular adaptations to physical training. *Annu Rev Physiol* 45:169–89, 1983
38. Clausen JP: Circulatory adjustments to dynamic exercise and effect of physical training in normal subjects and in patients with coronary artery disease. *Prog Cardiovasc Dis* 18:459–95, 1976
39. Paterson DH, Shephard RJ, Cunningham D, Jones NL, Andrew G: Effects of physical training on cardiovascular function following myocardial infarction. *J Appl Physiol* 47:482–89, 1979
40. Redwood DR, Roring DR, Epstein SE: Circulatory and symptomatic effects of physical training in patients with coronary artery disease and angina pectoris. *N Engl J Med* 286:959–65, 1972
41. Ghilarducci LE, Holly RG, Amsterdam EA: Effects of high resistance training in coronary artery disease. *Am J Cardiol* 64:866–70, 1989
42. Hurley BF, Hagberg JM, Goldberg AP, Seals DR, Ehsani AA, Brennan RE, Holloszy JO: Resistive training can reduce coronary risk factors without altering VO_{2max} or percent body fat. *Med Sci Sports Exerc* 20:150–54, 1988
43. Hurley BF, Kokkinos PF: Effects of weight training on risk factors for coronary artery disease. *Sports Med* 4:231–38, 1987
44. Jennings G, Nelson L, Nestel P, Esler M, Korner P, Burton D, Bazelmans J: The effects of changes in physical activity on major cardiovascular risk factors, hemodynamics, sympathetic function, and glucose utilization in man: a controlled study of four levels of activity. *Circulation* 73:30–40, 1986
45. O'Connor GT, Buring JE, Yusuf S, Goldhaber SZ, Olmstead EM, Paffenbarger RS Jr, Hennekens CH: An overview of randomized trials of rehabilitation with exercise after myocardial infarction. *Circulation* 80:234–44, 1989

46. Mittleman MA, Maclure M, Tofler GH, Sherwood JB, Goldberg RJ, Muller JE: Triggering of acute myocardial infarction by heavy physical exertion. *N Engl J Med* 329:1677–83, 1993
47. American Heart Association Writing Group: Exercise standards: a statement for health professionals from the American Heart Association (Special Report). *Circulation* 91:580–615, 1995
48. Pollock ML, Wilmore JH (Eds.): *Exercise in Health and Disease: Evaluation and Prescription of Exercise for Prevention and Rehabilitation.* 2nd ed. Philadelphia, Saunders, 1990, p. 105
49. American College of Sports Medicine: *Guidelines for Exercise Testing and Prescription.* 4th ed. Philadelphia, Lea & Febiger, 1991
50. Butler RM, Beierwaltes WH, Rogers FJ: The cardiovascular response to circuit weight-training in patients with cardiac disease. *J Cardiopulm Rehab* 7:402–409, 1987
51. Blackburn H: Physical activity and hypertension. *J Clin Hypertens* 2:154–62, 1986
52. Seals DR, Hagberg JM: The effect of exercise on human hypertension: a review. *Med Sci Sports Exerc* 16:207–15, 1984
53. Martin JE, Dubert PM, Lushman WC: Controlled trial of aerobic exercise in hypertension. *Circulation* 81:1560–67, 1990
54. Krotkiewski M, Lonnroth P, Mandroukas K, Wroblewski Z, Rebuffe-Scrive M, Holm G, Smith U, Bjorntorp P: The effects of physical training on insulin secretion and effectiveness and on glucose metabolism in obesity and type 2 (non-insulin-dependent) diabetes mellitus. *Diabetologia* 28:881–90, 1985
55. Leon AS: Effects of exercise conditioning on physiologic precursors of coronary heart disease. *J Cardiopulm Rehab* 11:46–57, 1991
56. Schneider SH, Khachadurian AK, Amorosa LF, Clemow L, Ruderman NB: Ten-year experience with an exercise-based outpatient lifestyle modification program in the treatment of diabetes mellitus. *Diabetes Care* 15:1800–10, 1992
57. Kahn J, Zola B, Juni J, Vinik A: Decreased exercise heart rate and blood pressure response in diabetic subjects with cardiac autonomic neuropathy. *Diabetes Care* 9:389–94, 1986
58. Hilsted J, Galbo H, Christensen N: Impaired cardiovascular responses to graded exercise in diabetic autonomic neuropathy. *Diabetes Care* 28:313–19, 1979
59. Nesto RW: Screening for asymptomatic coronary artery disease in diabetes. *Diabetes Care* 22:1393–95, 1999

60. American Diabetes Association: Consensus development conference on the diagnosis of coronary heart disease in people with diabetes. *Diabetes Care* 21:1551–59, 1998
61. van Hoeven KH, Factor SM: A comparison of the pathological spectrum of hypertensive, diabetic, and hypertensive-diabetic heart disease. *Circulation* 82:848–55, 1990
62. Grossman E, Messerli FH: Diabetic and hypertensive heart disease. *Ann Intern Med* 125:304–10, 1996
63. Eichhorn EJ, Kosinski E, Lewis SM, Hill TC, Emond LH, Leland OS: Usefulness of dipyridamole-thallium-201 perfusion scanning for distinguishing ischemic from nonischemic cardiomyopathy. *Am J Cardiol* 62:945–51, 1988
64. Holley JL, Fenton RA, Arthur RS: Thallium stress testing does not predict cardiovascular risk in diabetic patients with end-stage renal disease undergoing cadaveric renal transplant. *Am J Med* 90: 563–70, 1991
65. Stevens MJ, Dayanikli F, Raffel DM, Allman KD, Sandford T, Feldman EL, Wieland DM, Corbett J, Schwaiger M: Scintigraphic assessment of regionalized defects in myocardial sympathetic innervation and blood flow regulation in diabetic patients with autonomic neuropathy. *J Am Coll Cardiol* 31:1575–84, 1998
66. Nahser PJ, Brown RE, Oskarsson H, Winniford MD, Rossen JD: Maximal coronary flow reserve and metabolic coronary vasodilation in patients with diabetes mellitus. *Circulation* 91:635–40, 1995
67. Dean JD, Jones CJH, Hutchison SJ, Peters JR, Henderson AH: Hyperinsulinaemia and microvascular angina (syndrome "X"). *Lancet* 337:456–57, 1991
68. Jaap AJ, Shore AC, Tooke JE: Relationship of insulin resistance to microvascular dysfunction in subjects with fasting hyperglycemia. *Diabetologia* 40:238–43, 1997
69. Van Camp SP: The safety of cardiac rehabilitation. *J Cardiopulm Rehab* 11:64–70, 1991

Sergio Waxman, MD, is from Harvard Medical School, Boston, MA.
Richard W. Nesto, MD, is from the Lahey Clinic, Burlington, MA.

25

Nephropathy: Early

CARL ERIK MOGENSEN, MD

Highlights

- Many diabetic patients have a normal albumin excretion rate (<20 μg/min). In some patients, moderate-intensity exercise provokes albuminuria, but whether exercise-induced albuminuria in these individuals predicts progression is not yet known.
- The major factors for progression from normo- to microalbuminuria are poor metabolic control and high normal albumin excretion rate (10–20 μg/min).
- Good metabolic control reduces exercise-induced albuminuria.
- In patients with microalbuminuria (20–200 μg/min), albuminuria increases considerably with light to moderate exercise.
- Increases in baseline albuminuria without exercise are related to blood pressure elevation. With physical exercise, acute increases in albuminuria are also related to acute increases in blood pressure.

- Antihypertensive treatment decreases not only baseline blood pressure but also exercise-induced blood pressure elevation and abnormal albuminuria.
- In overt diabetic renal disease (albumin excretion >200 µg/min), there are marked changes in blood pressure at baseline. These changes are further aggravated by physical exercise, during which blood pressure may reach high levels.
- In the clinical setting, pragmatic guidelines are proposed. Patients with diabetes, especially with microalbuminuria and overt renal disease, should probably perform only moderate-intensity exercise; severe and erratic exercise may have a deleterious effect not only on metabolic control but also on vascular and renal disease, although such adverse effects have not been documented in clinical trials.

The existence of exercise proteinuria has been known for many years. There are early descriptions of the phenomenon, but the first published report was that of Collier in 1907,[1] describing "functional albuminuria" in athletes. Since then, many articles on this topic related to normal renal physiology have been published.[2–20] The first to describe comprehensively the hemodynamic effects of exercise on such parameters as heart rate and blood pressure in patients with diabetes was published in 1966 by the Swedish investigator T. Karlefors.[21] A new era began around 1970 after the introduction of radioimmunoassay and other immunobased techniques[22,23] as exact measurements of urinary albumin excretion rate.

Regular physical exercise is usually recommended as part of the clinical care of diabetic patients. Apart from its benefits, exercise may also have important implications for vascular function and disease. Diabetic nephropathy eventually may develop in about one-third of patients with type 1 diabetes[24,25] and in a considerable number of patients with type 2 diabetes. Patients with incipient and overt diabetic nephropathy are known to manifest generalized vascular complications, which could be exaggerated or complicated by the impact of exercise. Antihypertensive treatment and good metabolic control seem to be the most effective intervention measures in postponing progression of early and late renal disease.[16,24] In this context, reducing exercise-induced blood pressure elevation during antihypertensive treatment is also important.[16,26–30]

Renal and Blood Pressure Response to Exercise in Healthy Individuals

Numerous studies have explored the acute and prolonged effects of exercise on renal hemodynamics, albuminuria, and blood pressure. Exercise (e.g., on a bicycle ergometer) considerably increases blood pressure in direct relation to the exercise load.[11,31,32] At the same time, exercise can cause pronounced changes in renal function.[33] An outline of an exercise test is shown in Fig. 25.1. With severe acute exercise, some decline in the glomerular filtration rate (GFR) and an even more pronounced reduction in renal plasma flow (RPF) occur. Thus, the filtration fraction is considerably increased,[33] and filtration pressure over the glomerular membrane is likely increased. The latter may lead to an increase in urinary albumin excretion rate, especially with severe or prolonged exercise, even in normal individuals.[32] Such exercise-induced changes in renal function are transient, and usually after 1 h at rest, the hemodynamic pattern is again reversed.[32,33] There are no

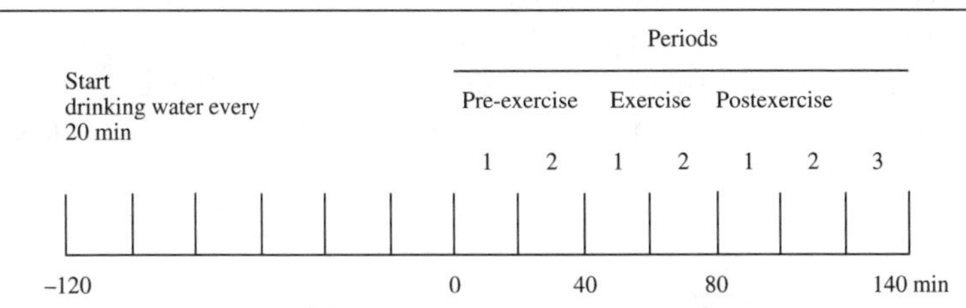

FIGURE 25.1 Experimental setup in the exercise provocation test on a bicycle ergometer. Heart rate was measured by counting the pulse rate, blood pressure by auscultatory technique, and urinary albumin excretion and urinary β_2-microglobulin excretion by radioimmunoassay; GFR/RPF was optional.

Reproduced from Mogensen CE, Christensen CK, Vittinghus E: The stages of diabetic renal disease with emphasis on the stage of incipient diabetic nephropathy. *Diabetes* 32 (Suppl. 2): 64–78, 1983.

reports indicating that exercise-induced changes in renal function in otherwise healthy individuals are deleterious in the long run. In other words, healthy individuals exposed to long-term exercise through their jobs or their sport activities do not appear to be more likely to develop renal disease.

Renal and Blood Pressure Response to Exercise in Type 1 Diabetic Patients

Karlefors,[21] many years ago, examined the hemodynamic response to exercise in diabetic individuals with complications. Since then, numerous studies have been performed to explore the renal and blood pressure response to exercise in diabetic individuals,[10–15,17,28,29,31–51] especially after it became possible to measure urinary proteins in small concentrations.[22,23] This chapter will focus on type 1 diabetes, because little information is available on the effect of exercise on renal function in patients with type 2 diabetes.[12,52,53]

Usually, the baseline urinary albumin excretion rate is increased in newly diagnosed type 1 diabetic patients, at least in those with poor glycemic control[31] (Fig. 25.2). This increase in albumin excretion rate is amplified by light and moderate physical exercise.[32] β_2-Microglobulin excretion, a marker of tubular proteinuria, is normal, suggesting that the changes are of glomerular origin.[10] It is also clear that glomerular hyperfiltration is often found at the time hyperglycemia is first diagnosed. With proper insulin treatment for a few weeks, these renal abnormalities are normalized, although some glomerular hyperfiltration usually persists. Most type 1 diabetic patients exhibit a normal baseline albumin excretion rate for the first 5 years after diagnosis,[25] although new studies suggest that this is not universally the case.[24]

Normoalbuminuric Diabetic Individuals

In normoalbuminuric type 1 diabetic individuals, changes in GFR and RPF in response to exercise are similar to those in healthy people without diabetes. As in people without diabetes, exercise causes a slight reduction in GFR during exercise and a more pronounced reduction in plasma flow, resulting in an increased filtration fraction. Usually, filtration fraction is already increased at baseline in type 1 di-

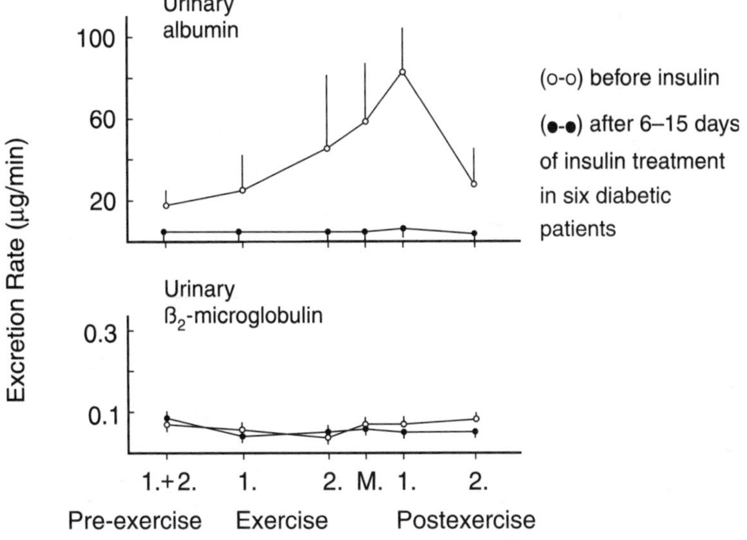

FIGURE 25.2 Urinary albumin and β_2-microglobulin excretion at the onset of type 1 diabetes in young patients, before and after insulin treatment, as described in Fig. 25.1. Urinary albumin excretion indicates glomerular proteinuria; β_2-microglobulin excretion indicates tubular proteinuria. The latter is not found.

Reproduced from Mogensen CE, Christensen CK, Vittinghus E: The stages of diabetic renal disease with emphasis on the stage of incipient diabetic nephropathy. *Diabetes* 32 (Suppl. 2): 64–78, 1983.

abetic patients, and this abnormality is amplified by exercise.[33] Therefore, exercise may lead to an increased albumin excretion rate in a considerable proportion of patients with type 1 diabetes (Fig. 25.3). Exercise-induced microalbuminuria in diabetes was first described in 1975.[11] Studies soon made clear that the greatest increase occurred immediately after exercise[10] (Fig. 25.2). Also apparent was that this increase in albumin excretion is of glomerular origin, because β_2-microglobulin excretion is not increased by exercise in these patients (Fig. 25.3). Thus, the exercise test reveals early glomerular changes or abnormalities.[10]

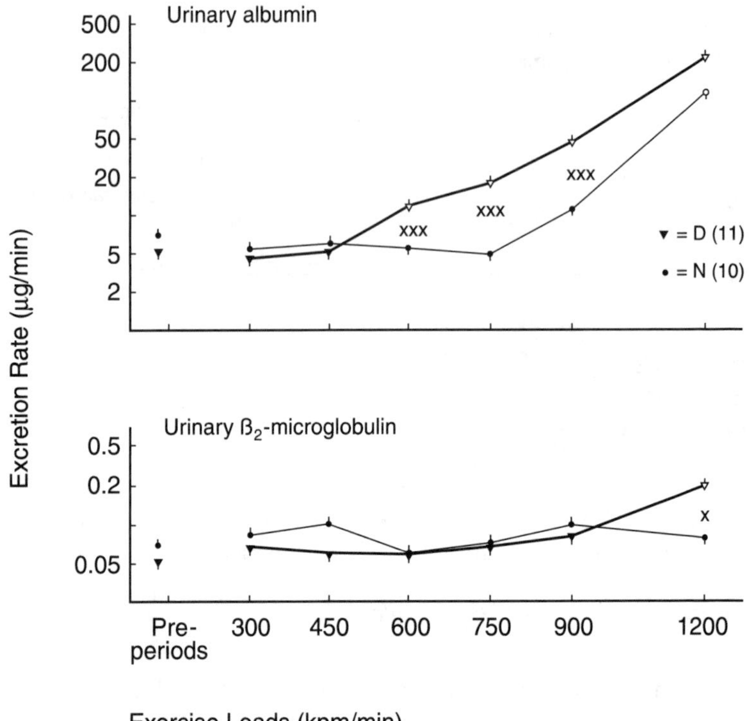

FIGURE 25.3 Graded exercise in diabetic (D) and normal (N) men; measurements of urinary proteins are in periods with increasing exercise. xxx, $P < 0.01$; x, $P < 0.05$.

Reproduced from Mogensen CE, Christensen CK, Vittinghus E: The stages of diabetic renal disease with emphasis on the stage of incipient diabetic nephropathy. *Diabetes* 32 (Suppl. 2): 64–78, 1983.

In some studies, exercise-induced albuminuria was not different in normoalbuminuric patients with type 1 diabetes and healthy control subjects.[37] This may reflect differences in diabetes duration and also the nature of the exercise test. Some investigators used a fixed exercise load, whereas others used a submaximal exercise load related to a calculated maximal exercise level.[37]

It has been suggested that exercise-induced albuminuria (in normoalbuminuric individuals) could be a predictor of the later development of microalbuminuria in type 1 diabetic patients. However, no proper prospective long-term study has been conducted to clarify this issue. Furthermore, the considerable variability in exercise-induced albuminuria in patients with normal baseline values suggests this test may not be a valid predictor. Resting baseline values (e.g., overnight collections or early-morning urine) show a gradual increase in albumin excretion with time in patients who progress to microalbuminuria or overt renal disease. For these reasons, longitudinal measurements of baseline values may provide more useful information than the exercise test, both in the clinical setting and in research projects. Baseline values for albumin excretion at rest may also show considerable variability; however, performing many repeated measurements is easy. Potentially, the exercise test might be used to study the response to antihypertensive treatment. A drug that not only protects against an exercise-induced blood pressure elevation but also ameliorates exercise-induced albuminuria may be considered beneficial.[27–30]

Because exercise may induce microalbuminuria in normoalbuminuric individuals, care should be taken that urine samples collected after exercise are not used in the clinical follow-up of patients; early-morning urine should be used instead.[24]

Microalbuminuric Diabetic Individuals

Type 1 diabetic patients with microalbuminuria (urinary albumin excretion rates >20 μg/min) or incipient diabetic nephropathy usually show some increase in blood pressure in the baseline resting situation. This increase is further aggravated by physical exercise, and usually there is a correlation between the albuminuria (Fig. 25.4) and the blood pressure increase (Fig. 25.5) induced by exercise.[31] As in patients with normoalbuminuria, exercise-induced albuminuria in patients with microalbuminuria at rest is of glomerular origin.[10,31,32] It is likely that the increased systemic blood pressure response in microalbuminuric individuals is to some extent transmitted to the glomerulus, inducing a stretching effect on the glomerular structure and thus producing an increased glomerular passage of plasma protein molecules, in particular, albumin.

Whether the increased albuminuria caused by this mechanism promotes further renal damage is unknown, although it has been proposed that albuminuria in its own right may contribute to renal structural damage.[24] To date, there is no evidence that short-term periods of exercise, by provoking proteinuria, cause renal damage. However, this possibility cannot be excluded.

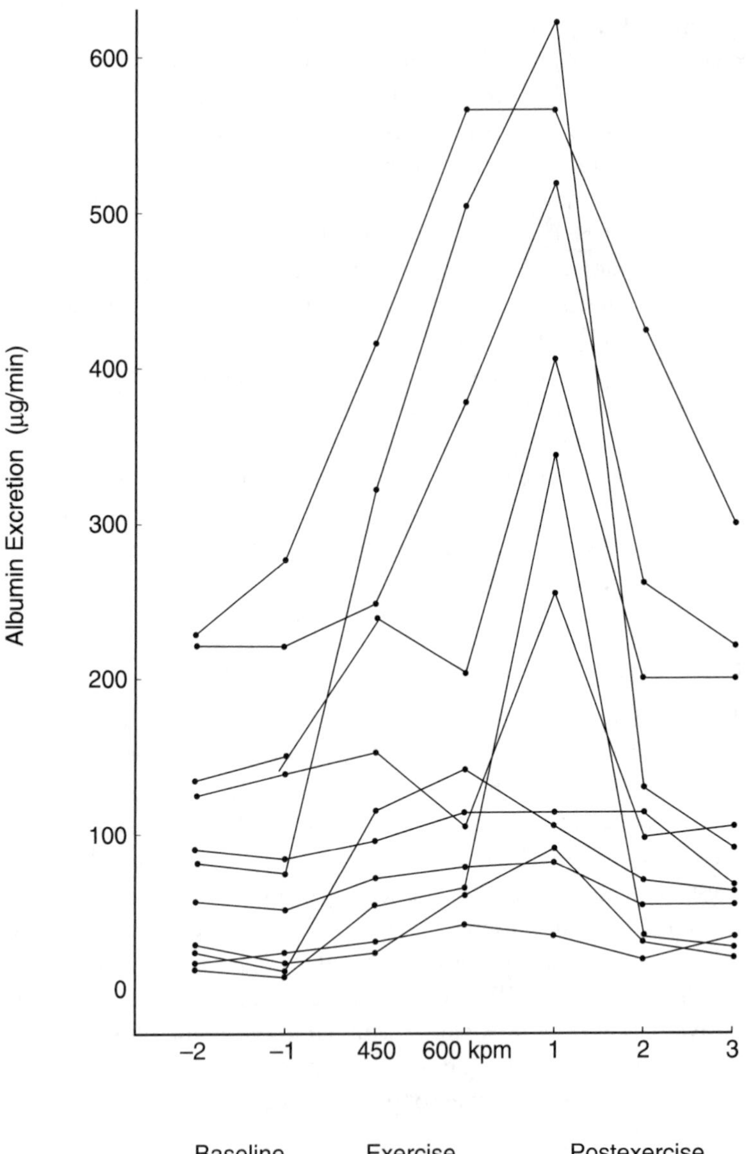

FIGURE 25.4 Urinary albumin excretion during exercise in young diabetic men with incipient diabetic nephropathy (baseline urinary albumin excretion at screening: 20–200 μg/min).

Reproduced from Mogensen CE, Christensen CK, Vittinghus E: The stages of diabetic renal disease with emphasis on the stage of incipient diabetic nephropathy. *Diabetes* 32 (Suppl. 2): 64–78, 1983.

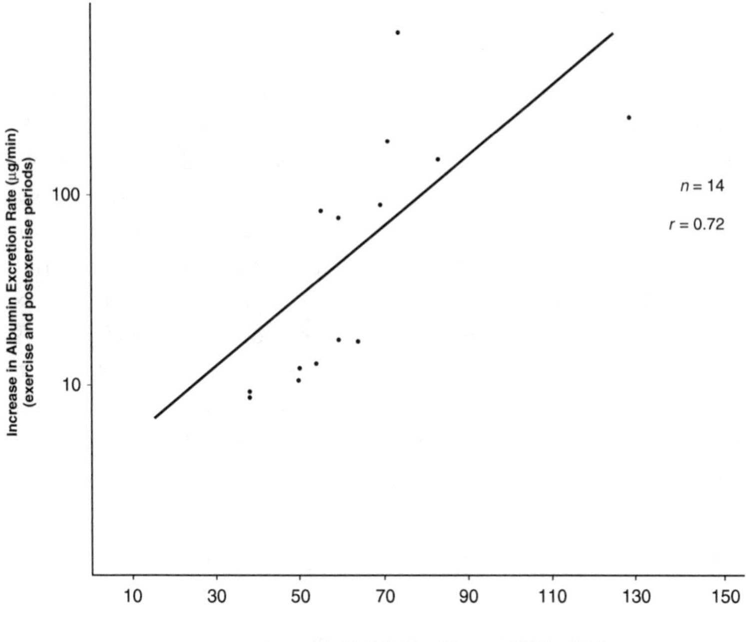

FIGURE 25.5 Increase in albumin excretion rate during exercise plotted against the increase in systolic blood pressure during exercise (600 kpm/min) (patients as shown in Fig 25.4).

Reproduced from Mogensen CE, Christensen CK, Vittinghus E: The stages of diabetic renal disease with emphasis on the stage of incipient diabetic nephropathy. *Diabetes* 32 (Suppl. 2): 64–78, 1983.

Individuals With Diabetes and Overt Proteinuria

Overt proteinuria is characterized by large increases in urinary albumin excretion to rates >200 µg/min. With the development of proteinuria, the decline in GFR usually starts. Exercise increases blood pressure abnormally in proteinuric diabetic individuals.[21] The clearance of large molecular dextran is also enhanced by exercise in these individuals.[34] This has been attributed to depletion of negative charges on the glomerular capillary wall; however, whether this phenomenon influences exercise-induced proteinuria is unknown. The influence of exercise on the clinical status of patients with overt nephropathy has been poorly investigated and warrants further study.

The Daily Life Exercise Situation and Renal Prognosis

As indicated, there may be a potential risk of more rapid progression of nephropathy in individuals who exercise intensively on a regular basis and thus have more exercise-induced albuminuria and blood pressure increases during their daily life situation. There are no definitive studies that address this important clinical issue. A study from Japan in a small series of patients suggests no difference in clinical outcome between individuals with diabetes who exercised to a limited extent and those who exercised heavily in their daily life situation.[54] Less questionable is the potential risk of severe exercise in patients with nephropathy who also have proliferative retinopathy. These patients may experience retinal hemorrhages as a result of substantial elevations in blood pressure (see Chapter 23).

Effect of Intervention Programs on Exercise-Induced Albuminuria

It has been documented that exercise-induced albuminuria can be reduced by good metabolic control in patients with type 1 diabetes.[32,44,49] Exercise-induced albuminuria in type 1 diabetic patients can also be reduced in the short term as well as in the long term by antihypertensive treatment.[27–29] An example is shown in Fig. 25.6. A similar effect of antihypertensive agents has also been observed in patients with essential hypertension.[16,26,30] Aspirin and dipyridamole may reduce exercise-induced albuminuria, but further studies are needed to confirm this finding.[41] A similar effect using picotamide in type 2 diabetic patients was obtained by Giustina et al.[55] Indomethacin seems also to reduce exercise-induced albuminuria.[56] New studies confirm the effect of antihypertensive treatment on albuminuria, including exercise-induced change.[57,58]

Pragmatic Exercise Recommendations in Patients With Type 1 Diabetes and Nephropathy

Whether or not specific exercise recommendations are needed for most patients with incipient or overt nephropathy is an open question. In patients with overt nephropathy, there is usually self-limitation because their exercise capacity is generally diminished. Clearly, however,

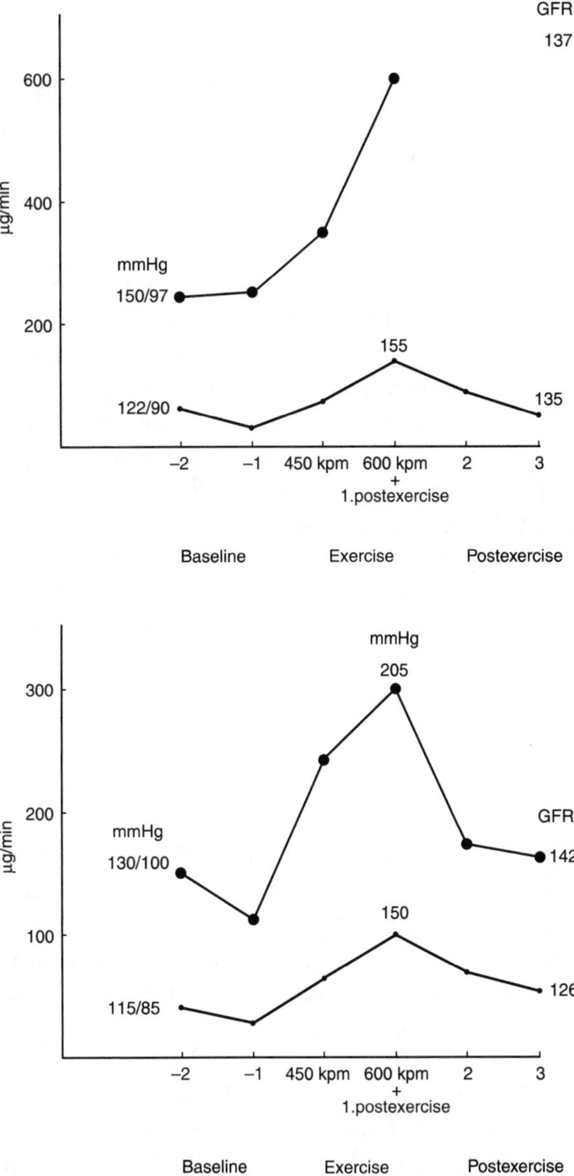

FIGURE 25.6 Albumin excretion before and after antihypertensive treatment. Data from exercise provocation tests.

Reproduced from Mogensen CE, Christensen CK, Vittinghus E: The stages of diabetic renal disease with emphasis on the stage of incipient diabetic nephropathy. *Diabetes* 32 (Suppl. 2): 64–78, 1983.

recommending severe exercise or excessive sport activities in these individuals would not be prudent. On the other hand, there is no reason light to moderate exercise should be excluded from the patient's usual daily activities. Such exercise may be useful for other reasons and is unlikely to have any harmful effect on renal function.

Notes Regarding Type 2 Diabetes

Only a few studies examine exercise-induced albuminuria in patients with type 2 diabetes.[13,52,53] Light to moderate exercise may induce microalbuminuria in these patients, and good control may ameliorate the abnormality.[13] However, moderate-intensity exercise can be of importance in the clinical management of type 2 diabetic patients, and no evidence suggests that it has an adverse effect on renal prognosis. Rather, exercise should be encouraged. In the long run, such an exercise program may reduce the associated hypertension, although there are no clinical trials in this area. Note that patients with type 2 diabetes are often quite sedentary, and as shown in the Diabetes Prevention Program in the U.S., it is usually more advisable to propose, rather than discourage, exercise.

References

1. Collier W: Functional albuminuria in athletes. *Br Med J* 1:4–6, 1907
2. Campanacci L, Faccini L, Englaro E, Rustia R, Guarnieri GF, Barat R, Carraro M, De Zotti R, Micheli W: Exercise-induced proteinuria. *Contrib Nephrol* 26:31–41, 1981
3. Castenfors J: Renal function during exercise with special reference to exercise proteinuria and the release of renin (Abstract). *Acta Physiol Scand* 70 (Suppl.):293, 1967
4. Clerico A, Giammattei C, Cecchini L, Lucchetti A, Cruschelli L, Penno G, Gregori G, Giampietro O: Exercise-induced proteinuria in well-trained athletes. *Clin Chem* 36:562–64, 1990
5. Houser MT, Jahn MF, Kobayashi A, Walburn J: Assessment of urinary protein excretion in the adolescent: effect of body position and exercise. *J Pediatr* 109:556–61, 1986
6. Houser MT: Characterization of recumbent, ambulatory, and postexercise proteinuria in the adolescent. *Pediatr Res* 21:442–46, 1987

7. Huttunen NP, Käär ML, Pietiläinen M, Vierikko P, Reinilä M: Exercise-induced proteinuria in children and adolescents. *Scand J Clin Lab Invest* 41:58–87, 1981
8. Kachadorian WA, Johnson RE: Renal responses to various rates of exercise. *J Appl Physiol* 28:748–52, 1970
9. Krämer BK, Kernz M, Ress KM, Pfohl M, Müller GA, Schmülling RM, Risler T: Influence of strenuous exercise on albumin excretion. *Clin Chem* 34:2516–18, 1988
10. Mogensen CE, Vittinghus E, Solling E: Abnormal albumin excretion after two provocative renal tests in diabetes: physical exercise and lysine injection. *Kidney Int* 16:385–93, 1979
11. Mogensen CE, Vittinghus E: Urinary albumin excretion during exercise in juvenile diabetes: a provocative test for early abnormalities. *Scand J Clin Lab Invest* 35:295–300, 1975
12. Dahlquist G, Aperia A, Carlsson L, Linne T, Persson B, Thoren C, Wilton P: Effect of metabolic control and duration on exercise-induced albuminuria in diabetic teenagers. *Acta Paediatr Scand* 72:895–902, 1983
13. Mohamed A, Wilkin T, Leatherdale BA, Rowe D: Response of urinary albumin to submaximal exercise in newly diagnosed non-insulin-dependent diabetes. *Br Med J* 288:1342–43, 1984
14. Nordgren H, Freyschuss U, Persson B: Blood pressure response to physical exercise in healthy adolescents and adolescents with insulin-dependent diabetes mellitus. *Clin Sci* 86:425–32, 1994
15. Osei K: Ambulatory and exercise-induced blood pressure responses in type 1 diabetic patients and normal subjects. *Diabetes Res Clin Pract* 3:125–34, 1987
16. Pedersen EB, Mogensen CE, Larsen JS: Effects of exercise on urinary excretion of albumin and β_2-microglobulin in young patients with mild essential hypertension without treatment and during long-term propranolol treatment. *Scand J Clin Lab Invest* 41:493–98, 1981
17. Poortmans J, Dorchy H, Toussaint D: Urinary excretion of total proteins, albumin, and β_2-microglobulin during rest and exercise in diabetic adolescents with and without retinopathy. *Diabetes Care* 5:617–23, 1982
18. Poortmans JR: Postexercise proteinuria in humans: facts and mechanisms. *JAMA* 253:236–40, 1985
19. Robertshaw M, Cheung CK, Fairly I, Swaminathan R: Protein excretion after prolonged exercise. *Ann Clin Biochem* 30:34–37, 1993

20. Taylor A: Some characteristics of exercise proteinuria. *Clin Sci* 19:209–17, 1960
21. Karlefors T: Circulatory studies during exercise with particular reference to diabetics. *Acta Med Scand* 180 (Suppl.):449, 1966
22. Keen H, Chlouverakis C: Urinary albumin excretion and diabetes mellitus. *Lancet* ii:1155–56, 1964
23. Miles DW, Mogensen CE, Gundersen HJG: Radioimmunoassay for urinary albumin using a single antibody. *Scand J Clin Lab Invest* 26:5–11, 1970
24. Mogensen CE: Definition of diabetic renal disease in insulin-dependent diabetes mellitus based on renal function tests. In *The Kidney and Hypertension in Diabetes Mellitus.* 5th ed. Mogensen CE, Ed. Boston, MA, Kluwer Academic Publishers, 2000, p. 13–28
25. Mogensen CE: Microalbuminuria, early blood pressure elevation, and diabetic renal disease. *Curr Opin Endocrinol Diabetes* 1:239–47, 1994
26. Christensen CK, Krusell LR: Acute and long-term effect of antihypertensive treatment on exercise-induced microalbuminuria in essential hypertension. *J Clin Hypertens* 3:704–12, 1987
27. Christensen CK, Mogensen CE: Acute and long-term effect of antihypertensive treatment on exercise-induced albuminuria in incipient diabetic nephropathy. *Scand J Clin Lab Invest* 46:553–59, 1986
28. Romanelli G, Giustina A, Bossoni S, Caldonaxxo A, Cimino A, Cravarezza P, Giustina G: Short-term administration of captopril and nifedipine and exercise-induced albuminuria in normotensive diabetic patients with early-stage nephropathy. *Diabetes* 39: 1333–38, 1990
29. Romanelli G, Giustina A, Cimino A: Short-term effect of captopril on microalbuminuria induced by exercise in normotensive diabetics. *Br Med J* 298:284–88, 1989
30. Samuelsson O, Rångemark C, Lind H, Lindholm L, Pennert K, Hedner T: Lisinopril lowers postexercise albuminuria more effectively than atenolol in uncomplicated, primary hypertension. *J Hypertens* 12 (Suppl. 3):S43, 1994
31. Christensen CK: Abnormal albuminuria and blood pressure rise in incipient diabetic nephropathy induced by exercise. *Kidney Int* 25:819–23, 1984

32. Vittinghus E, Mogensen CE: Graded exercise and protein excretion in diabetic man and the effect of insulin treatment. *Kidney Int* 21:725–29, 1982
33. Vittinghus E, Mogensen CE: Albumin excretion and renal haemodynamic response to physical exercise in normal and diabetic man. *Scand J Clin Lab Invest* 41:627–32, 1981
34. Ala-Houhala I: Effects of exercise on glomerular passage of macromolecules in patients with diabetic nephropathy and in healthy subjects. *Scand J Clin Lab Invest* 50:27–33, 1990
35. Brouhard BH, Allen K, Sapire D, Travis LB: Effect of exercise on urinary N-acetyl-β-D-glucosaminidase activity and albumin excretion in children with type 1 diabetes mellitus. *Diabetes Care* 8:466–72, 1985
36. Chase HP, Garg SK, Harris S, Marshall G, Hoops S: Elevation of resting and exercise blood pressures in subjects with type 1 diabetes and relation to albuminuria. *J Diabetes Complications* 6:138–42, 1992
37. Feldt-Rasmussen B, Baker L, Deckert T: Exercise as a provocative test in early renal disease in type 1 (insulin-dependent) diabetes: albuminuric, systemic and renal haemodynamic responses. *Diabetologia* 28:389–96, 1985
38. Garg SK, Chase HP, Harris S, Marshall G, Hoops S, Osberg I: Glycemic control and longitudinal testing for exercise microalbuminuria in subjects with type 1 diabetes. *J Diabetes Complications* 4:154–58, 1990
39. Groop L, Stenman S, Groop PH, Mäkipernaa A, Teppo AM: The effect of exercise on urinary excretion of different size proteins in patients with insulin-dependent diabetes mellitus. *Scand J Clin Lab Invest* 50:525–32, 1990
40. Hermansson G, Ludvigsson J: Renal function and blood-pressure reaction during exercise in diabetic and non-diabetic children and adolescents. *Acta Paediatr Scand* 283 (Suppl.):86–94, 1980
41. Hopper AH, Tindall H, Urquhart S, Davies JA: Reduction of exercise-induced albuminuria by aspirin-dipyridamole in patients with diabetes mellitus. *Horm Metab Res* 19:210–13, 1987
42. Huttunen NP, Käär ML, Puukka R, Åkerblom HK: Exercise-induced proteinuria in children and adolescents with type 1 (insulin-dependent) diabetes. *Diabetologia* 21:495–97, 1981

43. Jefferson JG, Greene SA, Smith MA, Smith RF, Griffin NKG, Baum JD: Urine albumin to creatinine ratio response to exercise in diabetes. *Arch Dis Child* 60:305, 1985
44. Koivisto VA, Huttunen NP, Vierikko P: Continuous subcutaneous insulin infusion corrects exercise-induced albuminuria in juvenile diabetes. *Br Med J* 282:778–79, 1981
45. Rubler S, Arvan SB: Exercise testing in young asymptomatic diabetic patients. *Angiology* 27:539–48, 1976
46. Torffvit O, Castenfors J, Bengtsson U, Agardh CD: Exercise stimulation in insulin-dependent diabetics, normal increase in albuminuria with abnormal blood pressure response. *Scand J Clin Lab Invest* 47:253–59, 1987
47. Townsend JC: Increased albumin excretion in diabetes. *J Clin Pathol* 43:3–8, 1990
48. Viberti GC, Jarrett RJ, McCartney M, Keen M: Increased glomerular permeability to albumin induced by exercise in diabetic subjects. *Diabetologia* 14:293–300, 1978
49. Viberti GC, Pickup JC, Bilous RW, Keen H, Mackintosh D: Correction of exercise-induced microalbuminuria in insulin-dependent diabetics after 3 weeks of subcutaneous insulin infusion. *Diabetes* 30:818–23, 1981
50. Watts GF, Williams I, Morris RW, Mandalia S, Shaw KM, Polak A: An acceptable exercise test to study microalbuminuria in type 1 diabetes. *Diabet Med* 6:787–92, 1989
51. Bognetti E, Meschi F, Pattarini A, Zoja A, Chiumello G: Postexercise albuminuria does not predict microalbuminuria in type 1 diabetic patients. *Diabet Med* 11:850–56, 1994
52. Fujita Y, Matoba K, Takeuchi H, Ishii K, Yajima Y: Anaerobic threshold can provoke microalbuminuria in non-insulin-dependent diabetics. *Diabet Res Clin Pract* 22:155–62, 1994
53. Inomata S, Oosawa Y, Itoh M, Inoue M, Masamune O: Analysis of urinary proteins in diabetes mellitus with reference to the relationship between microalbuminuria and diabetic renal lesions. *J Jpn Diabetic Soc* 30:429–35, 1987
54. Matsuoka K, Nakao T, Atsumi Y, Takekoshi H: Exercise regimen for patients with diabetic nephropathy. *J Diabetes Complications* 5:98–100, 1991
55. Giustina A, Bossoni S, Cimino A, Comini MT, Gazzoli N, Leproux GB, Wehrenberg WB, Romanelli G, Giustina G: Picotamide, a dual

TXB synthetase inhibitor and TXB receptor antagonist, reduces exercise-induced albuminuria in microalbuminuric patients with NIDDM. *Diabetes* 42:178–82, 1993

56. Rudberg S, Sätterström G, Dahlquist R, Dahlquist G: Indomethacin but not metoprolol reduces exercise-induced albumin excretion rate in type 1 diabetic patients with microalbuminuria. *Diabet Med* 10:460–64, 1993
57. Poulsen PL, Ebbehøj E, Nosadini R, Fioretto P, Deferrari D, Crepaldi D, Mogensen CE: Early ACE-i intervention in microalbuminuric patients with type 1 diabetes: effects on albumin excretion, 24 h ambulatory blood pressure, and renal function. *Diabete Metab* 27:123–28, 2001
58. Poulsen PL, Ebbehøj E, Mogensen CE: Lisinopril reduces albuminuria during exercise in low grade microalbuminuric type 1 diabetic patients: a double blind randomized study. *J Intern Med* 249:433–40, 2001

Carl Erik Mogensen, MD, is from Aarhus Kommunehospital, Aarhus, Denmark.

26

Nephropathy: Advanced

SAMUEL A. HEADLEY, PHD,
MICHAEL J. GERMAIN, MD,
AND GREGORY L. BRADEN, MD

Highlights

- Of dialysis patients, 40.3% have diabetes.
- Dialysis patients have functional capacities that are 50% those of sedentary age-matched control subjects.
- Exercise capacity in dialysis patients is limited by both central and peripheral factors.
- Exercise testing should be performed in all patients before initiation of an exercise program.
- A program of endurance training is highly recommended in appropriately screened dialysis and transplant patients because cardiovascular disease is the major cause of death in these populations.
- Exercise can be performed safely during the first 2 h of a dialysis treatment or during off-dialysis days.
- A low-resistance, high-repetition resistance training program is recommended for appropriately screened patients.

Within the past 2 decades, there has been a substantial increase in the number of individuals with diabetes who require renal replacement therapy (RRT).[1] Based on the data reported by the United States Renal Data System, 40.3% of individuals who are currently receiving RRT (i.e., hemodialysis) are individuals with diabetes.[2] In 1988, this number was 27% and in 1992, it was 36%.[3] It is also now apparent that individuals with type 2 diabetes, who actually comprise the vast majority of the diabetic population, are at great risk of developing renal complications due to their disease.[1] In fact, 28.7% of end-stage renal disease (ESRD) patients are individuals who have type 2 diabetes, whereas 11.6% have type 1 diabetes.[2]

Although no specific studies of exercise capacity in diabetic, dialysis-dependent, or renal transplant patients have been performed, exercise studies in nondiabetic, dialysis, and transplant patients are useful in developing safe and beneficial exercise programs for individuals with diabetes and renal disease. Researchers have found that hemodialysis patients, in general, have functional capacities that are about 50% those of sedentary, age-matched, healthy control subjects.[4,5] Physical inactivity, in addition to chronic uremia, may be responsible for the low functional capacity that characterizes ESRD patients. Painter[6] described a "spiral of deconditioning" that is common among ESRD patients. Prolonged periods of bed rest and inactivity have been shown to have wide-ranging negative physiological effects on patients, including decreased glucose tolerance.[7]

Functional Capacity in ESRD Patients

ESRD patients have lower cardiac outputs than healthy age-matched individuals.[5] In addition, the maximal obtainable cardiac output in patients on dialysis has been reported as 16 l/min, which is well below that seen in normal sedentary individuals (range 25–30 l/min).The lower cardiac output is caused by a blunted heart rate response, because stroke volume is not drastically different from normal.[5] Typically, the maximum heart rate of ESRD patients is 75% of their age-predicted maximum value.[5] The reason for this blunted maximum heart rate is currently unknown, and furthermore, we do not know if ESRD patients with diabetes have a different heart rate response than other ESRD patients. This may be the case because nearly all patients with advanced diabetic nephropathy have grossly abnormal autonomic tests, and 50% have symptomatic autonomic neuropathy.[8]

The measurement of peak oxygen consumption (VO_{2peak}) is considered to be the "gold standard" for aerobic fitness. ESRD patients have VO_{2peak} values that range from 14.4 to 28.3 ml · kg^{-1} · min^{-1} compared with those of normal sedentary individuals, which range from 30 to 40 ml · kg^{-1} · min^{-1}.[6] Such a low aerobic capacity makes it difficult for ESRD patients to perform a significant amount of physical work on a daily basis, and therefore, many are unemployed. Although submaximal exercise in diabetic patients is clearly beneficial, even a 25% increase in VO_{2peak} does not increase exercise capacity enough in most dialysis patients to allow for more rigorous daily activities, such as washing windows, painting, or snow shoveling.[6] The low aerobic capacity is caused by reductions in the oxygen-carrying capacity of blood (central factors) and by impaired oxygen extraction by peripheral tissues (i.e., peripheral factors).[5]

Before the introduction of human recombinant erythropoietin (EPO), researchers believed that anemia was the main reason for the observed low functional capacity in ESRD patients. However, although EPO administration improves peak oxygen uptake (by 18%), the magnitude of the improvement is not proportional to the increase in hematocrit (58%).[5] As a result, it has become quite clear that skeletal muscle dysfunction plays a significant role in the reduced exercise tolerance observed among ESRD patients.[5] Diesel et al.[9] found a significant correlation ($r = 0.66–0.68$, $P < 0.05$) between isokinetic muscular strength and peak oxygen uptake in a sample of ESRD patients. However, they did not find as strong a relationship with hemoglobin concentration, total blood hemoglobin content, or hematocrit ($r = 0.33–0.54$, $P > 0.05$), indexes of oxygen transport capacity.[9] In addition, studies measuring arterial-venous oxygen difference during exercise in dialysis patients, either at low or near-normal hematocrits, show that A-VO_2 difference does not increase as hematocrit increases because of decreased tissue oxygen use.[5]

Decrements in the expression of muscular strength have consistently been found among ESRD patients. Although results were preliminary, Bohannon et al.[10] observed that ESRD patients with diabetes had the most significant strength impairment compared with other ESRD patients. The reason for the fatigue and muscle weakness observed among ESRD patients has not been conclusively established.

However, researchers have proposed a number of reasons, including muscle wasting, atrophy of type II fibers, corticosteroid use, malnutrition, peripheral neuropathy, ischemic myopathy, hyperparathyroidism, a deficiency in carnitine, sedentary living, excitation-contraction coupling abnormalities, abnormalities in aerobic and anaerobic metabolism, slow muscle relaxation, and reduced skeletal muscle blood flow due to impaired vasodilation.[11–13]

Predialysis: Benefits of Starting an Exercise Program Early and Starting Dialysis Early

Dialysis patients who start dialysis with a glomerular filtration rate <10 ml/min and uremic symptoms are more likely to be hospitalized, malnourished, and have a more sedentary lifestyle than patients who start dialysis earlier. The late-start patients may have great difficulty starting or continuing an exercise program. Early initiation of dialysis (i.e., a healthy start) may allow maintenance of an exercise program promoting a sense of well-being. Because diabetic patients have such a high incidence of ESRD, and exercise has been shown to be beneficial in ESRD patients, it would be logical to initiate an exercise program as early as possible in the course of the patient's disease.

Benefits of Aerobic Exercise in ESRD Patients and Transplant Recipients

Exercise training is highly recommended in appropriately screened ESRD patients and transplant recipients because cardiovascular disease is the major cause of death within this patient population. Coronary artery disease (CAD) accounts for 14–50% of deaths after renal transplantation.[14] Diabetes increases the risk of cardiovascular complications in ESRD patients and transplant recipients.[14] Individuals with diabetes, who comprise the highest proportion of individuals with advanced renal disease, can benefit significantly from chronic endurance training. Chronic endurance training is likely to increase functional capacity, reduce body fat, increase lean body mass, improve blood pressure control, reduce triglyceride-rich very-low-density lipoproteins (VLDLs), improve glycemic control, and enhance insulin sensitivity in patients with renal disease and in transplant recipients .[4,15,16]

Benefits of Intradialytic Exercise

The previously mentioned benefits of chronic exercise training primarily refer to exercise on off-dialysis days. Intradialytic exercise, or exercise conducted during a hemodialysis session, has been shown to be both safe and effective, particularly during the first 2 h of a dialysis treatment.[17] Exercising during hemodialysis offers a number of benefits, such as improved patient compliance to exercise, reduced boredom, ease of patient supervision, less muscle cramping, and less hypotensive episodes.[18,19] Moreover, some researchers believe that intradialytic exercise may improve urea clearance and reduce the postdialysis urea rebound that occurs.[20] Furthermore, Fitts[16] claims that the safest time for the diabetic ESRD patient to exercise is during the hemodialysis session because blood glucose is "clamped" during that time and the possibility of exercise-induced hyperkalemia is reduced. Recently, Cappy et al.[21] reported a 12% reduction in phosphorus levels after a 12-month in-center exercise program. However, they reported a nonsignificant reduction in plasma glucose and glycosylated hemoglobin after the 12-month exercise program in their diabetic patients.[21]

Peritoneal Dialysis

Because peritoneal dialysis is usually done continuously, fluid and electrolytes are kept at a steady state. This should be an ideal situation in terms of tolerability and safety of exercise. Peritoneal dialysis is usually a home treatment so exercise can be prescribed at home or in an outpatient exercise facility. There may be some limitations to very strenuous exercise because of abdominal distension from the peritoneal fluid in the abdomen. Recently, Lo et al.[22] demonstrated that a 12-week endurance training program was safe and led to an improvement in both exercise tolerance (16.2% increase in VO_{2peak}) and quality of life measures.

Transplant Patients

Kidney transplantation leads to an increase in aerobic capacity within about 6–8 weeks after surgery in patients previously on hemodialysis.[6] This improvement in exercise capacity is due, in part, to the correction of anemia. However, increases in VO_{2peak} in renal transplant patients do not fully correlate with increases in hematocrit, and other factors, such as correction of uremic myopathy, may be important.[23]

Transplant patients with diabetes have a 20-fold greater chance of dying from cardiovascular disease than normal patients, whereas the nondiabetic transplant recipient has a 6-fold greater risk.[14] Some of the side effects associated with the use of immunosuppressive drugs in the treatment of transplant recipients include hypertension, hyperlipidemia, glucose intolerance, and steroid-induced diabetes. Chronic endurance training can favorably alter these risk factors for CAD.

Screening

Before the initiation of an exercise program, whether intradialytic or during off-dialysis days, the dialysis patient should have a thorough medical examination. Such an examination is essential to determine if the benefits of exercise for a specific patient outweigh the risks involved. The physician needs to screen the patient for evidence of macro- and microvascular complications that may be associated with diabetes.[15] In individuals with diabetes, it is important to assess the level of cardiac function and to screen for subclinical CAD (see Chapters 13–15, 24) because diabetes, hypertension, hyperlipidemia, and the uremic milieu are all associated with accelerated atherosclerosis. Virtually all patients with advanced diabetic nephropathy have retinopathy, with blindness being five times more common in diabetic subjects with nephropathy versus those without. Stroke, CAD, and peripheral vascular disease are two to five times more common.[8]

A physician-supervised graded exercise stress test is recommended before exercise participation. Such a test helps to evaluate the cardiovascular response to exercise, including any evidence of ischemia, dysrhythmias, hemodynamic abnormalities, and left ventricular dysfunction, and gives an objective measure of exercise tolerance. Patients with documented contraindications to exercise, as defined by organizations such as the American College of Sports Medicine (ACSM) or the American Heart Association, should not be allowed to participate in an exercise program.[24,25] For example, type 1 diabetic subjects with fasting plasma glucose levels >240 mg/dl and evidence of ketosis from a blood sample, or plasma glucose levels in excess of 300 mg/dl, should not exercise.[24] In such cases, the risks involved with exercise outweigh the benefits.

Aerobic Exercise Prescription

As previously stated, whether doing intradialytic exercise or exercise on off-dialysis days, it is ideal to perform some graded exercise test before the initiation of an exercise program. Information from this test can be used to help develop the initial exercise prescription and to chart patient progress over time. Intradialytic exercise sessions should be conducted during the first 2 h of a hemodialysis treatment.[17] Patients with arm grafts can perform exercise with a cycle placed in front of their dialysis chair. Initially, most hemodialysis patients are unable to exercise continuously for a prolonged period of time; therefore, an interval training method is recommended. Work periods from as little as 3 min interspersed with 2-min rest periods can be used. Over time, as the patient adapts to exercise, the work period can be increased and the rest interval decreased. The goal is to have the patient exercise continuously for at least 20–40 min, three times each week, at a work rate that elicits a rating of perceived exertion (RPE) of fairly light[11] to somewhat hard[13] using the Borg scale, which is a 15-point Likert scale used to document perceived exertion.[24] Each session should consist of a warm-up at a low work rate, a conditioning period at the target work rate as previously specified, and a cooldown (see Chapter 14).

With a few exceptions, the ESRD patient with diabetes who exercises on off-dialysis days needs to follow similar exercise guidelines that have been established for other individuals with diabetes (see Chapter 14).[15,24,25] Because of their hemodialysis schedule, most ESRD patients with diabetes will only be able to exercise three to four times each week. Individuals with type 1 diabetes should not exercise unless they are in good metabolic control. Both types of diabetic patients should begin each exercise session with a 5- to 10-min warm-up using aerobic-type activities followed by a brief period of static stretching. The conditioning period should last from 20 to 60 min per session at a work rate that corresponds to an RPE of 11–13 on the Borg scale (a more detailed discussion on RPE and the Borg scale can be found in Chapter 14 and 27). A 5- to 10-min cooldown period should follow. During this time, the patient should perform static stretching, focusing primarily on those muscle groups used during the activity.

To avoid hypoglycemic episodes, ESRD patients with type 1 diabetes should monitor plasma glucose levels before, during, and after exercise.[24] They will also need to adjust the dose and timing of their insulin injection relative to each exercise session. Patients should be educated about the warning signs of hypoglycemia, and they should always have some easily digestible carbohydrate available to them when they exercise. The ACSM also recommends that patients with diabetes exercise with a partner.[24]

Like other diabetic patients, ESRD patients with diabetes need to be cautious about their footwear and be cognizant of the impact of their medications on plasma glucose levels.[24] However, unlike other individuals with diabetes who exercise, ESRD patients with diabetes need to be conservative in their consumption of fluids, even when exercising in the heat. The ESRD patient should gain no more than 1–2 kg of fluid between hemodialysis sessions. This restriction may put them at risk of dehydration and developing some form of heat-related illness. Consequently, ESRD patients with diabetes should avoid exercising in excessively hot conditions and, in general, should avoid exercising in extreme environmental conditions.

Resistance Exercise

Dynamic aerobic exercise has traditionally been used in the management of individuals with diabetes. Because ESRD patients are known to have poor muscular strength, which may affect their ability to perform activities of daily living, a properly designed and supervised resistance training program may be beneficial in appropriately screened individuals (see Chapter 16). A program of resistance exercise should increase muscular strength, muscular endurance, and bone mass.[26] However, because ESRD patients are at an increased risk of experiencing some form of musculoskeletal injury, they should follow established guidelines aimed at minimizing such injuries.[27] In addition, some accommodation may need to be made for the presence of the fistula.

At the commencement of a resistance training program, ESRD patients should be taught proper weight-lifting techniques, including correct body positioning, avoidance of breath holding to minimize the effect of the Valsalva maneuver, and the use of full range of motion exercise.[26] The ACSM recommends the use of light weights during a resistance training program for individuals with diabetes. Weights that can be lifted 10–15 times per set are recommended.[25] The RPE associated with the chosen resistances should be <15 (i.e., hard). The progression should be slow, involving an increase in resistance used of about 2–5 lb (upper body) to 5–10 lb (lower body) when 15 repetitions can be comfortably completed.[26] Finally, to realize the benefits of resistance training, ESRD patients should perform resistance exercise involving 8–10 different exercises (i.e., one exercise for each major muscle group) at least two times per week.[28]

During hemodialysis sessions, dumbbells and therobands (i.e., elastic bands that offer resistance when stretched) can be used with discretion. Although the research evidence documenting the specific benefits of this type of activity in ESRD patients with diabetes is lacking, patients are likely to improve strength and flexibility if they perform this type of exercise on a regular basis.

There are no published studies documenting the optimal exercise program for diabetic transplant recipients; this is also the case in ESRD patients with diabetes. Until such specific guidelines are developed, it seems prudent to follow the recommendations that have been used by other diabetic patients.[14]

Location of Exercise

If the dialysis facility does not have an in-center exercise program, patients will need to be referred to community programs such as those associated with their work, the Young Men's Christian Association (YMCA), the Jewish Community Center (JCC), or health clubs. Ideally, the dialysis center should provide a renal rehabilitation program, with exercise being performed during hemodialysis using a modified bicycle ergometer. The success of the rehabilitation program will depend on the coordinated efforts of skilled and supportive staff, including enthusiastic physicians, nurses, physical therapists, and exercise physiologists. Patients on home dialysis should have their programs designed for use either at home or at a facility in the community.

The diabetic dialysis patient may be particularly prone to hyperkalemia because of potassium shifts from the intracellular space due to hyperglycemia and acidosis. Submaximal exercise has been shown to result in acute elevations of serum potassium in the noncritical range. Therefore, exercise may be somewhat safer in the hemodialysis patient when done during a dialysis treatment when potassium is being removed.[16]

Conclusions

ESRD patients with diabetes and diabetic transplant recipients have an elevated risk of dying from cardiovascular disease compared with non-diabetic ESRD patients and age-matched individuals without renal disease. As a result, a program of endurance exercise that has been shown to favorably alter many of the CAD risk factors is highly recommended for this patient population. A program of resistance exercise should also be followed to help offset some of the musculoskeletal deconditioning that is associated with advanced renal disease. Exercise should be incorporated into the outpatient care plan for all patients. At the present time, because there are no specific guidelines available for exercising ESRD patients with diabetes, it seems prudent to follow, with modification, guidelines that have been established by the American Diabetes Association and the ACSM for exercising individuals with diabetes.

References

1. Ritz E, Rychlik I, Locatelli F, Halimi S: End-stage renal failure in type 2 diabetes: a medical catastrophe of worldwide dimensions. *Am J Kidney Dis* 34:795–808, 1999
2. United States Renal Data System: *The 1999 Annual Data Report.* http://www.usrds.org/1999_adr.htm
3. Rychlik I, Miltenberger-Miltenyi G, Ritz E: The drama of the continuous increase in end-stage renal failure in patients with type II diabetes mellitus. *Nephrol Dial Transplant* 13 (Suppl. 8):6–10, 1998
4. Johansen KL: Physical functioning and exercise capacity in patients on dialysis. *Adv Ren Replace Ther* 6:141–48, 1999
5. Painter P, Moore GE: The impact of recombinant human erythropoietin on exercise capacity in hemodialysis patients. *Adv Ren Replace Ther* 1:55–65, 1994
6. Painter P: The importance of exercise training in rehabilitation of patients with end-stage renal disease. *Am J Kidney Dis* 24:S2–S9, 1994
7. Krasnoff J, Painter P: The physiological consequences of bed rest and inactivity. *Adv Ren Replace Ther* 6:124–32, 1999
8. Brenner BM: *The Kidney.* Philadelphia, PA, W.B. Saunders, 2000, p. 1742–43

9. Diesel W, Noakes TD, Swanepoel C, Lambert M: Isokinetic muscle strength predicts maximum exercise tolerance in renal patients on chronic hemodialysis. *Am J Kidney Dis* 16:109–14, 1990
10. Bohannon RW, Hull D, Palmeri D: Muscle impairments and gait performance deficits in kidney transplantation candidates. *Am J Kidney Dis* 24:480–85, 1994
11. Bradley J, Anderson JR, Evans DB, Cowley AJ: Impaired nutritive skeletal muscle blood flow in patients with chronic renal failure. *Clin Sci* 79:239–45, 1990
12. Clyne N, Esbjornsson M, Jansson E, Jogestrand T, Lins L, Pehrsson SK: Effects of renal failure on skeletal muscle. *Nephron* 63:395–99, 1993
13. Fahal IH, Bell GM, Bone JM, Edwards RHT: Physiological abnormalities of skeletal muscle in dialysis patients. *Nephron Dial Transplant* 12:119–27, 1997
14. Painter P: Exercise after renal transplantation. *Adv Ren Replace Ther* 6:159–64, 1999
15. American Diabetes Association, American College of Sports Medicine: Diabetes mellitus and exercise (joint Position Statement). *Med Sci Sports Exerc* 29:i–vi, 1997
16. Fitts SS: Physical benefits and challenges of exercise for people with chronic renal disease. *J Ren Nutr* 7:123–28, 1997
17. Moore GE, Painter PL, Brinker KR, Stay-Gundersen J, Mitchell JH: Cardiovascular response to submaximal stationary cycling during hemodialysis. *Am J Kidney Dis* 31:631–37, 1998
18. Painter PL, Nelson-Worel JN, Hill MM, Thornbery DR, Shelp WR, Harrington AR, Weinstein AB: Effects of exercise training during hemodialysis. *Nephron* 43:87–92, 1986
19. Moore GE, Brinker KR, Stray-Gundersen J, Mitchell JH: Determinants of VO2peak in patients with end-stage renal disease: on and off dialysis. *Med Sci Sports Exerc* 25:18–23, 1993
20. Germain M, Belliveau S, Mulhern J, O'Shea M, Braden G: Effect of intradialytic exercise on urea kinetics and rebound. *J Am Soc Nephrol* 6:599, 1995 (presented at the 28th Annual Meeting of the American Society of Nephrology, San Diego, CA, 1995)
21. Cappy CS, Jablonka J, Schroeder ET: The effects of exercise during hemodialysis on physical performance and nutrition assessment. *J Ren Nutr* 9:63–70, 1999

22. Lo CY, Li L, Lo WK, Chan ML, So E, Tang S, Yuen MC, Cheng IK, Chan TM: Benefits of exercise training in patients on continuous ambulatory peritoneal dialysis. *Am J Kidney Dis* 32:1011–18, 1998
23. Kempeneers BS, Noakes TD, van Zyl-Smit R, Myburg KH, Lambert M, Adams B, Wiggins T: Skeletal muscle limits the exercise tolerance of renal transplant recipients: effects of a graded exercise training program. *Am J Kidney Dis* 16:57–65, 1990
24. American College of Sports Medicine: *Guidelines for Exercise Testing and Prescription.* 6th ed. Philadelphia, Williams & Wilkins, 2000
25. American College of Sports Medicine: *American College of Sports Medicine Resource Manual for Guidelines for Exercise Testing and Prescription.* 3rd ed. Philadelphia, Lippincott Williams and Wilkins, 1998
26. Soukup JT, Maynard TS, Kovaleski JE: Resistance training guidelines for individuals with diabetes mellitus. *Diabetes Educ* 20: 129–37, 1994
27. Copley JB, Lindberg JS: The risks of exercise. *Adv Ren Replace Ther* 6:165–71, 1999
28. Feigenbaum MS, Pollock ML: Prescription of resistance training for health and disease. *Med Sci Sports Exerc* 31:38–45, 1999

Samuel A. Headley, PhD, is from Springfield College, Springfield, MA. Michael J. Germain, MD, and Gregory L. Braden, MD, are from Tufts University School of Medicine, Springfield, MA.

27

Neuropathy

AARON I. VINIK, MD, PhD, FCP, FACP, FACE,
AND TOMRIS ERBAS, MD

Highlights

- Neuropathy complicates the management of diabetes.
- Somatic neuropathy (calluses and warm insensate feet) with loss of reflexes or vibration perception increases susceptibility to ulcers, Charcot joint destruction, and limb loss.
- Autonomic nerve dysfunction impairs the ability to exercise because of *1*) decreased systolic and diastolic cardiac function, *2*) postural hypotension and nocturnal/supine hypertension, *3*) impaired cutaneous blood flow and sweating, *4*) impaired pupillary reaction and night vision, and *5*) gastroparesis with irregular fuel delivery.
- Preferred exercises are non–weight-bearing.
- Rate of perceived exertion is a safer guide for exercise intensity than heart rate.

- A paradigm for exercise in patients with cardiovascular autonomic neuropathy is provided.
- Foot care education reduces risk of ulcers and gangrene by one-third.

Diabetic neuropathy may have an impact on the risks and benefits of exercise in a number of untoward ways. Although there is good reason to believe that exercise is beneficial to people with diabetes in general, exercise programs for patients with diabetic neuropathy should be carefully managed to avoid adverse and possibly serious consequences. It is quite appropriate to acknowledge the fact that exercise complicates diabetes management once neuropathy is present. Even though significant risks are associated with exercise for diabetic patients with neuropathy, these can be decreased by initial evaluation and recommendations. Before providing specific recommendations for exercise in people with diabetic neuropathy, it is useful to review certain aspects of the different kinds of diabetic neuropathy.

Types of Neuropathy

Somatic Neuropathy

Neuropathy is the most common and troublesome complication of diabetes.[1–4] Diabetic neuropathy comprises a number of different syndromes, each with a range of clinical neurological disturbances. These include *1*) subclinical neuropathy determined by abnormalities in electrodiagnostic and quantitative sensory or autonomic function testing, *2*) diffuse clinical neuropathy with distal symmetric sensorimotor and autonomic syndromes, and *3*) focal syndromes.[5] The spectrum of clinical neuropathic syndromes described in patients with diabetes includes dysfunction of almost every segment of the somatic peripheral and autonomic nervous system.[6]

Small-Fiber Dysfunction

The small unmyelinated nerve fibers (C-fibers) subserve thermal and pain sensations, and the small autonomic fibers affect sweating and vascular control. Damage to small fibers has the greatest impact on survival and quality of life, producing initial symptoms such as pain, numbness, anhidrotic skin with disordered blood flow (predisposing to foot ulcers), infection, gangrene, and limb loss. Small-fiber neuropathy affects both the somatic and autonomic nervous systems. Abnormalities in small nerve fibers are thought to be responsible for the early occurrence of pain and heat hyperalgesia and the late hypoalgesia, impairment of warm thermal perception, and impaired skin blood flow in diabetic neuropathy.[7–9] Initially, when there is ongoing damage to the nerves, the patient experiences pain of the burning, dysesthetic type often accompanied by hyperalgesia and allodynia. Contact with clothes or objects, as well as disturbance of hair follicles, may be excruciating. The pain is distinct from that found with large-fiber damage, in which case, it is often deep-seated and gnawing in character.

Large-Fiber Dysfunction

Large-fiber neuropathies are manifested by reduced vibration and position sense, weakness, muscle wasting and depressed tendon reflexes, ataxia, and poor coordination. Exercise that requires coordination skills, such as golf and tennis, may be difficult for the patient with neuropathy. Most diabetic peripheral neuropathy is mixed, with both large and small nerve fiber involvement. In our own outpatient population, only 15% of patients with symptoms of electrophysiologically confirmed neuropathy had no objective signs, and 63.7% of patients with signs had no symptoms.[10] Thus, it is important to carry out thorough physical examinations before the patient enters an exercise program. A small proportion of patients show "pure" small nerve or large nerve fiber deficit. Sensory neuropathy can be detected by a variety of sensitive quantitative tests, but several studies show that vibration perception thresholds are an effective indicator of risk of foot ulceration, with thresholds >25 V indicating significant risk.[11,12] The population-attributable risk (that proportion of the neuropathic population in whom ulceration and limb loss can be attributed to loss of large-fiber function) is significant because of the frequency (78%) of loss of vibration perception in this population of subjects. Sensory neuropathy permits minor repeated trauma causing skin ulcerations due to unperceived pressure. Absence of patella reflexes may also predict ulceration and limb loss.[13] The finding of calluses in peripheral insensitivity confers an 11-fold increase in likelihood of limb loss.[14]

Studies have shown that education can reduce the risk of ulceration and amputation.[15–17] Failure to educate patients with regard to foot care in the presence of peripheral neuropathy increases risk 3.2-fold for ulcers and subsequent limb loss.[18] The presence of unilateral foot swelling, redness, heat, or discomfort after exercising or walking should alert the health care provider to the possibility of a Charcot foot. Charcot foot may present acutely with severe pain, a warm to hot foot with increased blood flow (despite decreased warm sensory perception and vibration detection), and clear evidence of acute osteopenia.[19–21] An important factor in the development of Charcot joints is equinovarus deformity caused by Achilles tendon shortening. The repetitive trauma in the Charcot foot increases osteoclastic activity coupled with increased blood flow and, consequently, osteopenia.[22] The osteopenia predisposes the small bones of the foot to minor fractures with minimal provocation, especially with the development of equinus.[6] People with severe Charcot joints (neuroarthropathy) should avoid weight-bearing exercises because they can result in multiple fractures and dislocation of the bones of the feet and ankle without the patient's awareness.

Diabetic Amyotrophies

Diabetic amyotrophy can be clinically identified based on the recognition of these common features: *1*) it primarily affects men >50 years of age, *2*) it has a gradual or abrupt onset, *3*) it begins with pain in the thighs and hips or buttocks and is *4*) followed by significant weakness of the proximal muscles of the lower limbs with the inability to rise from a sitting position (positive Gower's maneuver), *5*) it begins unilaterally and is spread bilaterally, *6*) it coexists with distal symmetric polyneuropathy, and *7*) it causes spontaneous muscle fasciculation or is provoked by percussion. Reflexes are diminished in proportion to the wasting, which can be quite profound. The condition may be part of a more generalized diabetic cachexia. Fortunately, it is self-limiting, and the patient usually recovers spontaneously within a year or two. Patients often cannot stand unsupported, climb stairs, or rise from the kneeling or sitting position. It is the one condition in which the exercise prescription should not demand the use of the proximal muscles. On the other hand, a well-designed rehabilitation program incorporating the use of weight training can hasten recovery from the amyotrophy. Since the condition occurs in older people with long-standing diabetes, a weight-training program must be evaluated in relation to the presence of retinopathy and other complications that limit the use of weights.

Mononeuropathies

Mononeuropathies are caused by vasculitis and subsequent ischemia or infarction of the nerve and can affect cranial, truncal, and peripheral nerves. These may involve cranial nerves 3, 4, 6, and 7, as well as the intercostals. Peripheral nerve mononeuropathies in diabetes include peroneal, sural, sciatic, femoral, ulnar, and median nerves. They occur primarily in the older population, their onset is generally acute and associated with pain, and their course is self-limiting, resolving within 6–8 weeks. These mononeuropathies are due to vascular obstruction, after which adjacent neuronal fascicles take over the function of those infarcted. In mononeuropathies, such as peroneal palsy, in which weakness is a prominent feature, physical therapy may be necessary to maintain good muscle tone and prevent permanent weakness and contractures. Based on our experience, a passive or active exercise program may facilitate return of motor function of the nerves involved and help to preserve whatever muscle function escaped the initial attack.[10]

Entrapment Syndromes

Entrapment syndromes are not usually uncovered by the physician unless they are far advanced or are gross. Common sites of nerve entrapment include the foot, where the medial and lateral plantar nerves are compressed, and the carpal tunnel, which compresses the median nerve. Carpal tunnel syndrome occurs twice as frequently in the diabetic population than the normal healthy population, and its increased prevalence in diabetes may be related to repeated undetected trauma, metabolic changes, or accumulation of fluid or edema within the confined space of the carpal tunnel. The ulnar nerve may also be compressed at the wrist or elbow and the lateral cutaneous nerves of the thigh under the inguinal ligament. Because these conditions do not respond to any form of metabolic intervention, it is important to recognize the entrapping nature of the condition. Exercise constitutes a hazard because repeated minor trauma accentuates the nerve compression and aggravates the symptoms.

Most people with diabetes have experienced a form of entrapment at some point in their lives and may seek surgery. The symptoms may be as mild as a little tingling in the fingers in carpal tunnel syndrome; however, the tingling may be deceptive, masking more extreme sensory symptoms that may spread to the remaining fingers and even up the arm into areas not supplied by the median nerve. The clinical picture, coupled with the signs of compression of the appropriate nerve, is usually clear enough to make the diagnosis. Confirmation can be obtained by electrophysiological study. Once recognized, the key to a successful response is the cessation of all activity, especially of the repetitive traumatic type, splinting of the affected limb for support, and salvage of residual function. Surgical decompression may be necessary in cases where the condition is progressing, followed by an exercise program to rehabilitate the affected muscles.[10]

Autonomic Neuropathy

The autonomic nervous system regulates all involuntary functions in the body, many of which are central to the consideration of an exercise program in the management of diabetes. The main groups of autonomic neuropathic disturbances in diabetes include *1*) subclinical autonomic neuropathy, determined by abnormalities in quantitative autonomic function tests, and *2*) clinical autonomic neuropathy, which presents with symptoms or signs.

In clinic- and hospital-based studies, the prevalence rates of diabetic autonomic neuropathy (DAN) reported range from 0 to 100%.[23] This dramatic variability in reported prevalence may reflect a lack of a standard, accepted definition of DAN, different diagnosis methods, variable study selection criteria, and referral bias. The prevalence of autonomic neuropathy is 47% in the EURODIAB IDDM Complications Study.[24] Involvement of the autonomic nervous system can occur as early as the first year after diagnosis, and major manifestations are cardiovascular, gastrointestinal, and genitourinary system dysfunction. Complications affecting these systems contribute greatly to the morbidity, mortality, and reduced quality of life and activities of daily living in the person with diabetes.[9] In some cases, autonomic dysfunction may be present at the time of diagnosis of both type 1 and type 2 diabetic patients.[25] However, clinical features of this form of neuropathy are often unsuspected and, without careful scrutiny, may go undetected. They include resting tachycardia with exercise intolerance, orthostatic hypotension, impaired sweating and cutaneous blood flow regulation, hypoglycemic unawareness, delayed gastric emptying, diarrhea alternating with constipation, bladder atony, and impotence in males. The precise coincidence of sensorimotor and autonomic neuropathies is variable, but they commonly coexist. In people with peripheral neuropathy, 50% will have asymptomatic autonomic neuropathy.[26]

The presence of autonomic complications is life-threatening, with estimates of mortality ranging from 25 to 50% within 5–10 years of diagnosis.[27–33] The 5-year mortality of patients with DAN is three times higher than that in diabetic patients without autonomic involvement.[34] Although this statistic emphasizes the need for early diagnosis and intervention, the causes of death are quite variable. They include sudden death for which no explanation has proved satisfactory, silent myocardial infarction with congestive failure or neuropathic cardiomyopathy, prolongation of QT intervals corrected for heart rate (QTc) with malignant ventricular arrhythmias, progressive renal failure, aspiration pneumonias with gastroparesis, and perioperative respiratory problems due to impaired hypoxia-induced respiratory drive.[35,36] Thus, the detection of autonomic neuropathy should alert physicians to the factors contributing to premature demise. In this way, these patients should be more assiduously assessed for worsening renal function, atypical features of coronary artery disease, and congestive failure. However, there is evidence that spironolactone, ACE inhibitors, calcium-channel blockers, and β-blockers reverse the loss of heart rate variability (HRV).[37–42] It remains to be established whether reduced mortality can be derived from intensification of vigilance in asymptomatic patients with abnormal autonomic function tests or use of these agents.

Cardiovascular Autonomic Neuropathy

Cardiovascular autonomic neuropathy (CAN) is a serious complication of diabetes that is associated with a poor prognosis. The development of sensitive, reproducible, and simple noninvasive cardiovascular reflex tests has allowed extensive evaluation of diabetic CAN. The prevalence rate of borderline or definite CAN is 8.5 or 16.8% among type 1 diabetic patients and 12.2 or 22.1% among type 2 diabetic patients, respectively.[43] In the EURODIAB IDDM Complications Study, 19.3% of the type 1 diabetic patients had abnormal HRV, and 5.9%

had postural hypotension.[24] Clinical symptoms of CAN generally do not occur until long after the onset of diabetes. The mean mortality rates over periods up to 10 years are 27% in diabetic patients with CAN compared with 5% in those without CAN.[27–32,34,44–49] In diabetic patients with asymptomatic CAN, exercise capacity, blood pressure, heart rate, and cardiac stroke volume are diminished. Abnormalities in autonomic function manifested by abnormal heart rate, blood pressure, or response could limit a patient's capability to perform exercise.[50] Exercise tolerance in the person with clinically significant DAN may be extremely limited because of the impaired sympathetic and parasympathetic nervous systems that normally augment cardiac output and redistribute blood flow to the working muscle.

In normal individuals during the early stages of exercise, there is a decrease in cardiac parasympathetic nervous system activity followed by an increase in vascular sympathetic nervous system activity. In diabetic patients evaluated by graded exercise, it was found that the worse the CAN, the more abnormal the cardiovascular performance, systemic peripheral resistance, and change in heart rate. Thus, cardiovascular autonomic nervous system neuropathy appears to contribute to the poor exercise tolerance observed in many diabetic patients.[51]

In cardiac autonomic neuropathic patients without postural hypotension, heart rate is excessive at rest and during the early phase of exercise; as the effort progresses, the normal activation of the sympathetic autonomic nervous system allows these patients to develop virtually normal hemodynamic responses. But, in diabetic patients with postural hypotension, the deficiency of the sympathetic autonomic nervous system outflow prevents an adequate response in terms of heart rate and systolic blood pressure increase during each phase of exercise.[52]

Diabetic patients with early CAN have resting tachycardia and loss of beat-to-beat variation in heart rate with deep breathing.[27,53] The highest resting heart rates are found in patients with parasympathetic dysfunction.[27] The heart rate may decline with combined vagal and sympathetic dysfunction but always remains above normal. A fixed heart rate that is unresponsive to mild exercise indicates nearly complete cardiac denervation in diabetic patients.

CAN and QTc. Diabetic patients with CAN have prolonged QTc intervals. In the EURODIAB IDDM Complications Study, the prevalence of an abnormally prolonged corrected QT is 16% in the whole population, 11% in males, and 21% in females.[54] Prolonged QTc interval is indicative of an imbalance between right and left ventricular sympathetic innervation. Diabetic patients with regional sympathetic imbalance and QTc interval prolongation also may be at greater risk for arrhythmias. Although vagal stimulation has little intrinsic effect on the excitability of the myocardium, intact vagal function does oppose the arrhythmogenic effects of sympathetic tone.[55] Exercise-induced hypoglycemia may activate the sympathetic nervous system and thus predispose the patient to arrhythmia. Because diabetic patients with CAN have vagal denervation, they may lose the protective vagal slowing influence on adrenergic-mediated tachyarrhythmias. These arrhythmias are nearly impossible to detect because they occur so rarely; protracted monitoring or provocative testing may be required. It is shown that in a meta-analysis, prolonged QTc interval predicted premature cardiovascular mortality.[56]

CAN and ventricular function. Diminished stroke volume at rest and with exercise has been observed in diabetic patients with CAN, and impaired ejection fraction responses have been noted.[57,58] Early radionuclide ventriculographic studies in diabetic patients who have been asymptomatic for a long period have demonstrated abnormal left ventricle ejection fraction responses to exercise.[59,60] However, the interpretation of left ventricle function studies in these patients was hindered by the possibility of underlying ischemic heart disease. Our group studied resting and exercise radionuclide ventriculograms from patients with long-standing diabetes who had no tomographic thallium scan evidence of ischemic heart disease.[58] Abnormal left ventricular systolic function at rest and during exercise was found in 37% of the diabetic patients. CAN was found in 91% of the diabetic patients with abnormal systolic function, and the incidence of abnormal systolic function was 59% in diabetic patients with CAN as opposed to 8% in those without CAN. Mean ejection fractions at rest and with maximal exercise were reduced in the patients with CAN when compared with those in patients without CAN. Thus, CAN contributes to diminished exercise tolerance.

We also examined left ventricular diastolic function in diabetic patients with CAN. Of the patients, 21% had abnormal test results. The diabetic patients with abnormal left ventricular diastolic function had more severe CAN than those with normal test results.[61] Thus,

CAN could contribute to abnormal ventricular function in a variety of ways. For instance, abnormal coordination of peripheral arterial resistance and blood flow into vascular beds, such as the splanchnic, skeletal, and venous capacitance, at rest and exercise, could change the loading conditions of cardiac chambers. This could lead to abnormal changes in left ventricular volumes, pressures, and ejection fractions during exercise testing. In addition, the uneven sympathetic denervation of the myocardium could significantly limit the ability to enhance inotropic (contractility) and diastolic (relaxation) function during exercise. Diabetic patients may have diminished cardiac reserve of catecholamines, further reducing the effects of sympathetic innervation to the heart.

CAN and coronary artery disease. Diabetes is an important risk factor for the development of coronary artery disease (CAD). The prevalence of both asymptomatic and symptomatic CAD is increased in diabetic patients.[62] Cardiac sympathetic denervation is common in both patients with painful CAD and patients with asymptomatic CAD, regardless of DAN. The cardiac sympathetic signals play an important role in modulating myocardial blood flow during exercise.[63] Diabetic subjects with evidence of cardiac sympathetic dysfunction have impaired sympathetically mediated dilatation of coronary resistance vessels. This vasomotor abnormality develops early in the course of DAN, and its severity is related to the degree of cardiac sympathetic nerve dysfunction. Coronary microvascular abnormalities and endothelial dysfunction have been reported in diabetic patients with normal left ventricular systolic function and angiographically normal coronary arteries.[64,65] Maximal coronary flow and flow reserve are impaired in young adult type 1 diabetic patients with or without minimal microvascular complications.[66]

Autonomic function testing. Because the cardiovascular system is a prime target of autonomic dysfunction in diabetic patients, a number of simple, objective tests of cardiovascular function and reflexes have been developed to aid in the diagnosis of CAN (Table 27.1). Nonetheless, the earliest and most sensitive clinical marker of CAN is the simple bedside point-of-care evaluation of HRV in response to metronomic breathing (Fig. 27.1).[53] Increased resting heart rate and loss of heart rate variation in response to deep breathing are primary indicators

TABLE 27.1 Diagnostic Tests of Cardiovascular Autonomic Neuropathy

Test	Method/Parameters
Resting heart rate	>100 beats/min is abnormal.
Beat-to-beat heart rate variation*	With the patient at rest and supine (no overnight coffee or hypoglycemic episodes), breathing six breaths per minute, with heart rate monitored by ECG or an ANSCORE device, a difference in heart rate of >15 beats/min is normal and <10 beats/min is abnormal; R-R inspiration/R-R expiration >1.17. All indexes of HRV are age-dependent.†
Heart rate response to standing*	During continuous ECG monitoring, the R-R interval is measured at beats 15 and 30 after standing. Normally, a tachycardia is followed by reflex bradycardia. The 30:15 ratio is normally >1.03.
Heart rate response to Valsalva maneuver*	The subject forcibly exhales into the mouthpiece of a manometer to 40 mmHg for 15 s during ECG monitoring. Healthy subjects develop tachycardia and peripheral vasoconstriction during strain and an overshot bradycardia and experience a rise in blood pressure with release. The ratio of longest R-R to shortest R-R should be >1.2.
Systolic blood pressure response to standing	Systolic blood pressure is measured in the supine subject. The patient stands, and the systolic blood pressure is measured after 2 min. Normal response is a fall of <10 mmHg, borderline is a fall of 10–29 mmHg, and abnormal is a fall of >30 mmHg with symptoms.
Diastolic blood pressure response to isometric exercise	The subject squeezes a handgrip dynamometer to establish a maximum. Grip is then squeezed at 30% maximum for 5 min. The normal response for diastolic blood pressure is a rise of >16 mmHg in the other arm.
ECG QT/QTc intervals	The QTc should be <440 ms.
Spectral analysis	VLF peak ↓ (sympathetic dysfunction) LF peak ↓ (sympathetic dysfunction) HF peak ↓ (parasympathetic dysfunction) LH/HF ratio ↓ (sympathetic imbalance)
Neurovascular flow	Using noninvasive laser Doppler measures of peripheral sympathetic responses to nociception.

*These can now be performed quickly (<15 min) in the practitioner's office, with a central reference laboratory providing quality control and normative values (ANSCORE; Boston Medical Technologies). †Lowest normal value of expiration/inspiration ratio: age 20–24 years: 1.17; 25–29 years: 1.15; 30–34 years: 1.13; 35–39 years: 1.12; 40–44 years: 1.10; 45–49 years: 1.08; 50–54 years: 1.07; 55–59 years: 1.06; 60–64 years: 1.04; 65–69 years: 1.03; 70–75 years: 1.02. ECG, electrocardiogram.

Perform two tests out of following three for CPT Code 95921: Metronomic Breathing, Valsalva, Standing 30:15. Valsalva and Standing are similar measures.				
# Of Tests Performed	**All Results Normal**	**1 Result Abnormal**	**2 Results Abnormal**	**3 Results Abnormal**
2	**Normal**	**Early-Intermediate AD**	**Intermediate-Advanced AD**	------------------
3	**Normal**	**Early AD**	**Intermediate AD**	**Advanced AD**
Heart rate typically starts normal and increases until advanced AD, when it may decrease.				

Symptoms due to AD may present at any stage of the disease but are more likely with advancing severity

← **Less Likely Symptomatic** — **More Likely Symptomatic** →

Diagnosis	**Normal**	**Early AD**	**Intermediate AD**	**Advanced AD**
Rx Considerations	**Retest in 1 Year**	**Stabilize / Reverse: Retest in 3 Months to Confirm Diagnosis or Show Reversal**	**Intensive Prevention / Treatment: Retest in 1 year**	**Intensive Prevention: Retest in 1 Year**

Prevalence/Consequences	**Symptoms**	**Treatment**	**Vigilance**
25–30% of diabetic subjects have DAN vs. 2.5% of the normal population, as diagnosed by HRV testing. Diabetic subjects with DAN stand roughly a 27% chance of death within a 5-year period compared with roughly a 5% chance for diabetic subjects without DAN. Causes of death may be treated or prevented, and include the following: ◆ Renal disease ◆ Myocardial infarction ◆ Sudden death Autonomic neuropathy sufferers also face a dramatically higher risk of the following: ◆ Heart failure ◆ Silent ischemia and silent myocardial infarction ◆ Retinopathy ◆ Amputation	DAN is a great mimic. The autonomic nervous system innervates every organ in the body, and thus symptoms can be varied and are often mistaken for symptoms of other disease (ulcer, benign prostate hypertrophy, and so forth). Common symptoms include the following: ◆ Orthostatic dizziness, tachycardia ◆ Exercise intolerance ◆ Dry skin ◆ Impotence, urinary urgency, or frequency or incontinence ◆ Anorexia, nausea, vomiting, bloating ◆ Diarrhea, constipation, fecal incontinence ◆ Pupillary abnormalities ◆ Sweating abnormalities ◆ "Brittle" diabetes ◆ Hypoglycemia unawareness and unresponsiveness	Systemic prevention ◆ Better glycemic control (HbA_{1c}<6.5%) ◆ Antioxidants (α-lipoic acid, vitamin E) ◆ Exercise (Caution: exercise is useful in pre- and early-DAN, but patients with DAN are at high risk of silent ischemia and have altered heart rate at VO_{2max}) End-organ prophylaxis ◆ ACE inhibitors (even normotensives) ◆ β-Blockers, aspirin ◆ Improved blood pressure and lipid control Symptomatic ◆ Gastroparesis ◆ Gastrointestinal: constipation, diarrhea ◆ Genitourinary: erectile dysfunction, urinary problems ◆ Cardiovascular: orthostasis, edema, impaired ventricular function ◆ Peripheral neurovascular: feet (dry, cracked, ulcers)	Pay close attention for signs of further end-organ damage ◆ Exercise stress test (detect silent ischemia, heart rate at VO_{2max}) ◆ Discuss silent myocardial infarction symptoms with patient ◆ Microalbuminuria tests ◆ Greater attention to feet ◆ Sleep apnea, hypoxia (sudden death) ◆ Care with intensification of glycemic control

FIGURE 27.1 Assessment and management of autonomic dysfunction (AD): understanding the HRV component.

of parasympathetic dysfunction. Tests for sympathetic dysfunction include measurements of heart rate and blood pressure responses to standing, exercise, and handgrip. Abnormalities in two or more assessments are required for a diagnosis of autonomic neuropathy. Both time domain and frequency domain indexes of HRV seem to be more sensitive than standard cardiovascular reflex tests.[67] Frequency domain analysis of HRV in the supine or standing position may provide a useful tool of autonomic dysfunction. In the frequency domain analysis, the very-low-frequency (VLF) heart rate fluctuations are thought to be mediated by the sympathetic system. The low-frequency (LF) heart rate fluctuations are under sympathetic control with vagal modulation, whereas the high-frequency (HF) fluctuations are under parasympathetic control. The balance between the sympathetic and parasympathetic components of autonomic nerve function can be assessed with the LF/HF ratio. The VLF, LF, and HF components have been demonstrated to be reduced in diabetic patients with advanced stages of CAN. The HF component is reduced in diabetic patients with vagal dysfunction. In diabetic patients with sympathetic dysfunction, VLF and LF components are reduced.[49] The 24-h recording of HRV gives insights into abnormal patterns of circadian rhythms regulated by sympathovagal activity. In diabetic patients, a reduced day-night rhythm in sympathovagal balance is due to reduction in nocturnal vagal activity.

Sympathetic innervation of the heart can be visualized and quantified by single-photon emission-computed tomography with [^{123}I]metaiodobenzylguanidine (MIBG). MIBG imaging is a valuable tool for the detection of early alterations in myocardial sympathetic innervation in diabetic patients. Diabetic CAN has been directly characterized by reduced or absent myocardial MIBG uptake.[68–70] The sympathetic innervation of the heart can also be visualized with positron emission imaging using carbon-11 hydroxyephedrine. Defects in carbon-11 hydroxyephedrine uptake have been correlated with CAN and impaired vasodilator response of coronary resistance vessels.[63]

Diabetic patients who are likely to have CAN should be strongly advised to have cardiac stress testing before undertaking an exercise program. Physicians should be aware that as a group, diabetic patients with long-standing disease, particularly those with CAN, have a high incidence of abnormal exercise radionuclide ventriculographic test results, even in the absence of coronary artery disease. Therefore, resting or stress thallium myocardial scintigraphy may be a more appropriate noninvasive diagnostic test for the presence and extent of coronary artery disease in these patients.[71]

Postural Hypotension

Postural hypotension is defined as a fall in systolic blood pressure >30 mmHg upon standing, accompanied by symptoms of dizziness, weakness, faintness, visual impairment, pain in the back of the head, and loss of consciousness. In some patients, postural hypotension may become disabling, but blood pressure fall may also be asymptomatic. Postural hypotension occurs in CAN as a result of abnormalities in baroreceptor function, poor cardiovascular reactivity, and impaired peripheral vasoconstrictor responses. The combination of decreased release of catecholamines with increased sensitivity to their vasoconstrictive effect is a cause for concern during exercise, which activates the autonomic nervous system.[72–74] During exercise, the catecholamine response to exercise is blunted in diabetic patients with CAN. Further compounding the problem with blood pressure regulation is the loss of the normal diurnal rhythm of blood pressure modulation in diabetic patients with autonomic neuropathy. In diabetic patients with CAN, blood pressure is characterized by an abnormal circadian rhythm with a rise during the night and a fall in the early morning. The abnormal circadian rhythm has been shown to correlate with orthostatic hypotension due to CAN.[75] Of particular relevance is the observation that many people with the symptom complex become hypotensive with eating or within 10–15 min of taking their insulin injection. The symptoms, which are not unlike those of hypoglycemia, are often incorrectly ascribed to the hypoglycemic action of insulin but occur too early and are actually due to a fall in blood pressure. Both the impaired vagal heart rate control and sympathetic nervous dysfunction exaggerate the hemodynamic effects of insulin in patients with diabetes and could contribute to insulin-induced hypotension.[76] Postural hypotension poses many treatment problems, especially involving the proximity of exercise to meals and insulin shots.

Sweating Disturbances

Hyperhidrosis of the upper body, often related to eating and anhidrosis of the lower body, is a characteristic feature of autonomic neuropathy. Loss of lower body sweating can cause dry, brittle skin that cracks easily and with loss of protective sensation, predisposes the patient to ulcer formation that can lead to loss of the limb. Special attention must be paid to foot care, especially when exercising.

Alterations in Cutaneous Blood Flow

Microvascular skin blood flow is under the control of the autonomic nervous system and is often compromised by autonomic neuropathy. Defective blood flow in the small capillary circulation is found in response to mental arithmetic, cold pressor, handgrip, and heating. The defect is associated with a reduction in the amplitude of vasomotion, which resembles premature aging.[77,78] There are differences in the glabrous and hairy skin circulations. In hairy skin, a functional defect is found before the development of neuropathy.[79] The clinical counterparts are dry skin, loss of sweating, and development of fissures and cracks that are portals of entry for microorganisms, leading to infectious ulcers and gangrene. The exercising diabetic must pay particular attention to appropriate footwear, padded socks, and hydrating creams.

Edema

Edema often complicates autonomic neuropathy. Swelling of feet predisposes them to exercise-induced injury and the risk of foot ulceration. It can be managed with elevation of the foot in bed at night, use of body stockings by day, and administration of ephedrine.[80] The effects of exercise on the edema are not known.

Gastroparesis Diabeticorum

Gastroparesis diabeticorum can be detected in 25% of patients with diabetes. It is usually clinically silent, although severe diabetic gastroparesis is one of the most debilitating of all gastrointestinal complications of diabetes. The most prevalent gastrointestinal complication is a motility disturbance of the viscera, which is generally the result of widespread autonomic neuropathy. Typical symptoms of diabetic gastroparesis are early satiety, nausea, vomiting, abdominal bloating, epigastric pain, and anorexia. Gastric emptying can be easily demonstrated by scintigraphic techniques. Even with mild symptoms, gastroparesis interferes with nutrient delivery to the small bowel and therefore disrupts the relationship between glucose absorption and exogenous insulin administration. These changes may result in wide swings of glucose levels and unexpected episodes of postprandial hypoglycemia and apparent "brittle diabetes."[81] Every attempt should be made to normalize gastric emptying using prokinetic agents, e.g., metoclopramide, and avoiding high-fiber and high-fat foods, and each patient should learn the vagaries of his or her own stomach with regard to fuel delivery before embarking on an exercise program. The belief that solid food will buffer the tendency toward exercise-induced hypoglycemia is not acceptable in gastroparesis. Rather, liquid supplements should be available during and after exercise because the rate of liquid emptying remains within normal limits in most individuals with gastroparesis.[82] Because emptying may take hours, no specific time to wait after a meal can be recommended, and the use of insulin lispro, according to prevailing postexercise glucose, not meal content, is advisable if exercise hypoglycemia is to be avoided.

Diarrhea

Diarrhea in autonomic neuropathy can be sudden, explosive, paroxysmal, nocturnal, seasonal, uncontrollable, and embarrassing.[81] Individuals prone to such episodes should prehydrate and make preparations for adequate hydration before and during exercise. The severe and intermittent nature of diabetic diarrhea makes it difficult to anticipate these events with any degree of certainty. Protective padding may be necessary to avoid embarrassment.

Respiratory Dysfunction

Respiratory reflexes may be impaired in diabetic patients with autonomic neuropathy. Chronic pulmonary autonomic denervation can induce alterations of the ventilatory response to exercise by influencing the breathing pattern and possibly by determining an abnormally high inspiratory drive. An increased chemosensitivity may actually contribute to sustaining the greater central inspiratory activity, leading to an excessively high ventilatory output during heavy exercise.[83] A temporal relationship between sudden cardiac arrest and interference with normal respiration by hypoxia, drugs, or anesthesia has been reported.[36] Sudden cardiopulmonary arrest in diabetic patients with CAN may be respiratory in origin because of the loss of hypoxic respiratory drive, but the effects of exercise are not clear.

Pupillary Abnormalities

The pupil in DAN reacts poorly to light and does not dilate appropriately in the dark.[84] This abnormality interferes with night vision and places subjects at risk of injury if exercise is performed at night. Patients should be warned about this possible hazard.

Exercise Prescription in Patients With Neuropathy

If, at the urging of the patient or in the opinion of the managing physician, exercise training is deemed appropriate, certain considerations pertaining to exercise in the diabetic patient with neuropathy must be addressed before the exercise program begins. Occult heart disease is a major concern, and repeated cardiac ischemia or arrhythmias may have serious consequences if not addressed. Symptoms of angina are not reliable indicators of important coronary artery disease in patients with DAN because of the higher frequency of silent myocardial ischemia and infarction in such patients.[85–87] A high frequency of abnormal radionuclide ventriculographic responses to exercise in diabetic patients with a low likelihood of coronary artery disease reflects diabetic cardiomyopathy, which may be due to autonomic neuropathy. Therefore, we advocate exercise thallium scintigraphy as the preferred screening technique for cardiac disease in this population.[58] Evidence of myocardial ischemia or important arrhythmias during supervised stress testing must postpone plans for initiating an exercise program.

CAN must be addressed before embarking on regular exercise training. As mentioned previously, diabetic patients with CAN have blunted maximal heart rate and blood pressure responses to maximal exercise, a finding that must be integrated into the exercise prescription.[50,88] There is a higher incidence of abnormal ventricular responses to exercise in patients with CAN, suggesting that slower progression and more careful monitoring of an exercise prescription are in order.[58] CAN is associated with prolongation of the QT interval, and concern over the predisposition to ventricular arrhythmias associated with long QT intervals >430 ms is prudent.[89]

We recommend that exercise programs for diabetic patients with CAN be closely supervised, with consideration given to the poor exercise tolerance associated with resting tachycardia, lower maximal heart rate, and abnormal blood pressure responses (usually decreased maximal blood pressure, but occasionally, severely exaggerated increased blood pressure).[90] Safe parameters have not been established.

Pay special attention to the feet of diabetic patients before starting them on an exercise program. Properly fitting shoes are of great importance. Nail care, regular removal of calluses, and aggressive treatment of edema become crucial. Careful examination of the feet before and after exercise must become routine. One hour of education reduces the risk of an ulcer and foot loss by one-third.[91] Pain may prevent patients from exercising. Superficial C-fiber pain can be reduced by topical application of capsaicin, use of body stockings to prevent movement of hair follicles, or use of clonidine. Deep pain can be ameliorated by insulin infusion or lidocaine. If these measures fail, try amitriptyline or clonazepam with or without fluphenazine.[92] Gabapentin monotherapy appeared to be efficacious for the treatment of pain and sleep interference associated with diabetic neuropathy.[93,94] Even minor pains cannot be ignored; we have seen patients continue to exercise for weeks on fractured feet, believing their injuries to be minor because of insensate feet.

Metabolic control must be assessed before beginning exercise. Regulation of fuel supply and demand to exercising muscles is complex; attempts at intensive management of diabetes center around the supply of insulin and glucose. Neuropathy results in major perturbations of the normal pattern of metabolic responses to exercise. In severely neuropathic patients with gastroparesis and with blood glucose values >240 mg/dl, inadequate insulin during exercise may result in decreased muscle uptake of glucose from the blood despite ongoing hepatic glycogenolysis and gluconeogenesis and inappropriate gut delivery of glucose, resulting in extreme elevations in serum glucose levels.[5] Therefore, if the patient's blood glucose level is >240 mg/dl, exercise is best left for another day.

Hypoglycemia is more frequently encountered in autonomic neuropathy during and after exercise and must be addressed before beginning a regular exercise program. Although insulin levels are normally suppressed during exercise, patients receiving exogenous insulin may, at times, be exercising in a high-insulin state, which suppresses hepatic glucose output. Couple that with failure of counterregulation and the result may be hypoglycemia during or soon after exercise.[95,96] Furthermore, after exercise, the muscle continues to take up increased amounts of glucose for up to 8–12 h, and delayed hypoglycemia may result because of irregular gut fuel delivery and impaired counter-regulatory hormone responses. Indeed, as little as 20 min of aerobic exercise in the early morning may be associated with hypoglycemia in the evening, and the association between the two could go unrecognized by the unwary patient or physician.

It has now become clear that strict glycemic control; a stepwise progressive management of hyperglycemia, lipids, and blood pressure; and use of antioxidant and ACE inhibitors slow progression of autonomic neuropathy.[97] The Diabetes Control and Complications Trial (DCCT) has shown without question the importance of attention to intensive insulin therapy in preventing the onset and progression of neuropathy. The DCCT demonstrated that autonomic dysfunction was reduced by 53% in patients with very intensive glycemic control.[98] Intensive therapy only slowed the deterioration of R-R variation and had no effect on Valsalva ratio. The R-R variation and the Valsalva ratio had significantly greater slopes of decline over time in the patients randomized to conventional therapy compared with those randomized to intensive therapy.[99] Burger et al.[100] showed the effect of strict glycemic control on HRV in type 1 diabetic patients with CAN. The response to improved glycemic control depends on the degree of autonomic dysfunction at the time therapy begins. In patients with early CAN, reversibility is evident by power spectral analysis of HRV as early as 1 year after institution of strict control.

Howorka et al.[101] reported the effects of regularly performed endurance training on HRV in diabetic patients with CAN. A 12-week training period increases the cumulative spectral power of the total frequency band but to a different extent with different degrees of autonomic neuropathy. Patients with the early form of CAN showed an increase of spectral power of both the HF and LF components, whereas those with severe CAN showed no changes after the training period. In diabetic patients with early CAN, regularly performed endurance training increased HRV due to improved sympathetic and parasympathetic supply, whereas in subjects with severe CAN, no effect on HRV could be demonstrated after this kind of training.

Exercise for Patients With Peripheral Neuropathy

Non–weight-bearing activities that improve tone, poise, balance, and awareness of the lower extremities are appropriate exercise choices for patients with peripheral neuropathy.[102] Recommended exercises include tai chi, swimming, bicycling, rowing, and upper-extremity (chair and arm) exercises (if they do not cause severe hypertension). Patients should begin with gentle pain-free stretching before exercise. More stretching can be done when the patient is fully warmed up. Patients with improved muscle function should be taught to stretch using props (e.g., a towel or stick). Although exercise cannot reverse the occurrence of peripheral neuropathy, it can help slow the rate of its development and prevent further loss of fitness associated with disuse. Range of motion activities for the major joints (i.e., the ankle, knee, hip, trunk, shoulder, elbow, and wrist) should be performed to prevent or minimize contractures.

Exercise for Patients With Autonomic Neuropathy

Patients with symptomatic autonomic neuropathy are at high risk for developing complications during exercise (Table 27.2). Sudden death and silent myocardial infarction have been attributed to autonomic neuropathy in diabetes, in which the heart has become unresponsive to nerve impulses. Hypotension and hypertension after vigorous exercise, particularly when starting an exercise program,[103] are more likely to develop in patients with autonomic neuropathy. The risk of hypotension is greater in patients with significant autonomic neuropathy who perform high-intensity exercises with rapid changes in body position.[104] There is also a strong correlation between autonomic neuropathy and microvascular disease.

Individuals with autonomic neuropathy can have difficulty in thermoregulation and are prone to dehydration. Therefore, they should avoid exercise in hot or cold environments and should be vigilant about adequate hydration. Because these patients are prone to hypoglycemia and may also have a reduced ability to detect hypoglycemia, they require more careful glucose monitoring.

Physicians should review the drug treatment list for their patients with postural hypotension and eliminate, if possible, those drugs potentially contributing to hypotension with exercise. Also, physicians

TABLE 27.2 Effects of Diabetic Autonomic Neuropathy on Exercise Risk

- Resting tachycardia and decreased maximal responsiveness
- Decreased HRV
- Postural hypotension with exercise
- Exaggerated blood pressure responses with supine position and exercise
- Loss of diurnal blood pressure variation
- Cardiovascular and cardiorespiratory instability
- Abnormal systolic ejection fractions at rest/exercise
- Abnormal diastolic filling rates/times at rest/exercise
- Silent myocardial ischemia
- Poor exercise tolerance
- Failure of pupil adaptation to darkness
- Gastroparesis and diabetic diarrhea
- Hypoglycemia
- Decreased hypoglycemia awareness
- Hypoglycemia unresponsiveness
- Heat intolerance due to defective sympathetic thermoregulation and sweating (prone to dehydration)
- Susceptibility to foot ulcers and limb loss due to disordered regulation of cutaneous blood flow
- Incontinence

Adapted from Vinik et al.[81]

should encourage the use of full-length supportive garments, such as body stockings, to increase venous return during exercise. Patients with postural hypotension should coordinate exercise with mealtimes and insulin shots and avoid administration of insulin immediately before beginning exercise.

For patients with autonomic neuropathy, a conservative approach to exercise is best. For example, if a patient is unable to talk or maintain pedaling frequency, the exercise should be terminated. Whether patients with asymptomatic abnormalities in autonomic function tests are at similar risk is unclear, but a prudent approach to their exercise programs may be in order.

Exercise and Blood Glucose Regulation in Patients With Neuropathy

The metabolic response to exercise in patients with diabetic neuropathy is highly variable and cannot be predicted for an individual.

Therefore, guidelines can only be viewed as approximate, and alterations must be tailored for each patient. Self-monitoring of blood glucose (SMBG) is the cornerstone of effective management. It is essential that patients master SMBG before exercise training begins. In the insulin-requiring patient, a set time for exercising each day is best to minimize the number of adjustments necessary. Patients should be educated about the duration and peak actions of various insulin preparations in relation to gastric emptying to avoid exercising at peak insulin levels and before the stomach delivers its nutrient contents. In an attempt to gain maximal benefit from the acute glucose-lowering effects of exercise, exercise may be planned each day around a meal to blunt the glycemic fluxes,[95,105] or it can occur at home when the tardy stomach is emptying. Patients must be made fully aware of the potential risk of early and delayed hypoglycemia. Patients should wear an identification bracelet or necklace that indicates the presence of diabetes and medications for use during exercise in the event of an emergency. Physicians should provide a prescription for syringes prefilled with 1 mg glucagon for emergency intramuscular administration and insist that the patient carry them. It is important to avoid injecting insulin into the exercising limbs. The abdomen is the preferred injection site, especially in patients with autonomic neuropathy who are more prone to insulin-induced hypotension, which tends to be worse in the morning and improves later in the day.[96] Exercise may thus have to be deferred.

Intensity of Exercise

Although gentle exercise for 20 min three times a week reduces the likelihood of foot loss, studies indicate that exercise at 50–75% of maximal oxygen uptake is required for improved cardiovascular fitness. The heart rate in non-neuropaths is a conveniently monitored reflection of maximal oxygen uptake and is used to guide management. A formula used with success to identify the target heart rate to be attained during exercise is 50–70% of the maximal heart rate minus the resting heart rate added to the resting heart rate, i.e., target heart rate = 0.5–0.7(maximum heart rate – resting heart rate) + resting heart rate. A more simple formula is to subtract the patient's age from 220 and multiply the result by 0.7. However, published tables of maximal expected heart rates must be avoided when preparing an exercise prescription, particularly in patients with CAN whose maximal levels are depressed. Rather, the rating of perceived exertion (RPE) scale (Fig. 27.2) should be used for determining exercise intensity for these patients. Patients should aim to achieve moderate-range RPEs gradually over 2–4 weeks. The intensity of the exercise should not be increased to compensate for an abbreviated exercise session. Isometric exercise in the patient with neuropathy may be in order, provided that it does not cause an excessive rise in blood pressure. Figure 27.3 is a suggested paradigm for exercise management of patients with autonomic neuropathy.

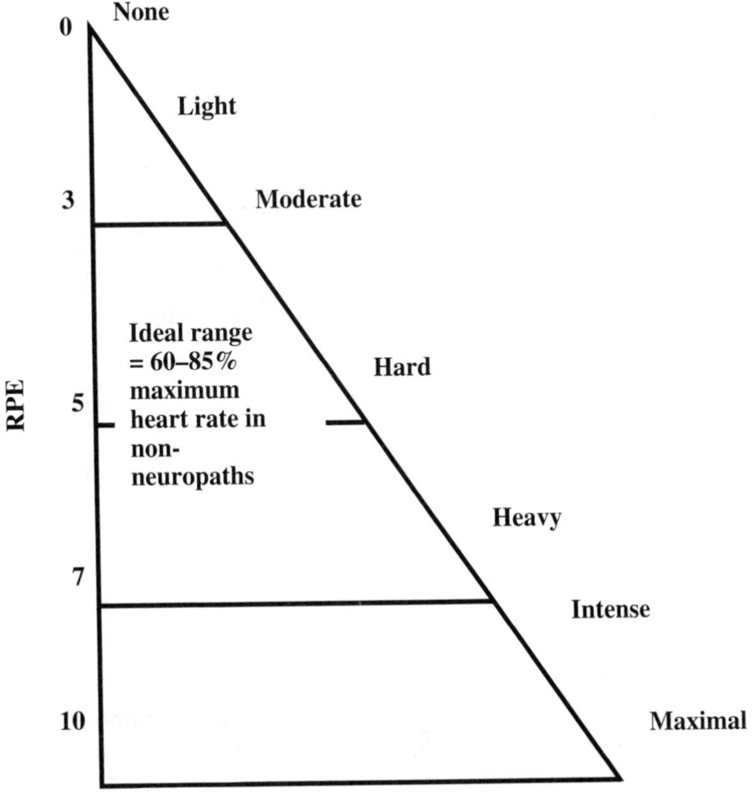

FIGURE 27.2 Suggested method for subjective evaluation of intensity of exercise in diabetic neuropathy.

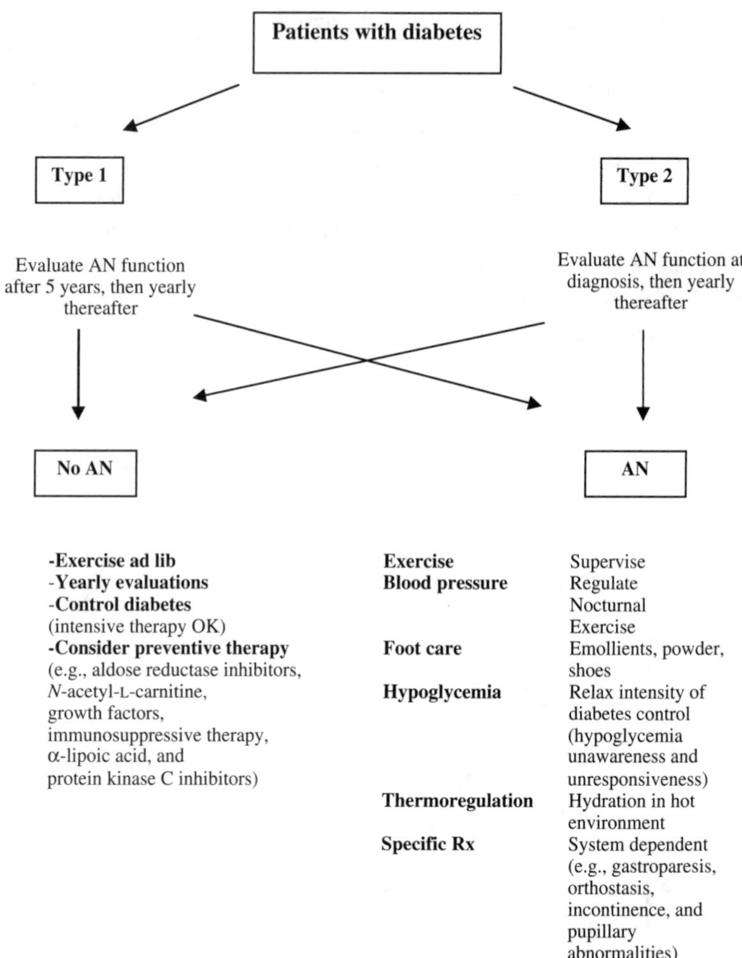

FIGURE 27.3 Suggested paradigm for exercise management of autonomic neuropathy (AN).

References

1. Young MJ, Boulton AJ, MacLeod AF, Williams DR, Sonksen PH: A multicentre study of prevalence of diabetic peripheral neuropathy in the United Kingdom hospital clinic population. *Diabetologia* 36:150–54, 1993
2. Tesfaye S, Stevens LK, Stephenson JM, Fuller JH, Plater M, Ionescu-Tirgoviste C, Nuber A, Pozza G, Ward JD: Prevalence of diabetic peripheral neuropathy and its relation to glycaemic

control and potential risk factors: the EURODIAB IDDM Complications Study. *Diabetologia* 11:1377–84, 1996

3. Adler AI, Boyko EJ, Ahroni JH, Stensel V, Forsberg RC, Smith DG: Risk factors for diabetic peripheral sensory neuropathy: results of the Seattle Prospective Diabetic Foot Study. *Diabetes Care* 20:1162–67, 1997
4. Franklin GM, Shetterly SM, Cohen JA, Baxter J, Hamman RF: Risk factors for distal symmetric neuropathy in NIDDM: the San Luis Valley Diabetes Study. *Diabetes Care* 17:1172–77, 1994
5. Consensus Statement: Report and recommendations of the San Antonio conference on diabetic neuropathy: American Diabetes Association American Academy of Neurology. *Diabetes Care* 11:592–97, 1988
6. Vinik AI: Diagnosis and management of diabetic neuropathy. *Clin Geriatr Med* 15:293–320, 1999
7. Dyck PJ: Small fiber neuropathy determination. *Muscle Nerve* 11:998–99, 1988
8. Hanson P, Schumacker P, Debugne TH, Clerin M: Evaluation of somatic and autonomic small fibers neuropathy in diabetes. *Am J Phys Med Rehabil* 71:44–47, 1992
9. Vinik AI, Erbas T, Stansberry KB, Pittenger GL: Small fiber neuropathy and neurovascular disturbances in diabetes mellitus. *Exp Clin Endocrinol Diabetes* 109 (Suppl. 2):444–66, 2001
10. Vinik AI, Holland MT, LeBeau JM, Liuzzi FJ, Stansberry KB, Colen LB: Diabetic neuropathies. *Diabetes Care* 15:1–50, 1992
11. Young MJ, Breddy JL, Veves A, Boulton AJ: The prediction of diabetic neuropathic foot ulceration using vibration perception thresholds: a prospective study. *Diabetes Care* 17:557–60, 1994
12. Coppini DV, Young PJ, Weng C, Macleod AF, Sonksen PH: Outcome on diabetic foot complications in relation to clinical examination and quantitative sensory testing: a case-control study. *Diabet Med* 15:765–71, 1998
13. Nelson RG, Gohdea DM, Everhart JE, Hartner JA, Zweiner FL, Pettit DJ: Lower extremity amputations in non-insulin-dependent diabetes: 12-year follow-up study in Pima Indians. *Diabetes Care* 11:8–16, 1988
14. Murray HJ, Young MJ, Hollis S, Boulton AJ: The association between callus formation, high pressures and neuropathy in diabetic foot ulceration. *Diabet Med* 13:979–82, 1996

15. Malone JM, Snyder M, Anderson G, Bernhard VM, Holloway GA Jr, Bunt TJ: Prevention of amputation by diabetic education. *Ann J Surg* 158:520–24, 1989
16. Thompson FJ, Veves A, Ashe H, Boulton AJM: A team approach to diabetic foot care: the Manchester experience. *Foot* 1:75–82, 1991
17. Litzelman DK, Slemenda CW, Langefeld CD, Hays LM, Welch MA, Bild DE, Ford ES, Vinicor F: Reduction of lower extremity clinical abnormalities in patients with non-insulin-dependent diabetes mellitus: a randomized, controlled trial. *Ann Intern Med* 119:36–41, 1993
18. Pecoraro RE, Reiber GE, Burgess EM: Pathways to diabetic limb amputation: basis for prevention. *Diabetes Care* 13:513–21, 1990
19. Young MJ, Marshall A, Adams JE, Selby PL, Boulton AJM: Osteopenia, neurological dysfunction and the development of Charcot neuroarthropathy. *Diabetes Care* 18:34–38, 1995
20. Gough A, Abraha H, Li F, Purewal TS, Foster AV, Watkins PJ, Moniz C, Edmonds ME: Measurement of markers of osteoclast and osteoblast activity in patients with acute and chronic diabetic Charcot neuroarthropathy. *Diabet Med* 14:527–31, 1997
21. Childs M, Armstrong DG, Edelson GW: Is Charcot arthropathy a late sequela of osteoporosis in patient with diabetes mellitus? *J Foot Ankle Surg* 37:437–39, 1998
22. Shapiro SA, Stansberry KB, Hill MA, Meyer MD, McNitt PM, Bhatt BA, Vinik AI: Normal blood flow response and vasomotion in the diabetic Charcot foot. *J Diabetes Complications* 12:147–53, 1998
23. Ziegler D, Gries FA, Spuler M, Lessmann F: Epidemiology of diabetic neuropathy: the diabetic cardiovascular autonomic neuropathy multicenter study group. *J Diabetes Complications* 6:49–57, 1992
24. Stephenson J, Fuller JH, EURODIAB IDDM Complications Study Group: Microvascular and acute complications in IDDM patients: the EURODIAB IDDM Complications Study. *Diabetologia* 37:278–85, 1994
25. Ziegler D, Dannehl K, Spuler M, Muhlen H, Gries FA: Prevalence of cardiovascular autonomic nerve dysfunction assessed by spectral analysis and standard test of heart rate variation in newly diagnosed IDDM patients. *Diabetes Care* 15:908–11, 1992

26. Vinik AI, Mitchell BD, Leichter SB, Wagner AL, O'Brian JT, Georges LP: Epidemiology of the complications of diabetes. In *Diabetes: Clinical Science in Practice.* Leslie RDG, Robbins DC, Eds. Cambridge, U.K., Cambridge University Press, 1994, p. 221–87
27. Ewing D, Campbell I, Clarke B: The natural history of diabetic autonomic neuropathy. *Q J Med* 49:95–108, 1980
28. Ewing DJ, Boland O, Neilson JMM, Cho CG, Clarke BF: Autonomic neuropathy, QT interval lengthening, and unexpected deaths in male diabetic patients. *Diabetologia* 34:182–85, 1991
29. Rathmann W, Ziegler D, Jahnke M, Haastert B, Gries FA: Mortality in diabetic patients with cardiovascular autonomic neuropathy. *Diabet Med* 10:820–24, 1993
30. Navarro X, Kennedy WR, Aeppli D, Sutherland DER: Neuropathy and mortality in diabetes: influence of pancreas transplantation. *Muscle Nerve* 19:1009–16, 1996
31. Orchard TJ, Lloyd CE, Maser RE, Kuller LH: Why diabetic autonomic neuropathy predict IDDM mortality? An analysis from Pittsburgh Epidemiology of Diabetes Complications Study. *Diabetes Res Clin Pract* 34 (Suppl.):S165–71, 1996
32. Levitt NS, Stansberry KB, Wynchank S, Vinik AI: The natural progression of autonomic neuropathy and autonomic function tests in a cohort of people with IDDM. *Diabetes Care* 19:751–54, 1996
33. Kahn JK, Sisson JC, Vinik AI: QT interval prolongation and sudden cardiac death in diabetic autonomic neuropathy. *J Clin Endocrinol Metab* 64:751–54, 1987
34. Hasslacher C, Bassler G: Prognose der kardialen autonomen neuropathie bei diabetikern. *Munch med Wschr* 125:375–77, 1983
35. Gonin JM, Kadrofske MM, Schmaltz S, Bastyr EJ, Vinik AI: Corrected Q-T interval prolongation as diagnostic tool for assessment of cardiac autonomic neuropathy in diabetes mellitus. *Diabetes Care* 13:68–71, 1990
36. Sobotka PA, Liss HP, Vinik AI: Impaired hypoxic ventilatory drive in diabetic patients with autonomic neuropathy. *J Clin Endocrinol Metab* 62:658–63, 1986
37. MacFadyen RJ, Barr CS, Struthers AD: Aldosterone blockade reduces vascular collagen turnover, improves heart rate variability and reduces early morning rise in heart rate in heart failure patients. *Cardiovasc Res* 35:30–34, 1997

38. Athyros VG, Didangelos TP, Karamitsos DT, Papageorgiou AA, Boudoulas H, Kontopoulos AG: Long-term effect of converting enzyme inhibition on circadian sympathetic and parasympathetic modulation in patients with diabetic autonomic neuropathy. *Acta Cardiol* 53:201–09, 1998
39. Kawano Y, Makino Y, Okuda N, Takishita S, Omae T: Effects of diltiazem retard on ambulatory blood pressure and heart rate variability in patients with essential hypertension. *Blood Press Monit* 5:181–85, 2000
40. Pinar E, Garcia-Alberola A, Llamas C, Vicente T, Lopez-Candel J, Rojo JL, Fernandez R, Valdes M: Effects of verapamil on indexes of heart rate variability after acute myocardial infarction. *Am J Cardiol* 81:1085–89, 1998
41. Kontopoulos AG, Athyros VG, Papageorgiou AA, Boudoulas H: Effect of quinapril or metoprolol on circadian sympathetic and parasympathetic modulation after acute myocardial infarction. *Am J Cardiol* 84:1164–69, 1999
42. Weber F, Schneider H, von Arnim T, Urbaszek W: Heart rate variability and ischaemia in patients with coronary heart disease and stable angina pectoris: influence of drug therapy and prognostic value: TIBBS Investigators Group: Total Ischemic Burden Bisoprolol Study. *Eur Heart J* 20:38–50, 1999
43. Ziegler D, Gries FA, Muhlen H, Rathmann W, Spuler M, Lessmann F, the DiaCAN Multicenter Study Group: Prevalence and clinical correlates of cardiovascular autonomic and peripheral diabetic neuropathy in patients attending diabetes center. *Diabete Metab* 19:143–51, 1993
44. Navarro X, Kennedy WR, Loewenson RB, Sutherland DER: Influence of pancreas transplantation on cardiorespiratory reflexes, nerve conduction, and mortality in diabetes. *Diabetes* 39: 802–06, 1990
45. Sampson MJ, Wilson S, Karagiannis P, Edmonds M, Watkins PJ: Progression of diabetic autonomic neuropathy over a decade in insulin-dependent diabetics. *Q J Med* 75:635–46, 1990
46. O'Brien IA, McFadden JP, Corral RJM: The influence of autonomic neuropathy on mortality in insulin-dependent diabetes. *Q J Med* 79:495–502, 1991
47. Jermendy G, Toth L, Voros P, Koltai MZ, Pogatsa G: Cardiac autonomic neuropathy and QT interval length: a follow-up study in diabetic patients. *Acta Cardiol* 46:189–200, 1991

48. Luft D, Rak R, Renn W, Konz K, Eggstein M: Diabetischeautonome neuropathie: verlauf und prognostische bedeutung kardiovaskularer reflexteste. *Diab Stoffw* 2:239–44, 1993
49. Ziegler D: Cardiovascular autonomic neuropathy: clinical manifestations and measurement. *Diabetes Reviews* 7:342–57, 1999
50. Kahn JK, Zola B, Juni JE, Vinik AI: Decreased exercise heart rate and blood pressure response in diabetic subjects with cardiac autonomic neuropathy. *Diabetes Care* 9:389–94, 1986
51. Pfeifer M: Cardiovascular assessment. In *Diabetic Neuropathy*. 2nd ed. Dyck PC, Thomas PK, Eds. Philadelphia, W.B. Saunders, 1999, p. 171–83
52. Bottini P, Tantucci C, Scionti L, Dottorini ML, Puxeddu E, Reboldi G, Bolli GB, Casucci G, Santeusanio F, Sorbini CA, Brunetti P: Cardiovascular response to exercise in diabetic patients: influence of autonomic neuropathy of different severity. *Diabetologia* 38:244–50, 1995
53. Ziegler D, Laux G, Dannehl K, Spuler M, Muhlen H, Mayer P, Gries FA: Assessment of cardiovascular autonomic function: age-related normal ranges and reproducibility of spectral analysis, vector analysis, and standard tests of heart rate variation and blood pressure responses. *Diabet Med* 9:166–75, 1992
54. Veglio M, Borra M, Stevens LK, Fuller JH, Perin PC, the EURODIAB IDDM Complications Study Group: The relation between QTc interval prolongation and diabetic complications. *Diabetologia* 42:68–75, 1999
55. Kolman BS, Verrier RL, Lown B: Effect of vagus nerve stimulation upon excitability of the canine ventricle. *Am J Cardiol* 37: 1041–45, 1976
56. Whitsel EA, Boyko EJ, Siscovick DS: Reassessing the role of QTc in the diagnosis of autonomic failure among patients with diabetes: a meta-analysis. *Diabetes Care* 23:241–47, 2000
57. Cryer PE: Normal and abnormal sympathoadrenal function in patients with insulin-dependent diabetes mellitus. *N Y State J Med* 82:886–91, 1982
58. Zola B, Kahn J, Juni J, Vinik A: Abnormal cardiac function in diabetics with autonomic neuropathy in the absence of ischemic heart disease. *J Clin Endocrinol Metab* 63:208–14, 1986
59. Mildenberger RR, Bar-Shlomo B, Druck MN, Jablonsky G, Morch JE, Hilton JD, Kenshole AB, Forbath N, McLaughlin PR: Clinically unrecognized ventricular dysfunction in young diabetic patients. *J Am Coll Cardiol* 4:234–38, 1984

60. Vered Z, Battler A, Sega P: Exercise-induced left ventricular dysfunction in young men with asymptomatic diabetes mellitus (diabetic cardiomyopathy). *Am J Cardiol* 54:633–37, 1984
61. Kahn JK, Zola B, Juni JE, Vinik AI: Radionuclide assessment of left ventricular diastolic filling in diabetes mellitus with and without cardiac autonomic neuropathy. *J Am Coll Cardiol* 7:1303–09, 1986
62. Airaksinen KEJ, Koistinen MJ: Association between silent coronary artery disease, diabetes, and autonomic neuropathy: fact or fallacy? *Diabetes Care* 15:288–92, 1992
63. Di Carli MF, Bianco-Batlles D, Landa ME, Kazmers A, Groehn H, Muzik O, Grunberger G: Effects of autonomic neuropathy on coronary blood flow in patients with diabetes mellitus. *Circulation* 100:813–19, 1999
64. Nahser PJ, Brown RE, Oskarsson H, Winniford MD, Rossen JD: Maximal coronary flow reserve and metabolic coronary vasodilatation in patients with diabetes mellitus. *Circulation* 91:635–40, 1995
65. Nitenberg A, Valensi P, Sachs R, Dali M, Aptecar E, Attali J-R: Impairment of coronary vascular reserve and ACh-induced coronary vasodilation in diabetic patients with angiographically normal coronary arteries and normal left ventricular systolic function. *Diabetes* 42:1017–25, 1993
66. Pitkanen OP, Nuutila P, Raitakari OT, Ronnemaa T, Koskinen PJ, Iida H, Lehtimaki TJ, Laine HK, Takala T, Viikari JS, Knuuti J: Coronary flow reserve is reduced in young men with IDDM. *Diabetes* 47:248–54, 1998
67. Ziegler D, Dannehl K, Muhlen H, Spuler M, Gries FA: Prevalence of cardiovascular autonomic dysfunction assessed by spectral analysis, vector analysis, and standard tests of heart rate variation and blood pressure responses at various stages of diabetic neuropathy. *Diabet Med* 9:806–14, 1992
68. Ziegler D, Weise F, Langen KJ, Piolot R, Boy C, Hubinger A, Muller-Gartner HW, Gries FA: Effect of glycaemic control on myocardial sympathetic innervation assessed by [123I]metaiodobenzylguanidine scintigraphy: a 4-year prospective study in IDDM patients. *Diabetologia* 41:443–51, 1998
69. Langen KJ, Ziegler D, Weise F, Piolot R, Boy C, Hubinger A, Gries FA, Muller-Gartner HW: Evaluation of QT interval length, QT dispersion and myocardial m-iodobenzylguanidine uptake

in insulin-dependent diabetic patients with and without autonomic neuropathy. *Clin Sci (Colch)* 93:325–33, 1997

70. Mantysaari M, Kuikka J, Mustonen J, Tahvanainen K, Vanninen E, Lansimies E, Uusitupa M: Noninvasive detection of cardiac sympathetic nervous dysfunction in diabetic patients using [123I]metaiodobenzylguanidine. *Diabetes* 41:1069–75, 1992
71. Kahn JK, Vinik AI: Exercise training in the diabetic patient. *Med Interne* 9:117–25, 1988
72. Hilsted J: Pathophysiology in diabetic autonomic neuropathy: cardiovascular, hormonal, and metabolic studies. *N Y State J Med* 82:892–903, 1982
73. Cryer PE, Silverberg AB, Santiago JV, Shah SD: Plasma catecholamines in diabetes: the syndromes of hypoadrenergic and hyperadrenergic postural hypotension. *Am J Med* 64:407–16, 1978
74. Abrahm DR, Hollingsworth PJ, Smith CB, Jim L, Zucker LB, Sobotka PA, Vinik AI: Decreased alpha 2-adrenergic receptors on platelet membranes from diabetic patients with autonomic neuropathy and orthostatic hypotension. *J Clin Endocrinol Metab* 63:906–12, 1986
75. Nakano S, Uchida K, Kigoshi T, Azukizawa S, Iwasaki R, Kaneko M, Morimoto S: Circadian rhythm of blood pressure to normotensive NIDDM subjects: its relationship to microvascular complications. *Diabetes Care* 14:707–11, 1990
76. Makimattila S, Mantysaari M, Schlenzka A, Summanen P, Yki-Jarvinen H: Mechanism of altered hemodynamic and metabolic responses to insulin in patients with insulin-dependent diabetes mellitus and autonomic dysfunction. *J Clin Endocrinol Metab* 83:468–75, 1998
77. Stansberry KB, Shapiro SA, Hill MA, McNitt PM, Meyer MD, Vinik AI: Impaired peripheral vasomotion in diabetes. *Diabetes Care* 19:715–21, 1996
78. Stansberry KB, Shapiro SA, Hill MA, McPitt PM, Meyer MD, Vinik AI: Impairment of peripheral blood flow responses in diabetes resembles an enhanced aging effect. *Diabetes Care* 20:1711–16, 1997
79. Stansberry KB, Peppard HR, Babyak LM, Popp G, McNitt PM, Vinik AI: Primary nociceptive afferents mediate the blood flow dysfunction in glabrous (hairy) skin of type 2 diabetes: a new model for the pathogenesis of microvascular dysfunction. *Diabetes Care* 22:1549–54, 1999

80. Edmonds M, Archer A, Watkins P: Ephedrine: a new treatment for diabetic neuropathic oedema. *Lancet* i:548–51, 1983
81. Vinik A, Erbas T, Stansberry K: Gastrointestinal, genitourinary, and neurovascular disturbances in diabetes. *Diabetes Reviews* 7:358–78, 1999
82. Barnett JL, Vinik AI: Gastrointestinal disturbances. In *Therapy for Diabetes Mellitus and Related Disorders.* Lebovitz HE, Ed. Alexandria, VA, American Diabetes Association, 1994, p. 288–96
83. Tantucci C, Bottini P, Dottorini ML, Pexeddu E, Casucci G, Scionti L, Sorbini CA: Ventilatory response to exercise in diabetic subjects with autonomic neuropathy. *J Appl Physiol* 81:1978–86, 1996
84. Levy DM, Rowley DA, Abraham RR: Portable infrared pupillometry using Pupilscan: relation to somatic and autonomic nerve function in diabetes mellitus. *Clin Autonom Res* 2:335–41, 1992
85. Janand-Delenne B, Savin B, Habib G, Bory M, Vague P, Lassmann-Vague V: Silent myocardial ischemia in patients with diabetes: who to screen. *Diabetes Care* 22:1396–1400, 1999
86. Lubaszewski W, Kawecka-Jaszcz K, Czarnecka D, Rajzer M, Stochmal A: Silent myocardial ischaemia in patients with essential arterial hypertension and non-insulin dependent diabetes mellitus. *J Hum Hypertens* 13:309–13, 1999
87. Valensi P, Sachs RN, Lormeau B, Taupin JM, Ouzan J, Blasco A, Nitenberg A, Metz D, Paries J, Talvard O, Leutenegger M, Attali JR: Silent myocardial ischaemia and left ventricle hypertrophy in diabetic patients. *Diabete Metab* 23:409–16, 1997
88. Radice M, Rocca A, Bedon E, Musacchio N, Morabito A, Segalinin G: Abnormal response to exercise in middle-aged NIDDM patients with and without autonomic neuropathy. *Diabet Med* 13: 259–65, 1996
89. Kahn J, Sisson J, Vinik A: QT interval prolongation and sudden cardiac death in diabetic autonomic neuropathy. *J Clin Endocrinol Metab* 64:751–54, 1987
90. Vinik AI, Suwanwalaikorn S: Autonomic neuropathy. In *Current Therapy of Diabetes Mellitus*. DeFronzo R, Ed. St. Louis, MO, Mosby, 1997, p. 165–76
91. Malone JM, Synder M, Anderson G, Bernhard VM, Holloway GA Jr, Bunt TJ: Prevention of amputation by diabetic education. *Ann J Surg* 158:520–24, 1989

92. Vinik AI, Park TS, Stansberry KB, Pittenger GL: Diabetic neuropathies. *Diabetologia* 43:957–73, 2000
93. Morello CM, Leckband SG, Stoner CP, Moorhouse DF, Sahagian GA: Randomized double-blind study comparing the efficacy of gabapentin with amitriptyline on diabetic peripheral neuropathy pain. *Arch Intern Med* 159:1931–37, 1999
94. Backonja MM: Gabapentin monotherapy for the symptomatic treatment of painful neuropathy: a multicenter, double-blind, placebo-controlled trial in patients with diabetes mellitus. *Epilepsia* 40 (Suppl. 6):S57–59, 1999
95. Zinman B: Comparison of the acute and long-term effects of exercise on glucose control in type I diabetes. *Diabetes Care* 7: 515–19, 1984
96. Berger M: Metabolic and hormonal effects of muscular exercise in juvenile type I diabetes. *Diabetologia* 13:355–65, 1977
97. Gaede P, Vedel P, Parving HH, Pedersen O: Intensified multifactorial intervention in patients with type 2 diabetes mellitus and microalbuminuria: the Steno Type 2 Randomised Study. *Lancet* 353:617–22, 1999
98. Diabetes Control and Complications Trial Research Group: The effect of intensive diabetes therapy on the development and progression of neuropathy. *Ann Intern Med* 122:561–68, 1995
99. Diabetes Control and Complications Trial Research Group: The effect of intensive diabetes therapy on measures of autonomic nervous system function in the Diabetes Control and Complications Trail (DCCT). *Diabetologia* 41:416–23, 1998
100. Burger AJ, Weinrauch LA, D'Elia JA, Aronson D: Effect of glycemic control on heart rate variability in type I diabetic patients with cardiac autonomic neuropathy. *Am J Cardiol* 84:687–91, 1999
101. Howorka K, Pumprla J, Haber P, Koller-Strametz J, Mondrzyk J, Schabmann A: Effects of physical training on heart rate variability in diabetic patients with various degrees of cardiovascular autonomic neuropathy. *Cardiovasc Res* 34:206–14, 1997
102. Graham C, Lasko-McCarthey P: Exercise options for persons with diabetic complications. *Diabetes Educ* 16:212–20, 1990
103. Vitug A, Schneider SH, Ruderman NB: Exercise and type I diabetes mellitus. *Exerc Sport Sci Rev* 16:285–304, 1988

104. Campaigne B, Lampman R: The clinical application of exercise in type I diabetes. In *Exercise in the Clinical Management of Diabetes.* Champaign, IL, Human Kinetics, 1994, p. 139–68

105. Caron D: The effects of postprandial exercise on meal-related glucose intolerance in insulin-dependent diabetes individuals. *Diabetes Care* 5:364–69, 1982

Aaron I. Vinik, MD, PhD, FCP, FACP, FACE, and Tomris Erbas, MD, are from the Strelitz Diabetes Institute, Norfolk, VA.

28

Musculoskeletal Disorders and Sports Injuries

RICHARD M. LAMPMAN, PhD

Highlights

- It is unknown whether an athlete with diabetes is at a greater risk for musculoskeletal injury than an athlete without this disease.
- Precautionary measures that alter or modify training methods, sports equipment, and/or mode of physical activity may reduce the risk of an athletic injury.
- Individuals with diabetes should be encouraged to participate in regular exercise involving competitive or recreational sports and/or physical fitness for enjoyment and health.

Routine exercise is engaged in for a variety of reasons. Many people exercise for relaxation and social camaraderie. Others participate for health, fitness, and recreational reasons. It is likely that age is a major determinant

TABLE 28.1 Activity Interests Associated With Age

Interest Level	Young	Middle-Aged	Elderly
1	Competitive sports	Health/fitness	Health/fitness
2	Recreational sports	Recreational sports	Recreational sports
3	Health/fitness	Competitive sports	Competitive sports

Interest level: 1 > 2 > 3.

of an individual's interest in and level of physical activity (Table 28.1). The young are more inclined to engage in competitive sports, whereas as an individual ages, recreation and health are usually given as the major reasons to exercise routinely. Enhanced cardiovascular fitness, weight control, and increased muscular strength are typically the exercise motivators of the middle-aged and older adult.

The more competitive the sport (especially those involving physical contact) and the higher the intensity of the activity, the more likely the chance for an athletic injury. The prevalence of musculoskeletal injuries attributable to participation in strenuous activities in diabetic individuals compared with nondiabetic individuals has not been well studied.

Individuals with diabetes are encouraged to exercise routinely because of the well-documented physical, metabolic, and psychological benefits.[1,2] Realistic goals and objectives can be established so that diabetic subjects can participate safely in competitive and recreational sports and exercise activities such as jogging, which have the potential to traumatize lower limbs, especially the feet. Diabetic subjects routinely exercising in their young and middle-age years may increase peak bone mineral density (BMD) in early years, maintain it through midlife, and delay or prevent the severity of osteoporosis and prevalence of fractures in later years. It is unknown whether diabetic individuals exercising routinely or participating in sports have a greater propensity for injury than people in the general population.

Injuries Associated With Exercise and Sports

Knowledge of preventive measures and their application can minimize musculoskeletal injuries associated with exercise and sports. Individuals should be cognizant of their physical and medical limitations and of their metabolic and physiological responses to exercise. In addition, they should be knowledgeable about appropriate exercise training regimens and injury prevention. Because many injuries result from inappropriate training techniques, poor or faulty equipment, or biomechanical abnormalities, these factors should be closely monitored.

Individuals Without Diabetes

All athletes who violate rules of training, including those with and without diabetes, are at increased risk for acute or overuse athletic injuries. A higher incidence of musculoskeletal injuries occurs with competitive sports. The demands of competitive sports often require a participant to perform maneuvers involving sudden accelerations and decelerations that can cause extreme biomechanical stresses resulting in musculoskeletal injuries. Traumatic injuries occur frequently in contact sports, whereas overuse injuries to soft tissues, ligaments, muscles, and bone occur with repetitive sports such as jogging and running.

Individuals With Diabetes

An individual with diabetes may be at a disadvantage when performing high-intensity sports because of altered glucose production and/or utilization.[3,4] However, whether this leads to athletic injuries secondary to abnormal muscle responses is unclear. It is theoretical that diabetic neuropathy and angiopathy may increase the chance or severity of trauma-related fractures or other complications, but little information exists supporting this contention.

An epidemiological study conducted over a 3-year period in middle-aged and older adults showed an association between sports-related, trauma-induced ankle fracture and being diabetic and obese.[5] Whether this relationship exists in diabetic subjects independent of obesity is unknown. Wolf[6] studied the prevalence of pedal fractures in 60 diabetic athletes compared with 60 nondiabetic athletes. Results showed an increased prevalence of fracture in this small number of diabetic athletes, especially if they had the disease >25 years. Diabetic men, but not diabetic women, were at a higher risk to develop a fracture than were nondiabetic individuals. However, no strong link was found between daily activity levels and the prevalence of fractures among diabetic subjects. Fracture sites found in the diabetic individuals were the proximal phalanges of the hallux and the second, third, and fifth digits. The second and fifth metatarsals were the most frequently reported fracture bones for both diabetic and normal individuals.

Other reports[7–10] have suggested a relationship between diabetes and stress fractures of the lower extremities. These fractures may be associated with neuropathic bone changes,[11] vascular disease,[7] or reduced bone mass.[12] Lower-limb fractures may occur even in the young diabetic patient with or without symmetric peripheral neuropathy. Case reports of two diabetic runners in their early 20s suggest that jogging may have increased their risk of bilateral calcaneal region stress fractures.[10]

Prevention of fractures in diabetic subjects, including sports-related fractures, is important because postsurgical complications may be elevated in individuals with this disease. After a closed ankle fracture, the risk of infection after either surgical or nonsurgical treatment was found to be 32% in 25 diabetic subjects, whereas it was only 8% for nondiabetic individuals.[13] In one study in which results of all ankle fractures treated surgically in patients with diabetes were retrospectively reviewed, the relative risk of postoperative complication was nearly three times greater in diabetic individuals than in nondiabetic individuals matched for age, sex, and fracture severity.[14] An increased risk of wound complication after surgical treatment of calcaneus fractures has also been reported.[15] In a study by Kristiansen,[16] an increased rate of wound infection was found in 10 diabetic patients after surgery for malleolar fractures, but no increased risk of fractures, no difference in the type of injury present, or delayed bone healing were found in this study. Whether the likelihood of wound complications after surgical treatment of fractures is the same in athletic diabetic subjects as in nondiabetic individuals has not been adequately studied.

What might be called diabetic osteopenia may occur in other areas of the body as well. In diabetic subjects studied prospectively over a 9-year period, women with type 1 or type 2 diabetes had a higher relative risk of hip fracture of 6.9 and 1.8, respectively, compared with women without diabetes.[17] BMD measurement in the lumbar spine, distal and proximal sites of the radius, and calcaneus in 26 diabetic patients showed that BMD was reduced only in the radius.[18] An increased incidence of osteoporotic fractures has also been reported in diabetic subjects with confounding medical conditions. The occurrence of spontaneous fractures in patients with type 1 diabetes after renal transplantation was 40% but only 11% in nondiabetic individuals, and most fractures occurred within 3 years after surgery.[19] This increased occurrence of fractures might be related to immunosuppressive medications and/or the lack of routine exercise to help prevent loss of bone mineral mass.

Upper-extremity injuries, especially of the glenohumeral joint, may also be more prevalent in diabetic individuals. Bridgeman[20] described an association of periarthritis (phases of severe pain, increasing stiffness, diminution in joint capacity, and slow recovery to normal) of the shoulder with diabetes. The incidence of this condition in 800 diabetic individuals was 10.8% and was significantly greater ($P < 0.005$) than the incidence of 2.3% found in nondiabetic subjects. Interestingly, 42% of diabetic patients had involvement of both shoulders, but this symmetrical problem appeared unrelated to polyneuropathy. Shoulder disease in Pima Indians (a population with a high prevalence of type 2 diabetes) was reported to be associated with type 2 diabetes.[21]

Prevention of Injuries

In general, a young person with diabetes should be encouraged to participate in exercise or sports (see Chapters 4, 13, 31).[1] Young athletes in good metabolic control need not be limited in their choice of recreational and competitive sports because no evidence exists to the contrary. The middle-aged to older individual with diabetes should be encouraged to lead a normal active lifestyle. The natural degeneration of muscles, bones, tendons, ligaments, and articular surfaces associated with aging may be accelerated with physical inactivity, and in the case of diabetes, may be more pronounced. Because they are often sedentary and may suffer from latent or overt metabolic and neurological abnormalities, some individuals with diabetes are potentially at greater risk for cardiac and musculoskeletal complications when exercising. Before beginning an exercise program, especially a high-intensity one, individuals should be thoroughly evaluated for any underlying medical problems that may put them at risk for injury.

Aerobic exercises such as walking, jogging, and running should be performed in ways that do not traumatize the feet. High-resistance exercises using free weights or machines may be appropriate for young diabetic individuals but not for those with long-term diabetes. Older adult diabetic individuals should be encouraged to perform low-resistance training by selecting an amount of weight just heavy enough to slightly fatigue the muscle group involved after performing 8–15 repetitions over the full range of muscle motion. Patients should be cautioned not to perform a Valsalva maneuver when performing resistant exercises. A simple approach is to have the patient maintain a normal breathing pattern. Progression of weight training can be accomplished by periodically increasing the amount of weight lifted by no more than 10% and by increasing to three sets of 8–15 repetitions per session. Circuit training is an effective method of resistance training and is performed by doing one resistance exercise followed by another (within 30 s) in a series of exercises. Systolic blood pressure, if monitored, should not go over 180 mmHg during exercise.[22] A bracelet or shoe tag indicating an individual has diabetes and other relevant medical information should always be worn while exercising.

Warm-Up and Cooldown

During an exercise session, the individual can help avoid musculoskeletal injuries by warming up thoroughly before the exercise session and stretching and cooling down adequately after it is completed. Whether patients with diabetes are exercising at a low or high intensity of physical exertion, it is recommended they begin their exercise session with a low-level exercise intensity for 2–5 min (warm-up) and perform a low-intensity activity again after their exercise session (cooldown). A warm-up period of easy physical activity allows for proper cardiovascular adjustments, may minimize the risk of exercise-induced cardiovascular complications (e.g., ischemia, arrhythmias), and reduces a patient's perception of fatigue. Warm-up activities might include slow walking or easy cycling and range of motion activities followed by easy static stretching of major muscle groups throughout the body. Static stretching involves slow and cautious extension of the muscle group to a tension just below the pain threshold and holding at this point for 10–30 s. This procedure should be repeated two to six times, with slightly more tension applied with each consecutive static stretch to reach the muscle's maximum range. Static stretching is believed to improve flexibility and may prevent athletic injuries. Also, during the postexercise period, a mild cooldown period of slow walking or slow cycling may eliminate the potential for ischemic or arrhythmic responses and allows the cardiovascular system to more slowly return to normal resting conditions. Because muscles are well warmed-up after an exercise session, static stretching or flexibility training may be effective at this time. These warm-up and cooldown sessions may not be as beneficial until a patient can perform at least 10–15 min of continuous exercise.

Overuse Injuries

Musculoskeletal injuries can result from chronic, repetitive, impact-related stresses rather than acute trauma. These injuries are referred to as overuse injuries. They are common when an individual progresses from one level of training to a higher level too quickly. The beginner is usually enthusiastic, is poorly conditioned, and often uses inferior equipment. Training overload by both inexperienced and competitive athletes can lead to musculoskeletal stresses sufficient to cause strains, sprains, and fractures. The causes of these injuries can be multifactorial and may involve training errors, biomechanical factors, and poor equipment. Diabetic patients should set realistic exercise training goals with respect to intensity of effort, duration of sustained activity, and frequency of exercise.[1] If minor joint or muscle pain persists or becomes more severe, the diabetic individual should rest these areas for a few days. Alternative training modes should be performed until this condition subsides.

Of major concern for diabetic patients with either peripheral vascular occlusive arterial disease and/or peripheral neuropathy is repetitive physical activity that may traumatize the feet, ankles, and/or lower leg. Patients with diabetic neuropathy may have a reduction in the sensation of pain and be unaware of excessive impact forces (see Chapters 22 and 27). They may also have a reduced proprioception, or joint position sense. This condition should be evaluated clinically because inadequate foot position awareness may not provide appropriate joint protection. Walking on uneven surfaces may increase abnormal joint position in individuals without protective proprioceptive input, leading to soft tissue injuries and possibly bone fractures. Individuals without reflex stabilization of the lower limb should be encouraged to participate in activities such as swimming or cycling on a stationary bicycle to reduce the potential for musculoskeletal injuries.

Unchecked forces associated with repetitive stresses in exercises such as brisk walking or jogging could place an individual at increased risk for lower-extremity stress fractures. Suitable shoe selection is important in the prevention of lower-limb athletic injuries. Shoes should have a built-up heel to absorb impact forces and a good arch support (firm but not rigid) to prevent excessive pronation. The midsoles of athletic shoes, if constructed with air or silica gel pockets, provide additional absorbency of shearing forces generated by impact with the ground. Shoes having these features can be beneficial to individuals with peripheral neuropathy and/or microvascular disease. A well-constructed and supportive athletic shoe, as described, can be obtained from sporting goods stores or stores specializing in name-brand athletic footwear.

Commercially available or specifically constructed orthotic devices may help prevent excessive pronation and eliminate other pathologic stresses and trauma. A tube-type sock should not be worn because it can easily fold in the shoe and cause abrasions and blisters. A hydrophobic (wicks water away from the feet) fiber blend (e.g., cotton/polyester, rayon/nylon/Lycra, or an acrylic fiber) sock having a constructed toe and heel design, preferably with a medium-density cushioning pad, is best for protection against shock, abrasions, and blisters. Proper foot care is important in individuals with diabetes to prevent blisters and possible infections. Daily inspection of the toes and plantar surfaces of the feet is essential because it is important to detect any abnormality early. Patients should be advised to see their physicians immediately should any changes occur in their feet. In the event of an overuse injury to the foot in a person with diabetes, special care to minimize the danger of more serious complications is recommended.[23]

Trauma Injuries

No major studies have demonstrated that individuals with diabetes are at greater risk for trauma injuries than those without diabetes. In the event of injury in the general population, evidence suggests a higher prevalence of later-life complications, such as reduced range of motion, bursitis, articular laxity, tendinitis, and synovitis.[24] Whether an individual with diabetes has a greater prevalence or severity of later-life sequelae associated with a previous athletic injury is unknown.

Conclusion

Additional scientific and clinical evidence is necessary before it can be determined whether an individual with diabetes is at increased risk for musculoskeletal injuries when exercising. Although accidental trauma injuries occur in many sports, overuse injuries may be more prevalent in individuals with diabetes. The occurrence of these events may relate to the method of training usually recommended to diabetic individuals—namely, endurance training programs involving activities such as brisk walking and jogging. Inadvertent overuse injuries may be avoided by taking appropriate precautions to minimize potential problems. During an exercise session, the individual can help avoid musculoskeletal injuries by warming up thoroughly before the exercise session and stretching and cooling down adequately after it is completed. Treatment and rehabilitation for injuries in diabetic subjects should be similar to that for people without diabetes, pending further clinical or experimental research findings.

It is reasonable to recommend caution to a person with diabetes who is planning to engage in a high-intensity, repetitive-impact activity, such as brisk walking, jogging, or running. In most cases, the risk for complications and injuries can be minimized with adequate medical screening, prudent approaches to exercise training, proper equipment, and coordination of exercise, diet, insulin and other hypoglycemic drug dosages, and hydration. Existing evidence suggests that the metabolic, physical, and psychological benefits of exercise training far outweigh the potential complications and risks of musculoskeletal injuries in this population. A person with diabetes should be encouraged, not discouraged or excluded, from athletics, sports, or health/fitness-related activities unless it can be determined that the risk-to-benefit ratio suggests otherwise.

References

1. Campaigne BN, Lampman RM: *Exercise in the Clinical Management of Diabetes*. Champaign, IL, Human Kinetics, 1994
2. Wallberg-Henriksson H: Exercise and diabetes mellitus. *Exerc Sport Sci Rev* 20:339–68, 1992
3. Bak JF, Jacobsen UK, Jorgensen FS, Pedersen O: Insulin receptor function and glycogen synthase activity in skeletal muscle biopsies

from patients with insulin-dependent diabetes mellitus: effects of physical training. *J Clin Endocrinol Metab* 69:158–64, 1989

4. Menon RK, Grace AA, Burgoyne W, Fonseca VA, James IM, Dandona P: Muscle blood flow in diabetes mellitus: evidence of abnormality after exercise. *Diabetes Care* 15:693–95, 1992
5. Daly PJ, Fitzgerald RH Jr, Melton LJ, Ilstrup DM: Epidemiology of ankle fractures in Rochester, Minnesota. *Acta Orthop Scand* 58:539–44, 1987
6. Wolf S: Diabetes mellitus and predisposition to athletic pedal fracture. *J Foot Ankle Surg* 37:16–22, 1998
7. Conventry MB, Rothacker GW Jr: Bilateral calcaneal fracture in a diabetic patient: a case report. *J Bone Joint Surg* 61A:462–64, 1979
8. Daffner RH: Stress fractures: current concepts. *Skeletal Radiol* 2:221–29, 1978
9. Heath H III, Melton LJ III, Chu CP: Diabetes mellitus and risk of skeletal fracture. *N Engl J Med* 303:567–70, 1990
10. Jones R, Johnson KA: Diagnostic problems: jogging and diabetes mellitus. *Foot Ankle* 1:362–64, 1981
11. El-Khoury GY, Kathol MH: Neuropathic fractures in patients with diabetes mellitus. *Radiology* 134:313–16, 1980
12. Levin ME, Bolsseau VC, Avioll LV: Effects of diabetes mellitus on bone mass in juvenile and adult-onset diabetes. *N Engl J Med* 294: 241–45, 1976
13. Flynn JM, Rodriguez-del Rio F, Piza PA: Closed ankle fractures in the diabetic patient. *Foot Ankle Int* 21:311–19, 2000
14. Blotter RH, Connolly E, Wasan A, Chapman MW: Acute complications in the operative treatment of isolated ankle fractures in patients with diabetes mellitus. *Foot Ankle Int* 20:687–94, 1999
15. Folk JW, Starr AJ, Early JS: Early wound complications of operative treatment of calcaneus fractures: analysis of 190 fractures. *J Orthop Trauma* 13:369–72, 1999
16. Kristiansen B: Results of surgical treatment of malleolar fractures in patients with diabetes mellitus. *Dan Med Bull* 30:272–74, 1983
17. Forsen L, Meyer HE, Midthjell K, Edna TH: Diabetes mellitus and the incidence of hip fracture: results from the Nord-Trondelag Health Survey. *Diabetologia* 42:920–25, 1999
18. Hirano Y, Kishimoto H, Hagino H, Teshima R: The change of bone mineral density in secondary osteoporosis and vertebral fracture incidence. *J Bone Miner Metab* 17:119–24, 1999

19. Nisbeth U, Lindh E, Ljunghall S, Backman U, Fellstrom B: Increased fracture rate in diabetes mellitus and females after renal transplantation. *Transplantation* 67:1218–22, 1999
20. Bridgeman JF: Periarthritis of the shoulder and diabetes mellitus. *Am Rheum Dis* 31:69–71, 1972
21. Jacobsson LT, Nagi DK, Pillemer SR, Knowler WC, Hanson RL, Pettitt DJ, Bennett PH: Low prevalences of chronic widespread pain and shoulder disorders among the Pima Indians. *J Rheumatol* 23:907–09, 1996
22. Bernbaum M, Albert SG, Cohen JD: Exercise training in individuals with retinopathy and blindness. *Arch Phys Med Rehabil* 70:605–11, 1989
23. Coughlin RR: Common injuries of the foot: often more than 'just a sprain.' *Postgrad Med* 86:175–79, 182, 185, 1989
24. Raskin RJ, Rebecca GS: Posttraumatic sports-related musculoskeletal abnormalities: prevalence in a normal population. *Am J Sports Med* 11:336–39, 1983

Richard M. Lampman, PhD, is from the St. Joseph Mercy Hospital, Ann Arbor, MI, and currently has an appointment at the University of Michigan Medical School, Ann Arbor, MI.

Exercise in Special Patient Groups

29

Women and Exercise

KRISTA BORNSTEIN, BA, AND
LOIS JOVANOVIC, MD

Highlights

Exercise and Pregnancy

- Exercise may not be efficacious for the pregestational woman with type 1 diabetes who is planning a pregnancy or is currently pregnant.
- Exercise in the form of arm ergometry has been documented to be safe for a sedentary, unfit pregnant woman and may be a helpful adjunctive therapy to medical nutritional therapy for a woman with gestational diabetes.
- Postpartum, if glucose control is maintained, the woman with diabetes should be able to return to an exercise program similar to that of a woman without diabetes.

Amenorrhea and Exercise

- The adolescent girl with diabetes who is amenorrheic needs intensive therapy to ensure that she does not develop accelerated retinopathy when glucose control is achieved. If amenorrhea persists beyond the age of 16, treatment with estrogen therapy to protect the bones is advised.

Osteoporosis and Exercise

- Women with diabetes should be offered a weight-bearing exercise program along with hormonal replacement therapy when they reach menopause. In addition, smoking cessation programs are recommended to improve bone mass status. Insulin dosing for the exercising menopausal woman who is taking hormonal replacement therapy is complicated; thus, a team that is expert in insulin therapy is needed as part of the exercise program.

Association of Exercise and Menstrual Disorders in Women With Diabetes

An important measure of pubertal development is an abrupt increase in growth velocity. This growth spurt occurs at a specific bone age rather than at a specific chronological age.[1] The rapid growth phase decelerates at mid-puberty and ceases as bony epiphyseal fusion occurs. A later growth spurt and later sexual maturation are associated with mild chronic illness and undernutrition. Exercise, as well as undernutrition, may have a profound effect on the pituitary-gonadal axis: delayed release of gonadotropins and subsequent delay in ovarian maturation in adolescent girls. Numerous studies have shown that menarche occurs later in athletes than in nonathletes.[2–4] Gonadotropin and steroid hormone patterns in amenorrheic athletic women show no monthly phasic elevations and no follicular or luteal development.[2] Lack of effective gonadotropin stimulation is indicated by a largely quiescent and disorganized pattern of luteinizing hormone secretion,[3] most likely the result of decreased activity of the gonadotropin-releasing hormone pulse generator in the hypothalamus of the brain. One study clearly showed that exercise per se is a cause of menstrual irregularities.[5] Women with normal cycles become amenorrheic within 2 months of the initiation of a strenuous exercise program. Despite the effort by these investigators to control for caloric intake and weight, exercise could not be implicated as the only variable causing amenorrhea. Some proposed hypotheses as to the mechanism for exercise-associated amenorrhea include low body fat composition, hyperandrogenism, hyperprolactinemia, psychological and physical stress, and premature menopause.[6] Two of these hypotheses seem to be most likely. The hypothalamic gonadotropin-releasing hormone pulse generator may be inhibited by an increase in adrenal hormone. Consistent with this hypothesis, most studies show mildly elevated cortisol levels in amenorrheic athletes.[5] The second hypothesis, which is equally likely, is that there is a net energy drain. Caloric intake is not adequate to supply energy needs, and the amenorrhea is starvation-induced.[7]

The American Association for Pediatrics[8] has suggested that low-dose oral contraceptives (50 μg estrogen equivalent per day) for amenorrheic girls over the age of 16 be prescribed to protect against skeletal demineralization. In addition, improved nutritional programs are needed to replace the increased energy needs of puberty and the energy costs of strenuous exercise. In the case of an amenorrheic athletic girl with type 1 diabetes, dietary instruction is paramount as part of the exercise program, not only as treatment of the exercise-induced menstrual disorder, but also to maintain as near-normal blood glucose levels as is safe and feasible, because chronic hyperglycemia delays puberty and is associated with short stature. Normalization of blood glucose initiates a growth spurt in pubescent adolescent girls, and menarche follows soon thereafter.[9] One concern associated with rapid normalization of blood glucose in the population of adolescents with diabetes is the risk of malignant diabetic retinopathy, postulated to be due to exaggerated growth hormone levels that aggravate a predisposed retina.[10,11] Thus, the diabetes management program for an amenorrheic, adolescent girl with diabetes whose blood glucose levels are less than optimal should be carried out by a skilled health care team to improve glucose control without aggravating retinal status.

Osteoporosis and the Woman With Diabetes: Utility of an Exercise Program

Currently, it is fashionable to define osteoporosis as a critical reduction in bone mass to the point that fracture vulnerability increases. In this sense, osteoporosis is analogous to anemia, defined as a low red blood cell mass. However, this definition is not strictly accurate. Osteoporosis consists not only of a reduction in bone mass but also of important changes in trabecular structure, such as trabecular perforation and loss of connectivity.[12] Osteoporosis and the associated fracture risk are major public health problems, especially for older women. Peak bone mass is attained by the second decade. There is then a marked acceleration of bone loss in women after menopause, especially during the immediate perimenopausal years.[13] By age 65, with aging, bone mass falls to a critical point, increasing the risk of fracture. Men too lose bone mass. However, because men reach a higher peak mass, the age at which they reach a critical fracture level is well into the seventh and eighth decade of life (Fig. 29.1).

The relationship between physical activity and bone mass has been well studied.[14] These investigations clearly show that bone responds to the physical stress of exercise. The observation that resistance exercise provides a superior stimulus for bone carries important therapeutic implications because weight-bearing exercise has been traditionally prescribed to maintain skeletal integrity. Regular physical activity is likely to boost peak bone mass in young women, to slow the decline in bone mineral density in middle-aged women, and may increase bone mineral density in patients with established osteoporosis. Although serious resistance training in an elderly, frail population is not feasible,

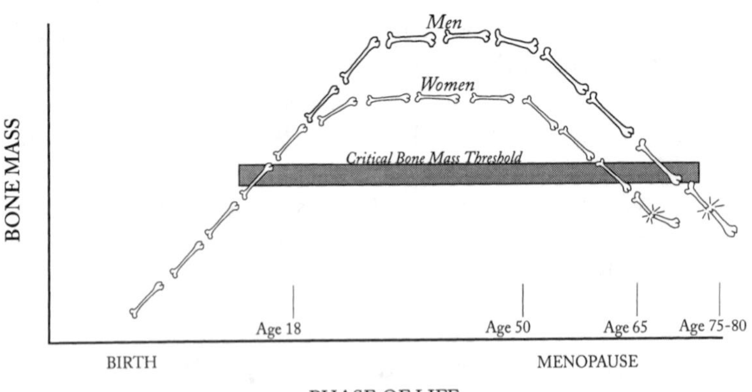

FIGURE 29.1 Schematic representation of bone mass accrual and bone mass loss to the point of critical levels that predispose to fracture. Men achieve a higher bone mass by early adulthood than women and thus have more reserves to forfeit before the critical level is achieved.

the benefits of high-intensity, progressive resistance training in some older subjects has been demonstrated. The reduction in risk of fracture in active women is highly significant compared with the relative risk in sedentary women (relative risk 0.76). Furthermore, active individuals have greater muscle mass and are stronger, which also decreases the risk of falling.[15,16] The adaptations in aging skeletal muscle to exercise training may prevent sarcopenia (muscle cell mass depletion), enhance the ease of carrying out the activities of daily living, and exert a beneficial effect on age-associated diseases to which diabetic women are predisposed: coronary artery disease, hypertension, osteoporosis, and obesity.[13,16,17] There has been an attempt to quantify the effectiveness of different exercises in increasing bone mass. Although these studies are indirect,[18] there appears to be the greatest bone response when women run or walk up and down steps. Non–weight-bearing exercises, such as cycling, produced relatively low bone responses.[19]

Although estradiol plays an important role in reproduction, this hormone can also exert physiological actions on a variety of nonreproductive tissues. Under certain conditions, estradiol can alter blood glucose levels by its effects on gluconeogenesis and glycogenolysis.[20] It can also alter plasma lipids by effects on their production and utilization. Thus, estrogens can reduce plasma cholesterol levels in postmenopausal women.[20] However, in some women with hypertriglyceridemia, estrogens may increase plasma triglycerides.

Many studies have shown that estrogens increase the bone mineral content in menopausal women.[21] Estrogen therapy also prevents bone loss in postmenopausal women who take it early in the postmenopausal period as well as later in life. If a woman stops taking estrogen after 7 years, however, when she reaches 75 years of age, bone density reveals only a minimal residual benefit.[22] Therefore, estrogen therapy should be continued for a lifetime. When a menopausal woman is advised about the benefits of hormonal replacement therapy, she should be told that there is a slight increase in the risk of cancer, which must be weighed in each case.[23,24] Also, women with either hypertension or cardiovascular disease need close monitoring if and when hormonal replacement therapy is started.

Poorly controlled diabetes is an independent risk factor for osteoporosis. In addition, end-stage kidney disease and associated secondary hyperparathyroidism also result in osteoporosis. Demineralization and pathological fractures are well-described complications of diabetes, along with Charcot joints and osteoarthropathies. These conditions result in disuse atrophy of the muscles and thus a higher risk of falls. Improvement in glycemic control has markedly decreased the prevalence of these problems.

Women with diabetes need exercise to maintain well-mineralized bones before menopause. Because estrogens have been reported to prevent bone loss and diminish the risk of cardiovascular disease, they are often recommended as part of the treatment of women with diabetes as long as they do not worsen glycemic control or markedly increase plasma triglycerides. Smoking decreases the effect of estrogen on the maintenance of bone density. Therefore, smoking cessation programs are mandatory for women with diabetes who are predisposed to osteoporosis. Postmenopausal women with diabetes not on hormonal replacement therapy will need to increase their insulin requirement ~20% when hormonal replacement therapy with estrogen and progesterone is started. Guidance from the health care team concerning the appropriate insulin adjustments is especially important. When an exercise program is combined with hormonal replacement therapy, the insulin regimen becomes especially challenging. Menopause also changes the diabetes program for women with type 2 diabetes. Unfortunately, because menopause is associated with a decrease in metabolic rate, fewer calories are needed to maintain body weight. If caloric intake is not reduced by at least 20% after menopause, weight gain is inevitable.[25] Adding exercise to the daily routine of a postmenopausal woman allows her to ingest more calories and avoid weight gain. An exercise program for women with type 2 diabetes not only prevents additional weight gain associated with menopause but also independently decreases insulin resistance. Thus, the hyperglycemia associated with the weight gain of menopause is minimized.

Exercise for the Pregestational Woman With Diabetes

The state of pregnancy may be considered a form of mild exercise: metabolic rate, minute ventilation, and respiratory exchange all increase to a level equal to mild to moderate exercise.[26] When counseling a woman with type 1 diabetes who is contemplating pregnancy, tight glucose control should be stressed. The risks of exercise to the pregnancy, including its sometimes negative impact on glucose control, should be emphasized. If exercise is undertaken in pregnancies complicated by diabetes,[27] insulin doses need constant surveillance to ensure the best possible control under the circumstances.[28] The utility of an exercise program as part of the glucose control protocol for the woman with pregestational diabetes, be it type 1 or type 2, is questionable. The paramount management goal for the best outcome of pregnancy is to achieve and maintain normoglycemia.[29] Exercise adds an additional variable that may make glucose control more difficult. The only study to investigate the use of exercise to manage type 1 diabetes in pregnancy used a walking program in women with type 1 diabetes[30] and found no improvement in after-dinner glucose levels. Exercise in the first trimester does not increase the risk of a spontaneous abortion. Women with type 1 diabetes have no increased risk of spontaneous abortion as long as their blood glucose levels are within 4 SDs of the mean of the levels of a pregnant woman without diabetes (equal to 7.12% in an assay standardized to the Diabetes Control and Complications Trial upper limits of normal of 6.01%). If the blood glucose levels of a woman with diabetes are above 4 SDs, then her risk of spontaneous abortion rises dramatically in direct relation to her degree of hyperglycemia.[31] Thus, exercise would only be a risk for a spontaneous abortion if the exercise program interfered with the maintenance of feasible near-normal glucose levels. If a woman with type 1 diabetes has vascular complications, then the recommendations for any type 1 diabetic patient who has vascular compromise should be followed, including restrictions of certain exercises for the patient with retinopathy. If a woman has preexisting or pregnancy-induced hypertension, then bed rest may be needed to manage blood pressure, and exercise cannot be performed. There are also obstetrical indications for bed rest during pregnancy that independently require that patients avoid exercise, such as vaginal bleeding due to placental previa or premature labor.

Exercise for the Woman With Gestational Diabetes

Gestational diabetes mellitus (GDM) is one form of diabetes occurring in pregnancy in which exercise may be a helpful adjunctive therapy.[32–34] Current management of GDM consists of medical nutritional therapy and careful monitoring of fasting and postprandial glucose levels. The goal of therapy is maintenance of euglycemia. When euglycemia is not achieved by diet alone, exercise can improve glucose intolerance and may obviate the need for insulin therapy.

The definition of GDM is diabetes with the onset or recognition in pregnancy.[35] GDM occurs in ~3.5% of all pregnancies and traditionally is diagnosed in someone who has had a history of diabetes in the family or has expressed macrosomia in previous pregnancies.[35] Women with GDM will mostly likely develop type 2 diabetes at a rate of ~10% per year. Therefore, it is likely that within 5 years, 50% of women who had GDM at one time will develop permanent diabetes.[36] This rate can be minimized if the patient begins an exercise program and a restrictive carbohydrate diet to reduce weight gain and increase insulin sensitivity, respectively.

Normal Pregnancy Compared With GDM

The normal pregnant woman will have a rise in insulin secretion throughout the pregnancy to meet the glucose needs of both mother and fetus during gestation. A normal pregnant woman will also produce anti-insulin hormones, which help to sustain an elevated postprandial glucose level so that the glucose will cross the placenta and the baby can use maternal glucose. In comparison, although insulin secretion increases in the patient with GDM (as a normal function of pregnancy), her blood glucose remains high because she is insulin-insensitive (Fig. 29.2). Over time, the pancreas will not be able to produce enough insulin to match gestational glucose needs (Fig. 29.3). Anti-insulin hormones (Table 29.1) produced during pregnancy further complicate GDM because these women have reduced insulin sensitivity and cannot use the glucose in their blood, which can lead to fetal weight gain (or macrosomia) and a number of other health risks for the baby.

Risks of GDM

GDM puts mother and child at risk for a number of related complications.[37] Also, the β-cell function in the pancreas becomes greatly diminished, resulting in glucose intolerance.[36] If untreated, GDM can lead to neonatal respiratory distress syndrome, hyperinsulinemia, hypoglycemia, and macrosomia. Macrosomia is the most common risk factor to the fetus.[36] A child's large birth weight contributes to a number

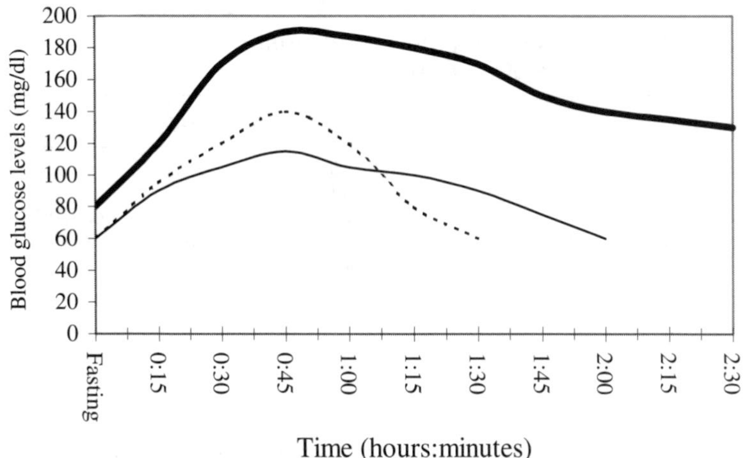

FIGURE 29.2 Comparison of blood glucose levels over time in nonpregnant women, normal pregnant women, and women with GDM. The dotted line represents nonpregnant women, the thin solid line represents normal pregnant women, and the thick solid line represents women with GDM.

of complications, the worst being birth trauma, possibly leading to fetal mortality. Macrosomia is associated with neonatal hyperinsulinemia, usually associated with maternal postprandial hyperglycemia.[36] Most cases of GDM occur in the last months of pregnancy. However, if a women has GDM before the eighth gestational week (the point at which organogenesis is complete) and it is not detected, high blood glucose

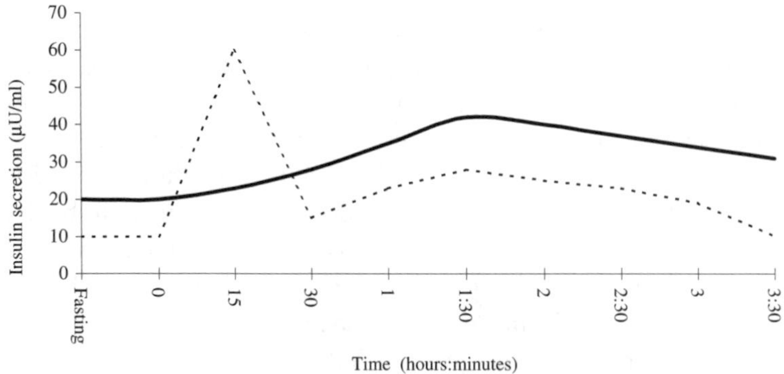

FIGURE 29.3 Comparison of meal-related insulin secretion over time in normal pregnant women and women with GDM. The dotted line represents normal pregnant women, and the solid line represents women with GDM.

TABLE 29.1 Diabetogenic Factors Related to Mother and Fetus

Mother	Fetus
Increased food consumption	Insulinase in the placenta
Increased weight gain	Anti-insulin hormones
Decreased exercise	■ Human chorionic gonadotropin (hCG)
Increased insulin requirement	■ 17-Hydroxy-progesterone (17-OHP)
Increased creatinine clearance	■ Estradiol (E_2)
Anti-insulin hormones	
■ Prolactin (PRL)	
■ Cortisol	

levels may have already begun to cause health risks to the mother and child. Risk of fetal malformations increase by 23% if the mother's hyperglycemia is >4 SDs above the mean of the normal population (>7.12% in an assay of HbA_{1c} standardized to the Diabetes Control and Complications Trial).[38]

Treatments for GDM

Diet can be an important factor in controlling GDM. Low carbohydrate intake is the first line of treatment for postprandial hyperglycemia. A recommended diet consists of 24–30 calories per kilogram of the present weight per day, of which 40% comes from carbohydrate.[36] A woman needs 24–25 kcal/kg/24 h during the first 8–10 weeks of gestation. After 10 weeks, she needs 30 kcal/kg/24 h of her present pregnant weight. Women who are greater than 120% over their ideal weight should eat ≤24 kcal/kg/24 h the entire pregnancy.[38] If diet proves insufficient in controlling blood glucose levels, before insulin is prescribed, exercise is recommended.[38] Exercise increases the rate at which meal-related glucose is taken into the body and may prove to be the perfect solution in preventing many risk factors, including macrosomia, that women with GDM face during pregnancy. Many health professionals prescribe insulin in conjunction with diet for GDM. Insulin therapy reduces hyperglycemia but may not correct the fundamental problem, which may involve hyperinsulinemia from peripheral insulin resistance.[39] A treatment plan, that reduces blood glucose and reduces peripheral insulin resistance, such as exercise, would be preferable for women with GDM. If diet and exercise have been prescribed and are still not sufficient in achieving euglycemia, then insulin therapy is recommended.[38]

Historical Problems With Starting Exercise Programs During Pregnancy

Exercise may prove to be a pleasant and productive alternative to insulin treatment; however, the literature has not always supported exercise during pregnancy. Several studies have found that premature labor and bradycardia were induced after exercise.[40–43] Initially, these studies raised concerns about maternal exercise during pregnancy. Women who develop GDM tend to be obese and sedentary, which complicates the risks involved with starting an exercise program during pregnancy. Artal et al.[44] studied the effect of maternal exercise on the fetus. They found that bradycardia occurred in three fetuses out of sixteen. A study by Collings and Curet[45] reported that fetal heart rate increased after maternal exercise. Tradeway and Young[46] found that maternal exercise decreases glucose uptake in the fetus.

However, the techniques used to assess fetal welfare have been crude and difficult to use while the mother is exercising.[39] In addition, ethics committees have placed restrictions on strenuous exercise during pregnancy, limiting investigators from testing exercise limits for pregnant mothers.[39] If exercise becomes the treatment of choice in lowering blood glucose levels, it would be imperative to choose the type and duration of exercise that does not cause sustained increase fetal heart rate, uterine activity, decreased fetal glucose uptake, or macrosomia.

Safety First

Recently, much attention has been given to the topic of exercise during pregnancy, and most of the literature shows that moderate-intensity exercise may actually be safe for the fetus and the mother.[36–39,47] Before 1985, sedentary, overweight women, including many women with GDM, were advised not to start an exercise program while pregnant. In 1985, the Second International Workshop-Conference on Gestational Diabetes Mellitus[48] sanctioned the concept that women who previously were using an exercise program could continue their program in pregnancy. They recommended that before beginning an exercise program, pregnant women should be screened with a physical examination and complete history. Health care providers should review their patient's type of diabetes, diabetic control, gestational age, chronological age, and long-term complications of diabetes to help determine the type and intensity of exercise that would most benefit mother and child. In 1991, the Third International Workshop-Conference on Gestational Diabetes Mellitus approved that women could start a moderate-intensity exercise program during pregnancy.[36] Subsequent studies have been organized to show the degree of exercise and the type of exercise that offer the best results for women with GDM.[49–52]

One case report followed a nondiabetic marathon runner with a twin pregnancy. The 33-year-old subject ran ~107 ± 19 km/week during her pregnancy. She delivered at 36 weeks by cesarean section. Both children were healthy, and the mother resumed her exercise program 8 days after delivery.[53] It is crucial to note that this woman did not begin marathon training during her pregnancy but had been training for some time before conception. Although she did not have diabetes, her data, along with research on diabetic subjects in gravidas, show that equal-intensity exercise programs preterm and during the first term of pregnancy is generally safe.

Veille[54] studied the prevalence of uterine contractions before and after exercise in women during the last 8 weeks of pregnancy. The subjects used either walking on an indoor track or riding a bicycle ergometer. Whereas neither fetal heart rate nor uterine activity was monitored during the 30-min exercise sessions, the researchers found no effect on fetal heart rate before or after exercise.[38]

As will be discussed in more detail later, Bung et al.[33] studied 17 patients with GDM who participated in an exercise program and found that there was no difference in maternal and fetal complications between the study and control groups. They concluded that a moderate-intensity exercise program is both safe for the fetus and effective in improving glucose tolerance in the mother. A follow-up study[47] tested the effects of moderate and strenuous exercise on fetal heart rate, long-term maternal complications, and fetal morbidity. The investigators found that in the absence of significant fetal heart rate changes and uterine activity, regular exercise was safe for the fetus. Assuming that moderate-intensity exercise is safe for the fetus, we can consider the question of whether exercise helps to lower blood glucose levels in gestational diabetic mothers.

Exercise and Blood Glucose

Studies indicate that exercise reduces the risk of hyperglycemia by increasing glucose uptake in the muscle.[55,56] Carpenter[57] pointed out that acute exertion, as opposed to chronic exertion, aids in increasing glucose uptake in the muscle to as much as 40 times its normal rate while exercising and that it also reduces insulin release in the pancreas, which increases the effects of exercise to stimulate lipolysis, glycogenolysis, and gluconeogenesis.[57] Individuals who exercise display improved insulin responses and glucose tolerance up to 40 h past the time they last exercised.[56] This study also demonstrated that sedentary individuals increased their glucose tolerance up to 14 h after a single exercise session. It appears that insulin-mediated glucose uptake is more significant in obese, sedentary subjects after exercising than in fit subjects.

Types of Exercise

Research suggests that exercise lowers blood glucose levels and decreases the need for insulin during pregnancy in women with diabetes.[49,58] Most research, however, is unclear as to which types of exercise are the most beneficial to mother and fetus. Bevier et al.[39] planned a study to test the effect of five different types of exercises on fetal distress, low birth weight, maternal hypertension, and uterine contractions. The investigators recruited fit pregnant women to test the effects of a standard bicycle, a recumbent bicycle, the walking treadmill, a rowing ergometer, and the upper arm ergometer on the parameters mentioned above. The standard bicycle proved to be the most strenuous on the mother and fetus, causing uterine contractions in 50% of the 25 sessions. The recumbent bicycle, on the other hand, did not cause uterine contractions but did produce hypotension in the mother. The walking treadmill was safe until the pace was increased to a jog, at which point 40% of the women experienced contractions. The rowing ergometer was relatively safe if the seat was secured and the arms did most of the work. Uterine contractions were detected in only 10% of the participants who used the rowing ergometer. The safest form of exercise, however, was the arm ergometer, associated with no uterine contractions or maternal hypotension with no fetal heart rate changes. The maternal heart rate was targeted to a pulse rate using the following algorithm: $(220 - \text{age}) \times (70\%\ VO_{2max})$. The researchers concluded that the safest forms of exercise are those that do not put stress on the trunk of the body but use the upper-body muscles.

Subsequently, Jovanovic-Peterson et al.[49] tested the use of arm ergometry as a means of increasing glucose tolerance in gestational diabetic women. In this 1989 study, 20 gestational diabetic women were split into two categories to test the effect of exercise on unfit women. Of the women, 10 were put on diets, and the other 10 were put on diets and an arm ergometry exercise program for 6 weeks. All 20 test subjects improved their glucose tolerance, yet the women put on the exercise and diet program showed a markedly greater decrease in blood glucose level compared with those who were on diet alone. The researchers also found that whereas exercising women had a decrease in their need for insulin, they increased the need for glucose. Birth outcomes were comparable for both groups.

Bung et al.[33] executed a similar study in 1991 with 41 gestational diabetic women. Of the women, 17 completed a bicycle training curriculum for roughly 1 h, three times a week. It was found that the women who were not on the exercise program required exogenous insulin, whereas the women who exercised did not. The two groups had comparable mean blood glucose levels throughout the study. The study reinforced the 1989 report of Jovanovic-Peterson et al.,[49] which showed that women with GDM could safely exercise during their term and inevitably increase insulin sensitivity. Bung et al.[33] found that when 41 gestational diabetic women were put on an exercise program and supervised three times a week, all subjects eliminated their exogenous insulin injections. These findings support the view that women with GDM can have significant benefit from supervised exercise. Bung et al. were able to show that the exercise and nonexercise groups demonstrated corresponding mean glucose values during their pregnancies.

A recent study by Poehlman et al.[51] examined the effect of aerobic endurance exercise (stationary bicycle) versus resistance training (weight lifting) in young, nonobese women. The study compared the insulin sensitivity in three groups of women: 14 women after endurance training, 17 women after resistance training, and 20 control subjects. The results indicated that both endurance and resistance training increased insulin sensitivity. Poehlman et al. also noted that women who performed endurance training augmented glucose disposal more than those who performed resistance training or the nonexercising control women. Although Poehlman et al. concluded that resistance training and endurance training used different mechanisms, both types of training increased glucose uptake in young, nonobese women. This study is good news for women with GDM who prefer resistance training to aerobic exercise.

Avery et al.[50] researched the effect of a moderate-intensity exercise program for gestational diabetic women. The exercise curriculum consisted of three or four 30-min exercise sessions a week (on a bicycle ergometer) for one group of GDM women, two of which were supervised by the investigator. The other group of GDM women did not exercise and served as control subjects. HbA_{1c} was tested, and subjects kept diaries on their fasting and 2-h after-meal blood glucose levels. The results showed that there was no difference between the control group and the exercised group in pre- and postprandial blood glucose, HbA_{1c}, and occurrence of newborn hypoglycemia. Avery et al. concluded that there was no decrease in blood glucose levels in the exercise group compared with the control group, but there was an increase in cardiorespiratory fitness in the exercise group.[50]

Avery et al.[50] asserts that exercise may acutely drop blood glucose levels as well as chronically lower blood glucose levels. The researchers go on to say that these outcomes have not been clearly confirmed in women with GDM. Avery et al. did not demonstrate significant differences in the exercise group in part because these women were not supervised for half of their exercise sessions per week. Although this method is a safe protocol, the women most likely did not keep up as strenuous of an exercise program at home as when supervised. The women with GDM in this study most likely experienced an acute drop in blood glucose but not prolonged euglycemia from light exercise. Avery et al. concluded that to experience a decrease in blood glucose levels, subjects might need more vigorous exercise over a longer period of time (Table 29.2).

What Studies Need to be Done

More research is needed to show which types of exercises are indeed safe and beneficial for pregnant women with GDM. Studies in the future need to examine the effects of different types of exercise on fetal physiology, maternal blood pressure, glucose tolerance, and fetal birth weight. Also, an algorithm for care should be developed that considers the age of the mother, the fitness of the mother before pregnancy,

TABLE 29.2 Comparison of the Effect of Exercise on Safety and Glucose Tolerance in Five Studies

Studies	Safe (for mother and fetus)	Unsafe (for mother and/or fetus)	Improved Glucose Tolerance
Bevier et al.[39] tested five types of exercises	Arm and rowing ergometers	Jogging on treadmill, recumbent bicycle, stationary bicycle	+
Jovanovic-Peterson et al.[49] tested arm ergometer on glucose tolerance	X		+
Bung et al.[33] tested bicycle training on glucose tolerance	X		+
Poehlman et al.[51] compared aerobic vs. resistance training	X		+
Avery et al.[50] tested moderate, partially supervised exercise	X		–

Plus sign (+) indicates improved glucose tolerance; minus sign (–) indicates no improvement in glucose tolerance. Recumbent and stationary bicycle, treadmill, and rower precipitated uterine contractions.

non-GDM complications, and screening techniques before a health care provider recommends the form of exercise to treat GDM. Women who are considering pregnancy may benefit from starting an exercise program before they are pregnant. They should also consider getting tested for GDM as soon as they learn they are pregnant to reduce the risks associated with hyperglycemia.

Postpartum Exercise Programs

Women should be encouraged to resume an exercise program as soon as they feel ready. Most women are able to exercise by 2 weeks after a vaginal delivery. After a cesarean delivery, it is recommended that 4–6 weeks pass before an exercise program is undertaken. As long as postpartum glucose levels are well controlled, women with diabetes recover at the same rate as women without diabetes. Thus, women with diabetes can safely return to an exercise program in the same time period as women without diabetes.[59]

References

1. Bullen BA, Skrinar GS, Beitins IZ, Von Mering G, Turnbull BA, MacArthur JW: Induction of menstrual disorders by strenuous exercise in untrained women. *N Engl J Med* 312:1349–53, 1985
2. Ding JH, Sheckter CB, Drinkwater BL, Soules MR, Bremner WJ, Shainholtz S, Southworth MB: High cortisol levels in exercise-associated amenorrhea. *Ann Intern Med* 108:530–34, 1988
3. Loucks AB, Mortola JF, Girton L, Yen SSC: Alterations in the hypothalamic-pituitary-ovarian and the hypothalamic-pituitary-adrenal axes in athletic women. *J Clin Endocrinol Metab* 68:402–11, 1989
4. Marcus R, Cann C, Madvig P: Menstrual function and bone mass in elite women distance runners: endocrine and metabolic features. *Ann Intern Med* 102:158–63, 1985
5. Louks AB, Vaitukaitis J, Cameron JL, Rogol AD, Skrinar G, Warren MP, Kendrick J, Limacher MC: The reproductive system and exercise in women. *Med Sci Sports Exerc* 24:S288–93, 1992
6. Warren MP: The effect of exercise on pubertal progression and reproductive function in girls. *J Clin Endocrinol Metab* 51:1150–57, 1980
7. Tanner JM, Davies SWD: Clinical longitudinal standards for height and height velocity for North American children. *J Pediatr* 107:317–29, 1985
8. Committee on Sports Medicine of the American Academy of Pediatrics: Amenorrhea in adolescent athletes. *Pediatrics* 84:394–95, 1989
9. Drash AL, Daneman D, Travis L: Progressive retinopathy with improved metabolic control in diabetic dwarfism (Mauriacís syndrome) (Abstract). *Diabetes* 29 (Suppl. 2):1A, 1980
10. Tamborlane WV, Puklin JE, Bergman M, Verdonk C, Rudolf MC, Felig P, Genel M, Sherwin R: Long-term improvement of metabolic control with the insulin pump does not reverse diabetic microangiopathy. *Diabetes Care* 5 (Suppl. 1):58–64, 1982
11. Marcus R, Drinkwater B, Dalsky G, Dufek J, Raab D, Slemenda C, Snow-Harter C: Osteoporosis and exercise in women. *Med Sci Sports Exerc* 24:5301–07, 1992
12. Snow-Harter C, Marcus R: Exercise, bone mineral density, and osteoporosis. In *Exercise and Sports Medicine Reviews.* Holloszy JO, Ed. Baltimore, MD, Williams & Wilkins, 1991, p. 606–18

13. Sorock GS, Bush TL, Golden AL, Fried LP, DeFronzo R: Increased insulin sensitivity and insulin binding to monocytes after physical training. *N Engl J Med* 301:1200–204, 1979
14. Talmage RV, Stinnett SS, Landwehr JT, Vincent LM, McCartney WH: Age-related loss of bone mineral density in non-athletic women. *Bone Miner* 1:115–25, 1986
15. Pocock NJ, Eisman J, Gwinn T: Muscle strength, physical fitness and weight but not age predict femoral neck bone mass. *J Bone Miner Res* 4:441–47, 1989
16. Tipton CM, Vailas AC, Bouchard C, Shephard RJ, Stephens T, Sutton H, McPherson B (Eds.): *Exercise, Fitness and Health: A Consensus of Current Knowledge.* Champaign, IL, Human Kinetics, 1990, p. 331–34
17. Dalsky GK, Stocke KS, Ehsani RG: Weight-bearing exercise training and lumbar bone mineral content in post-menopausal women. *Ann Intern Med* 108:824–28, 1988
18. Rodgers MA, Evans WJ: Changes in skeletal muscle with aging: effects of exercise training. *Exerc Sport Sci Rev* 21:65–102, 1993
19. Woodward MI, Cunningham JL: Skeletal accelerations measured during different exercises. *J Engineer Med* 2017:79–85, 1993
20. van der Mooren MJ, de Graaf J, Demacker PN, de Haan AF, Rolland R: Changes in the low density lipoprotein profile during 17 beta-estradiol-dydrogesterone therapy in post-menopausal women. *Metab Clin Exp* 43:799–802, 1994
21. Bunt JC: Metabolic actions of estradiol: significance for acute and chronic exercise responses. *Med Sci Sports Exerc* 22:286–90, 1990
22. Felson DT, Zhang Y, Hannan MT, Kiel DP, Wilson PWF, Anderson J: The effect of post-menopausal estrogen therapy on bone density in elderly women. *N Engl J Med* 329:1141–46, 1993
23. Baker VL, Leitman D, Jaffe RB: Selective estrogen receptor modulators in reproductive medicine and biology (Abstract). *Obstet Gynecol Surv* 55 (Suppl. 2):S21–47, 2000
24. Nanda K, Bastian LA, Hasselblad V, Simel DL: Hormone replacement therapy and the risk of colorectal cancer: a meta-analysis (Abstract). *Obstet Gynecol* 93:880–88, 1999
25. Reilly JJ, Lord A, Bunker VW, Prentice AM, Coward WA, Thomas AJ, Briggs RS: Energy balance in healthy elderly women. *Br J Nutr* 69:21–27, 1993

26. Bonen A, Campagna P, Gilchrist L, Young DC, Beresford P: Substrate and endocrine responses during exercise at selected stages of pregnancy. *J Appl Physiol* 73:134–42, 1992
27. Artal R: Exercise in gestational diabetes. In *Controversies in Diabetes and Pregnancy.* Jovanovic L, Ed. New York, Springer-Verlag, 1988, p. 101–11
28. Artal R, Wiswell RA, Drinkwater BL, St. John-Repovich WE: Exercise guidelines in pregnancy. In *Exercise in Pregnancy.* 2nd ed. Artal R, Wiswell RA, Drinkwater BL, Eds. Baltimore, MD, Williams & Wilkins, 1991, p. 87–99
29. Jovanovic L, Druzin M, Peterson CM: The effect of euglycemia on the outcome of pregnancy in insulin dependent diabetics as compared to normal controls. *Am J Med* 71:92–97, 1981
30. Hollingsworth DR, Moore TR: Postprandial walking exercise in pregnant insulin-dependent (type 1) diabetic women: reduction of plasma lipid levels but absence of a significant effect on glycemic control. *Am J Obstet Gynecol* 157:1359–63, 1987
31. Mills JL, Simpson JL, Driscoll SG, Jovanovic-Peterson L, Van Allen M, Aarons JH, Metzger BE, Bieber FR, Knopp RH, Holms LB, Peterson CM, Withiam-Wilson M, Brown Z, Ober C, Harley E, Macpherson TA, Duckles AE, Mueller-Heubach E, The National Institutes of Child Health and Human Development: Diabetes In Early Pregnancy Study: incidence of spontaneous abortion among normal women and insulin-dependent diabetic women whose pregnancies were identified within 21 days of conception. *N Engl J Med* 319:1617–23, 1988
32. Horton ES: Exercise in the treatment of NIDDM: applications for GDM? *Diabetes* 40 (Suppl. 2):175–78, 1991
33. Bung P, Artal R, Khodufuian N, Kjos S: Exercise in gestational diabetes: an optional therapeutic approach? *Diabetes* 40 (Suppl. 2): 182–85, 1991
34. Jovanovic-Peterson L, Peterson CM: Is exercise safe or useful for gestational diabetic women? *Diabetes* 40 (Suppl. 2):179–81, 1991
35. Hare JW: *Diabetes Complicating Pregnancy: The Joslin Clinic Method.* New York, Alan R. Liss, 1989
36. Jovanovic L: Role of diet and insulin treatment of diabetes in pregnancy. *Clin Obstet Gynecol* 43:46–55, 2000

37. Carpenter M: The role of exercise in pregnant women with diabetes mellitus. *Clin Obstet Gynecol* 43:56–64, 2000
38. Jovanovic L, Peterson C: Diabetes mellitus in women over the life phases and in pregnancy. In *Textbook of Women's Health.* Wallis LA, Kasper AS, Reader GG, Barbo DM, Brown W, Etingin OR, Nadelson CC, Eds. Philadelphia, Lippincott-Raven, 1998, p. 533–43
39. Bevier WC, Jovanovic-Peterson L, Peterson CM: Pancreatic disorders of pregnancy: diagnosis, management, and outcome of gestational diabetes. In *Endocrine Disorders of Pregnancy: Endocrine Clinics of North America.* Jovanovic-Peterson L, Peterson CM, Eds. Philadelphia, W.B. Saunders, 1995, p. 103–38
40. Lotgering FK, Gilbert RD, Longo LD: Exercise responses in pregnant sheep: oxygen consumption, uterine blood flow, and blood volume. *J Appl Physiol* 55:834–41, 1983
41. Clapp JF: Acute exercise stress in the pregnant ewe. *Am J Obstet Gynecol* 136:489–93, 1986
42. Pernoll ML, Metcalfe J, Paul M: Fetal cardiac response to maternal exercise. In *Fetal and Newborn Cardiovascular Physiology.* Vol. 2. Longo LD, Reneau DD, Eds. Philadelphia, Praeger, 1978, p. 12–23
43. Erkkola R: The physical work capacity of the expectant mother and its effect on pregnancy, labor, and the newborn. *Int J Gynecol Obstet* 14:153–59, 1976
44. Artal R, Romem Y, Paul RH, Wiswell R: Fetal bradycardia induced by maternal exercise (Abstract). *Lancet* ii:258–60, 1984
45. Collings C, Curet LB: Fetal heart rate response to maternal exercise. *Am J Obstet Gynecol* 151:498–501, 1985
46. Tradeway JL, Young JC: Decreased glucose uptake in the fetus after maternal exercise. *Med Sci Sports Exerc* 21:140–44, 1989
47. Bung P, Bung C, Artal R, Khodiguian N, Fallenstein F, Spatling L: Therapeutic exercise for insulin-requiring gestational diabetics: effects on the fetus: results of a randomized prospective longitudinal study (Abstract). *J Perinat Med* 21:125–37, 1993
48. Sandoval-Rodriguez T, Partida-Hernandez CG, Arreola-Ortiz F: Diabetes mellitus: exercise and pregnancy (Abstract). *Ginecol Obstet Mex* 65:478–81, 1997
49. Jovanovic-Peterson L, Durak EP, Peterson CM: Randomized trial of diet versus diet plus cardiovascular conditioning on glucose levels in gestational diabetes. *Am J Obstet Gynecol* 161: 415–19, 1989

50. Avery MD, Leon AS, Kopher RA: Effects of a partially home-based exercise program for women with gestational diabetes. *Obstet Gynecol* 89:10–15, 1997
51. Poehlman ET, Dvorak RV, DeNino WF, Brochu M, Ades PA: Effects of resistance training and endurance training on insulin sensitivity in nonobese, young women: a controlled randomized trial. *J Clin Endocrinol Metab* 85:2463–68, 2000
52. Jovanovic-Peterson L: Women and exercise. In *The Health Professional's Guide to Diabetes and Exercise.* Ruderman N, Devlin JT, Eds. Alexandria, VA, American Diabetes Association, 1995, p. 207–16
53. Davies B, Bailey DM, Budgett R, Sanderson DC, Griffin D: Intensive training during a twin pregnancy: a case report. *Int J Sports Med* 20:415–18, 1999
54. Veille JC: Maternal and fetal cardiovascular response to exercise during pregnancy. *Semin Perinatol* 20:250–62, 1996
55. Felig P, Wahren J: Role of insulin and glucagon in the regulation of hepatic glucose production during exercise. *Diabetes* 28 (Suppl. 1): 71–75, 1979
56. Mikines KJ, Sonne B, Farrell PA: Effect of physical exercise on sensitivity and responsiveness to insulin in humans. *Am J Physiol* 254:E248–59, 1988
57. Carpenter MW: The role of exercise in pregnant women with diabetes mellitus. *Clin Obstet Gynecol* 43:56–64, 2000
58. Bogardus C, Ravussin E, Robbins DC, Wolfe RR, Horton ES, Sims EA: Effects of physical training and diet therapy on carbohydrate metabolism in patients with glucose intolerance and non-insulin-dependent diabetes mellitus. *Diabetes* 33:311–18, 1984
59. American College of Obstetricians and Gynecologists: *Home Exercise Programs.* Washington, DC, American College of Obstetricians and Gynecologists, 1986

Krista Bornstein, BA, and Lois Jovanovic, MD, are from Sansum Medical Research Institute, Santa Barbara, CA.

30

Exercise and Gestational Diabetes

THOMAS A. BUCHANAN, MD

Highlights

- Exercise can play an important role in attaining and maintaining target levels of glycemia during pregnancy in women with gestational diabetes mellitus (GDM).
- Regular, light exercise (e.g., walking for 20–30 min daily) is a rational component of the initial management regimen regardless of maternal glycemia.
- Intensification of the exercise prescription (e.g., to 25–40 min of exercise at 50% of calculated maximal aerobic capacity three times per week) can help to achieve safe levels of glycemia when diet and light exercise fail to do so.
- Pregnancy-induced hypertension, preterm rupture of membranes, preterm labor in current or past pregnancies, incompetent cervix, persistent vaginal bleeding, or evidence for intrauterine growth retardation are contraindications to exercise during pregnancy.

- Women with a history of GDM are at high risk for developing diabetes, especially type 2 diabetes, after pregnancy.
- Insulin resistance appears to be an important component of and risk factor for progression to type 2 diabetes.
- Recommendations for behaviors, such as regular exercise, that reduce insulin resistance and help in attaining ideal body weight are an important part of postpartum management in women with GDM.

Overview

There are two major considerations for the care of women who develop gestational diabetes mellitus (GDM). The first is optimizing the growth and development of their babies during pregnancy. The second is minimizing the risk that the mother will develop diabetes after pregnancy. Exercise has a potential role in each setting.

What is GDM?

Simply stated, GDM is glucose intolerance that is first detected during pregnancy.[1] The diagnosis is based on a three-step process.[1] First, women are assessed for clinical characteristics that indicate some risk of GDM. Women with no clinical risk factors (for practical purposes, lean young white women with no personal or family history of diabetes) require no further testing or treatment. All other women have a relatively simple 50-g glucose challenge test. This test is usually performed between 24 and 28 weeks' gestation. It may be performed earlier in women with high-risk characteristics, such as obesity, glycosuria, a strong family history of diabetes, or a prior personal history of GDM. If the 50-g challenge test reveals little or no risk of GDM (i.e., a 1-h plasma glucose level <140 mg/dl), no further testing is indicated. Women with a higher 1-h glucose result have the final test, a 3-h oral glucose tolerance test, which either makes or excludes the diagnosis of GDM. This process identifies ~5–7% of pregnant women (higher in some ethnic groups) with the worst glucose tolerance during pregnancy. They have a spectrum of hyperglycemia ranging from slightly greater than normal to overt diabetes with fasting plasma glucose concentrations ≥126 mg/dl. The women impart risks of perinatal and long-term morbidities to their offspring that are loosely correlated to the degree of maternal hyperglycemia during gestation. The women themselves are at increased risk for developing diabetes when they are not pregnant. The discussion that follows pertains primarily to women who do not have overt fasting hyperglycemia. Other women should be managed as if they had preexisting diabetes before pregnancy; the role of exercise in that management is largely undefined.

Exercise and the Antepartum Management of GDM

GDM Antepartum: Significance for the Baby

Maternal hyperglycemia during the second and third trimesters, when most cases of GDM are diagnosed, increases the chances that infants will grow excessively in utero. The growth is most likely related to the delivery of excess calories from the mother, which both overnourish the fetus and stimulate excessive fetal insulin secretion. Without appropriate treatment, newborns of women with GDM tend to be larger and fatter than newborns of mothers without GDM. They also tend to have somewhat higher insulin concentrations when born. These changes that develop in utero may lead to birth trauma, a need for cesarean delivery, and, in the first 1–2 days of life, neonatal hypoglycemia. Neonatal jaundice and increased hematocrit may occur as well, although the mechanisms for those two complications are poorly understood. Two concepts underlie current approaches to the antepartum management of GDM: *1*) the risk of complications related to fetal overnutrition and excessive growth increase gradually and continuously with increasing maternal glycemia, and *2*) over the range of glycemia most often encountered in GDM, most infants will not manifest excessive growth or perinatal complications.[2,3] It is also important to note that overnutrition in utero may result in metabolic "imprinting" that leads to an increased risk of obesity and glucose intolerance during childhood and adolescence.[4,5] Those long-term risks have been correlated to the degree of fetal hyperinsulinism in one study.[5]

Rationale for Antepartum Exercise Therapy

The logical approach to prevention of complications of GDM in offspring is to normalize maternal glucose levels, either in all women or in those whose babies show signs of excessive growth. The effects of exercise on glucose metabolism are detailed elsewhere in this book (see Chapter 4). The main rationale for applying exercise to the antepartum treatment of GDM resides in the ability of exercise to lower circulating glucose concentrations. GDM appears to result from limited capacity of pancreatic β-cells to compensate for insulin resistance.[6] Theoretically, increasing insulin sensitivity with exercise could improve the balance between insulin secretion and sensitivity in women with GDM, thereby lowering maternal glucose levels and mitigating fetal overnutrition. In reality, the effects of chronic physical conditioning on insulin sensitivity in pregnancy have not been studied directly. Information that is available is limited to small reports of the effects of exercise on maternal glucose levels.

The Evidence: Effects of Exercise on Maternal Glycemia and Perinatal Outcomes

Three groups have reported the effects of chronic physical conditioning on maternal glucose levels in GDM. Jovanovic-Peterson et al.[7] studied 20 women with diet-treated GDM and fasting plasma glucose concentrations of 81–107 mg/dl. During the third trimester, half of the women did no structured exercise. The other half performed arm ergometry under the supervision of the researchers for 20 min/day, 3 days/week for 6 weeks. The intensity of the exercise was set at ~50% of maximal aerobic capacity, as estimated by heart rate [0.7 × (220 – age in years) beats per minute],[8] up to a maximum of 140 beats per minute. Fasting plasma glucose concentrations in the diet only group fell slightly but not significantly, from 97 to 88 mg/dl during the 6-week study. Fasting glucose in the exercising group fell significantly, from 101 to 70 mg/dl over 6 weeks. Weekly measurements revealed that the fall in fasting glucose in the exercising group did not begin until the third week of the exercise program but continued thereafter to week 6. Birth weights and gestational ages at delivery were not different in the two groups, and no cases of perinatal morbidity were reported. Thus, exercise had an effect to lower maternal glucose levels compared with diet therapy alone. However, there was no detectable effect on infant birth weights in this small study.

Bung et al.[9] studied 41 women with GDM whose fasting plasma glucose levels in the third trimester were in a range often used as an indication for insulin therapy (i.e., 105–130 mg/dl after initiation of diet therapy). Half of the women were placed on insulin therapy. The other half participated in a 4-week exercise program that consisted of recumbent bicycle ergometry at 50% of maximum aerobic capacity (assessed by heart rate) for 45 min (three 15-min sessions of exercise with 5-min rests in between), 3 days each week. Seventeen women in each treatment group completed the trial; none of the exercise group received insulin therapy. Means of fasting plasma glucose concentrations during the 4-week study were similar in the insulin and exercise groups (94 ± 5 vs. 89 ± 6 mg/dl, respectively). More importantly, the groups had similar birth weights and low rates of perinatal complications. Thus, treatment with a supervised exercise program produced outcomes that were comparable to treatment with insulin. However, the study was too small to have meaningful power to compare rates of perinatal morbidity, which overall are generally low in GDM.

Avery et al.[10] studied 31 women with diet-treated GDM, randomized to either no change in usual activities or three to four 30-min sessions of exercise per week at 70% of estimated maximal heart rate (two sessions per week supervised, others at home). There was no difference in self-monitored fasting or postprandial glucose concentrations between the groups, despite a documented training effect in the exercise group.

Thus, two of three studies demonstrated clear effects of supervised exercise programs to either lower maternal glucose levels compared with diet therapy alone or maintain maternal glucose in the same range achieved with insulin therapy. A third study found no effect of a mixture of supervised and unsupervised exercise on blood glucose levels. None of the studies was of sufficient size to provide meaningful information about the effects of exercise on perinatal outcomes. Finally, no studies have been conducted to assess the impact of antepartum exercise therapy on long-term rates of obesity or diabetes in the offspring of women with GDM.

Recommendations

Therapy for GDM is generally administered in two steps. Initially, all women are given instructions in nutritional self-management. A summary of approaches has been prepared by Fagen et al.[11] Once nutritional therapy is implemented, patients are evaluated to identify those in need of additional treatment to minimize the risk of perinatal complications. Two general approaches have been used for this second step. The more common approach is to have patients perform self-monitoring of blood glucose four to seven times each day. Women whose glucose levels are >90–95 mg/dl before meals or >120 mg/dl 2 h after meals are assigned additional therapy to lower their glucose concentrations below those thresholds.[1] An alternative approach[12] involves laboratory measurements of blood glucose levels at 1- to 2-week intervals, combined with measurement of the fetal abdominal circumference (AC) by ultrasound at ~30 weeks' gestation. Women who have very-high-risk glycemia (i.e., fasting plasma glucose >105 mg/dl) despite diet therapy are assigned to intensified therapy regardless of the fetal AC. Women who maintain fasting plasma glucose levels <105 mg/dl are assigned to intensified therapy only if the fetal AC is ≥70th percentile.

Intensification of therapy beyond nutritional management has generally consisted of exogenous insulin to lower maternal glucose levels in at-risk pregnancies. Those studies have generally revealed a beneficial effect of insulin therapy on perinatal outcomes.[13–15] Those studies have generally revealed a beneficial effect on perinatal outcome. Glyburide has recently been reported as a safe and effective alternative to insulin therapy.[16] The study by Bung et al.[9] suggests that a program of supervised aerobic exercise can be used to achieve maternal glycemic goals when dietary management fails to do so. Whether exercise will also optimize perinatal outcomes remains to be tested, although outcomes were good in that study. Larger studies are needed, particularly because perinatal morbidities are infrequent in GDM in general and they are not determined solely by maternal glucose levels.

Given the beneficial effects of exercise on maternal glycemia in at least two studies, it seems prudent to recommend some degree of regular physical activity as part of treatment for GDM. Recommendations for light exercise (e.g., walking for 20–30 min daily) can be made part of initial therapy, along with the initial dietary prescription. Although there are no clinical trials to evaluate the impact of this type of exercise, anecdotal experience (S.L. Kjos, unpublished data) suggests that it may lessen postprandial hyperglycemia, a risk factor for fetal macrosomia.[17,18] When patients participating in a glycemia-based management program fail to achieve target glucose levels with initial therapy, the addition of more intensive exercise may help to achieve the glycemic targets. Based on the studies of Jovanovic-Peterson et al.[7] and Bung et al.,[9] the exercise prescription should include 20–45 min of exercise at least 3 days/week at ~50% of calculated maximal aerobic capacity. The optimal form of intensified exercise has not been determined. The American College of Obstetricians and Gynecologists[19] does not prohibit any specific form of exercise during pregnancy other than activities that carry a risk of abdominal trauma. However, given that women with GDM are generally starting rather than continuing an exercise program during pregnancy, a focus on non–weight-bearing, low-impact activities such as recumbent bicycle[8] or arm ergometry[7] seems prudent. Based on the study of Jovanovic-Peterson et al.,[7] it may take 2–3 weeks before a detectable change in glycemia occurs once the intensified exercise has begun. Patients with the following conditions should not be considered candidates for an intensified exercise program: pregnancy-induced hypertension, preterm rupture of membranes, preterm labor (current or past pregnancies), incompetent cervix, persistent vaginal bleeding, or evidence of intrauterine growth retardation.[19]

Exercise and Postpartum Management of GDM

Rationale

Insulin resistance develops progressively during the second half of gestation,[20] reaching by the third trimester levels akin to those observed in people with type 2 diabetes.[21] Insulin secretion is increased in normal women to compensate for this insulin resistance.[22] Most studies indicate that insulin secretion is not increased appropriately in women who develop GDM.[20,22,23] These women develop insulin deficiency relative to the increased needs of pregnancy, resulting in hyperglycemia. A minority (2–15%) of women with GDM have antibodies to pancreatic antigens, suggesting evolving type 1 diabetes as a cause for β-cell dysfunction. The majority of patients do not have such antibodies. Studies in those women indicate that they not only have poor insulin secretion, they also have insulin resistance compared with women who have never had GDM.[24–26] Moreover, weight gain[27,28] or an additional pregnancy[27] increases the risk of type 2 diabetes after GDM. These findings suggest that a large proportion of women with GDM have as their defining metabolic abnormality a defect in pancreatic β-cell function that is caused or worsened by insulin resistance. Intervention to minimize insulin resistance is a logical approach to the postpartum management of such women. No strong rationale for this type of intervention exists in women with evidence of evolving type 1 diabetes.

The Evidence: Effects of Exercise on Risk of Diabetes

No controlled trials have been conducted to test the effectiveness of exercise in preventing or delaying the onset of diabetes after GDM. Nonetheless, two types of evidence suggest that exercise may be useful in this regard, particularly in women with evolving type 2 diabetes. Epidemiologic data from the Nurses Health Study[29] revealed that lean and obese women age 34–59 years who exercised vigorously at least once a week were significantly less likely to develop diabetes than women who did not exercise weekly. A subsequent analysis[30] revealed that protection from diabetes was closely associated with the total amount of energy expended rather than with the intensity of the physical activity. Exercise has also been linked epidemiologically to a reduced risk of GDM itself,[31] although the protective effect was limited to women with a prepregnancy BMI >30 kg/m^2. Two intervention studies have tested the effectiveness of exercise in the prevention of type 2 diabetes in men and women with impaired glucose tolerance. Women were not specifically selected or excluded on the basis of a history of GDM. In the Da Qing Study,[32] moderate-intensity physical activity (e.g., fast walking for 20–40 min/day) reduced the 6-year cumulative incidence of type 2 diabetes from 68% (control group) to 41%. A similar reduction was seen in a dietary intervention group and in a group receiving both interventions. In the Finnish Diabetes Prevention Study,[33] moderate-intensity exercise and dietary interventions were combined to reduce the 6-year incidence of type 2 diabetes by 58% compared with a group receiving no intervention. Thus, exercise has been associated with a reduced risk of diabetes in both observational and interventional studies, although not specifically in women with a history of GDM. Nonetheless, the similarities between the pathogenesis of type 2 diabetes after GDM and in other settings[3] suggests that exercise interventions will be useful in delaying or reducing the development of type 2 diabetes after GDM. Exercise has also been associated with a reduced risk of cardiovascular disease,[34] which may be important in women who have had GDM.[35]

Recommendations

The general approach to management of women with a history of GDM should include three components: education regarding behaviors that will reduce insulin resistance, regular follow-up visits to detect diabetes in its earliest stages should it develop, and contraception to allow a degree of glycemic control in any future pregnancy that will minimize the risk of birth defects in the baby. Regular physical activity is a logical, albeit unproven, part of the first component. Based on the information from the observational Nurses Health Study[29,30] and the interventional Da Qing[32] and Finnish[33] studies, prescription of brisk walking or other comparable exercise for 20–40 min each day is a reasonable approach. More prolonged or vigorous activities may further minimize the risk of diabetes in women who elect to pursue them. Exercise interventions should be combined with nutritional recommendations that are designed to obtain and maintain ideal body weight. Direct studies of specific types and intensities of exercise in women with prior GDM will be required to support any more specific recommendations.

Summary

GDM is a common condition among young women. There is indirect evidence to support the concept that programs of regular physical activity can improve pregnancy outcomes and the long-term health of the mother. However, rigorous and direct studies of exercise in women with GDM or a history thereof are lacking. In the absence of ideal evidence, recommendations for moderate-intensity physical activity as part of programs for both antepartum and postpartum GDM are logical and appear likely to have important health benefits.

References

1. Metzger BE, Coustan DM, the Organizing Committee: Summary and recommendations of the Fourth International Workshop-Conference on Gestational Diabetes Mellitus. *Diabetes Care* 21 (Suppl. 2):B161–67, 1998
2. Sermer M, Naylor CD, Gare DJ, Kenshole AB, Ritchie JWK, Farine D, Cohen HR, McArthur K, Holzapfel S, Biringer A, Chen E, Cadesky KI, Greenblatt EM, Leyland NA, Morris HS, Bloom JA, Abells YB: Impact of increasing carbohydrate intolerance on maternal fetal outcomes in 3637 women without gestational diabetes. *Am J Obstet Gynecol* 173:146–56, 1995
3. Magee MS, Walden CE, Benedetti TJ, Knopp RH: Influence of diagnostic criteria on the incidence of gestational diabetes and perinatal morbidity. *JAMA* 269:609–15, 1993
4. Pettitt DJ, Bennett PH, Knowler WC, Baird HR, Aleck KA: Gestational diabetes mellitus and impaired glucose tolerance during pregnancy: long-term effects on obesity and glucose tolerance in the offspring. *Diabetes* 34 (Suppl. 2):119–22, 1985
5. Silverman BL, Rizzo T, Green OC, Cho N, Winter RJ, Ogata ES, Richards GE, Metzger BE: Long-term prospective evaluation of offspring of diabetic mothers. *Diabetes* 40 (Suppl. 2):121–25, 1991
6. Buchanan TA, Catalano PM: The pathogenesis of gestational diabetes mellitus: implications for diabetes following pregnancy. *Diabetes Reviews* 3:584–601, 1995
7. Jovanovic-Peterson L, Durak E, Peterson CM: Randomized trial of diet versus diet plus cardiovascular conditioning on glucose levels in gestational diabetes. *Am J Obstet Gynecol* 161:415–19, 1989
8. Jovanovic L, Kessler A, Peterson CM: Human maternal and fetal response to graded exercise. *J Appl Physiol* 58:1719–22, 1985
9. Bung P, Artal R, Khodiguiab N, Kjos S: Exercise in gestational diabetes: an optional therapeutic approach? *Diabetes* 40 (Suppl. 2): 182–85, 1991
10. Avery MD, Leon AD, Kopher RA: Effects of a partially home-based exercise program for women with gestational diabetes. *Obstet Gynecol* 89:10–15, 1997
11. Fagen C, King DJ, Erick M: Nutritional management in women with gestational diabetes: a review by ADA's Diabetes Care and Education Dietetic Practice Group. *J Am Diet Assoc* 95:460–67, 1995

12. Buchanan TA, Kjos SL, Schaefer U, Peters RK, Xiang A, Byrne J, Berkowitz K, Montoro M: Utility of fetal measurements in the management of gestational diabetes. *Diabetes Care* 21 (Suppl. 2): B99–106, 1998
13. Langer O, Rodriguez DA, Xenakis MJX, McFarland MB, Berkus MD, Arredondo F: Intensified vs conventional management of gestational diabetes. *Am J Obstet Gynecol* 170:1036–47, 1994
14. Kitzmiller JL, Elixhauser A, Carr S, Major CA, DeVeciana M, Dang-Kilduff L, Weschler JM: Assessment of costs and benefits of management of gestational diabetes mellitus. *Diabetes Care* 21 (Suppl. 2):B123–130, 1998
15. Jovanovic-Peterson L, Bevier W, Peterson CM: The Santa Barbara County Health Care Services program: birth weight change concomitant with screening for and treatment of glucose-intolerance of pregnancy: a potential cost-effective intervention? *Am J Perinatol* 14:221–28, 1997
16. Langer O, Conway DL, Berkus MD, Xenakis EM, Gonzales O: A comparison of glyburide and insulin in women with gestational diabetes mellitus. *N Engl J Med* 343:1134–38, 2000
17. Jovanovic-Peterson L, Peterson C, Reed GF, Metzger BE, Mills JL, Knopp RH, Aarons JH, the National Institute of Child Health and Human Development-Diabetes in Early Pregnancy Study: Maternal postprandial glucose levels and infant birth weight: the Diabetes in Early Pregnancy Study. *Am J Obstet Gynecol* 164:103–11, 1991
18. Combs CA, Gunderson E, Kitzmiller JL, Gavin LA, Main EK: Relationship of fetal macrosomia to maternal postprandial glucose control during pregnancy. *Diabetes Care* 15:1251–57, 1992
19. American College of Obstetricians and Gynecologists: *Exercise During Pregnancy and the Postpartum Period.* ACOG Technical Bulletin 189. Washington, DC, American College of Obstetricians and Gynecologists, 1994
20. Catalano OM, Tzyzbir ED, Wolfe RR, Cales J, Roman NM, Amini SB, Sims EAH: Carbohydrate metabolism during pregnancy in control subjects and women with gestational diabetes. *Am J Physiol* 264:E60–67, 1993
21. Bergman RN: Toward a physiological understanding of glucose tolerance: minimal model approach. *Diabetes* 38:1512–28, 1989
22. Buchanan TA, Metzger BE, Freinkel N, Bergman RN: Insulin sensitivity and B-cell responsiveness to glucose during late pregnancy

in lean and moderately obese women with normal glucose tolerance or mild gestational diabetes. *Am J Obstet Gynecol* 162:1008–14, 1990

23. Fisher PM, Sutherland HW, Bewsher PD: The insulin response to glucose infusion in gestational diabetes. *Diabetologia* 19:10–14, 1980
24. Ward WK, Johnston CLW, Beard JC, Benedetti TJ, Halter JB, Porte D: Insulin resistance and impaired insulin secretion in subjects with a history of gestational diabetes mellitus. *Diabetes* 34:861–69, 1985
25. Ryan EA, Imes S, Liu D, McManus R, Finegood DT, Polonsky KS, Sturis J: Defects in insulin secretion and action in women with a history of gestational diabetes. *Diabetes* 44:506–12, 1995
26. Xiang AH, Peters RK, Trigo E, Kjos SL, Lee WP, Buchanan TA: Multiple metabolic defects during late pregnancy in women at high risk for type 2 diabetes. *Diabetes* 48:848–54, 1999
27. Metzger BE, Cho NH, Roston SM, Rodvany R: Prepregnancy weight and antepartum insulin secretion predict glucose tolerance five years after gestational diabetes mellitus. *Diabetes Care* 16:1598–1605, 1993
28. Peters RK, Kjos SL, Xiang A, Buchanan TA: Long-term diabetogenic effect of a single pregnancy in women with prior gestational diabetes mellitus. *Lancet* 347:227–30, 1996
29. Manson JE, Rimm EB, Stampfer MJ, Colditz GA, Willett WC, Krolewski AS, Rosner B, Hennekens CH, Speizer FE: Physical activity and incidence of non-insulin-dependent diabetes mellitus in women. *Lancet* 338:774–78, 1991
30. Hu FB, Sigal RJ, Rich-Edwards JW, Colditz GA, Solomon CG, Willett WC, Speizer FE, Manson JE: Walking compared with vigorous physical activity and risk of type 2 diabetes in women: a prospective study. *JAMA* 282:1433–39, 1999
31. Dye TD, Knox KL, Artal R, Wojtowycz MA: Physical activity, obesity and diabetes in pregnancy. *Am J Epidemiol* 146:961–65, 1997
32. Pan XR, Li GW, Hu YH, Wang JX, Yang WY, An ZX, Hu ZX, Lin J, Xiao JZ, Cao HB, Liu PA, Jiang XG, Jiang YY, Wang JP, Zheng H, Zhang H, Bennett PH, Howard BV: Effects of diet and exercise in preventing NIDDM in people with impaired glucose tolerance: the Da Qing IGT and Diabetes Study. *Diabetes Care* 20:537–44, 1997

33. Tuomilehto J, Lindstrom J, Eriksson JG, Valle TT, Hamalainen H, Ilanne-Parikka P, Keinanen-Kiukaanniemi S, Laakso M, Louheranta A, Rastas M, Salminen V, Uusitupa M: Prevention of type 2 diabetes mellitus by changes in lifestyle among subjects impaired glucose tolerance. *N Engl J Med* 344:1343–50, 2001
34. Manson JE, Hu FB, Rich-Edwards JW, Colditz GA, Stampfer MJ, Willett WC, Speizer FE, Henneken CH: A prospective study of walking as compared with vigorous exercise in the prevention of coronary heart disease in women. *N Engl J Med* 341:650–58, 1999
35. Mestman JH: Follow-up studies in women with gestational diabetes mellitus. In *Gestational Diabetes.* Weiss PAM, Coustan DR, Eds. New York, Springer-Verlag, 1988, p. 191–98

Thomas A. Buchanan, MD, is from the LAC+USC Medical Center and the University of Southern California Keck School of Medicine, Los Angeles, CA.

31

Children and Adolescents

MICHAEL C. RIDDELL, PhD,
AND ODED BAR-OR, MD

Highlights

- Children and adolescents with type 1 diabetes may have a number of health- and fitness-related impairments, including lowered physical working capacity, reduced maximal aerobic power, impaired skeletal muscle blood flow, and elevated perceived exertion, particularly if they are in poor metabolic control.

- Physical training can improve many of these impairments, and youth with diabetes should be encouraged to participate in regular physical activity.

- Children and adolescents with type 1 diabetes should delay participation in physical activity if blood glucose levels are <60 mg/dl (<3.5 mmol/l) or >270 mg/dl (>15.0 mmol/l) with detectable urine ketones. Exercise is also contraindicated in the event that a child or adolescent has not taken, or will not take, any insulin on the day of the activity.

- Blood glucose responses to exercise are highly individualized, and levels can either decrease (particularly when plasma insulin levels are elevated after subcutaneous injection) or increase (if plasma insulin levels are low or if the activity is of a particularly strenuous nature).
- Hypoglycemia frequently occurs up to 6–10 h after the cessation of exercise in children with type 1 diabetes, and extra complex carbohydrates may be necessary, particularly at bedtime, to prevent nocturnal hypoglycemia.

The management of physical activity in youth with diabetes is challenging for patients, parents, and health care providers. Education, preparation, and ultimately experience are necessary for the successful care of these individuals so that they may enjoy all the benefits of a physically active lifestyle. This chapter describes the physiological responses to exercise in children and adolescents with diabetes and the rationale for incorporating physical activity into a child's daily activities. In addition, strategies for maximizing the benefits, while reducing the potential risks, of exercise in this special patient population are described.

Type 1 Diabetes

Aerobic Fitness and Cardiorespiratory Responses to Exercise

Children and adolescents with type 1 diabetes may have a number of impaired fitness-related components and alterations in their cardiorespiratory responses to exercise. A majority of studies indicate that maximal aerobic power ($\dot{V}O_{2max}$)[1–6] and physical work capacity[1,7–10] are impaired in young people with type 1 diabetes, especially if they have fair to poor metabolic control. It is currently unclear, however, if the observed lower aerobic performance is a function of a reduced level of habitual activity,[2,10] a small body stature,[10,11] or an impairment in cardiorespiratory function. Inactivity likely contributes to decreased performance and lower fitness status because, when matched for age, body size, and habitual activity, adolescents with type 1 diabetes have similar cardiac function and $\dot{V}O_{2max}$ as control adolescents.[12–15]

Children with type 1 diabetes have been shown to have higher systolic blood pressure,[5,16] lower O_2 pulse ($\dot{V}O_2$/heart rate),[1] a thickening of capillary basal membrane in skeletal muscle,[17–19] and impairments in the regulation of skeletal muscle blood flow.[20–22] In addition, adolescent boys with type 1 diabetes who exercise at a similar relative intensity as control subjects have elevated ratings of perceived exertion[23] and impaired carbohydrate utilization[24] despite being well insulinized. Therefore, it is important to consider that cardiorespiratory, metabolic, and perceptual effort may be altered in individuals with diabetes, which may impair their exercise performance. However, it is conceivable that well-motivated youth with type 1 diabetes who are in good metabolic control can compete in physical activities on equal ground with their peers. In fact, individuals with type 1 diabetes can reach world-class excellence in sports.

Blood Glucose Responses to Acute Exercise

The blood glucose response to acute exercise in children and adolescents with type 1 diabetes depends on several factors, such as metabolic state before exercise; food intake; type, timing, and site of insulin injection; and the intensity and duration of the activity. Even if these variables are similar among children, it appears that the glycemic response has a high level of interindividual variation.[25,26] Fortunately, however, blood glucose changes during exercise have some degree of reproducibility for youth, as long as the exercise conditions and pre-exercise insulin dose and diet are consistent.[25] These observations indicate that individualized strategies to limit excursions in blood glucose levels caused by exercise are necessary and may be implemented with some predictability.

Hypoglycemia During and After Exercise

A majority of children and adolescents with type 1 diabetes who exercise for prolonged periods (i.e., >30 min) 1–3 h after insulin injection have a significant drop in blood glucose levels, which leads to hypoglycemia.[5,25–28] The cause of hypoglycemia during exercise appears to be a failure in hepatic glucose production to match the increased glucose utilization by the working muscles, likely as a result of relative hyperinsulinemia or a failure in counterregulation during exercise. Hypoglycemia is not restricted to those individuals who begin exercise with lower glycemic levels because there appears to be a strong positive correlation between the drop in glycemia and the pre-exercise value.[26] In addition, severe postexercise late-onset hypoglycemia (i.e., up to 36 h after exercise) may be particularly prevalent in active children with type 1 diabetes,[29–33] possibly because proper strategies are not adopted to replace muscle and liver glycogen stores. It is important to mention that based on the investigations cited above, it appears that the maximal risk of postexercise hypoglycemia is within 6–10 h after the cessation of exercise. Therefore, patients and parents should be particularly cautious if exercise is performed before bedtime. Strategies to limit the possibility of hypoglycemia caused by exercise are provided under GUIDELINES FOR MODIFICATIONS IN INSULIN AND CARBOHYDRATE INTAKE TO LIMIT HYPOGLYCEMIA.

Hyperglycemia During and After Exercise

As in adults with type 1 diabetes, youth with type 1 diabetes who exercise while deprived of insulin and who are producing ketone bodies may experience a further deterioration of metabolic control and exaggerated hyperglycemia.[34] In addition, a small portion of individuals may experience increases in blood glucose levels during and immediately after prolonged moderate-intensity exercise, even though insulin has been administered before the activity.[35] During high-intensity exercise (pulse rate >170 beats per minute), blood glucose levels may increase dramatically, even in well-insulinized children[36] and young adults[37] with type 1 diabetes, possibly because of exaggerated sympathetic adrenergic activity.

Thus, the major challenge for active youth with type 1 diabetes is the delicate balance of food, insulin, and physical activity to continuously limit blood glucose excursions caused by exercise. A well-organized plan to avoid and treat hypo- and hyperglycemia should be developed and conveyed to the child's or adolescent's coaches, teachers, friends, guardians, and siblings. Children and adolescents with type 1 diabetes should delay participation in physical activity if blood glucose levels are <60 mg/dl (<3.5 mmol/l) or >270 mg/dl (>15.0 mmol/l) with detectable urine ketones. In addition, if for any reason a child has not taken insulin on the day of the activity, then exercise is contraindicated. Hypoglycemia, followed by successful treatment, should not limit the child's ability to return to the activity.

Guidelines for Modifications in Insulin and Carbohydrate Intake to Limit Hypoglycemia

From the above discussion, it is evident that physical activity requires modifications in food intake and/or insulin administration, particularly in active children and adolescents who attempt to resume, or wish to adopt, an active lifestyle after diagnosis. A major difficulty exists in determining adjustments in either insulin or diet, particularly in the child whose activities are spontaneous and of an unpredictable nature. Below are guidelines for children and adolescents that can be used to develop strategies to prevent exercise-induced hypoglycemia.

In tightly controlled individuals, short-duration (i.e., <30 min), postprandial exercise often does not result in hypoglycemia.[38] In addition, if exercise is performed after an overnight fast, the risk of hypoglycemia would be minimal.[39] During these occasions, blood glucose monitoring should be encouraged and carbohydrate snacks made available in the event that hypoglycemia develops. Typically, it is activities that last >30 min that cause exercise-induced or postexercise late-onset episodes of hypoglycemia, likely because proper strategies have not been implemented. In addition, days that include prolonged bursts of physical activity (e.g., field day at school, basketball or field hockey tournament, or hiking) require major alterations in either insulin and/or carbohydrate intake to limit hypoglycemia.

Insulin

The increased use of intensive insulin therapy has provided individuals with the flexibility to make insulin dose adjustments, usually in the bolus insulin, for planned increases in physical activity. For anticipated prolonged activities (i.e., >30 min) of moderate-intensity exercise (pulse rate of 130–160 beats/min), a 50–100% reduction in the usual bolus insulin requirement is recommended if the activity occurs 1–3 h after a meal and after administration of regular short-acting insulin.[27] The exact reduction in insulin dosage for each individual may be learned from blood glucose measurements made after the insulin adjustments. Patients should be particularly cautioned to monitor blood glucose levels after insulin adjustments and have additional carbohydrates available. Hypoglycemia during postprandial exercise is a particular threat because plasma insulin levels may be two to three times higher than those in nondiabetic youth.[24] On the other hand, fasted exercise and exercise performed in a postabsorptive state (>3 h after insulin administration and meal) may be performed with no insulin modifications, but additional carbohydrate may be required.[40,41]

Although decreasing the amount of insulin injected before and after exercise may have an advantage over altering dietary intake (because it mimics the normal response to physical activities and may help to promote weight loss), it may have some subtle disadvantages. Often, activities are spontaneous and of an unpredictable duration and intensity, particularly in youth. Therefore, alterations in insulin administration in anticipation of these activities are particularly difficult. In addition, it may be unwise to reduce the amount of insulin injected before the activity because pre-exercise hyperglycemia may occur. Thus, increasing the amount of carbohydrate ingested before and during the activity is an appropriate alternative to insulin adjustments.

Carbohydrate

In general, increasing carbohydrate ingestion before, during, and/or after physical activity is commonly recommended to prevent hypoglycemia. However, to be able to adjust the carbohydrate intake according to the child's activities, an estimate should be made of the calories expended during the child's activity.[42] Matching carbohydrate ingestion with total carbohydrate utilization attenuates the drop in blood glucose during exercise in children and adolescents with type 1 diabetes.[26] The intermittent ingestion of carbohydrate beverages matched with total carbohydrate utilization clearly attenuates the drop in blood glucose during exercise in youth who begin exercise with either high or moderate pre-exercise blood glucose concentrations (Fig. 31.1).[26] Therefore, the amount of carbohydrate intake depends on the type, intensity, and duration of the activity, as well as the child's body mass. Table 31.1 lists the caloric equivalents of common activities, each performed for 10 min. The table is subdivided into body mass groups to show how many calories a given activity is worth

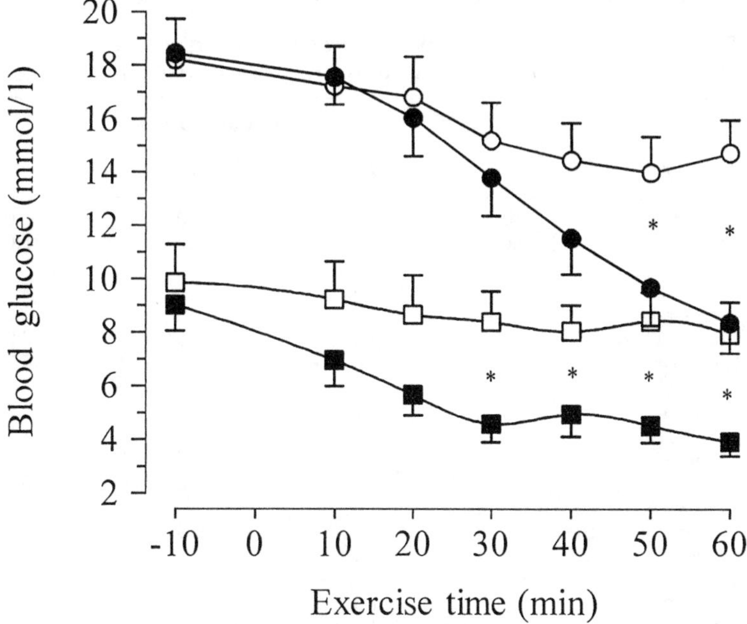

FIGURE 31.1 Blood glucose concentrations before, during, and immediately after 60 min of moderate-intensity exercise (55% $\dot{V}O_{2max}$) during either water ingestion (●, ■) or exogenous glucose ingestion (○, □) in children with type 1 diabetes. Exercise was performed ~90 min after breakfast and the usual insulin injection. Participants were subdivided into one of two classifications based on their pre-exercise blood glucose concentration: ≥15 mmol/l (○, ●) or <15 mmol/l (□, ■). Eight of the nine participants who began exercise with blood glucose ≥15 mmol/l completed 60 min of exercise in both trials; five of the eleven who began exercise with blood glucose <15 mmol/l completed 60 min of exercise with water ingestion compared with eight of eleven with glucose ingestion. *Water ingestion trial lower than glucose ingestion trial at <0.05.

for a particular child. From these data, tables of estimated "exercise exchanges" can be developed to estimate carbohydrate utilization for a variety of activities for children and adolescents who vary in body mass from 20 to 60 kg (Table 31.2). For a given activity, the child should ingest the recommended amount of carbohydrate 15–20 min before and every 15–20 min throughout the activity. The total amount of carbohydrate ingested should be as close as possible to the estimated carbohydrate expenditure for the given activity and body mass (Table 31.2). However, these tables are guidelines only, and individual blood glucose responses to exercise and carbohydrate intake vary

TABLE 31.1 Energy Expenditures (kcal/min) of Various Activities in Children of Various Body Masses

	Body Mass (kg)		
Activity	**20**	**40**	**60**
Basketball (game)	5.0	10.0	15.0
Cross-country skiing (leisure)	2.3	4.7	7.0
Cycling			
10 km/h	1.5	2.5	4.0
15 km/h	2.2	4.0	6.0
Figure skating	4.0	8.0	12.0
Ice hockey (ice time)	5.0	10.0	15.0
Running			
8 km/h	3.7	6.7	9.0
12 km/h	—	9.0	12.3
Snow shoeing	3.3	6.7	10.0
Soccer	3.7	7.2	10.7
Swimming			
30 m/min breast stroke	3.0	6.0	11.5
Tennis	2.5	4.3	6.3
Walking			
4 km/h	1.9	2.6	3.4
6 km/h	2.6	3.4	4.3

considerably among children and adolescents.[25,26] In addition, less carbohydrate may be consumed if individuals wish to allow a lower blood glucose toward euglycemic levels. The type of carbohydrate provided should be fast-acting (e.g., sports drink, candy, or juice) if it is consumed just before and during the activity. Indeed, carbohydrate beverages consisting of 6% carbohydrate may be useful in maintaining glycemic levels, providing additional fuel for utilization, and enhancing performance in healthy children and children with type 1 diabetes.[24,43] Alternatively, nutritionally complete fluids that contain fat and protein may be effective in preventing late-onset postexercise hypoglycemia if they are consumed during and immediately after the activity.[44]

Blood Glucose Monitoring

Frequent blood glucose monitoring is essential and should be encouraged to help reduce the risks of hypoglycemia and hyperglycemia

TABLE 31.2 Exercise Exchanges of 100 kcal (420 kJ) in Children of Various Body Masses

	Body Mass (kg)		
Activity	**20**	**40**	**60**
Basketball (game)	30	15	10
Cross-country skiing	40	20	15
Cycling			
10 km/h	65	40	25
15 km/h	45	25	15
Figure skating	25	15	10
Ice hockey (ice time)	20	10	5
Running			
8 km/h	25	15	10
12 km/h	—	10	10
Snow shoeing	30	15	10
Soccer	30	15	10
Swimming			
30 m/min breast stroke	55	25	15
Tennis	45	25	15
Walking			
4 km/h	60	40	30
6 km/h	40	30	25

Values shown are the estimated number of minutes that a certain activity should be sustained to be equivalent to one exercise exchange. Assuming that, on average, 60% of total energy is provided by carbohydrate, one exchange is equivalent to 60 kcal or 15 g carbohydrate.

during and after exercise. Although adolescents with type 1 diabetes may indicate that they are able to estimate their glucose concentrations, evidence indicates that glycemic awareness is particularly poor in these individuals.[45] Indeed, it appears that during exercise, many children tend to overestimate their blood glucose level when they are hypoglycemic and underestimate it when they are hyperglycemic (Fig. 31.2).

Benefits of Exercise

The benefits of exercise for the child or adolescent with type 1 diabetes are numerous. Insulin sensitivity is increased during and for several hours after an exercise session. In addition, the glycemic response to carbohydrate ingestion is blunted considerably both during and after

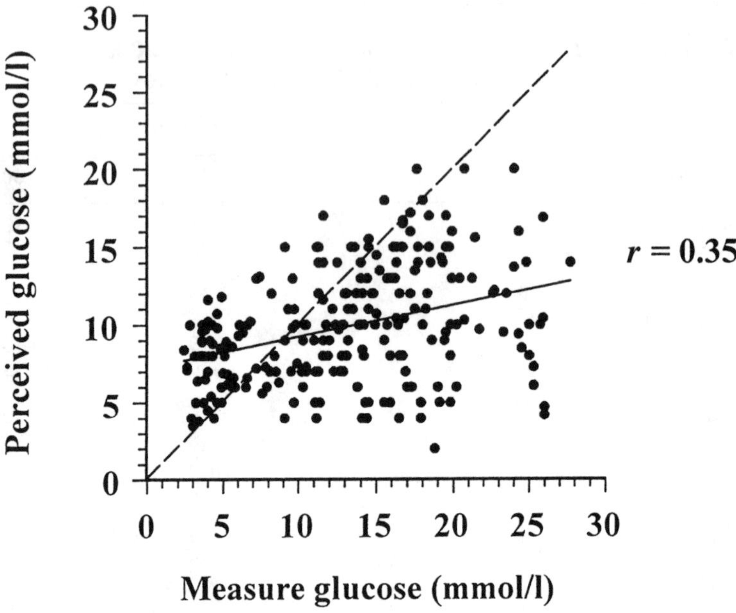

FIGURE 31.2 Measured versus perceived blood glucose levels during exercise in adolescents with type 1 diabetes: individual data. The dotted line is the line of identity. Subjects were asked to guess their blood glucose levels during exercise and were blinded to the actual values until the end of the experiment. Exercise consisted of 60 min of cycling at 55–60% of the individuals' predetermined $\dot{V}O_{2max}$.

physical activity. Regular physical activity may also decrease the insulin resistance that is commonly found in children and adolescents with type 1 diabetes, possibly by increasing glucose transport protein content. In addition to the beneficial effect on glucose disposal and insulin action, regular exercise may lower resting heart rate and blood pressure as well as maintain lean body mass and aid in weight reduction in children and adolescents both with and without type 1 diabetes.[41] As a further benefit, children and adolescents with type 1 diabetes may improve their self-esteem and self-confidence with regular participation in physical activities.

There appears to be a positive association between glycemic control and $\dot{V}O_{2max}$[6,9,46,47] or reported physical activity[48] in youth with type 1 diabetes. When subjects are stratified according to their participation, metabolic control is significantly better among youth with type 1 diabetes who frequently participate than among those who participate infrequently, regardless of the type of activity.[46] These relationships may indicate that glycemic control is better among children who are motivated to participate in any kind of program related to the treatment of their disease.

Despite the positive associations between $\dot{V}O_{2max}$ and glycemic control in the above cross-sectional studies, the influence of exercise training on metabolic control is inconsistent in clinical trials. Indeed, the influence of regular exercise on improving blood glucose control in children and adolescents with type 1 diabetes is almost equivocal, with some studies showing an improvement in blood glucose control[12,49,50] and others showing no change.[3,4,51,52] It would appear from these studies that training may decrease HbA_{1c} levels and fasting glycemia in some adolescents, particularly if they are in poor glycemic control (i.e., HbA_{1c} >10%) before the training period.[12,49] Adolescents and children who are already in good to fair metabolic control may not be expected to improve their blood glucose levels with training.[51,52] Nevertheless, physical training increases insulin sensitivity in these individuals and often reduces insulin requirements.[51] It is likely that carbohydrate ingestion to prevent or treat hypoglycemia may counter the beneficial effects of exercise on glycemic control in some individuals. Clearly, the goal of regular exercise should be to increase insulin sensitivity and improve the overall cardiovascular and psychological profile of the child with type 1 diabetes, regardless of any potential benefits to blood glucose management.

Adolescents with type 1 diabetes who undergo aerobic training appear to improve their cardiorespiratory endurance and muscle strength similar to those of nondiabetic control subjects.[3,46,53] In addition, seasonal diabetes camps that increase regular physical activities are beneficial in improving metabolic control, increasing fitness, and educating children in how to modify dietary intake or daily insulin dosage to prevent hypoglycemia.[54,55]

Epidemiologic evidence that regular physical activity increases longevity in individuals with type 1 diabetes[56] should be a powerful stimulus for health care providers to encourage youth with type 1 diabetes to participate in regular physical activity. In addition, there should be few restrictions placed on youth with diabetes who wish to participate in physical activities. Patients, guardians, and health care providers need to be aware, however, of the potential challenges that children and adolescents may face with exercise.

Dietary Requirements for the Active Child/Athlete With Type 1 Diabetes

Nutritional management of the young athlete with diabetes requires a delicate balance of diet, insulin, and exercise. The child with diabetes should eat a well-balanced diet of roughly 55% complex carbohydrate, 25% fat, and 20% protein (0.8 g/kg/day for maintenance or 1.2–1.5 g/kg/day for growth and training).[57] Ideally, the meal should be provided to the child 3 h before the activity to achieve euglycemia. The site of insulin injection should be distal to the exercising muscles, particularly if the insulin is administered up to 3 h before the time of competition. At any athletic event, the child should have and should be instructed to ingest extra carbohydrate in the form of fruit, bread, or candy, as well as fluid to prevent dehydration. Carbohydrate-containing sports beverages may also be useful in providing extra carbohydrate and fluid during the activity. The amount of carbohydrate supplement will vary according to body size and the intensity of the activity (Table 31.2). Most importantly, individuals should be encouraged to measure their blood glucose levels before, during (if possible), and after exercise to help guard against hypo- and hyperglycemia. This information not only helps to protect against hypoglycemia but also allows the individual to learn his or her own blood glucose response to exercise, which has been shown to have some degree of reproducibility.[25] Finally, the child and/or guardian should be particularly aware that hypoglycemia attributed to exercise may occur 6–10 h after the completion of exercise.[30,58] The above recommendations represent guidelines only, and individual cases clearly depend on the patient's exercise intensity, daily insulin requirement and sensitivity, degree of metabolic control, and pubertal development.

Exercise Prescription

With some degree of education and preparation, children and adolescents with type 1 diabetes can participate on equal ground with their peers. Recommended sports are those with predictable energy expenditures, such as running, cycling, and swimming.[33,57] Sports incorporating short, intense energy spurts with unpredictable energy expenditures are more difficult to standardize[57] but may be managed by frequent blood glucose measuring and a fine-tuning of the individual's insulin and dietary intake. Finally, it is essential that the child's or adolescent's coach (or supervisor) be aware of the medical condition and be educated on how to recognize and deal with hypoglycemia swiftly and effectively.

Type 2 Diabetes

Although the incidences of obesity, insulin resistance, and type 2 diabetes are on the rise in a number of adolescent populations,[59] surprisingly, there is a paucity of data in the literature that describe the benefits of regular physical activity and the metabolic responses to exercise in this patient group.

Clearly, inactivity, along with diet and heredity, contribute to obesity and to the etiology of type 2 diabetes in children and adolescents.[60] Indeed, physical inactivity is considered an independent risk factor for the development of type 2 diabetes in adolescents.[61] Given the recent increases in the prevalence of obesity among North American youth,[62,63] it should not be surprising if type 2 diabetes becomes a major pediatric problem in the coming years. There is certainly a tendency for overweight children to become overweight adults[64] because adiposity is a relatively stable characteristic throughout a life span.[65] This indicates that the recent surge of obesity in childhood will likely contribute to escalation in the percentage of adults who become obese and develop insulin resistance. In addition, there is some evidence that certain aspects of childhood participation in physical activity are predictive of adulthood activity levels,[66] which will likely translate to our inactive youth becoming inactive adults, further increasing the risk of a type 2 diabetes epidemic in our population. It is clear that both obesity and physical inactivity are independent risk factors for a variety of chronic diseases, including type 2 diabetes, and both are associated with considerable economic health care cost.[67,68] These observations strongly suggest that major interventions are required to curtail the decrease in physical activity patterns in youth, thereby helping limit the increased prevalence of obesity and type 2 diabetes in the North American population. Intervention programs that include physical activity as a treatment modality may be beneficial in improving body composition and blood glucose control and are currently under investigation.[69] It would seem prudent to promote, rather than to de-emphasize, regular physical education for youth in schools and to promote increased participation in after-school activities, perhaps through governmental intervention. Special attention should be given to early adolescents (e.g., ages 11–13 years), in which there is a precipitous reduction in spontaneous physical activity. This is particularly so among females.

Youth with type 2 diabetes may benefit more from participation in regular physical activity than their peers with type 1 diabetes. Indeed, exercise training, alone or combined with dietary changes and behavior modification, is known to decrease body weight,[70,71] fat percentage,[72] and resting blood pressure[70] in overweight children and adolescents. In addition, exercise training should increase insulin sensitivity, as has been shown in adults with type 2 diabetes.[73] Finally, and perhaps most importantly, regular exercise improves an overweight child's body image, self-esteem, and ability to socialize with his or her peers.[74,75]

Unless insulin therapy is used in the treatment of individuals with type 2 diabetes, acute exercise does not appear to cause exercise-induced or late exercise post-onset hypoglycemia in these individuals. In addition, because glucose transport into muscle occurs independent of insulin activation during exercise, physical activity should facilitate the oxidation of blood-borne glucose.

Conclusion

Regular physical activity should be considered an important component in the management of youth with diabetes. Children and adolescents with type 1 diabetes require daily management skills, which need to be learned and implemented successfully. Education and implementation of insulin administration and nutritional strategies as well as frequent blood glucose monitoring are crucial for successful management in these individuals. Youth with type 2 diabetes benefit considerably from regular exercise and should be encouraged to participate. Few limitations should be placed on active children with diabetes so that they may derive the social and physiological benefits of a physically active lifestyle.

References

1. Baraldi E, Monciotti C, Filippone M, Santuz P, Magagnin G, Zanconato S, Zacchello F: Gas exchange during exercise in diabetic children. *Pediatr Pulmonol* 13:155–60, 1992
2. Baran D, Dorchy H: Physical fitness in diabetic adolescents. *Bull Eur Physiopathol Respir* 18:51–58, 1982

3. Larsson Y, Persson B, Sterky G, Thoren C: Functional adaptation to vigorous training and exercise in diabetic and nondiabetic adolescents. *J Appl Physiol* 19:629–35, 1964
4. Larsson YAA, Sterky GCG, Ekengren KEK, Möller TGHO: Physical fitness and the influence of training in diabetic adolescent girls. *Diabetes* 11:109–17, 1962
5. Persson B, Thoren C: Prolonged exercise in adolescent boys with juvenile diabetes mellitus: circulatory and metabolic responses in relation to perceived exertion. *Acta Paediatr Scand Suppl* 283: 62–69, 1980
6. Poortmans JR, Saerens P, Edelman R, Vertongen F, Dorchy H: Influence of the degree of metabolic control on physical fitness in type I diabetic adolescents. *Int J Sports Med* 7:232–35, 1986
7. Austin A, Warty V, Janosky J, Arslanian S: The relationship of physical fitness to lipid and lipoprotein(a) levels in adolescents with IDDM. *Diabetes Care* 16:421–25, 1993
8. Barkai L, Peja M, Vamosi I: Physical work capacity in diabetic children and adolescents with and without cardiovascular autonomic dysfunction. *Diabet Med* 13:254–58, 1996
9. Huttunen NP, Kaar ML, Knip M, Mustonen A, Puukka R, Akerblom HK: Physical fitness of children and adolescents with insulin-dependent diabetes mellitus. *Ann Clin Res* 16:1–5, 1984
10. Sterky G: Physical work capacity in diabetic schoolchildren. *Acta Paediatr Scand* 52:1–10, 1963
11. Draminsky PH, Korsgaard B, Deckert T, Nielsen E: Growth, body weight and insulin requirement in diabetic children. *Acta Paediatr Scand* 67:453–57, 1978
12. Dahl-Jorgensen K, Meen HD, Hanssen KF, Aagenaes O: The effect of exercise on diabetic control and hemoglobin A1 (HbA1) in children. *Acta Paediatr Scand Suppl* 283:53–56, 1980
13. Hagan RD, Marks JF, Warren PA: Physiologic responses of juvenile-onset diabetic boys to muscular work. *Diabetes* 28:355–65, 1979
14. Rowland TW, Martha PMJ, Reiter EO, Cunningham LN: The influence of diabetes mellitus on cardiovascular function in children and adolescents. *Int J Sports Med* 13:431–35, 1992
15. Rutenfranz J, Mocellin R, Bauer J, Herzig W: Studies on the physical working capacity of healthy and sick adolescents. II. The physical working capacity of children and adolescents with diabetes mellitus. *Z Kinderheilkd* 103:133–56, 1968

16. Nordgren H, Freyschuss U, Persson B: Blood pressure response to physical exercise in healthy adolescents and adolescents with insulin-dependent diabetes mellitus. *Clin Sci (Colch)* 86:425–32, 1994
17. Raskin P, Marks JF, Burns HJ, Plumer ME, Siperstein MD: Capillary basement membrane width in diabetic children. *Am J Med* 58:365–72, 1975
18. Raskin P, Pietri AO, Unger R, Shannon WAJ: The effect of diabetic control on the width of skeletal-muscle capillary basement membrane in patients with type I diabetes mellitus. *N Engl J Med* 309:1546–50, 1983
19. Sosenko JM, Miettinen OS, Williamson JR, Gabbay KH: Muscle capillary basement-membrane thickness and long-term glycemia in type I diabetes mellitus. *N Engl J Med* 311:694–98, 1984
20. Ewald U, Tuvemo T: Reduced vascular reactivity in diabetic children and its relation to diabetic control. *Acta Paediatr Scand* 74:77–84, 1985
21. Ewald U, Tuvemo T, Rooth G: Early reduction of vascular reactivity in diabetic children detected by transcutaneous oxygen electrode. *Lancet* i:1287–88, 1981
22. Kobbah M, Ewald U, Tuvemo T: Vascular reactivity during the first year of diabetes in children. *Acta Paediatr Scand Suppl* 320: 56–63, 1985
23. Riddell MC, Bar-Or O, Gerstein HC, Heigenhauser GJ: Perceived exertion with glucose ingestion in adolescent males with IDDM. *Med Sci Sports Exerc* 32:167–73, 2000
24. Riddell MC, Bar-Or O, Hollidge-Horvat M, Schwarcz HP, Heigenhauser GJ: Glucose ingestion and substrate utilization during exercise in boys with IDDM. *J Appl Physiol* 88:1239–46, 2000
25. McNiven-Temple MY, Bar-Or O, Riddell MC: The reliability and repeatability of the blood glucose response to prolonged exercise in adolescent boys with IDDM. *Diabetes Care* 18:326–32, 1995
26. Riddell MC, Bar-Or O, Ayub BV, Calvert RE, Heigenhauser GJF: Glucose ingestion matched with total carbohydrate utilization attenuates hypoglycemia during exercise in adolescents with IDDM. *Int J Sport Nutr* 9:24–34, 1999
27. Schiffrin A, Parikh S: Accommodating planned exercise in type I diabetic patients on intensive treatment. *Diabetes Care* 8:337–42, 1985
28. Sills IN, Cerny FJ: Responses to continuous and intermittent exercise in healthy and insulin-dependent diabetic children. *Med Sci Sports Exerc* 15:450–54, 1983

29. Aman J, Karlsson I, Wranne L: Symptomatic hypoglycaemia in childhood diabetes: a population-based questionnaire study. *Diabet Med* 6:257–61, 1989
30. Bell DS, Cutter G: Characteristics of severe hypoglycemia in the patient with insulin-dependent diabetes. *South Med J* 87: 616–20, 1994
31. MacDonald MJ: Postexercise late-onset hypoglycemia in insulin-dependent diabetic patients. *Diabetes Care* 10:584–88, 1987
32. Shehadeh N, Kassem J, Tchaban I, Ravid S, Shahar E, Naveh T, Etzioni A: High incidence of hypoglycemic episodes with neurologic manifestations in children with insulin dependent diabetes mellitus. *J Pediatr Endocrinol Metab* 11 (Suppl. 1):183–87, 1998
33. Tupola S, Rajantie J, Maenpaa J: Severe hypoglycaemia in children and adolescents during multiple-dose insulin therapy. *Diabet Med* 15:695–99, 1998
34. Dorchy H, Poortmans J: Sport and the diabetic child. *Sports Med* 7:248–62, 1989
35. Caron D, Poussier P, Marliss EB, Zinman B: The effect of postprandial exercise on meal-related glucose intolerance in insulin-dependent diabetic individuals. *Diabetes Care* 5:364–69, 1982
36. Yasar SA, Tulassay T, Madacsy L, Korner A, Szucs L, Nagy I, Szabo A, Miltenyi M: Sympathetic-adrenergic activity and acid-base regulation under acute physical stress in type I (insulin-dependent) diabetic children. *Horm Res* 42:110–15, 1994
37. Purdon C, Brousson M, Nyveen SL, Miles PD, Halter JB, Vranic M, Marliss EB: The roles of insulin and catecholamines in the glucoregulatory response during intense exercise and early recovery in insulin-dependent diabetic and control subjects. *J Clin Endocrinol Metab* 76:566–73, 1993
38. Trovati M, Carta Q, Cavalot F, Vitali S, Passarino G, Rocca G, Emanuelli G, Lenti G: Continuous subcutaneous insulin infusion and postprandial exercise in tightly controlled type I (insulin-dependent) diabetic patients. *Diabetes Care* 7:327–30, 1984
39. Ruegemer JJ, Squires RW, Marsh HM, Haymond MW, Cryer PE, Rizza RA, Miles JM: Differences between prebreakfast and late afternoon glycemic responses to exercise in IDDM patients. *Diabetes Care* 13:104–10, 1990
40. Nathan DM, Madnek SF, Delahanty L: Programming pre-exercise snacks to prevent post-exercise hypoglycemia in intensively treated insulin-dependent diabetics. *Ann Intern Med* 102:483–86, 1985

41. Schiffrin A, Parikh S, Marliss E, Desrosiers MM: Metabolic response to fasting exercise in adolescent insulin-dependent diabetic subjects treated with continuous subcutaneous insulin infusion and intensive conventional therapy. *Diabetes Care* 7:255–60, 1984
42. Bar-Or O: *Pediatric Sports Medicine for the Practitioner: From Physiologic Principles to Clinical Applications.* New York, Springer-Verlag, 1983
43. Riddell MC, Bar-Or O, Wilk B, Parolin ML, Heigenhauser GJF: Substrate utilization during exercise with glucose and glucose plus fructose ingestion in boys ages 10–14 years. *J Appl Physiol* 90: 903–11, 2001
44. Hernandez JM, Moccia T, Fluckey JD, Ulbrecht JS, Farrell PA: Fluid snacks to help persons with type 1 diabetes avoid late onset postexercise hypoglycemia. *Med Sci Sports Exerc* 32:904–10, 2000
45. Nurick MA, Johnson SB: Enhancing blood glucose awareness in adolescents and young adults with IDDM. *Diabetes Care* 14:1–7, 1991
46. Huttunen NP, Lankela SL, Knip M, Lautala P, Kaar ML, Laasonen K, Puukka R: Effect of once-a-week training program on physical fitness and metabolic control in children with IDDM. *Diabetes Care* 12:737–40, 1989
47. Ludvigsson J: Physical exercise in relation to degree of metabolic control in juvenile diabetics. *Acta Paediatr Scand Suppl* 283:45–49, 1980
48. Sackey AH, Jefferson IG: Physical activity and glycaemic control in children with diabetes mellitus. *Diabet Med* 13:789–93, 1996
49. Campaigne BN, Gilliam TB, Spencer ML, Lampman RM, Schork MA: Effects of a physical activity program on metabolic control and cardiovascular fitness in children with insulin-dependent diabetes mellitus. *Diabetes Care* 7:57–62, 1984
50. Stratton R, Wilson DP, Endres RK, Goldstein DE: Improved glycemic control after supervised 8-wk exercise program in insulin-dependent diabetic adolescents. *Diabetes Care* 10:589–93, 1987
51. Landt KW, Campaigne BN, James FW, Sperling MA: Effects of exercise training on insulin sensitivity in adolescents with type I diabetes. *Diabetes Care* 8:461–65, 1985
52. Rowland TW, Swadba LA, Biggs DE, Burke EJ, Reiter EO: Glycemic control with physical training in insulin-dependent diabetes mellitus. *Am J Dis Child* 139:307–10, 1985

53. Mosher PE, Nash MS, Perry AC, LaPerriere AR, Goldberg RB: Aerobic circuit exercise training: effect on adolescents with well-controlled insulin-dependent diabetes mellitus. *Arch Phys Med Rehabil* 79:652–57, 1998
54. Akerblom HK, Koivukangas T, Ilkka J: Experiences from a winter camp for teenage diabetics. *Acta Paediatr Scand Suppl* 283:50–52, 1980
55. Braatvedt GD, Mildenhall L, Patten C, Harris G: Insulin requirements and metabolic control in children with diabetes mellitus attending a summer camp. *Diabet Med* 14:258–61, 1997
56. Moy CS, Songer TJ, LaPorte RE, Dorman JS, Kriska AM, Orchard TJ, Becker DJ, Drash AL: Insulin-dependent diabetes mellitus, physical activity, and death. *Am J Epidemiol* 137:74–81, 1993
57. Hough DO: Diabetes mellitus in sports. *Med Clin North Am* 78:423–37, 1994
58. Campaigne BN, Wallberg-Henriksson H, Gunnarsson R: Glucose and insulin responses in relation to insulin dose and caloric intake 12 h after acute physical exercise in men with IDDM. *Diabetes Care* 10:716–21, 1987
59. Fagot-Campagna A, Burrows NR, Williamson DF: The public health epidemiology of type 2 diabetes in children and adolescents: a case study of American Indian adolescents in the Southwestern United States. *Clin Chim Acta* 286:81–95, 1999
60. Cook VV, Hurley JS: Prevention of type 2 diabetes in childhood. *Clin Pediatr (Phila)* 37:123–29, 1998
61. Pinhas-Hamiel O, Standiford D, Hamiel D, Dolan LM, Cohen R, Zeitler PS: The type 2 family: a setting for development and treatment of adolescent type 2 diabetes mellitus. *Arch Pediatr Adolesc Med* 153:1063–67, 1999
62. Tremblay MS, Willms JD: Secular trends in the body mass index of Canadian children. *Can Med Assoc J* 163:1429–33, 2000
63. Troiano RP, Flegal KM, Kuczmarski RJ, Campbell SM, Johnson CL: Overweight prevalence and trends for children and adolescents: The National Health and Nutrition Examination Surveys, 1963 to 1991. *Arch Pediatr Adolesc Med* 149:1085–91, 1995
64. Whitaker RC, Wright JA, Pepe MS, Seidel KD, Dietz WH: Predicting obesity in young adulthood from childhood and parental obesity. *N Engl J Med* 337:869–73, 1997

65. Katzmarzyk PT, Perusse L, Malina RM, Bouchard C: Seven-year stability of indicators of obesity and adipose tissue distribution in the Canadian population. *Am J Clin Nutr* 69:1123–29, 1999
66. Taylor WC, Blair SN, Cummings SS, Wun CC, Malina RM: Childhood and adolescent physical activity patterns and adult physical activity. *Med Sci Sports Exerc* 31:118–23, 1999
67. Birmingham CL, Muller JL, Palepu A, Spinelli JJ, Anis AH: The cost of obesity in Canada. *Can Med Assoc J* 160:483–88, 1999
68. Katzmarzyk PT, Gledhill N, Shephard RJ: The economic burden of physical inactivity in Canada. *Can Med Assoc J* 163:1435–40, 2000
69. Macaulay AC, Paradis G, Potvin L, Cross EJ, Saad-Haddad C, McComber A, Desrosiers S, Kirby R, Montour LT, Lamping DL, Leduc N, Rivard M: The Kahnawake Schools Diabetes Prevention Project: intervention, evaluation, and baseline results of a diabetes primary prevention program with a native community in Canada. *Prev Med* 26:779–90, 1997
70. Brownell KD, Kelman JH, Stunkard AJ: Treatment of obese children with and without their mothers: changes in weight and blood pressure. *Pediatrics* 71:515–23, 1983
71. Epstein LH, Wing RR, Koeske R, Ossip D, Beck S: A comparison of lifestyle change and programmed aerobic exercise on weight reduction and fitness changes in obese children. *Behav Ther* 13: 651–65, 1982
72. Moody DL, Wilmore JH, Girandola RN, Royce JP: The effects of a jogging program on the body composition of normal and obese high school girls. *Med Sci Sports* 4:210–13, 1972
73. DeFronzo RA, Ferrannini E, Koivisto V: New concepts in the pathogenesis and treatment of noninsulin-dependent diabetes mellitus. *Am J Med* 74:52–81, 1983
74. Peckos PS, Spargo JA, Heald FP: Program and results of a camp for obese adolescent girls. *Postgrad Med* 27:527–33, 1960
75. Stanley EJ, Glaser HH, Levin DG, Adams PA, Coley IL: Overcoming obesity in adolescents: a description of a promising endeavor to improve management. *Clin Pediatr (Phila)* 9:29–36, 1970

Michael C. Riddell, PhD, is from York University, Toronto, Ontario, Canada. Oded Bar-Or, MD, is from McMaster University, Hamilton, Ontario, Canada.

32

Exercise and Aging

WILLIAM J. EVANS, PhD

Highlights

- The primary aspects of body composition that change with advancing age are decreased skeletal muscle mass, termed "sarcopenia," and increased body fatness.
- Sarcopenia results in muscle weakness, which has been associated with late-life disability and risk of falling among elderly people.
- Muscle weakness may limit activities of daily living in many older individuals. Therefore, strength training should be the primary recommendation for elderly people. Strength training has a number of positive benefits, including increased muscle strength and size, improved bone health, increased energy requirements, and increased levels of physical activity.
- Strength training is safe for almost all elderly people and has been demonstrated to be highly effective, even into the tenth decade of life.

- Relatively low-intensity aerobic exercise (~55% VO_{2max}) has been demonstrated to improve insulin action in older people.

Advancing age is associated with a remarkable number of changes in body composition. Reductions in lean body mass have been well characterized. This decreased lean body mass occurs primarily as a result of losses in skeletal muscle mass. This age-related loss in muscle mass has been termed "sarcopenia." Loss in muscle mass accounts for the age-associated decreases in basal metabolic rate, muscle strength, and activity levels, which in turn cause decreased energy requirements in the elderly. In sedentary individuals, the main determinant of energy expenditure is fat-free mass, which declines by ~15% between the third and eighth decade of life. It also appears that declining caloric needs are not matched by an appropriate decline in caloric intake, ultimately resulting in increased body fat content with advancing age. Increased body fatness and increased abdominal obesity are thought to be directly linked to the greatly increased incidence of type 2 diabetes among the elderly.

Sarcopenia is a direct cause of the age-related decrease in muscle strength. Frontera et al.[1] examined muscle strength and mass in 200 healthy 45- to 78-year-old men and women and concluded that muscle mass (not function) is the major determinant of the age- and sex-related differences in strength. This relationship was independent of muscle location (upper vs. lower extremities) and function (extension vs. flexion). Reduced muscle strength in the elderly is a major cause of increased prevalence of disability. Strength is defined as the amount of force produced by a muscle contraction; however, power is the product of force generation and speed of muscle contraction. Although many older individuals have lost strength, power may decline even more rapidly with advancing age. With advancing age and the low activity levels seen in the very old, muscle strength and power is a critical component of walking ability.[2] Bassey et al.[2] demonstrated that among frail nursing home residents, leg muscle power is more important than strength for performing daily activities such as stair climbing, rising from a chair, and walking. Older men and women who require the use of aids to perform these tasks have 42–54% less leg extensor power than those who could complete these tasks without assistance. The ability to rapidly generate force is a critical component of ambulation. Preservation of strength and prevention of sarcopenia, while important, may not result in a preservation in the ability to perform mobility-related activities of daily living. Indeed, muscle quality defined as the amount of force production per unit of muscle is decreased with advancing age,[3] and muscle power decreases to a greater extent than muscle strength.[4] Whereas sarcopenia has been demonstrated to be a predictor of disability in older people,[5] the strongest predictor of late-life mobility-related disability appears to be body fatness.[6–8] Although a number of studies have indicated that low body weight or weight loss is associated with an increase in the risk of hip fracture,[9–11] increased body weight and body fat have also recently been shown to increase the risk for a hip fracture in older white women.[12] This may be explained by the greatly reduced ability to generate power with increased amounts of body fat. Reduced muscle quality and decreased power production are also risk factors for hip fractures among older people.[13]

To what extent are these changes inevitable consequences of aging? Whereas it is difficult to determine the exact contribution of reduced levels of physical activity and biological aging, inactivity is an important contributor to sarcopenia and age-related body composition changes. Decreased testosterone levels in older men have been associated with sarcopenia,[14] increased body fatness, and increased waist-to-hip ratio.[15] However, physical activity does play a prominent role in age-related body compositional changes. By examining endurance-trained men, we saw that body fat stores and maximal aerobic capacity were not related to age, but rather were related to the total number of hours these men were exercising per week.[16] Even among sedentary individuals, energy spent in daily activities explains >75% of the variability in body fatness among young and older men.[17] These data and the results of other investigators indicate that levels of physical activity are important in determining energy expenditure and ultimately body fat accumulation.

Aerobic Exercise

Maximal aerobic capacity (VO_{2max}) declines with advancing age.[18] This age-associated decrease in VO_{2max} has been shown to be ~1% per year between the ages of 20 and 70 years. This decline is likely due to a number of factors, including decreased levels of physical activity, changing cardiac function (including decreased maximal cardiac output), and reduced muscle mass. Flegg and Lakatta[19] determined that skeletal muscle mass accounted for most of the variability in VO_{2max} in men and women above the age of 60 years. A number of studies have demonstrated that the age-related decline in VO_{2max} is ameliorated by physical activity.[20–23] Bortz and Bortz[24] reviewed world records of master athletes up to age 85 years for endurance events and noted that the decline in performance occurred at a rate of 0.5% per year. They concluded that this decline of 0.5% per year may represent the effects of age (or "biological" aging) on VO_{2max}, and the remainder of the decline may be the result of an increasingly sedentary lifestyle. However, Rosen et al.[25] examined predictors of this age-associated decline in VO_{2max} and concluded that VO_{2max} declines at the same rate in athletic and sedentary men and that 35% of this decline is due to sarcopenia.

Aerobic exercise has long been an important recommendation for the prevention and treatment of many of the chronic diseases typically associated with old age. These include type 2 diabetes (and impaired glucose tolerance), hypertension, heart disease, and osteoporosis. Regularly performed aerobic exercise increases insulin action. The responses of initially sedentary young (age 20–30 years) and older (age 60–70 years) men and women to 3 months of aerobic conditioning (70% of maximal heart rate, 45 min/day, 3 days per week) were examined by Meredith et al.[26] They found that the absolute gains in aerobic capacity were similar between the two age-groups. However, the mechanism for adaptation to regular submaximal exercise appears to be different between old and young people. Muscle biopsies taken before and after training showed a more than twofold increase in oxidative capacity of the muscles of the older subjects, whereas that of the young subjects showed smaller improvements. In addition, skeletal muscle glycogen stores in the older subjects, which were significantly lower than those of the young men and women initially, increased significantly. The degree to which the elderly demonstrate increases in maximal cardiac output in response to endurance training is still largely unanswered. Seals et al.[27] found no increases after 1 year of endurance training, whereas, more recently, Spina et al.[28] observed that older men increased maximal cardiac output, whereas healthy older women demonstrated no change in response to endurance exercise training. If these sex-related differences in cardiovascular response are real, it may explain the lack of response in maximal cardiac output when older men and women are included in the same study population.

Aerobic Exercise and Carbohydrate Metabolism

Etiology of Impaired Glucose Tolerance and Aging

The 2-h plasma glucose level during an oral glucose tolerance test (OGTT) increases by an average of 5.3 mg/dl per decade, and fasting plasma glucose increases by an average of 1 mg/dl per decade.[29] The Second National Health and Nutrition Examination Survey demonstrated a progressive increase of ~0.4 mmol/l (7.2 mg/dl) per decade of life in mean plasma glucose value 2 h after a 75-g OGTT ($n = 1{,}678$ men and 1,892 women).[30] Shimokata et al.[31] examined glucose tolerance in community-dwelling men and women ranging from age 17 to 92 years. By assessing level of obesity, pattern of body fat distribution, activity levels, and fitness levels, they attempted to examine the independent effect of age on glucose tolerance. They found no significant differences between the young and middle-aged groups; however, the elderly groups had significantly higher glucose and insulin values (after a glucose challenge) than young or middle-aged groups. Shimokata et al. concluded that "the major finding of this study is that the decline in glucose tolerance from the early-adult to the middle-age years is entirely explained by secondary influences (fatness and fitness), whereas the decline from mid-life to old age still is also influenced by chronological age. This finding is unique. It is also unexplained." However, it must be pointed out that anthropometric determination of body fatness becomes increasingly less accurate with advancing age and does not reflect the intra-abdominal and intramuscular accumulation of fat that occurs with aging.[32] The results of this study may be due more to an underestimate of true body fat levels than age per se. These age-associated changes in glucose tolerance can result in type 2 diabetes and the broad array of associated abnormalities. It has been estimated that 13% of men and women between the ages of 60 and 74 years have impaired glucose tolerance and an additional 17% have type 2 diabetes.[33] Recently, in a large population of elderly men and women (≥55 years of age), serum glucose and fructosamine levels were higher in subjects with retinopathy than in those without,[34] and within the groups with retinopathy, serum glucose was significantly associated with the number of hemorrhages. These relationships were independent of body composition, abdominal obesity, or the presence of type 2 diabetes.

The relationship between aging, body composition, activity, and glucose tolerance was also examined in 270 female and 462 male factory workers aged 22–73 years, none of whom were retired.[35] Plasma glucose levels, both fasting and after a glucose load, increased with age, but the correlation between age and total integrated glucose response after a glucose load was weak: in women, only 3% of the variance could be attributed to age. When activity levels and drug use were factored in, age accounted for only 1% of the variance in women and 6.25% in men.

Aging is associated with reduced glucose tolerance, decreased insulin action, and altered pancreatic morphology and secretory capacity.[36] It is unresolved if all or any of these factors are caused by age, per se, rather than changing body composition and reduced levels of physical activity. However, many individuals live long lives with no changes in glucose homeostasis.[37] The fact that many centenarians have normal glucose tolerance and demonstrate no impaired insulin action argues against a primary effect of aging and strongly points to lifestyle or genetic factors as the major influence on glucose homeostasis.

Aerobic exercise has significant effects on skeletal muscle, which may help explain its importance in the treatment of glucose intolerance and type 2 diabetes. Seals et al.[38] found that a high-intensity training program showed greater improvements in the insulin response to an oral glucose load than lower-intensity aerobic exercise. However, their subjects began the study with normal glucose tolerance. Kirwan et al.[39] found that 9 months of endurance training at 80% of the maximal heart rate (4 days/week) resulted in reduced glucose-stimulated insulin levels; however, no comparison was made to a lower-intensity exercise group. Hughes et al.[40] demonstrated that regularly performed aerobic exercise without weight loss resulted in improved glucose tolerance, an improved rate of insulin-stimulated glucose disposal, and increased skeletal muscle GLUT4 levels in older glucose-intolerant subjects. In this investigation, a moderate-intensity aerobic exercise program was compared with a higher-intensity program (50 vs. 75% of maximal heart rate reserve, 55 min/day, 4 days/week, for 12 weeks). Both moderate- and high-intensity exercise produced significant improvements in glucose tolerance, insulin sensitivity, and muscle GLUT4 (the glucose transporter protein in skeletal muscle) levels, with no difference between exercise intensities. This suggests that a prescription of moderate-intensity aerobic exercise should be recommended for older men or women with type 2 diabetes or a high risk for type 2 diabetes to help ensure compliance to the program.

Elderly and young men and women respond to aerobic exercise with similar absolute increases in maximal aerobic capacity. Increased fitness levels are associated with reduced mortality and increased life expectancy and have helped prevent the occurrence of type 2 diabetes in individuals at the greatest risk for developing this disease.[41] Thus, regularly performed aerobic exercise is important for older people who wish to improve their glucose tolerance.

Aerobic exercise is generally prescribed as an important adjunct to a weight loss program. When combined with weight loss, aerobic exercise has been demonstrated to increase insulin action to a greater extent than weight loss through diet restriction alone. In the study by Bogardus et al.,[42] diet therapy alone improved glucose tolerance, mainly by reducing basal endogenous glucose production and improving hepatic sensitivity to insulin. On the other hand, aerobic exercise training increased carbohydrate storage rates, and, therefore, "diet therapy plus physical training produced a more significant approach toward normal."[42] However, aerobic exercise (as opposed to resistance training) combined with a hypocaloric diet resulted in a greater reduction in resting metabolic rate than diet alone.[43] Heymsfield et al.[44] found that aerobic exercise combined with caloric restriction did not preserve fat-free mass and did not further accelerate weight loss when compared with diet alone. This lack of an effect of aerobic exercise may have been due to a greater decrease in resting metabolic rate in the exercising group. In perhaps the most comprehensive study of its kind, Goran and Poehlman[45] examined components of energy metabolism in older men and women engaged in regular endurance training. They found that endurance training did not increase total daily energy expenditure because of a compensatory decline in physical activity during the remainder of the day. For example, when elderly subjects participated in a regular walking program, they rested more; therefore, activities outside of walking decreased, and 24-h calorie expenditure was unchanged. However, older individuals who had been participating in endurance exercise for most of their lives had a greater resting metabolic rate and total daily energy expenditure than age-matched sedentary control subjects.[46] Ballor et al.[47] compared the effects of resistance training to that of diet restriction alone in obese women. They found that resistance exercise training results in increased strength and gains in muscle size as well as a preservation of fat-free mass during weight loss.

Increasing Levels of Physical Activity in the Elderly

It is never too late to begin exercising. Individuals with diabetes should consult their physician before beginning an exercise program. The following questionnaire was written for those individuals about to begin a moderate- or low-intensity exercise program. You should not begin training without consulting a physician if you answer "yes" to any of the following questions.

Pretraining Program Questionnaire

The American College of Sports Medicine recommends a physician-supervised stress test for anyone over the age of 35 years who wants to begin a vigorous training program. However, if the general recommendation for the patient is to simply walk, this test is not necessary. However, the following questions should be used to determine if the individual should be carefully examined by a physician.

- Do you get chest pains while at rest and/or during exertion?

If you answered "yes" to the above question, have you seen a physician to diagnose the cause of the pains?

- Have you ever had a heart attack?

If you answered "yes" to the above question, was your heart attack within the last year?

- Do you have high blood pressure?

If you do not know the answer to the above question, was your last blood pressure reading >150/100?

- Are you short of breath after extremely mild exertion, at rest, or at night in bed?

- Do you have any ulcerated wounds or cuts on your feet that do not seem to heal?
- Have you lost ≥10 lb in the past 6 months without trying and to your surprise?
- Do you get pain in your buttocks or the back of your legs (thighs and calves) when you walk?
- While at rest, do you frequently experience fast, irregular heartbeats or, at the other extreme, very slow beats? (Although a low heart rate can be a sign of an efficient and well-conditioned heart, a very low rate can also indicate a nearly complete heart block).
- Are you currently being treated for any heart or circulatory condition, such as vascular disease, stroke, angina, hypertension, congestive heart failure, poor circulation to the legs, valvular heart disease, blood clots, or pulmonary disease?
- As an adult, have you ever had a fracture of the hip, spine, or wrist?
- Did you fall more than twice in the past year (no matter what the reason)?

Advancing age results in increased muscle stiffness and reduced elasticity of connective tissue. For this reason, proper warm-up and stretching can have a greater effect in reducing the risk of an orthopedic injury in the elderly than in young men and women. A 5-min warm-up (exercise at a reduced intensity) followed by 5–10 min of slow stretching is highly recommended.

Cooling down after exercise is important in older individuals. You should never finish a workout by immediately jumping into a hot shower. End your exercise session with a slow walk and more stretching. Your postexercise stretching will be more effective than the stretching you did before the exercise. This is because your muscles have warmed up and, along with tendons and ligaments, are much more elastic.

Find a friend to exercise with. The more people you exercise with, the more likely you are to stay with the exercise. This is a perfect opportunity for sons and daughters to spend time with their older parents, to the benefit of both generations.

Strength Training

Whereas endurance exercise has been the more traditional means of increasing cardiovascular fitness, the American College of Sports Medicine currently recommends strength or resistance training as an important component of an overall fitness program. This is particularly important in the elderly, in whom loss of muscle mass and weakness are prominent deficits.

In strength conditioning or progressive resistance training, the resistance against which a muscle generates force is progressively increased over time. Progressive resistance training involves few contractions against a heavy load. This type of exercise is distinctly different from endurance exercise, which involves repetitive contractions against little resistance. The metabolic and morphological adaptations to these two different types of exercise are very different. Muscle strength has been shown to increase in response to training between 60 and 100% of the one-repetition maximum (1RM). 1RM is the maximum amount of weight that can be lifted with one contraction. Strength conditioning will result in an increase in muscle size, which is largely the result of increased contractile proteins. The mechanisms by which the mechanical events stimulate an increase in RNA synthesis and subsequent protein synthesis are not well understood. Lifting weight requires that a muscle shorten as it produces force. This is called a concentric contraction. Lowering the weight, on the other hand, forces the muscle to lengthen as it produces force. This is an eccentric muscle contraction. These lengthening muscle contractions have been shown to produce ultrastructural damage that may stimulate increased muscle protein turnover.

Our laboratory examined the effects of high-intensity resistance training of the knee extensors and flexors (80% of 1RM, 3 days/week) in older men (age 60–72 years). The average increase in knee flexor and extensor strength was 227 and 107%, respectively. Computed tomography (CT) scans and muscle biopsies were used to determine muscle size. Total muscle area by CT analysis increased by 11.4%, whereas the muscle biopsies showed an increase of 33.5% in type I fiber area and 27.5% in type II fiber area. In addition, lower-body VO_{2max} increased significantly, whereas upper-body VO_{2max} did not, indicating that increased muscle mass can increase maximal aerobic power. It appears that the age-related loss in muscle mass may be an important determinant in the reduced maximal aerobic capacity seen in elderly men and women.[19] Improving muscle strength can enhance the capacity of many older men and women to perform many activities, such as stair climbing, carrying packages, and even walking.

We applied this same training program to a group of frail, institutionalized elderly men and women (mean age 90 ± 3 years, range 87–96). After 8 weeks of training, the 10 subjects in this study increased muscle strength by almost 180% and muscle size by 11%. Fiatarone et al.[48] used a similar intervention on frail nursing home residents that demonstrated not only increases in muscle strength and size, but increased gait speed, stair-climbing power, and balance. In addition, spontaneous activity levels increased significantly, whereas the activity of the nonexercised control group was unchanged. It should be pointed out that this was a very old, very frail population with diagnoses of multiple chronic diseases. More recently, muscle biopsies taken from these subjects revealed that the exercise intervention resulted in a significant increase in type II muscle fiber size and an almost fivefold increase in muscle insulin-like growth factor I, a result not observed in the nonexercised control subjects.[49] An increase in overall levels of physical activity has been a common observation in our studies.[48,50,51] Because muscle weakness is a primary deficit in many older individuals, increased strength may stimulate more aerobic activities such as walking and cycling.

In addition to its effect on increasing muscle mass and function, resistance training can also have an important effect on energy balance in elderly men and women.[52] Men and women participating in a resistance training program of the upper- and lower-body muscles required ~15% more calories to maintain body weight after 12 weeks of training compared with their pretraining energy requirements. This increase in energy need resulted from an increased resting metabolic rate, the small energy cost of the exercise, and what was presumed to be an increase in the energy cost of increased protein metabolism. Because resistance training can preserve or even increase muscle mass during weight loss, this type of exercise may be of genuine benefit for those older men and women who must lose weight. Although endurance training has been demonstrated to be an important adjunct to weight loss programs in young men and women by increasing their daily energy expenditure, its utility in treating obesity in the elderly may not be great. This is because many sedentary older men and women do not spend many calories when they perform endurance exercise because they have low fitness levels. A session of 30–40 min of exercise may increase energy expenditure by only 100–200 kcal, with little residual effect on calorie expenditure. Aerobic exercise training will not preserve lean body mass to any great extent during weight loss. Strength training has been demonstrated to cause improved glucose tolerance in elderly subjects.[53] By improving bone density, muscle mass, strength, balance, and overall levels of physical activity, resistance training has been recently[50] demonstrated to be an important way to decrease the risk of osteoporotic bone fracture in postmenopausal women. Resnick and Greenspan[54] have argued that pharmacological treatment of bone in elderly people with osteoporosis may do little to prevent a bone fracture, and preventive strategies should focus on improving balance and decreasing the risk of a fall. Resistance exercise and balance training should play an important role is such a strategy.

Muscle Strength Training in the Elderly

Muscle strength training can be accomplished by virtually anyone. Many health care professionals have directed their patients away from strength training in the mistaken belief that it can cause undesirable elevations in blood pressure. If proper technique is used, the systolic pressure elevation during aerobic exercise is far greater than that during resistance training. Muscle strengthening exercises are rapidly becoming a critical component to cardiac rehabilitation programs as clinicians realize the need for strength as well as endurance for many activities of daily living.

Guidelines for Resistance Exercise Prescription in Elderly People

Candidates

- Adults of all ages are candidates for this type of exercise.
- Elderly, hypertensive patients should be carefully evaluated before beginning a strength training program.
- Instead of a treadmill stress test, use a weight-lifting stress test. Have the patient perform three sets of eight repetitions

at ~80% of the 1RM. Monitor electrocardiogram and blood pressure responses during the exercise.

- Patients with rheumatoid or osteoarthritis may also participate. Patients with a limited range of motion should train within the range of motion that is relatively pain free. Most patients will see a dramatic improvement in the pain-free range of motion as a result of resistance training.

Exercises

- Resistance training should be directed at the large muscle groups that are important in everyday activities, including the shoulders, arms, spine, hips, and legs.
- Each repetition is performed slowly through a full range of motion, allowing 2–3 s to lift the weight (concentric contraction) and 4–6 s to lower the weight (eccentric contraction).
- Performing the exercise more quickly will not enhance strength gains and may increase the risk of injury.

Training Intensity and Duration

- A high-intensity resistance training program has been shown to have the most dramatic effects at all ages. This is a training intensity that will approach or result in muscular fatigue after the weight has been lifted and lowered with proper form 8–12 times. A weight that can be lifted 20 or more times will increase muscular endurance but will not result in much gain in strength or muscle mass.
- The amount of weight that is lifted should increase as strength builds. This should take place about every 2–3 weeks. In our research studies, we have seen a 10–15% increase in strength per week during the first 8 weeks of training.
- We have seen significant gains in muscle strength and mass as well as an improvement in bone density with only 2 days/week of training.

Breathing Technique

- Inhale before a lift, exhale during the lift, and inhale as the weight is lowered to the beginning position.
- You should avoid performing the Valsalva maneuver (holding your breath during force production).
- With proper breathing technique, the cardiovascular stress of resistance exercise is minimal.
- Heart rate and blood pressure should rise only slightly above resting values in the elderly who follow these guidelines.

Equipment

- Any device that provides sufficient resistance to stress muscles beyond levels usually encountered may be used.
- Weight stack or compressed air resistance machines may be found at many community fitness facilities or purchased for home use.
- Simple weight-lifting devices might include Velcro-strapped wrist and ankle bags filled with sand or lead shot; heavy household objects, such as plastic milk jugs filled with water or gravel; or food cans of various sizes.

Conclusion

There is no other group in our society that can benefit more from regularly performed exercise than the elderly. Whereas both aerobic and strength conditioning are highly recommended, only strength training can stop or reverse sarcopenia. Increased muscle strength and mass in the elderly can be the first step toward a lifetime of increased physical activity and a realistic strategy for maintaining functional status and independence.

References

1. Frontera WR, Hughes VA, Evans WJ: A cross-sectional study of upper and lower extremity muscle strength in 45–78 year old men and women. *J Appl Physiol* 71:644–50, 1991

2. Bassey EJ, Fiatarone MA, O'Neill EF, Kelly M, Lipsitz LA, Evans WJ: Leg extensor power and functional performance in very old men and women. *Clin Sci* 82:321–27, 1992
3. Lynch NA, Metter EJ, Lindle RS, Fozard JL, Tobin JD, Roy TA, Fleg JL, Hurley BF: Muscle quality. I. Age-associated differences between arm and leg muscle groups. *J Appl Physiol* 86:188–94, 1999
4. Izquierdo M, Ibanez J, Gorostiaga E, Garrues M, Zuniga A, Anton A, Larrion JL, Hakkinen K: Maximal strength and power characteristics in isometric and dynamic actions of the upper and lower extremities in middle-aged and older men. *Acta Physiol Scand* 167:57–68, 1999
5. Baumgartner RN, Koehler KM, Gallagher D, Romero L, Heymsfield SB, Ross RR, Garry PJ, Lindeman RD: Epidemiology of sarcopenia among the elderly in New Mexico. *Am J Epidemiol* 147: 755–63, 1998 (published erratum appears in *Am J Epidemiol* 149: 1161, 1999)
6. Visser M, Langlois J, Guralnik JM, Cauley JA, Kronmal RA, Robbins J, Williamson JD, Harris TB: High body fatness, but not low fat-free mass, predicts disability in older men and women: the Cardiovascular Health Study. *Am J Clin Nutr* 68:584–90, 1998
7. Visser M, Harris TB, Langlois J, Hannan MT, Roubenoff R, Felson DT, Wilson PW, Kiel DP: Body fat and skeletal muscle mass in relation to physical disability in very old men and women of the Framingham Heart Study. *J Gerontol A Biol Sci Med Sci* 53:M214–21, 1998
8. Zamboni M, Turcato E, Santana H, Maggi S, Harris TB, Pietrobelli A, Heymsfield SB, Micciolo R, Bosello O: The relationship between body composition and physical performance in older women. *J Am Geriatr Soc* 47:1403–08, 1999
9. Stewart A, Walker L, Porter RW, Reid DM, Primrose WR: Predicting a second hip fracture. *J Clin Densitom* 2:363–70, 1999
10. Turner LW, Wang MQ, Fu Q: Risk factors for hip fracture among southern older women. *South Med J* 91:533–40, 1998
11. Mussolino ME, Looker AC, Madans JH, Langlois JA, Orwoll ES: Risk factors for hip fracture in white men: the NHANES I Epidemiologic Follow-up Study. *J Bone Miner Res* 13:918–24, 1998
12. Langlois JA, Visser M, Davidovic LS, Maggi S, Li G, Harris TB: Hip fracture risk in older white men is associated with change in

body weight from age 50 years to old age. *Arch Intern Med* 158:990–96, 1998

13. Phillips SK, Woledge RC, Bruce SA, Young A, Levy D, Yeo A, Martin FC: A study of force and cross-sectional area of adductor pollicis muscle in female hip fracture patients. *J Am Geriatr Soc* 46:999–1002, 1998
14. Baumgartner RN, Waters DL, Gallagher D, Morley JE, Garry PJ: Predictors of skeletal muscle mass in elderly men and women. *Mech Ageing Dev* 107:123–36, 1999
15. Vermeulen A, Goemaere S, Kaufman JM: Testosterone, body composition and aging. *J Endocrinol Invest* 22:110–16, 1999
16. Meredith CN, Zackin MJ, Frontera WR, Evans WJ: Body composition and aerobic capacity in young and middle-aged endurance-trained men. *Med Sci Sports Exerc* 19:557–63, 1987
17. Roberts SB, Young VR, Fuss P, Heyman MB, Fiatarone M, Dallal GE, Cortiella J, Evans WJ: What are the dietary energy needs of elderly adults? *Int J Obes Relat Metab Disord* 16:969–76, 1992
18. Buskirk ER, Hodgson JL: Age and aerobic power: the rate of change in men and women. *Fed Proc* 46:1824–29, 1987
19. Flegg JL, Lakatta EG: Role of muscle loss in the age-associated reduction in VO_{2max}. *J Appl Physiol* 65:1147–51, 1988
20. Dehn MM, Bruce RA: Longitudinal variations in maximal oxygen intake with age and activity. *J Appl Physiol* 33:805–07, 1972
21. Pollock ML, Foster C, Knapp D, Rod JL, Schmidt DH: Effect of age and training on aerobic capacity and body composition of master athletes. *J Appl Physiol* 62:725–31, 1987
22. Dill DB, Robinson S, Ross JC: A longitudinal study of 16 champion runners. *J Sports Med Phys Fitness* 7:4–27, 1967
23. Rogers MA, Hagberg JM, Martin WH, Ehsani AA, Holloszy JO: Decline in VO_{2max} with aging in master athletes and sedentary men. *J Appl Physiol* 68:2195–99, 1990
24. Bortz WM IV, Bortz WM II: How fast do we age? Exercise performance over time as a biomarker. *J Gerontol* 51:M223–25, 1996
25. Rosen MJ, Sorkin JD, Goldberg AP, Hagberg JM, Katzel LI: Predictors of age-associated decline in maximal aerobic capacity: a comparison of four statistical models. *J Appl Physiol* 84:2163–70, 1998
26. Meredith CN, Frontera WR, Fisher EC, Hughes VA, Herland JC, Edwards J, Evans WJ: Peripheral effects of endurance training in young and old subjects. *J Appl Physiol* 66:2844–49, 1989

27. Seals DR, Hagberg JM, Hurley BF, Ehsani AA, Holloszy JO: Endurance training in older men and women. I. Cardiovascular responses to exercise. *J Appl Physiol* 57:1024–29, 1984
28. Spina RJ, Ogawa T, Kohrt WM, Martin WH III, Holloszy JO, Ehsani AA: Differences in cardiovascular adaptation to endurance exercise training between older men and women. *J Appl Physiol* 75:849–55, 1993
29. Davidson MB: The effect of aging on carbohydrate metabolism: a review of the English literature and a practical approach to the diagnosis of diabetes mellitus in the elderly. *Metabolism* 28:688–705, 1979
30. Hadden WC, Harris MI: *Prevalence of Diagnosed Diabetes, Undiagnosed Diabetes, and Impaired Glucose Tolerance in Adults 20–74 Years of Age: United States, 1976–1980.* Washington, DC, U.S. Govt. Printing Office, 1987 (DHHS PHS publ. no. 87-1687)
31. Shimokata H, Muller DC, Fleg JL, Sorkin J, Ziemba AW, Andes R: Age as independent determinant of glucose tolerance. *Diabetes* 40:44–51, 1991
32. Borkan GA, Hultz DE, Gerzoff AF: Age changes in body composition revealed by computed tomography. *J Gerontol* 38:673–77, 1983
33. Harris MI, Hadden WC, Knowler WC, Bennett PH: Prevalence of diabetes and impaired glucose tolerance and plasma glucose levels in U.S. population aged 20–74 yr. *Diabetes* 36:523–34, 1987
34. Stolk RP, Vingerling JR, de Jong PT, Dielemans I, Hofman A, Lamberts SW, Pols HA, Grobbee DE: Retinopathy, glucose, and insulin in an elderly population: The Rotterdam Study. *Diabetes* 44:11–15, 1995
35. Zavaroni I, Dall'Aglio E, Bruschi F, Bonora E, Alpi O, Pezzarossa A, Butturini U: Effect of age and environmental factors on glucose tolerance and insulin secretion in a worker population. *J Am Geriatr Soc* 34:271–75, 1986
36. Evans WJ, Farrell PA: The aging pancreas: the effects of aging on insulin secretion and action. In *The Handbook of Physiology*. Jefferson JS, Cherrington AD, Eds. Oxford, U.K., Oxford University Press, 2001, p. 969–99
37. Paolisso G, Gambardella A, Ammendola S, D'Amore A, Balbi V, Varricchio M, D'Onofrio F: Glucose tolerance and insulin action in healthy centenarians. *Am J Physiol* 270:E890–94, 1996

38. Seals DR, Hagberg JM, Hurley BF, Ehsani AA, Holloszy JO: Effects of endurance training on glucose tolerance and plasma lipid levels in older men and women. *JAMA* 252:645–49, 1984
39. Kirwan JP, Kohrt WM, Wojta DM, Bourey RE, Holloszy JO: Endurance exercise training reduces glucose-stimulated insulin levels in 60- to 70-year-old men and women. *J Gerontol* 48:M84–90, 1993
40. Hughes VA, Fiatarone MA, Fielding RA, Kahn BB, Ferrara CM, Shepherd P, Fisher EC, Wolfe RR, Elahi D, Evans WJ: Exercise increases muscle GLUT 4 levels and insulin action in subjects with impaired glucose tolerance. *Am J Physiol* 264:E855–62, 1993
41. Helmrich SP, Ragland DR, Leung RW, Paffenbarger RS Jr: Physical activity and reduced occurrence of non-insulin-dependent diabetes mellitus. *N Engl J Med* 325:147–52, 1991
42. Bogardus C, Ravussin E, Robbins DC, Wolfe RR, Horton ES, Sims EAH: Effects of physical training and diet therapy on carbohydrate metabolism in patients with glucose intolerance and non-insulin-dependent diabetes mellitus. *Diabetes* 33:311–18, 1984
43. Phinney SD, LaGrange BM, O'Connell M, Danforth E Jr: Effects of aerobic exercise on energy expenditure and nitrogen balance during very low calorie dieting. *Metabolism* 37:758–65, 1988
44. Heymsfield SB, Casper K, Hearn J, Guy D: Rate of weight loss during underfeeding: relation to level of physical activity. *Metabolism* 38:215–23, 1989
45. Goran MI, Poehlman ET: Endurance training does not enhance total energy expenditure in healthy elderly persons. *Am J Physiol* 263:E950–57, 1992
46. Withers RT, Smith DA, Tucker RC, Brinkman M, Clark DG: Energy metabolism in sedentary and active 49- to 70-year-old women. *J Appl Physiol* 84:1333–40, 1998
47. Ballor DL, Katch VL, Becque MD, Marks CR: Resistance weight training during caloric restriction enhances lean body weight maintenance. *Am J Clin Nutr* 47:19–25, 1988
48. Fiatarone MA, O'Neill EF, Ryan ND, Clements KM, Solares GR, Nelson ME, Roberts SB, Kehayias JJ, Lipsitz LA, Evans WJ: Exercise training and nutritional supplementation for physical frailty in very elderly people. *N Engl J Med* 330:1769–75, 1994
49. Singh MA, Ding W, Manfredi TJ, Solares GS, O'Neill EF, Clements KM, Ryan ND, Kehayias JJ, Fielding RA, Evans WJ:

Insulin-like grow factor I in skeletal muscle after weight-lifting exercise in frail elders. *Am J Physiol* 277:E135–43, 1999

50. Nelson ME, Fiatarone MA, Morganti CM, Trice I, Greenberg RA, Evans WJ: Effects of high-intensity strength training on multiple risk factors for osteoporotic fractures. *JAMA* 272:1909–14, 1994
51. Frontera WR, Meredith CN, O'Reilly KP, Evans WJ: Strength training and determinants of VO_{2max} in older men. *J Appl Physiol* 68:329–33, 1990
52. Campbell WW, Crim MC, Young VR, Evans WJ: Increased energy requirements and body composition changes with resistance training in older adults. *Am J Clin Nutr* 60:167–75, 1994
53. Miller JP, Pratley RE, Goldberg AP, Gordon P, Rubin M, Treuth MS, Ryan AS, Hurley BF: Strength training increases insulin action in healthy 50- to 65-yr-old men. *J Appl Physiol* 77:1122–27, 1994
54. Resnick NM, Greenspan SL: 'Senile' osteoporosis reconsidered. *JAMA* 261:1025–29, 1989

William J. Evans, PhD, is from the University of Arkansas for Medical Sciences and the VA Medical Center, Little Rock, AR.

33

Patients on Various Drug Therapies

OM P. GANDA, MD, FACE

Highlights

- Patients with diabetes frequently take medications or other chemical agents in addition to insulin or oral hypoglycemic agents.
- Many commonly used drugs may cause significant alterations in the metabolic and nonmetabolic responses to exercise, sometimes affecting exercise performance.
- More commonly used drugs with potential significance in patients with diabetes include diuretics, β-adrenergic blockers, calcium-channel blockers, angiotensin-converting enzyme inhibitors, glucocorticoids, anabolic steroids, lipid-lowering agents, salicylates, and non-steroidal analgesics.
- Patients with chronic complications, such as cardiovascular disease, hypertension, autonomic neuropathy, peripheral vascular disease, and nephropathy,

are particularly vulnerable to the adverse effects of pharmacological agents.

- Prudent choice of drugs in individual situations can minimize adverse effects in regularly exercising diabetic patients.

Patients engaged in exercise or endurance training programs should be aware that certain drugs or chemical agents may cause significant alterations in the metabolic, cardiovascular, or hemodynamic responses to exercise. In such patients, therefore, the anticipated clinical effects of exercise on blood glucose, glucose counter-regulation, and cardiovascular risk factors may be appreciably different. The effects of different commonly used drugs for carbohydrate metabolism[1,2] are summarized in Table 33.1. In patients with certain chronic complications, such as cardiovascular disease, peripheral vascular disease, autonomic neuropathy, and renal disease, many pharmacological agents can potentially modify and limit physical performance during exercise. The following is a brief discussion of the multiple sites of action of commonly used agents in patients with diabetes or impaired glucose tolerance. The interaction of exercise with actions of insulin and glucose regulation in insulin-treated patients will not be discussed here (see Chapters 4, 20 and 21). Similarly, note that exercise can enhance the hypoglycemic effects of sulfonylureas (see Chapter 20).

Diuretics

The hyperglycemia induced by high doses of diuretic agents, particularly thiazides and chlorthalidone, is well known. This effect is produced via multiple mechanisms, including decreased insulin secretion and impaired insulin sensitivity. Hypokalemia, caused by these agents, is at least partially responsible for this effect. Patients engaging in regular exercise may be more at risk if fluid and electrolyte balance is not maintained. Other metabolic effects of thiazides and related diuretics include decreased sodium and magnesium levels, increased uric acid levels, modest increases in LDL cholesterol and

TABLE 33.1 Commonly Used Drugs or Agents Capable of Inducing Changes in Glucose Homeostasis

	Mechanism of Action		
	Insulin Secretion	**Glucose Disposal**	**Comments**
Potentially raise blood glucose			
Diuretics (thiazides, chlorthalidone, furosemide, metolazone)	↓	↓	K^+ depletion, other effects
β-Adrenergic antagonists (propranolol, nadolol, timolol)	0, ↓	0, ↓	More likely with noncardioselective agents
Calcium-channel blockers (dihydropyridine derivatives)	0	0, ↓	Effect rarely significant
Glucocorticoids	↑	↓	Cause marked insulin resistance
Anabolic steroids	0	↓	Cause major lipid effects
Growth hormone	↑	↓	A major insulin antagonist
Niacin	↑	↓	Particularly with high dosage
Cyclosporine	↓	↓	Often used with glucocorticoids
Tacrolimus	↓	?	Hyperglycemia more frequent than with cyclosporine
Potentially lower blood glucose			
α-Adrenergic antagonists (prazosin, doxazosin, terazosin)	0, ↑	0, ↑	Rarely significant
ACE inhibitors	0	0, ↑	
β-Adrenergic antagonists (propranolol, nadolol, timolol)			May impair recovery from hypoglycemia
Salicylates	0, ↑	0	With high dosage
Alcohol	0, ↑	↑	May cause hyperglycemia in the long term
Pentamidine	↑	0	May cause hyperglycemia in the long term
Quinine	↑	0, ↑	May cause severe hypoglycemia

triglyceride levels, and lower HDL cholesterol levels.[3,4] In general, all of the adverse effects are more prominent after prolonged use at a higher dosage.[4]

β-Adrenergic Antagonists

β-Adrenergic antagonists are frequently used in patients with angina or after myocardial infarction. They may decrease exercise capacity, lower peak heart rate and blood pressure, and improve myocardial ischemic changes on stress tests. Some patients with angina may experience better work capacity because of the relief of symptoms.

β-Adrenergic antagonists have complex effects on metabolic pathways involving insulin secretion, hepatic and peripheral glucose disposal, lipolysis, and lipoprotein metabolism.[4,5] In all of these respects, noncardioselective agents (e.g., propranolol, nadolol, and timolol) have greater activity than cardioselective agents (e.g., atenolol and metoprolol). By inhibiting insulin secretion and glucose disposal, β-blockers may worsen hyperglycemia.[1,2] In a large prospective study of subjects with hypertension, β-blockers use over 3–6 years were associated with a 28% increased risk for developing diabetes after adjustment of other risk factors.[6] However, the relationship with the type of β-blocker was not assessed in that study. More frequently, in patients with insulin-requiring diabetes, β-blockers may induce hypoglycemia by inhibiting muscle and hepatic glycogenolysis. Furthermore, β-blockers are known to impair the recovery from hypoglycemia, which is critically dependent on the β_2-adrenergic hepatic effects of epinephrine. This is especially relevant in patients with type 1 diabetes who frequently fail to release glucagon in response to hypoglycemia. In addition, these agents mask the adrenergic symptoms of hypoglycemia by altering the glycemic threshold for symptoms.[7] In this regard, it is of interest that one adrenergic symptom, sweating, is increased rather than decreased because it is mediated by a cholinergic mechanism.

β-Adrenergic antagonists might have adverse effects on the lipid profile, i.e., elevation of triglycerides and lowering of HDL cholesterol. However, these effects are also more frequent with nonselective agents.[5] In relation to exercise and diabetes, other pertinent adverse effects include worsening of symptoms of peripheral vascular disease, increased fatigue, and impairment of exercise tolerance. Finally, β-blockers, by impairing cellular potassium uptake, may promote exercise-induced hyperkalemia, particularly in patients with underlying renal insufficiency or patients on nonsteroidal analgesics. It would therefore be prudent to use only cardioselective β-blockers in patients with either type 1 or type 2 diabetes.

Despite some of the potential adverse effects of β-blockers described above, the use of atenolol for hypertension in patients with type 2 diabetes in the U.K. Prospective Diabetes Study was associated with a 32% reduction in diabetes-related mortality.

Angiotensin-Converting Enzyme Inhibitors, Calcium-Channel Blockers, and α-Adrenergic Antagonists

The newer classes of antihypertensive agents, including angiotensin-converting enzyme (ACE) inhibitors, calcium-channel blockers, and α-adrenergic antagonists, have more favorable metabolic effects in general and have been recommended by the American Diabetes Association as the preferred agents for control of hypertension in diabetic patients.[8] Calcium-channel blockers improve exercise capacity and ischemia in patients with coronary artery disease. From the glycemic point of view, there appears to be some heterogeneity of responses with different types of calcium-channel blockers. Drugs like verapamil and diltiazem have no significant effect on glycemic control, but some members of the dihydropyridine class, such as nifedipine, may impair insulin sensitivity,[9] and others, such as amlodipine, may improve glucose tolerance and enhance insulin sensitivity.[10] On the other hand, α-adrenergic antagonists and ACE inhibitors have been shown to improve insulin sensitivity.[9] The improvement of insulin sensitivity in response to an ACE inhibitor may persist after addition of low-dose thiazides.[9] These favorable responses in insulin sensitivity have now been shown for several agents belonging to the ACE inhibitor family, suggesting a class effect. In a case-control study, hospitalization due to hypoglycemia was 2.8 times more likely in patients with diabetes on ACE inhibitors.[11] However, certain adverse effects, such as dyspnea and postural hypotension leading to light-headedness, are not uncommon when α-blockers are used for hypertension or benign prostatic hypertrophy. Regarding their effects on lipids, calcium-channel blockers and ACE inhibitors have no significant adverse effects, whereas α-blockers have been shown to moderately raise HDL cholesterol levels and lower triglycerides in several studies.[4,12] The long-term renoprotective effects of ACE inhibitors in patients with type 1 diabetes and either microalbuminuria or clinical proteinuria have been recently demonstrated in prospective randomized studies.[13,14] Finally, several recent long-term trials have shown enhanced exercise capacity and prolonged survival rates after myocardial infarction in the presence or absence of impaired left ventricle function in patients on ACE inhibitors.[15–17] The long-term benefits and comparability of various angiotensin II receptor antagonists are currently being studied.

Despite the favorable metabolic effects of α-blockers mentioned above, few long-term outcome data are available regarding the safety of these agents. In ALLHAT (Antihypertensive and Lipid-Lowering Treatment to Prevent Heart Attack Trial), an ongoing trial involving >40,000 patients, recent interim analysis at 3.3 years revealed an increased incidence of stroke and congestive heart failure (relative risk 1.19 and 2.04, respectively) with the use of doxazosin versus chlorthalidone as the initial agent.[18] However, there was no difference in total mortality.

Glucocorticoids and Anabolic Steroids

It is well known that glucocorticoids, in supraphysiological and pharmacological doses, cause insulin resistance and compensatory hyperinsulinemia in nondiabetic individuals or in subjects with impaired glucose tolerance. Increasing the dosage of glucocorticoids progressively worsens preexisting hyperglycemia via multiple effects on liver, adipose tissue, and muscle.[1,2] Glucocorticoids, after prolonged use, also alter adipose tissue distribution and cause skin changes, leading to the typical cushingoid appearance, as well as to proximal muscle weakness due to steroid myopathy. These diverse effects may considerably impair physical performance. By inducing insulin resistance and increased lipogenesis, glucocorticoids can cause significant lipid changes (typically hypertriglyceridemia). Even more striking adverse changes in lipids may result from prolonged use of oral anabolic steroids, usually seen in young athletes. In a review of multiple studies evaluating the effects of different oral anabolic steroids, an average reduction of 52% in HDL cholesterol and an average rise of 36% in LDL cholesterol were consistently observed.[19] Because these effects were not observed by parenteral administration, it appears quite likely that the lipid alterations are mediated via hepatic effects of these agents. A marked increase in premature atherogenesis can be anticipated from the striking lipid effects of these agents. Moreover, other serious adverse effects, particularly with the use of 17-α alkylated androgens (e.g., methyltestosterone, oxandrolone, and stanozol), include hepatotoxicity, impaired spermatogenesis leading to infertility, and hirsutism and virilization in women.[20] The touted benefits of anabolic steroids in improving muscle strength or athletic performance should be weighed against these potential adverse effects.

Growth Hormone

Growth hormone, like glucocorticoids, is a classic diabetogenic hormone with diverse effects on carbohydrate, lipid, and protein metabolism. The levels of growth hormone and insulin-like growth factor I gradually decline with age and may be related to the decreases in muscle and bone mass and the increased adiposity in older individuals. Therefore, growth hormone treatment has been proposed in debilitated elderly people, in those with osteoporosis or sepsis, and in those in posttraumatic or postsurgical states.[21,22] However, the safety and efficacy of growth hormone have not yet been proven. In a placebo-controlled trial, growth hormone was administered to healthy elderly men, 70–85 years of age, over 6 months.[23] Even though lean tissue mass increased and fat mass decreased, muscle strength and systemic endurance were unaltered. Similarly, the efficacy of short-term growth hormone in improving athletic performance has not been documented to be different than training alone.[21] Potential adverse effects of long-term growth hormone treatment, besides cost, include accelerated atherosclerosis, hypertension, insulin resistance, degenerative arthropathy, and possibly increased incidence of tumors. At the present time, use of growth hormone to improve functional parameters is not recommended except in individuals with growth hormone deficiency. Some patients with AIDS and associated wasting and cachexia may also benefit from its effects on body composition.

Lipid-Lowering Drugs

Fibric acid derivatives, such as clofibrate and, less often, gemfibrozil and fenofibrate, may on rare occasions cause an acute or subacute muscular syndrome characterized by severe muscle pain, tenderness, and weakness generally involving shoulders, hips, and calves.[24] Muscle necrosis may result in markedly elevated creatinine phosphokinase, aldolase, and even myoglobinuria. Patients with underlying renal disease or hypothyroidism and patients taking hydroxymethylglutaryl coenzyme A (HMG-CoA) reductase inhibitors (statins) are more susceptible to this complication. Other drugs known to increase the risk of myosites in patients on fibrates include erythromycin, cyclosporine, and azole antifungals.[25]

Niacin (nicotinic acid), another commonly used lipid-lowering agent, can lead to hyperglycemia by inducing insulin resistance, particularly when β-cells are unable to adapt because of limited reserves, e.g., in patients with impaired glucose tolerance or overt type 2 diabetes.[26] However, this effect is usually not clinically significant unless the dose exceeds 1.0 g daily.[27]

Cyclosporine and Tacrolimus

Cyclosporine, a widely used immunosuppressant in patients with organ transplants and autoimmune disorders, may precipitate diabetes or glucose intolerance by direct effects on β-cells as well as on peripheral insulin sensitivity.[1,2,28] This effect is probably independent of the glucocorticoids[28,29] often used simultaneously in such patients. African-Americans may be more susceptible to the hyperglycemic effect of cyclosporine.[30] Patients on cyclosporine who engage in strenuous physical activity should be aware that they may be more susceptible to myositis and even rhabdomyolysis and acute renal failure if they are concurrently taking fibric acid derivatives or HMG-CoA reductase inhibitors (statins). In view of the high incidence of this adverse effect (up to 30% of patients on lovastatin),[25,31] the statins should be cautiously used in patients on cyclosporine. Recent evidence suggests that pravastatin (pravachol) may be associated with a lower incidence of toxicity in patients on cyclosporine because it is not metabolized by the cytochrome P-450 system.[25] The use of Tacrolimus (FK-506) is also associated with an increased incidence of diabetes as well as a worsening of previously diagnosed diabetes.[29,32]

Salicylates and Nonsteroidal Anti-Inflammatory Drugs

Salicylates and aspirin, in higher dosages (4–6 g/day), may induce hypoglycemia.[1] However, in usual dosages, there are no significant effects on glucose or insulin secretion. Nonsteroidal anti-inflammatory drugs (NSAIDs) (e.g., acetaminophen, ibuprofen, naproxen, and piroxicam) have the potential of causing renal injury and inducing hyperkalemia in older patients with type 2 diabetes or any patient with underlying renal disease.

Alcohol

Long-term moderate intake of alcohol (one to three drinks daily) has been reported to be cardioprotective in several epidemiological studies.[33,34] Recent studies suggest an enhanced insulin sensitivity in light to moderate drinkers (those who drink one to three drinks a day) compared with nondrinkers.[35] However, these salutary effects of alcohol need to be considered in light of other long-term effects of heavy alcohol intake, which include weight gain, elevated triglycerides, liver toxicity, and an increased incidence of cancer.

Pentamidine

Pentamidine is frequently used in the prophylaxis or treatment of Pneumocystis pneumonia in patients with AIDS. Its chemical structure is similar to the well-known diabetogenic agents alloxan and streptozotocin. A survey of patients with AIDS receiving intravenous pentamidine revealed a 14% incidence of acute hypoglycemic episodes (blood glucose <55 mg/dl).[36] A few of these episodes were fatal. An increased incidence of type 1 diabetes has been reported after prolonged therapy and in patients with underlying renal impairment.[37] However, aerosolized pentamidine, which has virtually replaced the intravenous route, has minimal effects on carbohydrate metabolism.

Quinine

Quinine is frequently used for the relief of muscle cramps. In patients with severe falciparum malaria, quinine was shown to induce severe hypoglycemia by multiple mechanisms, including an enhanced insulin release. Quinine, even in a modest dosage, may occasionally precipitate symptomatic hypoglycemia in healthy individuals.[38] Patients on endurance exercise programs and sulfonylurea therapy may conceivably be more susceptible to quinine-induced hypoglycemia.

Table 33.2 summarizes some important clinical considerations for patients on exercise programs.

TABLE 33.2 Potential Consequences of Certain Commonly Used Drugs in Exercising Patients With Diabetes or Impaired Glucose Tolerance

	Caveats During and After Exercise	Adverse Effects (Long-Term)
Diuretics	Electrolyte imbalance Dehydration	May precipitate gout Worsening glucose control (high dosage)
β-Blockers	Monitor heart rate May decrease exercise capacity Hypoglycemia unawareness Impaired recovery from hypoglycemia	May worsen hyperglycemia
α-Adrenergic antagonists	Postural hypotension	Increased risk of stroke and coronary heart failure (reported with Dexazosin)
Oral anabolic steroids		Liver toxicity Dyslipidemia (↓ HDL cholesterol, ↑ LDL cholesterol) Infertility
Fibric acid agents	Myalgia	Myositis
NSAIDs/high-dose salicylates	Hypoglycemia	Renal injury Hyperkalemia

References

1. Pandit MK, Burke J, Gustafson AB, Minocha A, Peiris AN: Drug-induced disorders of glucose tolerance. *Ann Intern Med* 118: 529–39, 1993
2. Ganda OP: Secondary forms of diabetes. In *Joslin's Diabetes Mellitus.* 13th ed. Kahn CR, Weir GC, Eds. Philadelphia, Lea & Febiger, 1994, p. 300–16
3. Lardinois CK, Neuman SL: The effects of antihypertensive agents on serum lipids and lipoproteins. *Arch Intern Med* 148:1280–88, 1988
4. Joint National Committee on Detection, Evaluation, and Treatment of High Blood Pressure: The fifth report of the Joint National Committee on Detection, Evaluation, and Treatment of High Blood Pressure. *Arch Intern Med* 153:154–83, 1993

5. Burris JF: β-Blockers, dyslipidemia, and coronary artery disease: a reassessment. *Arch Intern Med* 153:2085–92, 1993
6. Gress TW, Nieto FJ, Shahar E, Wofford MR, Brancati FL. Hypertension and antihypertensive therapy as risk factors for type 2 diabetes mellitus. *N Engl J Med* 342:905–12, 2000
7. Hirsch IB, Boyle PJ, Craft S, Cryer PE: Higher glycemic thresholds for symptoms during β-adrenergic blockade in IDDM. *Diabetes* 40:1177–86, 1991
8. American Diabetes Association: Treatment of hypertension in diabetes (Consensus Statement). *Diabetes Care* 16:1394–1401, 1993
9. Berne C, Pollare T, Lithell H: Effects of antihypertensive treatment on insulin sensitivity with special reference to ACE inhibitors. *Diabetes Care* 14 (Suppl. 4):39–47, 1991
10. Beer NA, Jakubowicz DJ, Beer RM, Nestler JE: The calcium-channel blocker amlodipine raises serum dehydroepiandrosterone sulfate and androstenedione, but lowers serum cortisol, in insulin-resistant obese and hypertensive men. *J Clin Endocrinol Metab* 76:1464–69, 1993
11. Herings RMC, de Boer A, Stricker BH, Leufkens HG, Porsius A: Hypoglycemia associated with use of inhibitors of angiotensin converting enzyme. *Lancet* 345:1195–98, 1995
12. Kasiske BL, Ma JZ, Kalil RSN, Louis TA: Effects of antihypertensive therapy on serum lipids. *Ann Intern Med* 122:133–41, 1995
13. Lewis EJ, Hunsicker LG, Bain RP, Rhode RD: The effect of angiotensin-converting enzyme inhibition on diabetic nephropathy. *N Engl J Med* 329:1456–62, 1993
14. ACE Inhibitors in Diabetic Nephropathy Trialists Group: Should all patients with type 1 diabetes mellitus and microalbuminuria receive angiotensin-converting enzyme inhibitors? A meta-analysis of individual patient data. *Ann Intern Med* 134:370–79, 2001
15. Gustafsson I, Torp-Pedersen C, Kober L, Gustafsson F, Hildebrandt P, on behalf of the Trace Study Group: Effect of the angiotensin-converting enzyme inhibitor tandolopril on mortality and morbidity in diabetic patients with left ventricular dysfunction after acute myocardial infarction. *J Am Coll Cardiol* 34:83–89, 1999
16. Heart Outcomes Prevention Evaluation (HOPE) Study Investigators: Effects of ramipril on cardiovascular and microvascular outcomes in people with diabetes mellitus: results of the HOPE study and MICRO HOPE substudy. *Lancet* 355:253–59, 2000

17. Feather MD, Yusuf Y, Kobeh L, Pfeffer M, Hall A, Murray G, Torp-Pedersen C, Ball S, Pogue J, Moye L, Braunwald E: Long-term ACE-inhibitor therapy in patients with heart failure or left-ventricular dysfunction: a systemic interview of data from individual patients. *Lancet* 355:1575–81, 2000
18. ALLHAT Officers and Coordinators for the ALLHAT Collaborative Research Group: Major cardiovascular events in hypertensive patients randomized to doxasosin vs. chlorthalidone. *JAMA* 283:1967–75, 2000
19. Glazer G: Atherogenic effects of anabolic steroids on serum lipid levels: a literature review. *Arch Intern Med* 151:1925–33, 1991
20. Wilson JD: Androgen abuse by athletes. *Endocr Rev* 9:181–99, 1988
21. Kaplan SL: The newer uses of growth hormone in adults. *Adv Intern Med* 38:287–301, 1993
22. Vance ML: Growth hormone for the elderly. *N Engl J Med* 323:52–54, 1990
23. Papadakis MA, Grady D, Black D, Tierney MJ, Gooding GAW, Schambelan M, Grunfeld C: Growth hormone replacement in healthy older men improves body composition but not functional ability. *Ann Intern Med* 124:708–16, 1996
24. Lane RJM, Mastaglia FL: Drug-induced myopathies in man. *Lancet* ii:562–65, 1978
25. Bottorff M, Hansten P: Long-term safety of hepatic hydroxymethyl glutaryl coenzyme A reductase inhibitors. *Arch Intern Med* 160:2273–80, 2000
26. Garg A, Grundy SM: Nicotinic acid as therapy for dyslipidemia in non-insulin-dependent diabetes. *JAMA* 264:723–26, 1990
27. Elam MB, Hunninghake DB, Darisk B, Garg R, Johnson C, Egan D, Kostis JB, Sheps DS, Bointon EA, for the ADMIT Investigators: Effect of niacin on lipid and lipoprotein levels and glycemic control in patients with diabetes and peripheral arterial disease. *JAMA* 284:1263–70, 2000
28. Teuscher AU, Seaquist ER, Robertson RP: Diminished insulin secretory reserve in diabetic pancreas transplant and nondiabetic kidney transplant recipients. *Diabetes* 43:593–98, 1994
29. European FK506 Multicenter Liver Study Group: Randomized trial comparing tacrolimus (FKJ06) and cyclosporin in prevention of liver allograft rejection. *Lancet* 344:423–28, 1994

30. Sumarini NB, Delaney V, Daskalaxis P, Davis R, Friedman EA, Hong JH, Sommer BG: Retrospective analysis of posttransplantation diabetes mellitus in black renal allograft recipients. *Diabetes Care* 14:760–62, 1991
31. Tobert JA: Rhabdomyolysis in patients receiving lovastatin after cardiac transplantation. *N Engl J Med* 318:47–48, 1988
32. Kawai T, Shimada A, Kasuga A: FK506-induced autoimmune diabetes (Letter). *Ann Intern Med* 132:511, 2000
33. Suh I, Shaten BJ, Cutler JA, Kuller LH: Alcohol use and mortality from coronary heart disease: the role of high-density cholesterol. *Ann Intern Med* 116:881–87, 1992
34. Ajani UA, Gaziano M, Lotufo PA, Liu S, Hennekens CH, Buring JE, Manson JE: Alcohol consumption and risk of coronary heart disease by diabetes status. *Circulation* 102:500–05, 2000
35. Facchini F, Chen Y-DI, Reaven GM: Light-to-moderate alcohol intake is associated with enhanced insulin sensitivity. *Diabetes Care* 17:115–19, 1994
36. Waskin H, Stehr-Green JK, Helmick CG, Sattler FR: Risk factors for hypoglycemia associated with pentamidine therapy for Pneumocystis pneumonia. *JAMA* 260:345–47, 1988
37. Assan R, Perronne C, Assan D, Chotard L, Mayaud C, Matheron S, Zuckman D: Pentamidine-induced derangements of glucose homeostasis: determinant roles of renal failure and drug accumulation. *Diabetes Care* 18:47–55, 1995
38. Limburg PJ, Katz H, Grant CS, Service FJ: Quinine-induced hypoglycemia. *Ann Intern Med* 119:218–19, 1993

Om P. Ganda, MD, FACE is from the Joslin Diabetes Center, Boston, MA.

34

Exercise in Diabetic Patients With Disabilities

JOEL STEIN, MD

Highlights

- Disability and diabetes commonly coexist. Diabetes is a risk factor for stroke, amputation, and neuropathy.
- Stroke is a common disabling condition in diabetic individuals. Exercise therapy is a key component of rehabilitation after stroke. Recent studies have provided increasing evidence that exercise can facilitate stroke recovery.
- The high prevalence of coronary artery disease in people with diabetes who sustain a stroke should be considered when prescribing exercise for these individuals.
- Both diabetes and stroke may be risk factors for carpal tunnel syndrome (CTS). Treatment of CTS may be complicated by coexisting disability (e.g., hemiparesis in the other arm).
- Leg amputation may occur as a complication of diabetes and imposes increased energy costs for ambulation. The energy requirements of walking with an

above-the-knee amputation are substantially higher than with a below-the-knee amputation.

- Neuropathy is an important cause of disability in individuals with diabetes. Ankle dorsiflexion weakness ("foot drop") may be effectively managed with the use of an ankle foot orthosis.
- In severe cases of neuropathy, a Charcot arthropathy may develop in the foot or ankle. This has a substantial impact on the ability to exercise and may result in amputation in some cases.
- Lower-extremity braces may be useful as a compensatory tool for individuals with leg weakness from stroke or neuropathy. Either plastic lightweight braces or metal braces attached to shoes may be appropriate in different situations. The least restrictive brace possible should generally be prescribed.

Disability and diabetes commonly coexist. In a number of disabling conditions, diabetes is a risk factor for the development of these disorders. Examples of these conditions include stroke, amputation, and peripheral neuropathy. In other cases, diabetes is a coincidental disorder, without substantial association. Examples of these conditions include major fractures, spinal cord injury, and traumatic brain injury. Finally, in a few cases, the presence of a disabling condition may contribute to the development of diabetes. An example of this would be an individual with multiple sclerosis who requires steroids to prevent progression of the disease and who, as a result of becoming sedentary, gains weight, thus precipitating symptomatic diabetes. This chapter will focus on those disabling conditions for which diabetes is known to be a risk factor, with some comments on recurring issues affecting individuals with diabetes who have non–diabetes-related disability.

Certain interactions between diabetes and disability are common to many disabling conditions. During the acute phase of a disabling injury or illness, glycemic control may be worsened. During the rehabilitation phase, reduced activity can contribute to increased blood glucose levels and lead to an increased need for insulin or oral hypoglycemic agents. As activity level increases during the rehabilitation process, however, there is often a need to gradually restore diabetic pharmacotherapy to baseline pre-illness levels. The ultimate level of activity and exercise achieved by an individual with diabetes and a disabling condition varies widely. Some disabled individuals are competitive athletes, participating in marathons and mountain climbing, whereas others may become sedentary as a result of their disability.

The ability of diabetic individuals to manage their diabetes may also be significantly affected by disability. Disorders affecting cognitive ability, such as stroke or traumatic brain injury, frequently limit the ability of the diabetic individual to monitor his or her blood glucose levels and self-administer medication. Limitations in motor control present in many neurological conditions can interfere with self-administration of insulin. Dysphagia may interfere with taking oral medications, as well as have an impact on diet and the prompt treatment of hypoglycemia.

Specific Disabling Conditions

Stroke

Stroke is the most common cause of acquired disability in adults in the U.S., with over 4 million stroke survivors alive in the U.S. today.[1] The relative risk of stroke attributable to diabetes is 1.4 for men and 1.7 for women.[2]

Exercise for Diabetic Patients After a Stroke

One of the most frequent manifestations of stroke is weakness of the affected side. The presence of hemiparesis or hemiplegia significantly affects a stroke survivor's ability to perform activities of daily living as well as engage in exercise. Therapeutic exercise constitutes a key portion of post-stroke rehabilitation, despite limited data on the optimal exercise programs for the stroke survivor. Over the course of rehabilitation, the ability to ambulate is often regained, but walking frequently requires the use of a brace and/or ambulatory aids such as a cane, four-pronged ("quad") cane, or hemiwalker. Because of the decreased efficiency of hemiplegic gait, reductions in walking speed and increased oxygen consumption typically result.[3] In patients who require the use of a brace, skin integrity should be monitored carefully, particularly in those with diabetic neuropathy or stroke-induced sensory loss. Further discussion of brace use in disabled diabetic individuals is provided below.

Therapeutic exercise post-stroke is used both to improve motor control and to increase independence in functional tasks. There are a variety of treatment approaches that have been advocated for therapeutic exercise post-stroke but little data to support the use of any specific approach over others. Multiple studies[4–11] have examined a variety of techniques, including proprioceptive neuromuscular facilitation (PNF) techniques, the Bobath (neurodevelopmental [NDT]) technique, and others, and have failed to demonstrate any meaningful benefits to these specialized techniques over "functionally oriented" therapeutic exercise. Most centers in the U.S. favor an ill-defined "standard approach," which is primarily functionally oriented and often draws variably from the other techniques (NDT, PNF, etc.) mentioned above. This approach emphasizes the provision of physical assistance and encouragement for the stroke patient during functional or prefunctional tasks, with gradual withdrawal of this support as the individual's ability to perform the task improves. This approach incorporates exercise in compensatory techniques to improve functional abilities during therapy sessions.

Some have theorized that a portion of the decreased function seen after stroke may be due to "learned disuse."[12] This hypothesis suggests that there is a learned behavior of distrusting the paretic limb because of severe weakness that develops early after a stroke. It also suggests that relearning to use the limb is incomplete because of these behavioral limitations, despite underlying improvement in neurological function. Several small studies[12–15] have demonstrated improved functional use of the paretic upper limb in chronic stable stroke patients by forcing use of the paretic limb through restraining the normal arm. Changes in brain activation have been demonstrated as a result of such training.[16] Animal studies have also demonstrated that motor activity enhances recovery after stroke.[17,18] Together, these studies have led to an increased interest in exercise as a means of improving neurological recovery rather than focusing on it exclusively as a means of compensation after a stroke. The ultimate implications of this research for the exercise prescription in stroke survivors remain to be determined.

Cardiovascular Considerations in Exercise After a Stroke

The shared risk factors between coronary artery disease (CAD) and stroke result in a prevalence of cardiovascular disease as high as 75% in individuals who sustain a stroke.[19] Of individuals with transient ischemic attack, stroke, or an asymptomatic carotid bruit, 35% had evidence of severe CAD (defined as >70% stenosis of one or more coronary arteries) in one series, with only 7% having normal coronary arteries.[20] Cardiac disease is the most common cause of death after stroke.[21] This high prevalence of CAD contributes to an increased likelihood that cardiac instability or ischemia will be precipitated by exercise carried out as part of a stroke rehabilitation program.[22] The increased prevalence of silent myocardial ischemia among diabetic individuals[23,24] raises the question of whether routine screening for exercise-induced cardiac ischemia should be undertaken for individuals undergoing intensive rehabilitation after a stroke (see Chapters 13–15, 24, and 39). Exercise stress testing has been proposed as a means of evaluating the presence and severity of CAD in post-stroke patients. A variety of adapted exercise testing techniques have been described that are suitable for use by hemiplegic individuals. These include arm, leg, or combined arm and leg ergometry, supine bicycle ergometry,[25] wheelchair ergometry, and low-velocity treadmill testing.[26] Cardiac monitoring during physical therapy has been used to monitor for exercise-induced ischemia or arrhythmia.[22] Dipyridamole thallium-201 testing or dobutamine echocardiography can be used to induce cardiac stress and identify ischemia without exercise. Despite the availability of these techniques, however, there have been no large-scale studies demonstrating improved outcomes as a result of routine cardiac testing in individuals after a stroke.

Deconditioning is often seen after a stroke because of the decreased ability of the patient to participate in walking and other forms of exercise. In lower-extremity ergometry tasks, stroke patients were unable to achieve the same workload as age-matched control subjects.[27] This deconditioning can be reduced through structured exercise programs designed to accommodate any residual physical disability. Increases in exercise duration, workload, and maximal O_2 consumption can result from aerobic training programs after a stroke.[28]

Complications of Exercise After a Stroke

There are reports suggesting an increased risk of median nerve entrapment at the wrist (carpal tunnel syndrome [CTS]) in hemiparetic stroke patients. This may be due to overuse of the neurologically intact upper extremity and wrist because of cane use.[29] Symptoms suggestive of CTS should be promptly evaluated in diabetic individuals after stroke because of the combined risk factors of stroke and diabetes. Treatment of CTS of the neurologically intact upper extremity in hemiparetic stroke survivors is complicated by difficulty in donning and doffing splints of the intact wrist and by the substantial temporary disability that results after carpal tunnel release surgery.

Amputation

Amputation remains a feared complication of diabetes despite improvements in foot care. Individuals with a unilateral, below-the-knee amputation (BKA) may be able to resume high levels of activity and exercise. The increased energy cost of ambulation associated with bilateral BKA is greater than that associated with unilateral BKA but less than that associated with a unilateral above-the-knee amputation (AKA) (Fig. 34.1).[3] Bilateral AKAs impose a high workload burden for prosthetic ambulation, and as a result, only a minority of individuals become successful prosthetic ambulators after bilateral AKA. It is important to recognize the energy efficiency of wheelchair mobility, which is superior to even a unilateral BKA.[3]

Gait velocity in individuals with BKA due to vascular disease is reduced by 44%, and oxygen consumption per unit distance is increased by 33%.[30] Individuals with shorter residual limbs have increased energy consumption than individuals with longer residual limbs.[31]

Exercise in diabetic individuals with leg amputation should take into account the high prevalence of vascular insufficiency and increased risk of injury to the intact leg. Claudication is common and may limit exercise tolerance. The intact leg should be monitored closely for any skin breakdown or evidence of ischemia to prevent progression to a more serious injury.

Neuropathy

Neuropathy is an important contributor to disability in individuals with diabetes. In cases that progress to motor weakness, there is a decreased ability to dorsiflex the ankles, resulting in "foot drop" and the need for ankle foot orthoses (AFOs) (see LOWER-EXTREMITY BRACES

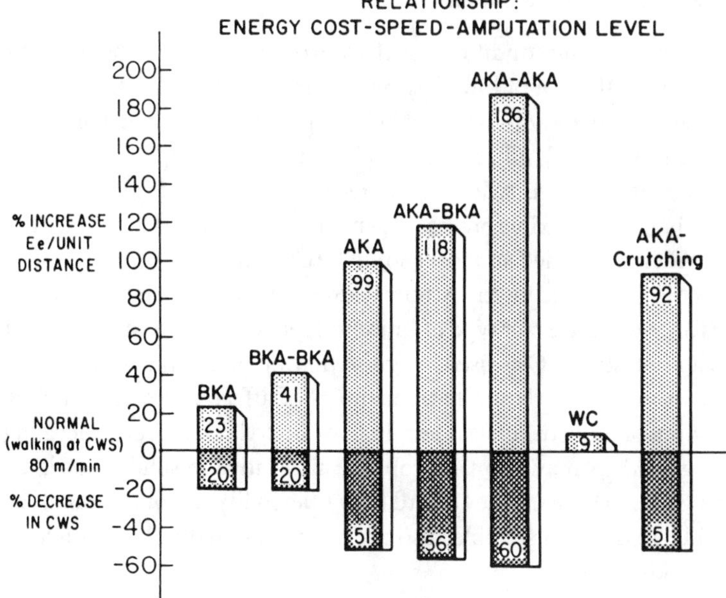

FIGURE 34.1 Energy cost of prosthetic ambulation. The energy cost of prosthetic ambulation is shown for BKA, AKA, and wheelchair propulsion (WC). The percentage increase in energy expenditure (Ee) per unit distance is shown, as is the percentage reduction at a comfortable walking speed (CWS).

Reproduced with permission from Gonzalez and Corcoran.[3]

below). Because of the associated loss of sensation, skin integrity must be monitored closely when braces are prescribed. Exercise programs must take into account the risk of skin breakdown when the level of physical activity is increased. Neuropathy may impair proprioception and balance. Compensation with ambulatory aids such as a cane or walker is often useful, with braces playing a role in treatment for any associated weakness.

In severe cases of diabetic neuropathy, a Charcot arthropathy may develop, typically in the foot and/or ankle. This is usually associated with substantial limitation in the ability to engage in lower-extremity exercise, although walking remains an option for some. In severe cases, Charcot arthropathy can lead to amputation, with its resulting impact on exercise abilities. Upper-extremity ergometry may be an alternative form of exercise for the motivated patient.

Lower-Extremity Braces

Certain disabling conditions, such as stroke and diabetic neuropathy, necessitate the use of lower-extremity braces. Typically, these braces are custom made and consist of lightweight plastics or metal braces attached to shoes. Unilateral braces have a smaller impact on exercise than bilateral braces. More rigid braces have a larger impact on exercise than more flexible braces. In general, the least restrictive brace that provides the needed support should be chosen.

Many specific lower-extremity exercises are limited by the use of braces, with the exact type of brace influencing the limitation. When a rigid plastic AFO is used, exercise that involves ankle movements may be significantly limited. Examples of affected exercises include walking on hilly or uneven terrain, Nordic style skiing, and bicycling. Hinged AFOs may be an appropriate alternative to solid AFOs in select patients because they afford better flexibility in dorsiflexion. Less solid AFOs, when suitable, also allow for more natural movement at the ankle joint.

Other General Rehabilitation Issues

As in stroke, CTS can develop in disabled individuals who use canes or other ambulatory aids and should be identified and treated before substantial nerve injury develops. Patients with diabetes may experience multiple disabling conditions concurrently, such as stroke and amputation or stroke and peripheral neuropathy. Exercise programs for such individuals need to be carefully individualized, with realistic goals set. Multidisciplinary rehabilitation programs are often useful to coordinate therapeutic exercise programs for any individual with a newly acquired disability and are particularly important for those with more than one disabling condition.

References

1. Anonymous: *Heart and Stroke Facts.* Dallas, TX, American Heart Association, 2000
2. Wolf PA, D'Agostino RB, Belanger AJ, Kannel WB: Probability of stroke: a risk profile from the Framingham Study. *Stroke* 22:312–18, 1991

3. Gonzalez EG, Corcoran PJ: Energy expenditure during ambulation. In *The Physiological Basis of Rehabilitation Medicine.* 2nd ed. Downey JA, Myers SJ, Gonzalez EG, Lieberman JS, Eds. Boston, MA, Butterworth-Heinemann, 1994, p. 431
4. Butefisch C, Hummelsheim H, Densler P, Mauritz K: Repetitive training of isolated movements improves the outcome of motor rehabilitation of the centrally paretic hand. *J Neurol Sci* 130:59–68, 1995
5. Dickstein R, Hocherman S, Pillar T, Shaham R: Stroke rehabilitation: three exercise therapy approaches. *Phys Ther* 66:1233–38, 1986
6. Hesse SA, Jahnke MT, Bertelt CM, Schreiner C, Lucke D, Mauritz KH: Gait outcome in ambulatory hemiparetic patients after a 4-week comprehensive rehabilitation program and prognostic factors. *Stroke* 25:1999–2004, 1994
7. Jongbloed L, Stacey S, Brighton C: Stroke rehabilitation: sensorimotor integrative treatment versus functional treatment. *Am J Occup Ther* 43:391–97, 1989
8. Logigian MK, Samuels MA, Falconer JF: Clinical exercise trial for stroke patients. *Arch Phys Med Rehabil* 64:364–67, 1983
9. Lord JP, Hall K: Neuromuscular reeducation versus traditional programs for stroke rehabilitation. *Arch Phys Med Rehabil* 67:88–91, 1986
10. Stern PH, McDowell F, Miller JM, Robinson M: Effects of facilitation exercise techniques in stroke rehabilitation. *Arch Phys Med Rehabil* 51:526–31, 1970
11. Wagenaar RC, Meijer OG, van Wieringen PC, Kuik DJ, Hazenberg GJ, Lindeboom J, Wichers F, Rijswijk H: The functional recovery of stroke: a comparison between neurodevelopmental treatment and the Brunnstrom method. *Scand J Rehab Med* 22:1–8, 1990
12. Taub E, Miller NE, Novack TA, Cook EW 3rd, Fleming WC, Nepomuceno CS, Connell JS, Crago JE: Technique to improve chronic motor deficit after stroke. *Arch Phys Med Rehabil* 74: 347–54, 1993
13. Kunkel A, Bopp B, Muller G, Villringer K, Villringer A, Taub E, Flor H: Constraint-induced movement therapy for motor recovery in chronic stroke patients. *Arch Phys Med Rehabil* 80:624–28, 1999
14. Miltner WHR, Bauder H, Sommer M, Dettmers C, Taub E: Effects of constraint-induced movement therapy on patients with chronic motor deficits after stroke: a replication. *Stroke* 30:586–92, 1999

15. Wolf SL, LeCraw DE, Barton LA, Jann BB: Forced use of hemiplegic upper extremities to reverse the effect of learned nonuse among chronic stroke and head-injured patients. *Exp Neurol* 104: 125–32, 1989
16. Liepert J, Bauder H, Miltner WHR, Taub E, Weiller C: Treatment-induced cortical reorganization after stroke in humans. *Stroke* 31:1210–16, 2000
17. Ohlsson A-L, Johansson BB: The environment influences functional outcome of cerebral infarction in rats. *Stroke* 26:644–49, 1995
18. Johansson BB: Functional outcome in rats transferred to an enriched environment 15 days after focal brain ischemia. *Stroke* 27: 324–26, 1996
19. Roth EJ: Heart disease in patients with stroke: incidence, impact, and implications for rehabilitation. I. Classification and prevalence. *Arch Phys Med Rehabil* 74:752–60, 1993
20. Hertzer NR, Young JR, Beven EG, Graor RA, O'Hara PJ, Ruschhaupt WF 3rd, deWolfe VG, Maljovec LC: Coronary angiography in 506 patients with extracranial cerebrovascular disease. *Arch Intern Med* 145:849–52, 1985
21. Matsumoto N, Whisnant JP, Kurland LT, Okazaki H: Natural history of stroke in Rochester, Minnesota, 1955 through 1969: an extension of a previous study, 1945 through 1954. *Stroke* 4: 20–29, 1973
22. Roth EJ, Mueller K, Green D: Cardiovascular response to physical therapy in stroke rehabilitation. *Neuro Rehabil* 2:7–15, 1992
23. Nesto RW, Phillips RT, Kett KG, Hill T, Perper E, Young E, Leland OS Jr: Angina and exertional myocardial ischemia in diabetic and nondiabetic patients: assessment by exercise thallium scintigraphy. *Ann Intern Med* 108:170–75, 1988
24. Zarich S, Waxman S, Freeman R, Mittleman M, Hegarty P, Nesto RW: Effect of autonomic nervous system dysfunction on the circadian pattern of myocardial ischemia in diabetes mellitus. *J Am Coll Cardiol* 24:956–62, 1994
25. Moldover JR, Daum MC, Downey JA: Cardiac stress testing of hemiparetic patients with a supine bicycle ergometer: preliminary study. *Arch Phys Med Rehabil* 65:470–76, 1984
26. Macko RF, Katzel LI, Yataco A, Tretter LD, DeSouza CA, Dengel DR, Smith GV, Silver KH: Low velocity graded treadmill stress testing in hemiparetic stroke patients. *Stroke* 28:988–92, 1997

27. Monga TN, Deforge DA, Williams J, Wolfe LA: Cardiovascular responses to acute exercise in patients with cerebrovascular responses to acute exercise in patients with cerebrovascular accidents. *Arch Phys Med Rehabil* 69:937–40, 1988
28. Potempa K, Lopez M, Braun LT, Szidon JP, Fogg L, Tincknell T: Physiological outcomes of aerobic exercise training in hemiparetic stroke patients. *Stroke* 26:101–05, 1995
29. Sato Y, Kaji M, Tsuru T, Oizumi K: Carpal tunnel syndrome involving unaffected limbs of stroke patients. *Stroke* 30:414–18, 1999
30. Waters RL, Perry J, Chambers R: Energy expenditure of amputee gait. In *Lower Extremity Amputation*. Moore WS, Malone JM, Eds. Philadelphia, W.B. Saunders, 1989, p. 250–60
31. Gonzalez EG, Corcoran PJ, Reyes RL: Energy expenditure in below knee amputees: correlation with stump length. *Arch Phys Med Rehabil* 55:111–19, 1974

Joel Stein, MD, is from the Spaulding Rehabilitation Hospital, Boston, MA.

Sports: Practical Advice and Experience

35

The Diabetic Athlete as a Role Model

PAULA HARPER, RN, CDE

Great accomplishments in the 2000 Olympic Games by athletes with diabetes underscore successes in the management of the disease in competitive sports. With advances in knowledge and technology over the last 25 years, high levels of athletic performance have been regularly achieved. Previously, active people with diabetes lacked sufficient guidelines for integrating training with diabetes management. Over and over, people who wanted to exercise had to learn by trial and error.

Today, with increased knowledge of the relationship between diabetes and exercise (see Chapters 14, 20, and 21), participating in regular physical activity is no longer like reinventing the wheel. Now, a bad knee injury is more likely to keep someone sidelined from a professional sport than is diabetes. This chapter highlights a few of the noted professional athletes and other amateur athletes with diabetes who paved the way. Often, the first concern of an athlete faced with a diagnosis of diabetes is "Will I still be able to play?"

Chris Dudley

"Will I be able to continue playing ball?" was professional basketball player Chris Dudley's first question to his doctor when he was diagnosed with type 1 diabetes during his sophomore year in high school. Dudley's physician told him he could continue to play basketball; his coaches were understanding and supportive.

Dudley, a 14-year veteran of the NBA, tests his blood glucose levels frequently because of his busy schedule. He adjusts his insulin and carbohydrate intake differently for game days, practice days, and travel days. Dudley reads nutrition labels, counts carbohydrates, and watches his food intake carefully, especially on the road.

As a role model for active kids with diabetes, Dudley spends time helping them realize they can play any sport they like, as long as they take care of themselves. He also enjoys scuba diving and spending time with his two children. Dudley currently is a member of the Phoenix Suns, and in 1999, played in the NBA finals with the New York Knicks.

Curt Fraser

Curt Fraser has spent the last 23 years in professional hockey, including his last two seasons as the Head Coach for the NHL's Atlanta Thrashers. He joined the Thrashers after a highly successful minor league coaching career and 12 years as a player with the Vancouver Canucks (1978–1983), Chicago Blackhawks (1983–1988), and Minnesota North Stars (1988–1990).

It was during his fifth NHL season in 1983 that Fraser was diagnosed with diabetes. After learning he had diabetes, Fraser was fortunate to be introduced to Bobby Clarke by a mutual friend. "That was the best thing that could have happened to me at that time," Fraser recalls. "Clarke, a player for the Philadelphia Flyers, had diabetes most of his life, and he told me exactly how he controlled it and how he managed it when he was playing. That eliminated a lot of the experimenting I would have had to do and I basically followed what he did."

Fraser was also fortunate that the Chicago Blackhawks, and especially general manager Bob Pulford, were solidly behind him when he was diagnosed with diabetes. Fraser recalls phoning Pulford not knowing what his reaction would be. "It was quite a relief when he told me that his brother had diabetes and to just make sure that I showed up to training camp in good shape."

Fraser's daily routine reflects how strongly he believes in self-monitoring of blood glucose. He checks his blood glucose four or five times a day to help maintain tighter control. After 18 years of taking shots, Fraser has recently changed to an insulin pump, which has made a significant difference in his daily routines and improved blood glucose control.

Fraser has served as the honorary chairman of Team Diabetes and hosted the Curt Fraser Golf Classic for 12 years to help raise funds to benefit diabetes research and kids' camps. He has served on the board of the Diabetes Exercise and Sports Association and continues to work with the American Diabetes Association and Canadian Diabetes Association to help raise awareness and funds for diabetes research and education.

Jonathan Hayes

Jonathan Hayes was diagnosed with type 1 diabetes in college. In his book, *Necessary Toughness*, he recounts, "I had always valued a healthy body, a strong physique, and I had been willing to pay the price to maintain it. Now the cost was going up. Now the cost included extra care about diet, extra attention during exercise, insulin shots, frequent finger pricks to check my sugar level. I would have to become the doctor of my own body, learning about its processes and fine-tuning my own lifestyle to accommodate it." He goes on to describe how he dealt with diabetes while pursuing a career in professional football.

Hayes spent 12 years playing professional football with the Kansas City Chiefs and the Pittsburgh Steelers. His professional football career included three AFC championship games and one Super Bowl. Currently, Hayes is the Special Teams Coordinator for the University of Oklahoma football team. In 2000, his team had a perfect 13-0 season and a National Championship victory in the Orange Bowl. In his spare time, Hayes enjoys spending time at his horse ranch and working part-time on radio and television.

Michelle McGann

LPGA golf pro Michelle McGann was diagnosed with type 1 diabetes at the age of 13. Golf has been a part of her life since she was 7 years old. McGann recalls, "Insulin became a life tool for me and my golf game at the beginning of my teenage years. Patience, perseverance, and a positive attitude have been goals in golf and with diabetic control." McGann is currently using an insulin pump and states that it "has been the immense tool that has provided continuous insulin infusion and has enabled my career to continue on a championship level."

McGann's successful golf career includes seven LPGA victories. In 1999, she posted her season-best finish of fourth place in the Sara Lee Classic. In 1998, McGann competed in 25 tournaments and recorded six top-10 finishes.

In her spare time, McGann enjoys traveling, shopping, ceramics, and working out. She also actively contributes to charitable organizations.

Bill Carlson

Bill Carlson has been insulin dependent for 24 years. As a teenager, he was so active in sports, his high school friends nicknamed him "jock." Like many of his peers, Carlson measured his self-worth and ability to persevere by his bench press maximum and his 2-mile split on the track. One day in February 1977, Carlson recalls, "The warm-up bench press weight felt like a one-rep maximum press. How could I possibly be this weak after a flu bug illness?" Later that day, in a rush visit to the doctor, Carlson was diagnosed with type 1 diabetes.

Throughout Carlson's life, he has had many athletic successes. In high school, he had a successful football career. In his 20s, he raced as a track professional and then as an amateur triathlete, competing in five Hawaiian Ironman Triathlons, among hundreds of other races. In his 30s, he ran more marathons and ultramarathons, clocking in at 2:38:01 in the Los Angeles Marathon in 1991—a record for an insulin-dependent athlete.

Carlson believes that attitude is critical to coping with diabetes. "Attitude is everything in your personal and professional life. I look at challenges not as insurmountable hurdles, but as goals or accomplishment opportunities."

Now 40, Carlson enjoys spending time with his wife and two children. He holds a master's degree in physical therapy and has a successful career marketing medical products and pharmaceuticals.

Pam Fernandes

Pam Fernandes was diagnosed with type 1 diabetes in 1965 at the age of 4. During her childhood, she managed her disease by taking one shot a day and testing her urine for excess sugar. At age 18, while undergoing a routine eye examination, Fernandes was told she had small hemorrhages in her eyes, and the doctor recommended that she see a specialist. She soon discovered that the condition was serious. After laser treatment in both eyes and five surgeries, Fernandes was declared legally blind at the age of 21. Within 1 year, she learned that her kidneys also were failing. Kidney dialysis began in 1982. In 1987, Fernandes decided to have a kidney transplant—a decision that dramatically changed her life.

Before her diabetic complications, Fernandes led a very active life, being involved in softball and basketball all through elementary and high school. After the transplant, she was eager to return to a physically active life. Fernandes started slowly in a hospital cardiac rehabilitation program. Within months, she was encouraged to join the local gym. After 6 months of working out, she tested in the top 10% in cardiovascular fitness for women her age.

Needing goals to keep her motivated, Fernandes became interested in fund-raising events like the American Diabetes Association's Tour de Cure. She's been hooked on tandem cycling ever since.

Fernandes's bike racing career started in 1993 with a humble beginning—in her first race, she and her partner finished dead last. Never giving up, Fernandes continued to compete with increasing success in her bike racing and in her diabetes management. She got stronger, leaner, and felt better.

Fernandes's persistence and dedication paid off. She is now one of the most well-known tandem cyclists in the U.S and one of the fastest in the world, earning at least one National Championship every year from 1993 through 2000. Her most recent and most impressive athletic accomplishment was at the 2000 Sydney Paralympic Games, where she and her partner astounded the world by bringing home the first Gold Medal in tandem cycling for the U.S. in Paralympic history.

Diabetes management is challenging for Fernandes. Her current regimen includes four shots per day. All insulin is adjusted on a sliding scale depending on her exercise, current blood glucose level, and carbohydrate intake. She tests her glucose level six to ten times per day and much more often during heavy training and competition.

Fernandes will race as long as she can. She also plans to continue educating those around her about diabetes and the need for fund-raising for research to find a cure.

W. Guyton Hornsby, Jr.

In 1973, W. Guyton Hornsby, Jr., remembers reading an article on running and diabetes in a popular running magazine in which the author stated that it was impossible for a person with diabetes to run farther than 8 miles. He immediately put down the magazine and went out and ran 10 miles. Hornsby recalls, "I became interested in finding out if there were limits to what could be accomplished in sports if you had diabetes. Since that time, I have devoted my life to the scientific study of diabetes and exercise."

Hornsby was diagnosed with type 1 diabetes in 1967 at the age of 15. Throughout his life, he has participated in many different sports. In high school, he competed in football, wrestling, and track and field, continuing football and track and field in college. After college, Hornsby participated in weight lifting (Olympic-style lifting) and marathon running. He coached track and field at the University of South Carolina while a graduate assistant, coached high school track and field, and coached the weight lifting and track and field teams at Louisiana State University. Currently, Hornsby participates in track and field, recreational running, and recreational weight lifting.

Hornsby developed diabetes when there was little blood glucose monitoring, and standard treatment was one shot of Lente or NPH insulin daily. This treatment was easy, but the only measure of control was urine glucose testing and a fasting blood glucose measurement every 3 months. Insulin doses rarely changed, and information on diabetes and exercise in general, let alone diabetes and competitive sports, was sparse.

Because Hornsby exercises almost daily, he makes no insulin adjustments for exercise and ingests extra carbohydrates to compensate for any drops in blood glucose. His HbA_{1c} has been in the normal range since 1984, and he has had no diabetic complications after 34 years with the disease.

In his spare time, Hornsby plays the guitar and draws and paints. He also coaches a local youth track program and does all he can to help other athletes with diabetes improve their performances. In his work as an exercise physiologist, Hornsby is studying weight training for people with type 2 diabetes and is researching ways to improve exercise compliance in these patients.

David Marrero

David Marrero has been an athlete all of his life. He participated in football and track and field in high school and attended college on a football scholarship. Currently, Marrero participates in karate and bicycling. In karate, he holds a sixth-degree black belt. He commutes to work on his bicycle (a 44-mile roundtrip) two to three times a week and occasionally participates in bicycle races.

In all of his sports activities, he considers diabetes to be an incidental issue and something that he can work with, but by no means considers diabetes a controlling factor. Marrero explains, "Exercise makes it easier for me to control my diabetes. I train the same as my friends who do not have diabetes; however, I do make some adjustments in order to avoid acute problems such as hypoglycemia. For example, I always test my blood sugar prior to a workout. Depending on the value, I eat some carbs and/or adjust my insulin. If I plan on a long-term event, such as a long bike ride, I will reduce my basal insulin and test during the ride. I always carry some type of rapid-acting glucose to raise my blood sugar if the need arises." After exercising, Marrero closely monitors his glucose levels to avoid postexercise hypoglycemia.

Marrero recalls, "Sports have taught me many valuable lessons: teamwork, setting goals, and the importance of proper training and hard work. These are lessons that apply to dealing with my diabetes as well. As any athlete will tell you, the only limits are the ones you place upon yourself."

Steve Prosterman

Steve Prosterman was diagnosed with type 1 diabetes in 1966 at the age of 9. He credits sports as being the reason he has always led a healthy and active life.

Prosterman's sports accomplishments center around scuba diving, and he has been instrumental in gaining acceptance for individuals with diabetes to scuba dive. At his adventure camp for adults in the U.S. Virgin Islands, Prosterman has developed protocols that are now used worldwide and accepted as the safest guidelines for diabetes and scuba diving. He has been on the cover of *Scuba Diving* magazine twice and is cited in many other dive and diabetes magazines. He has also participated in triathlons and other running and bike races, is an avid windsurfer, and enjoys basketball, ocean swimming, weight training, and sea kayaking.

Prosterman's insulin regimen consists of multiple injections of Humalog before meals and NPH at bedtime. He does six to eight blood tests per day and more if participating in certain activities. For instance, before diving or windsurfing, he does three tests within an hour to determine not only his blood glucose level, but the direction of his glucose level (whether it is going up or down). If the level is going down, he eats a carbohydrate snack before proceeding.

Prosterman hopes to continue his camp in the U.S. Virgin Islands. He recently received his master's degree in educational counseling and hopes to get a degree in school psychology. He believes that diabetes has never held him back, although he feels the disease must be taken care of properly to enable a person to participate in any sports activity.

Conclusion

Today, many athletes successfully manage their diabetes. All maintain that self-monitoring of blood glucose is essential, that teammates and coaches are supportive, and that diabetes does not need to adversely affect their performance. These athletes serve as extraordinary role models; they are examples of the success to which an athlete with diabetes can aspire.

Paula Harper, RN, CDE, is founder of the International Diabetic Athletes Association and is currently Nashville, TN, coordinator of the VA Study, Glycemic Control and Complications in Diabetes Mellitus Type 2.

In Remembrance

The following is a glimpse at the life of the late Bill Talbert, a legendary tennis doubles champion who lived 70 years with diabetes. His life is truly inspirational and should be recognized and remembered.

NEIL RUDERMAN, MD, DPHIL
Editor-in-Chief

Bill Talbert, a legendary doubles champion who defied diabetes and went on to gain 33 national titles over 6 decades of tennis prominence, died February 28, 1999, at the age of 80. Talbert had been in declining health since sustaining a broken shoulder and pelvis, and later undergoing hip-replacement surgery, as the result of a mugging at a La Guardia Airport taxi stand in 1992 while on his way home from the United States Tennis Association's annual board meeting.

Talbert, who was diagnosed with diabetes at the age of 10, had been warned away from the playing fields but became fixated on the noncontact sport of tennis as a teenager. He was a singles finalist at the United States Championships, as the United States Open was then known, in 1944 and 1945, losing each time to Frank Parker. But he went on to claim eight doubles titles at that event, and he became the Open's tournament director from 1971 to 1975 and from 1978 to 1987. As an official, Talbert was instrumental in the adoption of the sudden-death tie breaker, an innovation that was initially unpopular with most players but received raves from spectators. "I never knew a player who bought a ticket," he said in defense of his successful lobbying for the tie breaker.

As a singles player, as a doubles partner, as a Davis Cup team member, and as the Davis Cup team captain for 5 years, Talbert was a stylish tactician of the sport that helped him transcend the lifelong limitations enforced by diabetes.

He was best known for playing the right side next to his favorite partner, the spirited Gardnar Mulloy. "He played the forehand, I played the backhand, and if I was the power behind the partnership, he was surely the stylist up front," said Mulloy, who reached six United States National doubles finals, one short of a team record, alongside Talbert. "Billy was the greatest doubles player we ever had, and he was a great friend; for 10 years there wasn't another American team that could beat us." Talbert and Mulloy captured four of the six United States finals they reached, claiming titles in 1942, 1945, 1946, and 1948.

Talbert collected nine major doubles titles, four of them in the United States mixed event with Margaret Osborne duPont, with whom he set a record by winning consecutive championships from 1943 to 1946. He won the French doubles championship in 1950 with the 20-year-old Tony Trabert, a fellow Cincinnatian for whom he served as mentor. Talbert's Davis Cup career as a player began in 1946 and concluded in 1952–1953, when he was the team's playing captain.

Talbert, a native of Cincinnati, entered the International Tennis Hall of Fame in 1967. He was also active in parlaying his tennis contacts into the business world, becoming executive vice president of the United States Banknote Corporation, a financial printing firm, in 1964. He remained with the company until his death.

36

Strength Training and Nutritional Supplements

ROBERT D. CHETLIN, MS, CSCS, AND
W. GUYTON HORNSBY, JR., PHD, CDE

Highlights

- Physicians and other health care professionals should be familiar with concepts associated with prescribing resistance exercise for athletes and should be able to advise patient athletes on training practices that may interfere with glycemic control or place these patients at unnecessary risk.
- There is no evidence that training with heavy or maximal loads is unsafe for fit diabetic patients without long-term complications.
- Sufficient protein intake should always be considered within the context of total energy intake. Resistance-trained individuals who consume adequate amounts of protein as part of a balanced diet do not generally require additional sources of protein.
- It is likely that taking creatine and carbohydrates together may require an adjustment in insulin therapy

that should take into account the carbohydrate amount, the creatine dose, and the training activity.

- Athletes with diabetes should avoid taking anabolic steroids and large amounts of steroid precursors.
- Use of nutritional supplements should always be discussed by the athlete with a physician or other qualified member of the diabetes health care team.

Although resistance exercise is predominantly used in diabetes management to attain health benefits such as increased muscular strength and flexibility, enhanced body composition, or reduced cardiovascular disease risk, exceptional patients may have goals that go far beyond general health and fitness. Strength training has an essential role in training for sports, especially those in which muscular power and/or size are important. Athletes with diabetes have achieved remarkable success in the competitive sports of weight lifting, power lifting, and body building. Isaac Berger was a two-time Olympic champion in weight lifting, and Tim Belknap won the Mr. America title and went on to become a highly regarded professional body builder.

Athletes are often willing to accept any training formula that may give them an extra advantage, no matter how bizarre or unfounded. Recent developments in athletic competition have heightened interest in nutritional supplementation. Physicians and other health care professionals should be familiar with concepts associated with prescribing resistance exercises for athletes and should be able to advise patient athletes on training practices that may place them at unnecessary risk or interfere with glycemic control.

Prescribing Training Programs

Training programs used by competitive athletes are very different from those used by fitness enthusiasts or recreational lifters. Program design depends on manipulation of resistance training variables: choice of exercise, order of exercise, resistance (intensity or load used), volume of exercise (number of sets and repetitions performed), and length of rest between exercises (see Chapter 16). Although specific principles of program design for athletes are beyond the scope of this book, excellent comprehensive texts are available for those who may be interested.[1,2] It may also be helpful to contact the National Strength and Conditioning Association for help in identifying a Certified Strength and Conditioning Specialist in a specific location (National Strength and Conditioning Association, 1955 N. Union Blvd., Colorado Springs, CO 80909. Tel: 800-815-6826).

High-Intensity Strength Training

Development of maximal strength and power requires the use of high-intensity resistance training. Very intense weight lifting has been associated with large acute increases in blood pressure. Whereas this may be potentially harmful for patients with cardiac or vascular complications, researchers have reported using high-intensity resistance training without detrimental effects in geriatric patients,[3] cardiac patients,[4] and in one patient after laser surgery for diabetic retinopathy.[5] Thorough pre-exercise screening is advisable for any patient involved in intense resistance training. There is no evidence that training with heavy or maximal loads is contraindicated in fit diabetic patients without long-term complications.

Glycemic Control

Research on the glycemic response to intense resistance exercise has been limited when compared with the same type of research involving aerobic activity. Investigations of chronic resistance training have demonstrated improvements in insulin sensitivity and/or glucose tolerance in both diabetic and nondiabetic subjects. The acute response to intense resistance exercise is typically a moderate increase in blood glucose (~20–40 mg/dl) during the exercise session, with reduced insulin requirements or delayed-onset hypoglycemia appearing many hours (perhaps as long as 48 h) after the session ends. Athletes should be advised to make appropriate adjustments in food intake or insulin dosage based on frequent self-monitoring of blood glucose.

Training Risks

Properly designed training programs can improve physical appearance and athletic performance, but quantity and quality of improvement are largely determined by genetic potential. Unreasonable expectations and a win-at-all-cost philosophy can cause some athletes to experiment with fraudulent, hazardous, and/or illegal training aids. Health care professionals should be able to advise athletes on proper nutrition[6] and the risks of using illegal anabolic-androgenic acids and dietary supplements.[7]

Nutritional Supplements

Interest in dietary strategies and nutritional supplementation by athletes has grown dramatically. The multitude of nutritional supplements available today is staggering, and all claim to offer certain performance or health benefits. The extent of misinformation conveyed through deceptive or false advertising for these products is quite alarming. The problems may become compounded for the athlete or health fitness enthusiast with diabetes. Unfortunately, little scientific research exists that addresses the specific physiological and performance effects in diabetic individuals. Use of nutritional supplements by the athlete should always be discussed with a physician or other qualified member of the diabetes health care team. Some of the more popular nutritional supplements currently being used are discussed below.

Protein/Protein Supplementation

Resistance-trained individuals, both competitive athletes and health and fitness enthusiasts, who consume adequate amounts of protein as part of a balanced diet do not generally require additional sources of protein. As part of a recent position statement concerning nutrition and athletic performance, the American College of Sports Medicine asserts that highly active people, particularly strength-trained individuals, may need to consume ~2 g protein/kg body wt/day to maintain their activity levels.[8] Typically, this protein intake can be met through diet alone by consuming a variety of whole reference proteins. These include highly digestible proteins, such as eggs, chicken, fish, and lean red meat, which contain all 10 essential amino acids.

Sufficient protein intake should always be considered within the context of total energy intake. For strength-trained athletes, both recreational and competitive, this means that enough total calories must be consumed to maintain body weight or to increase lean body mass. Highly trained individuals may need to ingest ≥50 calories/kg body wt/day to meet the goal of maintaining or increasing muscle mass.[8] This caloric intake should be balanced and should be consistent with the nutritional recommendations and principles for people with diabetes.[9]

In the case where protein supplements may be indicated, it is recommended that these be taken in hydrolysated form (i.e., partially predigested), contain all 10 essential amino acids, and not contain proportionally more fillers (especially fat). The use of individual amino acids has been a popular practice in the weight-trained community, but scientific studies have been inconclusive regarding their effectiveness. It is recommended, therefore, that if protein supplements are chosen, they should contain an abundance of amino acids, including all the essential amino acids.

Strength-trained individuals with diabetes require adequate amounts of protein intake just like all other individuals engaged in resistance exercise. Large amounts of protein, however, place additional stress on the kidneys. Individuals in poor control or who suffer diabetic complications involving the kidneys should consult their diabetes health care team before altering the protein composition of their diet.

Creatine Monohydrate

Creatine has become the most popular nutritional supplement. It is relatively inexpensive compared with most other supplements and has demonstrated performance improvements under certain conditions. Creatine is a naturally occurring biochemical compound that is synthesized in the liver, kidney, and pancreas from the amino acids arginine, glycine, and methionine. Creatine phosphate maintains cellular ATP balance, and phosphocreatine availability is the rate-limiting factor in short, maximal exertion. With intense maximal bouts of exercise, phosphocreatine depletion is associated with fatigue. Studies have demonstrated that both trained and untrained individuals ingesting creatine monohydrate increased their plasma creatine concentration and muscle creatine pool, delayed fatigue, improved recovery (by increasing the amount of phosphocreatine resynthesis), and increased levels of performance in various repeated bouts of maximal voluntary exercise.[10] It must be stated, however, that these positive results have been consistently demonstrated in laboratory investigations and not in competitive athletic environments.

Recent studies have demonstrated that creatine supplementation increased lean body mass (up to 9 lb), although it is uncertain if such an increase was due completely to an actual increase in lean tissue or if the effect was contributed to by an increase in intracellular water. However, a reasonable amount of evidence indicates that some of the weight gain may be due to an increase in protein synthesis. One recent study demonstrated that the combined effects of creatine and resistance training had a greater effect on increases in lean body mass and changes in body composition than either training or supplementation alone.[11]

Increases in plasma creatine concentration and the muscle creatine pool appear greatest in those subjects with the lowest initial creatine volume and less in individuals with high creatine content, although concurrent carbohydrate consumption appears to improve muscle saturation regardless of initial creatine levels.[12] Creatine entry into muscle is a saturable process, with uptake greatest during the first supplemental bouts. Muscle creatine remains elevated, however, with high-dose supplementation (20 g/day for 5 days) followed by a maintenance dose (2–5 g/day). Virtually identical saturation effects occur if 5 g/day is consumed without the high-dose ("loading" dose) portion, although this typically takes 2–3 weeks longer to achieve.[13] Recently, claims have been made that creatine ingested in various concoctions, including liquid form, promotes improved absorption into cells, although no scientific study corroborates such an effect.

Creatine may be taken into cells without insulin because of its association with a specific transporter. There is some evidence, however, that creatine combined with carbohydrates heightens insulin's effect on creatine transport.[12] This may enable saturation of the tissues to a level greater than that of taking creatine alone. There is no evidence to indicate how the concurrent administration of carbohydrates and creatine would affect levels of exogenous insulin taken by individuals with diabetes. It is therefore not advisable to attempt this regimen without consulting a physician or certified diabetes educator. It is quite likely that taking creatine and carbohydrates together may require an adjustment in insulin administration that should take into account the carbohydrate amount, the creatine dose, and the expected level and proximity of training activity.

Advertisers' claims that creatine monohydrate is a strength inducer for short-term, repeated maximal efforts appear to have some merit.[14] No ergogenic response was observed when low-dose regimens were used (<2 g/day), prolonged recovery was permitted (5–25 min) between exercise bouts, or endurance exercise was used.[10] No adverse effects have been cited in the scientific literature, although anecdotal reports to the Food and Drug Administration have included cramping, rash, shortness of breath, vomiting, gastrointestinal distress, nervousness, migraine, and fatigue. Long-term effects have gained the attention of the scientific community but have yet to be established. Investigations to date have shown no ill effect of creatine on renal, hepatic, or cardiovascular function. Creatine monohydrate has proven useful under certain clinical conditions in which specific diseases, such as chronic heart failure, inborn metabolic errors, and muscular dystrophies, are associated with defects in creatine metabolism.[14–17]

Androstenedione

Androstenedione, an androgen produced by the adrenal glands and gonads, has been used in Europe as a nasal spray and is available in the U.S. in tablet or capsule form. It has been described in the mass media as an anabolic steroid, but it is more appropriately described as a steroid precursor. Androstenedione has little activity that resembles that of anabolic steroids or testosterone. Its biochemical transformation occurs one step after dehydroepiandrosterone (DHEA) production and represents the immediate precursor to estrogen and testosterone.

Although huge exogenous doses of testosterone may increase nitrogen retention, muscle mass, and strength, the transient increases in testosterone observed with oral androstenedione appear to be insufficiently sustained to produce performance-enhancing effects. Androstenedione possesses little intrinsic activity and is largely reduced and conjugated before reaching peripheral tissues. Furthermore, androstenedione's metabolic fate upon mega-dose ingestion is similar to that of its sister metabolite, DHEA. Two independent scientific investigations found that oral androstenedione has no effect on protein metabolism, serum testosterone, or skeletal muscle morphology in recreationally active or weight-trained men. Androstenedione ingestion did, however, result in increased serum estradiol concentration in both studies. Furthermore, consumption of the supplement for 8 weeks resulted in a significant reduction in HDL cholesterol, and this decline represented an increased risk for cardiovascular disease.[18,19]

In men, increases in estrogen represent a negative effect on the accretion of lean muscle mass. This would likely represent a decline in strength-associated performance. Long-term effects of androstenedione are unknown, although adverse effects of elevated testosterone are well known, including heart, liver, and vascular problems. Because anabolic steroids and large amounts of steroid precursors could present physiological problems, which may magnify complications of diabetes, it is recommended that individuals with diabetes avoid these compounds. Furthermore, androstenedione has been added to the International Olympic Committee (IOC) and National Collegiate Athletic Association (NCAA) lists of banned substances. Competitive athletes, diabetic or not, must be aware of the consequences for consuming this supplement.

DHEA

Like its more popular counterpart androstenedione, DHEA is a weak adrenal androgen. It is the predominant androgen in women, where it functions to stimulate the libido. In men, DHEA's function is less clear, although recent evidence indicates it may play a role in immune function. DHEA is an intermediate in endogenous/synthetic testosterone production but does not raise testosterone levels by itself, because at high levels, DHEA will inhibit luteinizing hormone and follicle-stimulating hormone secretion. Oral consumption of DHEA in small doses (~50 mg) may cause transient increases in serum testosterone, but large doses are subject to first-pass metabolism in the liver and ultimately metabolized without effect on the circulating testosterone pool. However, DHEA supplementation has proven effective in both animals and humans when endogenous DHEA production slows or ceases completely.[20]

Additionally, at increased levels, DHEA can aromatize and lead to elevation of serum estrogen. No available investigation of oral supplementation with DHEA has demonstrated any clear ergogenic benefit in healthy, weight-trained individuals. No studies have been done involving the use of DHEA in individuals with diabetes. It is suggested that athletes with diabetes avoid DHEA (e.g., androstenedione) as well as other established steroid precursors.

α-Ketoisocaproate and β-hydroxy β-methylbutyrate

α-Ketoisocaproate (KIC) and β-hydroxy β-methylbutyrate (HMB) are catabolites of leucine, a branched-chain amino acid. KIC is the carbon "skeleton" of leucine. It has demonstrated anti-catabolic, anabolic effects in growing lambs and in hemodialysis patients.[21] HMB is also a leucine derivative. Animal studies using HMB have shown no anabolic effect with regard to body weight gain, and this supplement appears to be less effective than other related compounds of leucine. One study has shown increases in muscular strength in human subjects, but under suspect methodology. Other investigations have demonstrated equivocal results with regard to muscle hypertrophy and/or strength in humans.[21] It is unknown what effects KIC or HMB would have in diabetic individuals. It is recommended, therefore, that use of this supplement be discussed with the diabetes health care team.

Vanadyl Sulfate

Vanadium is a trace mineral, but it is not known if it is essential. The supplement has demonstrated insulin-like properties in liver and muscle preparations (in situ) as well as in experimental animals with induced diabetes.[22] Nondiabetic animals, however, show virtually no such insulin-like response. Vanadium exists in two oxidation states (cationic and anionic), but the state most relevant to insulin-like action remains undetermined. Advertisers claim it is an "anabolic inducer"; however, no scientific studies on weight-trained athletes have reported any ergogenic effect. In fact, one study found that not only did vanadyl sulfate produce no gains in strength or lean mass, it actually resulted in increases in body fat.[23] Only anecdotal evidence supports claims of anabolic potential.

Although no studies have been done in diabetic individuals taking vanadly sulfate, this particular supplement may pose greater dangers for diabetic subjects because of its demonstrated insulin-like properties. It is possible that if taken with exogenous insulin, an additive effect may result that could produce a deleterious hypoglycemic response. Great caution should be exercised in consuming this supplement.

Chromium Picolonate

Trivalent chromium is an essential dietary trace mineral required for normal carbohydrate and lipid metabolism and is also a cofactor to insulin action. Insufficient chromium may facilitate an increase in blood cholesterol and decrease sensitivity to insulin. Therefore, inadequate chromium is a likely risk factor for type 2 diabetes and cardiovascular disease. As an ergogenic (anabolic) aid, chromium picolonate may enhance muscle mass in two respects: first, if an athlete is chromium-deficient, the supplement may improve amino acid uptake within skeletal muscles via increased insulin action. Second, increased chromium may promote supra-normal amino acid uptake in athletes who train intensely because increased exercise intensity releases chromium from the tissues into the blood, resulting in chromium loss through excretion.[24] Circumstances may suggest a planned and prudent use of chromium where chromium deficiencies are present or likely. Chromium deficiency may complicate problems with insulin sensitivity in individuals with diabetes. Thus, it would be wise to thoroughly discuss with the diabetes health care team the use of chromium to correct a chromium-deficient situation.

Advertisers claim chromium picolonate can increase muscle size and strength by increasing normal insulin action; however, no studies have satisfactorily supported such claims. Furthermore, adequate amounts of chromium can be readily obtained through a sound diet that includes green vegetables, dairy products, nuts, and some fruits.

Fat Burners, Thermogenic Enhancers, and Energy Boosters

Fat burners, thermogenic enhancers, and energy boosters have been heavily advertised in various media forms, especially infomercials on television. They claim to either reduce body fat or increase amounts of available energy. These supplements usually contain one or more of the following constituents: pyruvate, ephedra, chitin, and medium-chain triglycerides.

Pyruvate is the end product of carbohydrate metabolism and is critical to oxidative metabolism. Advertisers claim pyruvate promotes fat loss, but this has only been demonstrated in obese subjects consuming a low-calorie diet. There is some evidence that pyruvate may improve certain types of endurance exercise, but it is unclear whether pyruvate promotes greater benefit to exercise than a high-carbohydrate pre-activity diet.[25] Although no evidence is available with regard to the effects of pyruvate and diabetic individuals, the exogenous insulin adjustment necessary for a high-carbohydrate meal may be complicated by concurrent consumption of pyruvate. If pyruvate does contribute to altered carbohydrate metabolism in some individuals, precautions should be taken to avoid complications.

Ephedra is the plant source for ephedrine, a stimulant of the central nervous system (CNS). CNS stimulants have gained contemporary notoriety because they have become popular weight loss remedies. They are also directly linked with cardiovascular problems, irritability, nervousness, and seizure disorders. Although stimulation of the CNS does promote fat metabolism, the risks of complications, especially for individuals with diabetes, far outweigh the benefits.

Chitin is an indigestible carbohydrate found predominately in the exoskeletons of insects. It is used in dietary supplements because of its ability to bind fat in the gastrointestinal system, thereby inhibiting its absorption and subsequent assimilation into the body. Like all "fat binders," chronic consumption of chitin and associated products prevents the absorption of essential fat and fat-soluble vitamins. The cumulative effects of such inhibition may compromise immune function, various metabolic pathways, and the integrity of skeletal and cardiac muscle.

Medium-chain triglycerides (MCTs) have also been promoted as "fat burners" because of their ability to be rapidly metabolized within the body, thus avoiding the possibility of being stored as fat. They have been used successfully in clinical realms for patients suffering from malabsorption or wasting diseases. Some studies have demonstrated small improvements in endurance exercise, although these results have been equivocal.[26] The effectiveness of MCTs in individuals with diabetes has not been explored.

All of these described metabolic "enhancers" pose specific problems. Pyruvate, chitin, and MCTs are all associated with various forms of gastrointestinal distress, including cramping and diarrhea. Ephedra and other CNS stimulants found in these types of products are linked to cardiac and nervous disorders.[27] None have produced validated evidence of improved training performance, especially with regard to resistance training. Furthermore, for the exercise enthusiast or athlete with diabetes taking exogenous insulin, they may cause unforeseen and detrimental consequences.

Summary

The availability of nutritional supplements in the fitness and athletic world is staggering. This compounds the dilemma that many individuals face in deciding which supplements are appropriate to consume. With specific reference to individuals with diabetes, many of the supplements on the market today may affect the body's sensitivity to insulin, macronutrient (carbohydrate, protein, and fat) metabolism, and response to exercise. It is strongly recommended, therefore, that consideration of using one or more of these or any other nutritional supplements should be thoroughly discussed with members of the diabetes health care team before experimentation.

References

1. Baechle TR, Earle RW, Eds. *Essentials of Strength Training and Conditioning.* 2nd ed. Champaign, IL, Human Kinetics, 2000
2. Fleck SJ, Kraemer WJ: *Designing Resistance Training Programs.* 2nd ed. Champaign, IL, Human Kinetics, 1997
3. Fiatarone MA, Marks EC, Ryan ND, Meredith CN, Lipsitz LA, Evans WJ: High-intensity strength training in nonagenarians. *JAMA* 263:3029–34, 1990
4. Ghilarducci LE, Holly RG, Amsterdam EA: Effects of high resistance training in coronary artery disease. *Am J Cardiol* 64:866–70, 1989
5. Durak EP, Jovanovic-Peterson L, Peterson CM: Randomized crossover study of effect of resistance training on glycemic control, muscular strength, and cholesterol in type I diabetic men. *Diabetes Care* 13:1039–43, 1990
6. Sargent RG, Hohn E: Protein needs for the athlete. *Natl Strength Cond Assoc J* 15:54–56, 1993
7. Lightsey DM, Attaway JR: Deceptive tactics used in marketing purported ergogenic aids. *Natl Strength Cond Assoc J* 14:26–31, 1992
8. American College of Sports Medicine: Nutrition and athletic performance (Position Statement). *Med Sci Sports Exerc* 32:2130–45, 2000
9. American Diabetes Association: Nutrition recommendations and principles for people with diabetes mellitus (Position Statement). *Diabetes Care* 24 (Suppl. 1):48–51, 2001

10. Kreider RB: Creatine supplementation: analysis of ergogenic value, medical safety, and concerns. *JEP_{online}* 1:7–18, 1998 (http://www.css.edu/users/tboone2/asep/jan3.htm)
11. Volek JS, Duncan ND, Mazzetti SA, Staron RS, Putukian M, Gomez AL, Pearson DR, Fink WJ, Kraemer WJ: Performance and muscle fiber adaptations to creatine supplementation and heavy resistance training. *Med Sci Sports Exerc* 31:1147–56, 1999
12. Green AL, Hultman E, MacDonald IA, Sewell DA, Greenhaff PL: Carbohydrate feeding augments skeletal muscle creatine accumulation during creatine supplementation in humans. *Am J Physiol* 271:E821–26, 1996
13. Greenhaff PL: Creatine and its application as an ergogenic aid. *Int J Sport Nutr* 5:S100–10, 1995
14. Volek JS, Kraemer WJ: Creatine supplementation: its effect on human muscular performance and body composition. *J Strength Cond Res* 10:200–10, 1996
15. Gordon A, Hultman E, Kaijser L, Kristjansson S, Rolf CJ, Nyquist O, Sylven C: Creatine supplementation in chronic heart failure increases skeletal muscle creatine phosphate and muscle performance. *Cardiovasc Res* 30:413–38, 1995
16. Stockler S, Hanefeld F, Frahm J: Creatine replacement therapy in guanidinoacetate methyltransferase deficiency, a novel inborn error of metabolism. *Lancet* 348:789–90, 1996
17. Tarnopolsky M, Martin J: Creatine monohydrate increases strength in patients with neuromuscular disease. *Neurology* 52:854–57, 1999
18. Brown GA, Vukovich MD, Reifenrath TA, Uhl NA, Parsons KA, Sharp RL, King DS: Effects of anabolic precursors on serum testosterone concentrations and adaptations to resistance training in young men. *Int J Sport Nutr Exerc Metab* 10:340–59, 2000
19. King DS, Sharp RL, Vukovich MD, Brown GS, Reifenrath TA, Uhl NL, Parsons KA: Effect of oral androstenedione on serum testosterone and adaptations to resistance training in young men. *JAMA* 281:2020–28, 1999
20. Blue JG, Lombardo JA: Steroids and steroid-like compounds. *Clin Sports Med* 18:667–89, 1999
21. Mero A: Leucine supplementation and intensive training. *Sports Med* 27:347–58, 1999

22. Kreider R: Dietary supplements and the promotion of muscle growth with resistance exercise. *Sports Med* 27:97–110, 1999
23. Fawcett JP, Farquhar SJ, Walker RJ, Thou T, Lowe G, Goulding A: The effect of oral vanadyl sulfate on body composition and performance in weight-training athletes. *Int J Sport Nutr* 6:382–90, 1996
24. Armsey TD, Green GA: Nutrition supplements: science vs. hype. *Phys Sports Med* 25:76–78;87–92, 1997
25. Sukala WR: Pyruvate: beyond the marketing hype. *Int J Sport Nutr* 8:241–49, 1998
26. Hawley JA, Brouns F, Jeukendrup A: Strategies to enhance fat utilization during exercise. *Sports Med* 25:241–57, 1998
27. Myers JB, Guskiewicz KM, Riemann BL: Syncope and atypical chest pain in an intercollegiate wrestler: a case report. *J Athletic Training* 34:263–66, 1999

Robert D. Chetlin, MS, CSCS, and W. Guyton Hornsby, Jr., PhD, CDE, are from the West Virginia University School of Medicine, Morgantown, WV.

37

Scuba Diving

DANIEL LORBER, MD, FACP, CDE

For many years, people with diabetes who used either insulin or sulfonylureas were essentially banned from scuba training in the U.S. and Great Britain. This proscription was due to a fear of hypoglycemia in the U.S. and U.K. and one reported case of paraplegia in the U.K. The British Sub-Aqua Club (BSAC) and the U.K. Sport Diving Medical Committee subsequently developed a protocol for safer diving techniques and for evaluating the level of fitness needed in diabetic divers.[1] In the past 5 years, collaborative efforts by the American Diabetes Association, the Undersea and Hyperbaric Medical Society, and the Divers Alert Network have resulted in further research into diabetes and diving and additional recommendations for diabetic divers.

Scuba diving is a high-risk sport that is not truly safe for people with diabetes, nor for anyone else. The diver is in a foreign environment and depends on technology to provide air or other breathing gas under appropriate pressure. If a diver misjudges the behavior of his or her breathing gas as pressure changes or is unable to return to the surface environment, accidents, often fatal ones, may happen. There are between 1 and 3 million certified scuba divers in the U.S., with another 250,000 being certified annually. In the past decade, there have been between three and nine deaths per year per 100,000 divers. In most cases, fatal diving accidents are due to human error; other causes include equipment failure or environmental factors. Inexperience, panic, and anxiety are significant risk factors; coronary artery disease is a cause or contributing factor in about one-third of cases. As divers and health professionals, we cannot make diving "safe." However, we can lessen the risks. It is important to point out that there is no evidence that diving accidents or deaths are more common in people with diabetes.

Diving Physiology

As the scuba diver descends, the ambient pressure increases by one atmosphere for every 33 ft of depth.[2] The greatest percentage increase occurs near the surface. Thus, breathing gases compress by 50% in the first 10 m, by another 17% between 10 and 20 m, and by another 8% as the diver reaches a depth of 30 m. To breathe at any depth greater than 1–2 ft underwater, the diver depends on his or her equipment to provide air at the ambient pressure. As the diver ascends, gases expand according to Boyle's law. It is these changes in the partial pressure of inert gases, particularly nitrogen, that lead to the physiological and pathophysiological changes seen in scuba diving.

Decompression Illness

Gas under pressure dissolves in liquid. In diving physiology, this means that nitrogen is dissolved in body fluids during the dive and comes out of solution with ascent. This change usually leads to small bubbles in the venous circulation, which are easily cleared by the lungs. If the ascent is too rapid, overcoming the body's ability to "off-gas," tissue bubbles may result, leading to decompression disease.[3] As the diver ascends, the exchange of inert gases from body tissues is limited by perfusion. Although there are no studies of this "off-gassing" phenomenon in diabetes, it is possible that microvascular disease may lead to diminished gas transfer and increased risk of decompression illness. The best known form of decompression illness is the "bends." Bends are characterized by bubbles in and around the joints, resulting in severe joint pain. In other cases, bubbles may cause skin rash and pruritis or may obstruct lymphatics, leading to localized lymphedema.

A more severe form of decompression illness occurs when gas enters the arterial circulation. This may occur in two ways. As the diver ascends, air in the lungs expands. Breath-holding during ascent may result in rupture of alveolar walls, allowing air to enter the arterial circulation. Bubbles act as foreign bodies, activating platelets, the coagulation cascade, and complement. The clinical presentation of this form of decompression illness depends on the location of arterial air emboli. The central nervous system (CNS) is affected in up to 80% of cases of air embolus; half of these individuals will have CNS symptoms at presentation. CNS signs of decompression illness may look remarkably similar to those of neuroglycopenia, including headache, blurred vision, diplopia, scotomata, dysarthria, vertigo, mental and personality changes, impaired consciousness, coma, ataxia, seizure, or death. Unlike hypoglycemia, spinal symptoms are common, including paresis, plegia, and urinary retention.

A similar syndrome of arterial gas embolism occurs when venous bubbles enter the arterial circulation through a patent atrial foramen ovale. Patent foramen ovale is present in ~20% of people; it has been found in 40% of cases of severe decompression illness.

Space limitations make a review of diving medicine impossible here. More detailed discussions of scuba physiology and medicine may be found elsewhere.[1–3]

What Are the Data Specific to Diabetes?

Fluid Metabolism

Scuba diving causes significant diuresis in normal adults. This fluid loss may be higher in divers with diabetes. In the study by Lerch et al.,[4] of ~70 dives by seven diabetic divers, subjects with diabetes had to drink an extra 1–2 liters of fluid a day to avoid an increase in hematocrit.

Glucose Metabolism

Scuba diving may entail significant exercise. Swimming with diving gear against a 1.3-knot current requires 13 metabolic equivalents. Although most divers don't usually encounter this level of exercise demand, it is not unknown.

Edge et al.[5] evaluated the effect of exercise under pressure on glucose metabolism in a study comparing moderate-intensity exercise at the surface with the same exercise in a pressure chamber at a simulated depth of 100 ft. There was no significant difference in blood glucose between the two environments.

In the BSAC survey of over 1,000 dives by diabetic divers, four people reported hypoglycemic episodes, with no fatalities (C.J. Edge, personal communication).

Uguccione et al.[6,7] from the Divers Alert Network studied 16 divers in a total of 131 dives. Divers began the dive with a mean blood glucose of 234 mg/dl. The average fall in blood glucose was between 51 and 56 mg/dl. Several divers had hypoglycemic episodes during nondive times; there were no episodes of clinical hypoglycemia during diving, and no dives were aborted for hypoglycemia. In three cases, capillary blood glucose was <80 mg/dl (47, 65, and 68 mg/dl). These episodes were easily treated with oral glucose.

Lerch et al.[4] studied seven divers in 10 dives, each to a maximum of 30 m over a 7-day period. Divers started with blood glucose levels between 180 and 220 mg/dl. Over the course of a 1-week dive trip, insulin requirements fell by between 33 and 60%. Although Lerch et al. reported no hypoglycemia, there was a greater tendency to dehydration among the diabetic divers.

What Don't We Know?

Although the data are encouraging, there are many gaps in our knowledge about diving physiology in diabetes. There are few controlled studies with published reports at this time, and the physiological effects of diving are only known in a small number of diabetic subjects. The Lerch and Uguccione studies took place under carefully controlled circumstances, with divers well controlled for glucose before diving. The BSAC survey, although largely based on self-report and follow-up of diabetic divers with letters and telephone calls, has collected a great deal of data on diving in various conditions, including greater depth, cold water, and special gas mixtures. In this series, the two documented deaths were due to a myocardial infarction and an unwitnessed death in a patient on a biguanide alone. Anecdotally, the recommendations of the BSAC have been well established for 9 years and have assisted many divers in controlling their diabetes so they can dive more safely. The risk for a diabetic diver in the U.K. appears to be less than that for a nondiabetic diver because of the attention to these precautions.[8]

Specific Recommendations

Who Is Fit to Dive?

- All divers need to be fit mentally and physically.[9]
- Divers with diabetes must have an excellent understanding of self-management, particularly regarding the effects of exercise.
- Divers with poor control (HbA_{1c} >9%) should not dive until they are in better control.
- Hypoglycemia unawareness or severe hypoglycemia (requiring the assistance of others) in the past year are contraindications to scuba diving.
- The diver with type 2 diabetes or long-standing type 1 diabetes is at greater risk for overt or clinical macrovascular disease, including myocardial infarction, coronary artery bypass grafts, congestive heart failure, cerebrovascular accident, or significant valvular disease. When present, these complications are contraindications to scuba diving. Even in the absence of documented vascular disease, the diver at high risk should have further evaluation, including an exercise stress test. The BSAC also recommends that a diabetes diving examination include a test for the presence of autonomic neuropathy. (The heart rate response to a Valsalva maneuver is a simple autonomic function test that can be performed in the office.)
- Until more is known about the effects of microvascular disease on gas behavior, it is inadvisable for individuals with significant diabetic retinopathy, neuropathy, or microalbuminuria to dive. Further, microalbuminuria and microvascular disease also indicate a higher risk for occult macrovascular disease.
- The BSAC also recommends that the medication regimen of the diabetic diver should not have been altered significantly in the last year.

General Recommendations for the Diabetic Diver

Before a Dive

- Have a complete physical examination annually. In the U.S., a physician's report is required only at the time of initial certification.
- Keep your diving skills and diabetes skills up to date.
- Make sure that both you and your buddy are fit and alert. Only one of a buddy pair should have diabetes.
- Your buddy should know the signs and treatment of hypoglycemia.
- Be sure you have access to capillary blood glucose equipment before and after your dive. Bring your testing kit onto the boat; make sure it is protected from sun and seawater.
- Inform the dive master of your diabetes.
- Be well hydrated before you dive (drink at least 2.5 liters of fluid).
- Carry glucose gel (at least two tubes on your person and have glucose and glucagon on the boat). Practice opening and ingesting glucose gel underwater.
- Wear a medical identification bracelet or neck charm.
- Carry flags or flares to attract attention (in case unexpected currents carry you away from the boat and your emergency kit).

During a Dive

- Start your dive hyperglycemic. The BSAC protocol, developed for diving in colder northern waters, recommends having a blood glucose level between 160 and 200 mg/dl. Steve Prosterman, who runs a diving camp in the U.S. Virgin Islands, recommends determining the direction of blood glucose change before diving (see Box 37.1).
- Stay in the water <2 h at a time.
- Limit your dive to <100 ft.

Box 37.1

Steve Prosterman, who teaches scuba diving in the Marine Science Department at the University of the Virgin Islands in St. Thomas and runs a 1-week activity camp for adults with diabetes (Camp DAVI; see RESOURCES at the end of this chapter), has developed techniques particularly applicable to beginning divers in calmer waters.

Prosterman suggests finding the direction of the blood glucose change. "This is really more important than knowing the level of the blood glucose at the beginning of an activity," he says. "It's especially important to find out if the blood glucose is dropping."

Prosterman instructs his pupils to do a series of three blood glucose tests within 1½ h (e.g., 1 h, 30 min, and 5–10 min) before an activity. "You should be able to see if the blood glucose is stable, dropping, or rising. If it is stable, aim for a 180–190 mg/dl minimum before beginning. If it is dropping, stabilize it before beginning. You may need an extra carbohydrate snack and two more tests to ensure the blood glucose level is acceptable. If blood glucose is rising, aim for a 120–130 mg/dl minimum before beginning. But do not dive until you have stabilized it." Prosterman also recommends testing after (or during, if possible) the activity. Dr. Edge of the BSAC points out that this approach may be applicable to the calm warm waters of the Virgin Islands but will be difficult in a "Zodiac in the North Sea" (C.J. Edge, personal communication). Thus, the BSAC recommends beginning your dive with a glucose level between 160 and 200 mg/dl.

In the unlikely event that a person experiences low blood glucose during scuba diving, Prosterman devised the "L" hand sign (using the thumb and index finger). If the sign is given, the buddy team and instructor begin a controlled ascent to the surface, inflate the buoyancy compensation device, and administer a fast-acting carbohydrate, such as a glucose gel. The BSAC recommends that divers treat hypoglycemia before the ascent as described above. Prosterman prefers Insta-Glucose (ICN Pharmaceuticals, Costa Mesa, CA) because the packaging holds up to the effects of the sun and ocean. "It is so important to avoid hypoglycemia while scuba diving or participating in any activity that may isolate you or that would make it difficult to treat."

- Schedule no more than 3 consecutive days of diving and no more than two dives a day.
- If you become hypoglycemic, signal your buddy (see Box 37.1) and prepare to end your dive. If necessary, glucose gel may be ingested underwater by inserting the nozzle of the glucose gel tube between the regulator mouthpiece and the corner of the mouth, allowing the gel to be squirted into the mouth without removing the regulator. This technique is commonly used by divers to drink during long decompression stops.

After a Dive

- Test your blood glucose immediately.
- Report any unusual symptoms to the dive master immediately.

Remember: Decompression illness or gas embolism can look like hypoglycemia, and hypoglycemia can look like decompression illness. Delay in treating either can result in severe injury or death. If you are unsure, treat both with glucose or glucagon and oxygen. Transport to a pressure chamber as soon as possible.

If a diabetic diver is undergoing hyperbaric oxygen treatment, capillary blood glucose measurement, which depends on glucose oxidase and atmospheric oxygen, may be inaccurate.

Conclusion

For many years, people with diabetes were excluded from the wonders of scuba diving because of fears of hypoglycemia. The advent of blood glucose self-monitoring and increased precision in diabetes management have reduced this worry for everyone with diabetes, including prospective divers. Although limited, research has not demonstrated any significant increase in risk of death or injury for divers with diabetes. The risk of hypoglycemia, while still present, can be minimized, and treatment can be easily administered in the water, on a boat, or at the shore. If a diver with diabetes follows certain logical guidelines, it appears that there is no significantly increased risk to his or her health as a result of diabetes. Nonetheless, what we don't know about the interactions of diabetes and the underwater environment clearly outweighs what we do know. There is a need for a great deal of further research in this area.

Acknowledgments

The author thanks Dr. Chris Edge of the BSAC for his editorial and scientific guidance.

References

1. Edge CJ, Linsday D, Wilmshurst P: The diving diabetic. *Diver* 37: 35–36, 1992
2. Bove AA: Medical aspects of sport diving. *Med Sci Sports Exerc* 28:591–95, 1996
3. Melamed Y, Shupak A, Bitterman H: Medical problems associated with underwater diving. *N Engl J Med* 326:30–35, 1992
4. Lerch M, Lutrop C, Thurm U: Diabetes and diving: can the risk of hypoglycemia be banned? *SPUMS J* 26:62–66, 1996
5. Edge CJ, Grieve AP, Gibbins N, O'Sullivan F, Bryson P: Effects of pressure on whole blood glucose measurements using the Bayer Glucometer 4 blood glucose meter. *Undersea Hyperbar Med* 23:221–24, 1996
6. Uguccione DM, Pollock NW, Dovenbarger JA, Dear G de L, Feinglos MN, Moon RE: Blood glucose response to single and repetitive dives in insulin-requiring diabetics: a preliminary report (Abstract). *Undersea Hyperb Med* 25 (Suppl.):52, 1998
7. Uguccione DM, Dear G de L, Dovenbarger JA, Feinglos M, Moon RE, Pollock NW: Plasma glucose response to recreational diving in insulin-requiring diabetics and controls (Abstract). *Undersea Hyperb Med* 27 (Suppl.):66, 2000
8. Edge CJ, Grieve AP, Gibbons N, O'Sullivan F, Bryson P: Control of blood glucose in a group of diabetic scuba divers. *Undersea Hyperb Med* 24:201–07, 1997
9. Edge CJ, Bryson P: Diabetes mellitus and SCUBA diving. In *Diving and Subaquatic Medicine.* 4th ed. Edmonds C, Lowry C, Pennefather J, Eds. Butterworth-Heinemann, Oxford, U.K. In press

Resources

Divers Alert Network (DAN)
Box 3823
Duke University Medical Center
Durham, NC 27710
www.diversalertnetwork.org

DAN is dedicated to safety, education, and research in the scuba diving community. DAN carries out research on diving with diabetes; provides guidelines, information, and insurance; and is overall a superb source of diving information and support.

British Sub-Aqua Club
Telford's Quay, Ellesmere Port
South Wirral, Cheshire, L65 4FY
U.K.
www.bsac.com
cjedge@diver.demon.co.uk

BSAC provides excellent medical and patient information, including a model patient questionnaire and medical guidelines.

Steve Prosterman
Camp DAVI, University of the Virgin Islands
P.O. Box 305511
St. Thomas, VI 00803-5511
www.diabetesnet.com/visle.html
E-mail: sproste@usvi.edu

Daniel Lorber, MD, FACP, CDE, is from the Diabetes Control Foundation, Flushing, NY, and Weill Medical College of Cornell University, New York, NY.

38

Mountain Hiking

JEAN-JACQUES GRIMM, MD

Mountains, like deserts and oceans, are relatively unaltered by human civilizations. They can sometimes be hostile to people, who nevertheless enjoy a sense of self-accomplishment from climbing them. Most hikers feel that they are doing more than simply exercising at high altitudes. Mountaineering is a complex experience; climbers are both exhilarated and challenged by the hazards of surviving in a demanding environment.

There are many mountain climbers with diabetes, such as the well-known Italian Vittorio Casirahgi. Their experience shows that even in this very strenuous activity, people with diabetes can still be active. However, they must take special care to monitor and manage their diabetes. There are some inherent dangers in mountaineering.

Hazards of Mountain Hiking

Dehydration

Sweating and high respiratory rates at high altitudes induce substantial fluid loss. Minimal water requirements are ~2–3 liters per day in these conditions. It is often difficult to melt snow because of wind, bad weather, and time constraints. Climbers usually find it more convenient to carry a daily quantity of water that they have prepared before starting each morning.

Sun Radiation

Ultraviolet (UV) radiation can be strong at high altitudes and increases even more in snow-covered areas. Climbers must protect their eyes with high-quality glasses and coat exposed skin areas, such as the nose, ears, neck, and scalp, with lotions offering high degrees of UV protection.

Frostbite and Hypothermia

Even the best footwear cannot prevent some moisture in the feet after a couple of hours of walking. Moisture exposes the toes and the heels to cold injuries, even when the temperature is above freezing. The same is true for fingers in wet gloves. The nose, ears, and other exposed parts of the face are also at risk in windy conditions. Abnormal skin sensitivity at the feet or circulatory insufficiency increases the danger of frostbite. Bivouacs are often unexpected or do not happen at the planned location. Protection from wind in a rock or ice cave is often lifesaving. Additional dry underwear and an aluminum emergency sheet should be available.

Avalanche

Drifted or recently fallen snow can be unstable on certain slopes. In some mountain ranges, good information about the risk of avalanche is available via a snow information telephone number, tourist information booths, or guide company offices. This danger should be taken into account when planning a hike during the winter or spring. Generally, starting early and returning in the early afternoon, before long sun exposure on the slopes, gives climbers some security.

Lightning

During the summer months, lightning is a common threat to climbers. Some exposed areas, such as ridges and summits, must be avoided when the risk for storms is high (usually in the late afternoon).

Mountain Sickness Syndrome

When lowlanders ascend to high altitudes (over 2,500 m/8,200 ft), they often experience headache, nausea, vomiting, insomnia, and lassitude. High-altitude pulmonary edema (HAPE) is a rare but potentially fatal complication of acute exposure to high altitudes.[1] Progressive acclimatization, over weeks, decreases the risk of these illnesses. No data are available for the prophylactic use of drugs (for example, acetazolamide) in people with diabetes. Nifedipine has proven to be helpful for the treatment of HAPE.

Insulin Conservation

Insulin is altered by high temperatures, light, excess agitation, and freezing.[2] At 45°C, for example, a loss of up to 15% of the biological activity can be expected after 1 month, depending on the type of insulin. Moreover, at high temperatures, degradation products with unwanted immunological effects (i.e., allergy) can appear. Excess agitation increases the risk of degradation with high temperatures.

When walking in the sun, it is advisable to store insulin in an insulated box in a nonexposed place in a backpack. With cold weather or at night, placing the insulin in a location close to the body—for example, a sleeping bag—can prevent it from freezing. If despite all care, the insulin freezes, a significant decrease in potency must be expected. This is particularly true for the long-acting preparations in which large aggregates are no longer soluble. Furthermore, these aggregates can also block the needle or the pump catheter. Table 38.1 provides insulin storage temperatures.

Self-Monitoring of Blood Glucose Equipment

All self-monitoring of blood glucose devices and their strips deliver acceptably accurate results as long as they work and are stored in the desired temperature, moisture, and oxygen pressure ranges.[3] For most of these devices, these ranges are about 10–30°C (59–86°F) for temperature and 20–80% for relative humidity. At high altitudes (4,350 m/14,272 ft), some systems underestimate the blood glucose results by as much as 45%, and others overestimate it up to 35%. It is hazardous to try to correct supposed under- or overestimated values.

TABLE 38.1 Insulin Storage

Temperature	Effect
<2°C (36°F; risk of freezing)	■ Short-acting insulin (soluble): usually no damage (no data are available for short-acting insulin analogs). Nevertheless, change to a new vial as soon as possible. ■ Long- or intermediate-acting insulin: probable loss of biological activity. Change to a new vial as soon as possible.
2–8°C (36–46°F)	■ Ideal storage temperature.
8–30°C (46–86°F)	■ No significant effect on insulin activity for 1 month.
30–45°C (86–113°F)	■ Acceptable for very short periods (days); loss of biological activity possible.

Check all insulins regularly for clumping or precipitation.

Diabetic Complications

Hypoglycemia

Exercising at high altitudes is a potent stimulation for the sympathetic nervous system, resulting in high heart rates and sweating. The recognition of hypoglycemia can be confusing in these conditions. Poor appetite and sometimes nausea are frequent at high altitudes and can compromise proper food and fluid intake, precipitating hypoglycemic attacks. Climbers must carefully plan drinking and eating schedules before getting started and monitor their blood glucose frequently. Hiking with at least one other person is helpful as well as safer in this regard.

Retinopathy

Retinal hemorrhages have been described in people without diabetes as part of the mountain sickness syndrome.[4] It seems likely that an untreated abnormal diabetic retina could be harmed by the same exposure to high altitudes. Whether a clinically normal diabetic retina is at high risk of damage is not yet known. A thorough retinal check should be performed before climbers with diabetes participate in high-altitude activities.

Neuropathy

Hikers with altered sensitivity in the lower extremities are prone to more frequent and severe foot injuries than would normally be expected. Even common blisters will be more severe because of the lack of sensation. The difficulties in maintaining adequate hygiene and, often, the necessity to continue to walk make wound healing a difficult challenge. Autonomic neuropathy can alter the heart rate and blood pressure adaptation to the effort and to the altitude.

Self-Management

If performed during good conditions, mountain hiking is an endurance sport. The exercise is aerobic and lasts many hours to several days. Under these circumstances, insulin needs usually decrease substantially, and carbohydrate consumption increases. Therefore, climbers should regularly monitor their blood glucose levels and keep a record of the duration and quality of their exercise in relation to their body's reactions. Access to aid stations may be difficult; rescue may not be available for several days. Therefore, careful self-management is essential.[5]

References

1. Tso EL, Wagner TJ: What's up in the management of high-altitude pulmonary edema? *Md Med J* 42:641–45, 1993
2. Brange J: *Stability of Insulin.* Boston, MA, Kluwer Academic, 1994
3. Banion CR, Klingensmith GJ: Performance of seven blood glucose testing systems at high altitude. *Diabetes Educ* 15:444–48, 1989
4. Frayser R, Houston CS, Bryan AC, Rennie ID, Gray G: Retinal hemorrhage at high altitude. *N Engl J Med* 282:1183–84, 1970
5. Auerbach PS (Ed.): *Wilderness Medicine: Management of Wilderness and Environmental Emergencies.* 3rd ed. St. Louis, MO, Mosby, 1995

Jean-Jacques Grimm, MD, is from the University Hospital, Lausanne, Switzerland.

39

Health/Fitness Facility Guidelines for Diabetes and Exercise

KYLE J. McINNIS, ScD, AND
GARY J. BALADY, MD

Highlights

- The projected increase in the prevalence of diabetes and the emerging trend of patients with chronic diseases joining health clubs suggest that substantially more individuals with diabetes will join the nearly 30 million U.S. adults who already exercise at fitness facilities.

- Appropriately prepared fitness staff at health clubs and fitness centers can be a resource for promoting physical activity and providing exercise leadership to individuals with diabetes.

- The incidence of a cardiovascular event during exercise among diabetic patients is greater than that among otherwise healthy individuals primarily because of the higher prevalence of coronary heart disease in these individuals.

- Potential medical complications associated with diabetes and exercise warrant special consideration for staff at health/fitness facilities that enroll individuals with this disease.

- To help health/fitness facility staff foster safe exercise participation for all members, the American Heart Association (AHA) and the American College of Sports Medicine (ACSM) have developed recommendations for cardiovascular screening, staffing, and emergency policies at health/fitness centers.
- These recommendations call for all facilities offering exercise equipment or services to conduct a cardiovascular screening of all new members and/or prospective users.
- A medical evaluation and supervised exercise test should be conducted for anyone identified as having diabetes. Written and active communication by facility staff with the individual's personal physician (or health care provider) is strongly recommended.
- Individuals with diabetes should be directed toward health/fitness facilities that have appropriately trained fitness staff who can prescribe safe exercise programs that adhere to accepted guidelines and who are knowledgeable about responding to possible adverse occurrences such as hypoglycemia.
- The AHA/ACSM recommendations call for all health/fitness facilities to have written emergency policies and procedures that are reviewed and practiced regularly.

The promotion of physical activity is an important focus of our national public health agenda. The attention now being given to exercise should lead to increased levels of regular physical activity throughout the U.S. population. This public health message of routine physical activity is likely to be heard by the ~16 million Americans who either have been diagnosed with diabetes (10.5 million) or are estimated to have the disease but whose condition remains undetected (5.5 million).[1,2]

Moderate (or higher) levels of physical activity and exercise are achieved in a number of settings, including >15,000 health/fitness facilities across the country. These facilities, which include public health clubs, work-site fitness centers, hospital-based facilities, and community exercise centers, are designed to provide participants with the opportunity to receive advice from professional staff, exercise in a stimulating environment, and have access to a variety of specialized equipment.

The number of health/fitness facilities and members is expected to expand significantly over the next decade. This expansion will prompt an increase in the 30 million men and women who already exercise at these facilities.[3] Whereas health club membership was once comprised primarily of young, healthy individuals, an aging population and general promotion of physical activity to the public will continue to broaden fitness facility demographics. Current market research indicates that 50% of health/fitness facility members are older than 35 years, and the fastest-growing segments of users are individuals older than 55 years and individuals aged 35–54 years.[3]

Specialty programs for older individuals and individuals with chronic diseases have been identified as popular programming trends at health clubs and fitness centers.[4] As the prevalence of diabetes continues to increase in the U.S., health clubs can provide important and needed opportunities for individuals with this disease to receive advice and guidance on physical activity, nutrition, and healthy lifestyle behaviors related to their disease management.

Benefits and Safety

Exercise or routine physical activity may protect against the development of diabetes and can improve this condition when it exists.[5,6] Many health benefits of regular exercise for individuals with diabetes are related to moderate levels of physical activity.[7] However, as in nondiabetic individuals, the benefits of exercise and exercise training are not without risks. Health/fitness facility personnel should be familiar with the complications of diabetes that may manifest during exercise. These complications are outlined in Table 39.1.[8] The valuable contribution of exercise for the treatment of diabetes and the risk-benefit ratio are discussed in Chapter 2.

TABLE 39.1 Exercise Complications That Can Be Observed in Diabetic Clients at Health/Fitness Facilities

Cardiovascular	Anginal chest discomfort Shortness of breath Dizziness Arrhythmias (may be silent) Excessive increments in blood pressure during exercise Postexercise orthostatic hypotension
Microvascular	Retinal hemorrhage
Metabolic	Worsening of hyperglycemia Hypoglycemia in patients on insulin or sulfonylurea therapy
Musculoskeletal and traumatic	Foot ulcers (especially in the presence of neuropathy) Orthopedic injury related to neuropathy Accelerated degenerative joint disease Eye injuries and retinal hemorrhage

Adapted with permission from the American Diabetes Association.[8]

Overall, the prevalence of cardiovascular disease is estimated to be three- to fourfold higher in men, and even higher in women, with diabetes.[9] Because of the high prevalence of neuropathy in these patients, symptoms of ischemic heart disease, such as angina pectoris, are often absent.[10] Precautions to minimize risk during exercise of moderate or higher intensity have been described for diabetes.[11] Although data from controlled clinical trials or other research studies are lacking, the incidence of a cardiovascular event during exercise in people with diabetes appears to be low when such precautions are followed, even in individuals with underlying occult or known cardiovascular disease.[12] Nevertheless, the incidence of a cardiovascular event in someone with heart disease is estimated to be 10 times that of otherwise healthy individuals.[9]

Health/Fitness Facility Guidelines

A higher incidence of coronary heart disease and silent myocardial ischemia in individuals with diabetes emphasizes the importance of adequate screening and evaluation before beginning exercise at moderate to vigorous levels. The potential for other medical risks, such as hypoglycemia, foot problems, or eye problems, in individuals with diabetes further substantiates the need for health/fitness facilities to be equipped with the resources to develop safe exercise programs and respond appropriately should an adverse event occur. The ability to provide general education about exercise for diabetic individuals should be considered a priority at facilities that enroll such individuals.

There is heightened concern that individuals at greater cardiovascular risk, such as those with diabetes, are exercising at fitness facilities that fail to provide adequate cardiovascular screening and emergency procedures outlined in previously published recommendations. A survey of 110 health/fitness facilities in Massachusetts found that efforts to screen new members at enrollment were limited and inconsistent.[4] Nearly 40% of responding facilities stated that they do not routinely use a screening interview or questionnaire to evaluate new members for symptoms or history of cardiovascular disease, and 10% stated that they conducted no initial cardiovascular health history screening at all. In this study, over two-thirds of the facilities, including the so-called "quality clubs," did not routinely practice emergency drills. Similar results were also reported in a study of nearly 200 clubs in the Midwest.[13]

During the last decade, several professional groups have published guidelines to address concerns regarding the safety, staffing, and programs at health clubs.[14–16] The latest and most explicit recommendations for safety measures at health/fitness facilities were developed by the American Heart Association (AHA) and the American College of Sports Medicine (ACSM).[17] These recommendations address preparticipation cardiovascular screening of all individuals (children, adolescents, and adults), staff qualifications, and emergency policies related to cardiovascular safety.

The existing AHA/ACSM recommendations[17] on cardiovascular screening, staffing, and emergency preparation at health/fitness facilities are highlighted in this chapter and supplemented with specific recommendations for individuals with diabetes. An overview of general recommendations for reducing complications related to exercise in diabetic subjects at health/fitness facilities is given in Table 39.2. These recommendations are intended to assist health/fitness facility staff to work in concert with health care providers to promote safe and effective physical activity/exercise. Other comprehensive guidelines for operating health/fitness facilities have been published by the ACSM.[15]

TABLE 39.2 General Recommendations to Reduce Diabetic Complications During Exercise at Health/Fitness Facilities

- Identify individuals with diabetes through proper preparticipation screening.
- Obtain medical evaluation and follow-up on all individuals identified as having diabetes.
- Design an individualized exercise program using information obtained from the medical evaluation.
- Educate clients and staff about safe exercise participation, such as knowing how to self-monitor blood glucose, adjust food intake and medication dosage, care for feet properly, and stay adequately hydrated. Written guidelines for diabetic clients may be helpful.
- Regularly check written records/diaries of self-monitored blood glucose levels and give feedback and/or make appropriate recommendations in concert with the primary health care provider.
- Ensure that all staff are properly trained to recognize and respond appropriately to early warning signs of hypoglycemia and other possible medical complications.
- Establish and routinely practice an emergency plan that includes factors related to diabetes and exercise, such as hypoglycemia, hyper- or hypotensive blood pressure responses, and cardiovascular emergencies.

Health/Fitness Facility Recommendations

Screening Prospective Members/Users

The primary purpose of preparticipation screening is to identify individuals known to be at risk for an adverse event during exercise and who need to undergo a medical evaluation before starting an exercise program. This involves identifying individuals with known cardiovascular disease, symptoms of cardiovascular disease, diabetes, and/or other risk factors for disease development. Screening also identifies individuals with known cardiovascular disease or other special medical needs who should not participate in an exercise program or who should participate at least initially in a medically supervised program.[17]

There is agreement among previously published guidelines, including the AHA/ACSM position stand, that all individuals joining a health/fitness facility should be screened before participation. (A complete copy of the AHA/ACSM joint position stand on cardiovascular screening, staffing, and emergency policies at health/fitness centers can be downloaded from the American Heart Association's website at http://www.americanheart.org. The steps to retrieve the article from the website include the following: *1*) click on "pubs" under the heading "Science and Professional," *2*) click on "AHA Scientific Statements," *3*) scroll down to the heading "exercise," and *4*) click on "Recommendations for Cardiovascular Screening, Staffing, and Emergency Policies at Health/Fitness Facilities." The article is also available in two different journals.[17]) Because the public health benefits of exercise are so great, it is important that a screening process not be so intensive that it serves to discourage participation. Simple questionnaires such as the Physical Activity Readiness Questionnaire (PAR-Q) (developed in Canada)[18] or a questionnaire developed by the American Heart Association[17] can often quickly identify problems that might pose a risk during exercise. At health/fitness facilities with minimum supervision, such as clubs with no professional staff or exercise rooms available in many hotels, screening can be accomplished with appropriately displayed signs for self-review. A summary of the AHA/ACSM recommendations for preparticipation cardiovascular screening for members joining a health/fitness facility is outlined in Table 39.3.

Specific Recommendations for Diabetes

The ACSM[14] and American Diabetes Association (ADA)[5] recommend a thorough physical examination by a qualified health care provider to assess the presence of macro- and/or microvascular complications in all individuals with diabetes who embark on an exercise program. Given the age of the person and duration of diabetes, the physician may recommend that an exercise test will need to be performed before the patient can safely participate in an exercise program. Such testing can be useful in identifying exercise-induced ischemic ST segment changes, hyper- or hypotensive blood pressure responses, or serious arrhythmias. Specifically, such testing should be performed in those individuals with diabetes who have known or suspected coronary heart disease. Exercise testing should be strongly considered in diabetic subjects who are >35 years old and in those who have had type 2 diabetes for >10 years, type 1 diabetes for >15 years, additional atherosclerotic risk factors for coronary heart disease, microvascular disease, peripheral vascular disease, or autonomic neuropathy.

Along with other specific recommendations from the health care provider, any abnormal findings from the exercise test should be documented by a qualified staff member of the health/fitness facility and

TABLE 39.3 Key Points on Recommendations From the AHA/ACSM on Preparticipation Cardiovascular Screening, Assumptions of Risks and Waivers, and Staffing for Health/Fitness Facilities

Preparticipation screening

- All facilities offering exercise equipment or services should conduct a cardiovascular screening of all new members and/or prospective users.
- The screening procedure should be simple, easy to perform, and not so intensive that it serves to discourage participation.
- Health appraisal forms should be interpreted by qualified staff (this can limit the number of unnecessary medical referrals and avoid barriers to participation).
- In view of the potential legal risk assumed by operators of fitness facilities, it is recommended that those facilities providing staff supervision document the results of screening.
- Individual facilities can determine the most cost-effective way to conduct and document preparticipation screening.

Assumptions of risk and waivers

- Individuals who fail to complete the health appraisal questionnaire upon request may be excluded from participation in a health/fitness facility exercise program to the extent permitted by law.
- Individuals without symptoms or a known history of cardiovascular disease who do not obtain recommended medical evaluations (when indicated) upon completing a health appraisal should be requested to sign an assumption of risk or a release/waiver where *1)* individuals who sign a waiver should be permitted to exercise and *2)* individuals who do not sign a waiver may be excluded from participation in a health/fitness facility to the extent permitted by law.
- Individuals with known cardiovascular disease who do not obtain recommended medical evaluations upon request may be excluded from participation in a health/fitness facility exercise program to the extent permitted by law.

Staffing

- Health/fitness facility personnel involved in the management or delivery of exercise programs must meet academic and professional standards and have the required experience as recommended by the AHA/ACSM.
- The levels of staff education and experience needed to foster program effectiveness and client safety vary with the health status of the clients.
- In all cases, an exercise leader must be trained in CPR.

Adapted from Balady et al.[17]

used to formulate a safe exercise prescription. Special considerations for evaluating individuals with diabetes who enroll at health/fitness facilities are shown in Table 39.4.[7]

Assumption of Risks

When appropriate guidelines are followed, it is likely that the potential benefits of physical activity will outweigh the risks for most men and women with diabetes.[5] To avoid possible barriers to participation in physical activity at fitness centers and to potentially reduce legal li-

TABLE 39.4 Diabetic Client Evaluation Before Starting an Exercise Program

Evaluate client knowledge regarding his or her diabetes and obtain diabetes history
- Type and duration of diabetes
- Diabetes medication: type, dose, and timing of administration
- Dietary habits, including timing of meals/snacks and fluids

Evaluate glycemic control in concert with health care provider
- Client may need modification of medication and/or carbohydrate ingestion if recurrent hypoglycemia is a problem
- Severe hyperglycemia may be worsened with intense exercise and warrants control

Evaluate for the presence of diabetic complications
- Is the subject known to have cardiovascular disease or is he or she at high risk?
- Is the subject at risk for injury due to peripheral neuropathy?
- Is diabetic renal disease present? High-intensity aerobic or resistance exercise may worsen progression.
- Does the subject have retinopathy that will be worsened by exercise activities that may increase ocular pressure?

Adapted from the American College of Sports Medicine.[7]

ability, the AHA/ACSM recommends that individuals without symptoms or a known history of cardiovascular disease who do not obtain the recommended medical evaluation after completing a health appraisal should be required to sign an assumption of risk or release/waiver.[17] However, individuals with known cardiovascular disease who do not obtain the recommended evaluation may be excluded from participation to the extent permitted by law. Although not specified in the guidelines,[17] it would be reasonable to use the same procedures on waivers for individuals with diabetes as used for individuals with cardiovascular disease. The release/waiver form may be legally recognized in the jurisdiction in which the facility is located. Specific recommendations from AHA/ACSM on assumptions of risk and waivers are outlined in Table 39.3.

Type of Facility

After evaluation by a qualified medical care provider, individuals with diabetes who are considered to be medically stable and without complicating risks are appropriate candidates for enrolling in non-medically supervised health/fitness facilities that have properly trained staff and emergency safety procedures. Clients with diabetes considered to be at moderate/high risk because of complicating medical

TABLE 39.5 Characteristics of Moderate-Risk/High-Risk Diabetic Patients, Such as American Heart Association Class C Patients With Cardiovascular Disease

Individuals at moderate to high risk for cardiac complications during exercise and/or unable to self-regulate activity or to understand recommended activity level includes individuals with the following diagnoses:

Coronary artery disease with the clinical characteristics outlined below:

- Valvular heart disease: excluding severe valvular stenosis or regurgitation with the clinical characteristics as outlined below.
- Congenital heart disease: risk stratification for patients with congenital heart disease should be guided by the 26th Bethesda Conference recommendations.[17]
- Cardiomyopathy: ejection fraction <30%; includes stable patients with heart failure with clinical characteristics as outlined below; not hypertrophic cardiomyopathy or recent myocarditis.

Class C clinical characteristics:

1. New York Heart Association class 3 or 4
2. Exercise test results
   - Exercise capacity <6 METs
   - Angina or ischemic ST depression at a work rate <6 METs
   - Fall in systolic blood pressure below resting levels during exercise
   - Nonsustained ventricular tachycardia with exercise
3. Previous episode of primary cardiac arrest, i.e., cardiac arrest that did not occur in the presence of an acute myocardial infarction or during a cardiac procedure
4. A medical problem that the physician believes may be life-threatening

Diabetic complications characterized by the clinical characteristics outlined below:

- Frequent episodes of hypoglycemia
- Erratic glycemic control
- Orthostatic hypotension
- Severe diabetic retinopathy
- Severe diabetic peripheral vascular disease
- Foot ulcers

Adapted from Fletcher et al.[16] and Balady et al.[17] MET, metabolic equivalent.

factors (Table 39.5) should be directed to facilities with specialized staff and emergency equipment or are not recommended to exercise unless their condition has been corrected or stabilized.[17]

Staffing

Exercise Training Leadership

Physical activity programs for individuals with diabetes without significant complications or limitations should include appropriate exercise for developing and maintaining cardiorespiratory fitness, body composition, and muscle strength and endurance.[7,19] Recommendations for physical activity and exercise programs for people with diabetes are discussed in Chapter 20.

Staff at health/fitness facilities involved in designing or leading exercise programs should take into consideration special precautions to enhance exercise safety for individuals with diabetes. It is particularly important that staff are properly educated to recognize and respond to possible diabetic complications of exercise (Table 39.1), particularly hypoglycemia (Table 39.6). At all staffed facilities, communication is important for identifying those individuals with diabetes who are involved in various aspects of health/fitness facility programs. Where appropriate, a creative identification system, such as color coding the client's exercise chart, can be used to enhance staff awareness of the presence of the disease. Use of identification bracelets should be encouraged in individuals with type 1 diabetes and type 2 diabetes who are prone to hypoglycemia.

Staff Qualifications

Health/fitness facility staff should have professional qualifications such as a degree in exercise science (or the equivalent) or certification from a nationally recognized society on the basis of a competency-based examination. However, the level of staff qualification will vary significantly depending on the type of participant accepted by the facility. Particularly in facilities that offer programs for individuals with diabetes, the staff should have special qualifications, such as an advanced

TABLE 39.6 Signs and Symptoms of Hypoglycemia

Dizziness
Shakiness
Sweating
Hunger
Headache
Irritability
Pale skin color
Sudden moodiness or behavior change
Clumsy or jerky movements
Difficulty paying attention or confusion
Tachycardia

clinically oriented certification from a nationally recognized professional society. In many of these facilities, other health care providers with specialized clinical skills may frequently be involved in formulating the exercise plan.[17]

Exercise leaders who work directly with program participants and provide instruction and leadership in specific modes of exercise to individuals with diabetes should have education and experience corresponding to that required by ACSM for certification as a health/fitness instructor or exercise specialist/clinical exercise physiologist. *In all cases, the exercise leader must be trained in CPR and should have prior supervised internship or work experience in the health/fitness industry.* Such leaders should have a working knowledge regarding the emergency management and triage of patients with acute complications of diabetes, particularly hypoglycemia and hypotension. Other specific recommendations from AHA/ACSM on staffing are shown in Table 39.3.[17]

Some health/fitness facilities provide services in allied health fields such as nutrition, stress management, and physical therapy. Personnel providing such services to individuals with diabetes should meet current accepted professional standards in those fields and should be certified, as recommended by relevant professional organizations, and licensed by or registered with the state, as required by law.[17]

Emergency Policies and Procedures

Health/fitness facilities must develop appropriate emergency response plans and must train their staff in appropriate procedures to provide assistance during a life-threatening emergency.[17] When an incident occurs, each staff member must perform the necessary emergency support steps in accordance with established procedures. It is important for everyone to know the emergency plan. Emergency drills should be practiced once every 3 months or more often with changes in staff; retraining and rehearsal are especially important. When new staff are hired, new team arrangements may be necessary. Because life-threatening cardiovascular emergencies are rare, constant vigilance by staff and familiarity with the plan and how to follow it are important. Specific recommendations on emergency plans at health/fitness facilities are shown in Table 39.7.[17]

The most common medical emergency at health/fitness facilities involving individuals with diabetes, particularly those on insulin ther-

TABLE 39.7 Key Points on Recommendations From the AHA/ACSM on Emergency Procedures at Health/Fitness Facilities

- All health/fitness facilities must have written emergency policies and procedures that are reviewed and practiced regularly.
- Emergency drills should be practiced once every 3 months. Such drills may be needed more often in facilities with a high staff turnover.
- All facilities must have a telephone that is readily accessible and available when emergency assistance is needed.
- The emergency plan must address transportation of victims to a hospital emergency room and must include telephone access to 911 or the local emergency unit access system.
- Health/fitness facility personnel should be familiar with emergency transport teams in the area so that access and location of the center are clearly identified.
- Staff should greet the emergency response team at the entrance of the facility so that they can be promptly guided to the site of the emergency.
- A staff member should remain with the victim at all times.
- Prompt emergency transport is optimized by free and ready access to the victim within the health/fitness facility and assistance by designated staff.

Adapted from Balady et al.[17]

apy, is hypoglycemia. Hypoglycemic reactions can occur in any diabetic individual taking medications that control glucose level (particularly insulin and/or sulfonylurea oral medications), especially when participating in unusually strenuous or prolonged exercise.[7] Precautionary measures to minimize the occurrence of hypoglycemia for exercisers with diabetes in the health/fitness facility should involve those outlined in this chapter and in Chapters 14 and 20.

In general, minimizing the risk of hypoglycemia involves measures to ensure safe levels of pre-exercise blood glucose, such as strategic timing and site of insulin injection; nutritional supplementation before, during, and/or after exercise; establishment of a consistent exercise time; and routine self-monitoring of blood glucose. Hypoglycemic reactions, when identified, should prompt immediate cessation of exercise, oral administration of easily absorbable carbohydrates in the alert conscious patient (e.g., orange juice, tube of cake frosting, or glucose tablets), and a call to the local emergency response system (e.g., 911) if lethargy, confusion, or altered consciousness is present. Facilities accepting diabetic clients should have a fresh supply of easily absorbable carbohydrates available for immediate use when needed.

Staff at health/fitness facilities can play an active role in minimizing risk for adverse events associated with diabetes and exercise. This involves the staff taking an active role in client education, diligent monitoring of individuals, and responding to a medical emergency in a timely and efficient manner. Such measures have been described previously in Table 39.2 and are outlined in detail elsewhere.[17]

Conclusions

The potential health benefits of physical activity for individuals with diabetes are great, but far too many people with this disease remain inactive. As the prevalence of diabetes continues to increase at a dramatic rate in the U.S., health/fitness facilities can serve as a resource to expand delivery of lifestyle-related programs on physical activity, nutrition, and health to individuals with this disease.

Potential medical complications associated with diabetes and exercise warrant special considerations for staff at health/fitness facilities that enroll individuals with this disease. Individuals with diabetes should be directed toward health/fitness facilities that have appropriately trained fitness staff who can prescribe a safe exercise program that adheres to accepted guidelines and who are knowledgeable about responding to possible adverse occurrences such as hypoglycemia. Recommendations from the AHA and ACSM for cardiovascular screening, staffing, and emergency policies at health/fitness centers are available[17] and should be reviewed in detail by health/fitness facility staff who accept diabetic patients in their facility.

Compliance with these broad principles of operation does not ensure that use of a health/fitness facility will be risk-free for all individuals with diabetes. However, the likelihood of exercise-related complications can be greatly reduced. Accordingly, a greater number of people with diabetes can enjoy the benefits of participating in the wide variety of exercise activities offered at today's health/fitness facilities at a reduced risk.

References

1. Burke J, Williams K, Gaskill S, Hazuda H, Haffner S, Stern M: Rapid rise in the incidences of type 2 diabetes from 1987 to 1996: results from the San Antonio Heart Study. *Arch Intern Med* 159:1450–57, 1999

2. King H, Aubert R, Herman H: Global burden of diabetes: 1995–2015: prevalence, numerical estimates and projections. *Diabetes Care* 21:1414–31, 1997
3. International Health, Racquet, and Sportsclub Association: *The State of the Health Club Industry.* Boston, MA, International Health, Racquet, and Sportsclub Association, 1999
4. McInnis KJ, Hayakawa S, Balady GJ: Cardiovascular screening and emergency procedures at health clubs and fitness centers. *Am J Cardiol* 80:380–83, 1997
5. American Diabetes Association: Diabetes mellitus and exercise (Position Statement). *Diabetes Care* 22 (Suppl. 1):S49–53, 1999
6. Albright AL: *American College of Sports Medicine: Exercise Management for Persons with Chronic Disease and Disabilities.* Champaign, IL, Human Kinetics, 1997, p. 94–98
7. American College of Sports Medicine: Exercise and type 2 diabetes. *Med Sci Sports Exerc* 32:1345–60, 2000
8. American Diabetes Association: Exercise and NIDDM (Technical Review). *Diabetes Care* 16 (Suppl. 2):54–58, 1993
9. American Heart Association: *Heart and Stroke Facts: 2000 Statistical Supplement.* Dallas, TX, American Heart Association, 2000
10. American Diabetes Association: Role of cardiovascular risk factors in prevention and treatment of macrovascular disease in diabetes (Consensus Statement). *Diabetes Care* 12:573–79, 1999
11. Zinker BA: Nutrition and exercise in individuals with diabetes. *Clin Sports Med* 18:585–606, 1999
12. Van Camp SP, Peterson RA: Cardiovascular complications of outpatient cardiac rehabilitation programs. *JAMA* 256:1160–63, 1986
13. McInnis K, Herbert W, Herbert D, Herbert J, Ribisl P, Franklin B: Low compliance with national standards for cardiovascular emergency preparedness at health clubs. *Chest* 120:283–88, 2001.
14. American College of Sports Medicine: *Guidelines for Exercise Testing and Prescription.* 6th ed. Franklin B, Ed. Baltimore, MD, Williams & Wilkins, 2000
15. Peterson JA, Tharrett SJ (Eds.): *American College of Sports Medicine Health/Fitness Facility Standards and Guidelines.* 2nd ed. Champaign, IL, Human Kinetics, 1997
16. Fletcher GF, Balady G, Froelicher VF, Hartley LH, Haskell WL, Pollock ML: Exercise standards: a statement from the American Heart Association. *Circulation* 91:580–615, 1995

17. Balady GJ, Chaitman B, Driscoll D, Foster C, Froelicher E, Gordon N, Pate R, Rippe J, Bazzarre T: Recommendations for cardiovascular screening, staffing, and emergency policies at health/fitness facilities. *Circulation* 97:2283–93, 1998 (also published in *Med Sci Sports Exerc* 30:1009–18, 1998)
18. Thomas S, Reading J, Shepard RJ: Revision of the Physical Activity Readiness Questionnaire (PAR-Q). *Can J Sport Sci* 17:338–45, 1992
19. American College of Sports Medicine: American College of Sports Medicine Position Stand: The recommended quantity and quality of exercise for developing and maintaining cardiorespiratory and muscular fitness, body composition, and flexibility in healthy adults. *Med Sci Sports Exerc* 30:975–91, 1998

Kyle J. McInnis, ScD, is from the University of Massachusetts, Boston, MA. Gary J. Balady, MD, is from the Boston University School of Medicine, Boston, MA.

Reimbursement and Resources

40

Medical Reimbursement and Managed Care Issues

ERIC DURAK, MSc, AND EMILY HILL, PA-C

Medical Billing

Although exercise has long been touted as part of the trilogy of treatment in diabetes, its use within the current health care system has been minimal at best. One reason for this is the lack of third-party reimbursement for health education or exercise therapy services. This chapter provides information on how exercise programs may be billed through physicians' offices, clinics, or hospitals.

In the past, payment for health care services was an issue between the patient and the health care professional. Insurance was a means for sharing the cost of health care between the patient and a third-party payer. With the emergence of health care reform, how we think about insurance is changing. Managed care, through its reimbursement policies, may influence the types and frequency of service that are performed. Exercise therapy is an example of a service that is often scrutinized by third-party payers.

Insurance companies typically recognize only licensed professionals in their credentialing process. The services of other providers may be reimbursed by reporting them under a physician's name and billing number. Payment policy dictates what services and what conditions are covered under the patient's benefit plan. In addition, providers must provide support for the medical necessity and appropriateness of the services for which they seek payment. Exercise therapy is not considered a covered service under most benefit plans. This does not mean that the service is provided free of charge. In most instances, once patients have been advised of their insurance company's payment policy, they can, and should be, held financially responsible for payment. It is important to use the proper current procedural terminology (CPT) and *International Classification of Diseases, Ninth Revision* (ICD-9) codes when reporting services to third-party payers, regardless of their payment policies. The services submitted for payment should be clearly and accurately reflected in the medical record documentation.

ICD-9 Clinical Modification Coding

The *International Classification of Diseases* manual organizes and classifies known causes of morbidity and mortality. Listed below are a few examples of diseases that are pertinent to exercise therapy. These examples are based on the 1999 edition.

250.0 Diabetes without mention of complication. This code requires the use of a fifth digit that more specifically describes the patient's condition. The options for the fifth digit are as follows:
- 0—Type 2 or unspecified type, not stated as uncontrolled
- 1—Type 1, not stated as uncontrolled
- 2—Type 2, or unspecified type, uncontrolled
- 3—Type 1, uncontrolled

251.2 Hypoglycemia, unspecified
278.00 Obesity, unspecified
278.01 Morbid obesity
390–398 Diseases of the circulatory system
401–405 Hypertensive disease
580–589 Nephritis (kidney disease)
646.1 Edema or excessive weight gain in pregnancy (requires a fifth digit that denotes the episode of care)
648.8 Abnormal glucose tolerance in pregnancy (gestational diabetes) (requires a fifth digit that denotes episode of care)
728.2 Muscular wasting and disuse atrophy, not elsewhere classified

In all of these examples, the code that most specifically describes the patient's condition or reason for the exercise therapy should be used.

This means selecting the highest number of available digits for the code category, such as using the fifth digit classifications noted above. Without the available fourth or fifth digit, the claim will most likely be denied by the insurance company. Coding most specifically also means selecting the most accurate code within a category. The ICD-9 codes help an insurer determine the medical necessity for the services performed.

CPT Coding

CPT codes are published by the American Medical Association for medical care provided by physicians and other health care professionals. They are used to describe the services provided to the patient and are associated with a unique fee in the insurer's database. Although medical groups may establish their own fee schedules, payment is dependent on the insurer's reimbursement methodology. Some insurance companies may pay the provider a percentage of the fees submitted. Increasingly, reimbursement is independent of the providers' fees and has its basis in the Resource Based Relative Value Scale. Under this method, the insurer sets a payment rate based on the relative value units assigned to the CPT codes by the Health Care Financing Administration. Although this is the same method used for Medicare payments, the payment rates generally are calculated differently, resulting in different payment amounts.

Many of the CPT codes used to describe services provided by exercise professionals are included in the Physical Medicine section of CPT. This section has been significantly revised over the last several years to more accurately describe the services and the supervision requirements. Some of the most common codes are highlighted below. Most of these codes are under the heading THERAPEUTIC PROCEDURE and require the physician or therapist to have direct one-on-one patient contact. Most are time-based and are used to report each 15 min of activity with the patient.

Therapeutic Procedure (97110)

This code describes exercises to develop strength and endurance, range of motion, and flexibility. It is used for a 15-min increment of activity, regardless of the number of body areas involved.

Aquatic Therapy With Therapeutic Exercises (97113)

In certain circumstances, therapeutic exercises may need to be performed in the water. This code describes hydrodynamics and ongoing progressive therapeutic exercise in an aquatic environment.

Therapeutic Activities (97530)

This code describes the use of dynamic activities to improve functional performance. The code is based on 15-min increments and requires one-on-one patient contact by the provider.

Self-Care Training (97535)

As with the other therapeutic activities, this service is reported in 15-min increments and requires direct contact with the provider. The code describes self-care/home management training, including meal preparation, instructions in use of adaptive equipment, and safety procedures.

Work Hardening/Conditioning (97545, 97546)

Code 97545 is for the initial 2 h of work with the provider. Code 97546 is for each additional hour of work with the patient. These codes are primarily used for patients whose work performance is impaired and who have not responded to other forms of therapy. An assessment of the patient's limitations and abilities is done before developing a program to address performance issues for work-related activities.

Performance Testing Code (97750)

This code describes the completion of a physical performance test or measurement of some aspect of the musculoskeletal system and requires the completion of a written report. The services are reported in units of 15 min, as measured by direct contact between the patient and provider.

After a medical evaluation, a physician may refer a patient to a health education specialist with expertise in lifestyle counseling. The counseling may include discussions on diet, exercise, stress reduction, etc. CPT codes 99401–99404 describe preventive medicine/risk factor reduction interventions to individual patients and are selected based on time. CPT codes 99411–99412 are used when these services are provided in a group setting.

Although lifestyle counseling can be a valuable intervention tool for some patients, many third-party payers, including Medicare, do not cover it under their benefit plans. As with other non-covered services, the patient is responsible for payment.

Changes in Health Care

There are negative and positive aspects to health care reform in the U.S. A government-regulated system is expensive, and quality of care is difficult to guarantee. However, many insurance companies are enacting their own reforms to provide more services to their customers and decrease overhead costs.

A managed care approach to health care payment has become the predominate form of reimbursement for health care services over the last decade. In many instances, this means a change in the types and frequency of services that are reimbursed. If quality exercise-related services can be provided to patients at a reasonable cost with positive outcomes, there may be an increase in the number of third-party payers willing to provide reimbursement.

Concluding Remarks

Although exercise is part of the trilogy of treatment of diabetes, it has been slow to make its way into the standards of diabetes care, even in the new millennium. To increase the likelihood of reimbursement in the near future, physicians and health care professionals should understand how to use existing coding for exercise services, having knowledge of individual state laws governing coding procedures. Health care professionals should also have an understanding of new trends in reimbursement, such as defined care, which allows for health promotion components in employee-based health plans. Exercise and health promotion benefits may become a key component in tomorrow's health plans. Exercise professionals should be persistent in obtaining referrals from physicians and be able to demonstrate quality outcomes in their programs. Changing one or more behaviors through exercise programming will make dramatic changes in insulin sensitivity and overall health and will improve health care expenditures.

Suggested Readings

Burrough DJ: Insurer and health clubs form partnership. *The Business Journal* (Phoenix). January 1995, p. 1

Curfman G: The health benefits of exercise. *N Engl J Med* 328:574–76, 1993

Durak EP, Shapiro AA: *The Ins and Outs of Medical Insurance Billing: A Resource Guide for the Fitness and Health Professional.* 3rd ed. Santa Barbara, CA, Medical Health & Fitness, 1999

Eisenberg DM, Kessler RC, Foster C, Norlock FE, Calkins DR, Delbanco TL: Unconventional medicine in the United States: prevalence, costs, and patterns of use. *N Engl J Med* 328:246–52, 1993

Graham, R. Foley/Graham Medicare Wellness Act of 2000. Complete Senate Bill 2232 found at: http://thomas.loc.gov

Hickey MS, Gavigan KE, McCammon MR, Tyndall GL, Porus WJ, Isreal RG, Houmard JA: Effects of seven days of exercise training on insulin action in morbidly obese men. *Clin Exerc Physiol* 1:24–28, 1999

Leaf A: Preventive medicine for our ailing health-care system. *JAMA* 269:616–18, 1993

Newport J: Only prevention can preserve us. *Healthcare Business.* March/April 2000, p. 104

Riddle C: Is the market ready for defined care? www.mcol.com. December 2000

Shephard RS, Corey P, Renzland P, Cox M: The impact of changes in fitness and lifestyle upon health-care utilization. *Can J Pub Health* 74:51–54, 1983

Young JC: Exercise: the missing link in diabetes management. *Am J Med Sports* 3:28–35, 2001

Eric Durak, MSc, is the president of Medical Health & Fitness, Santa Barbara, CA. Emily Hill, PA-C, is the president of Hill & Associates, Wilmington, NC.

Resources

American Diabetes Association Council on Exercise

The Council on Exercise is one of 12 Professional Section Councils of the American Diabetes Association (ADA). ADA Professional Section Council members serve on policy-making committees and task forces, write technical reviews and position statements, and act as liaisons and representatives to other organizations. Council members may also write, review, and/or edit professional and consumer books.

Professional Section Councils meet each year at the ADA Scientific Sessions and are responsible for organizing and chairing Scientific Symposia and reviewing submitted abstracts for presentation at the meeting.

ADA professional members with a clinical or research interest in exercise therapy and exercise physiology may become members of the Council on Exercise. The Council on Exercise provides a forum for professional members to do the following:

- Discuss the benefits, risks, and practical problems associated with exercise in patients with diabetes and related disorders.
- Disseminate new information about the effects of exercise to both medical and general communities.

- Establish standards for the development of safe and effective exercise programs.
- Foster a greater research interest in the physiology and pathophysiology of exercise and its use in the treatment of diabetes and its complications.

American College of Sports Medicine

The American College of Sports Medicine (ACSM) is the largest sports medicine and exercise science organization in the world. ACSM's mission is to promote and integrate scientific research, education, and practical applications of sports medicine and exercise science to maintain and enhance physical performance, fitness, health, and quality of life.

ACSM members, who work in diverse medical specialties, allied health professions, and scientific disciplines, are committed to the diagnosis, treatment, and prevention of sports-related injuries and the advancement of the science of exercise.

Professional Membership Benefits and Services

The three main categories of professional membership in ACSM are medicine, basic and applied science, and education and allied health. Benefits and services to professional members include subscriptions to *Medicine & Science in Sports & Exercise,* ACSM's monthly scientific journal, and *Sports Medicine Bulletin,* ACSM's quarterly magazine. Each year, members also receive access to an electronic membership directory and a quarterly review of current research topics in exercise science published in *Exercise and Sport Sciences Reviews.* ACSM also offers a category of membership appropriate for the health and fitness professional: ACSM's Alliance of Health & Fitness Professionals. Members of this category receive many of the benefits noted above but receive ACSM's *Health & Fitness Journal* instead of *Medicine & Science in Sports & Exercise.* In addition, ACSM members receive discounts on meeting registration fees, certification examinations, and other products and services.

Professional Education and Certification

ACSM offers professional education programs in sports medicine and exercise science. Nearly 5,000 people attend ACSM's Annual Meeting, where more than 2,000 research studies are presented. In addition, the ACSM Team Physicians[SM] Course enhances the medical skills of physicians working with athletic teams and individual athletes.

Seeking to increase the competency of individuals involved in health and fitness and cardiovascular rehabilitative exercise programs, ACSM offers professional certification. For certification, professionals must meet specific prerequisites and successfully pass both a written and a practical examination. Under review every 4 years, certified individuals must provide proof of continuing education to remain certified by ACSM.

For certification information, schedules, and applications, contact the ACSM Certification Resource Center at 1-800-486-5643 or www.lww.com/acsmcrc.

Physician and Patient Information

ACSM provides educational videos and brochures to physicians and patients. Summaries of official ACSM Pronouncements covering a variety of topics, including anabolic steroids, youth fitness, and weight loss programs, are also available. A complete list of educational materials may be obtained on request.

Research Grants

Research grants are available each year through the ACSM Foundation to students and professional members. Specific areas of funding include the effects of nutrition on human performance, exercise and cardiovascular disease risk factors, and physical activity epidemiology.

For more information about ACSM or any of these programs, contact the following:

American College of Sports Medicine
P.O. Box 1440
Indianapolis, IN 46206-1440
Tel: 317-637-9200
Fax: 317-634-7817
www.acsm.org

Diabetes Exercise and Sports Association

The Diabetes Exercise and Sports Association (DESA) is a nonprofit service organization dedicated to encouraging an active lifestyle for people with diabetes. Members include individuals with diabetes who participate in fitness activities at all levels, health care professionals, and everyone interested in the relationship between (or special problems of) diabetes and sports.

DESA's mission is to enhance the quality of life for people with diabetes through exercise. To accomplish its mission, DESA does the following:

- Educates people with diabetes and their health care providers about the role of exercise in enhancing health.
- Creates opportunities for those with diabetes to participate in a broad range of recreational, sport, and athletic activities.
- Enhances self-care and self-management skills among sports-minded individuals with diabetes.
- Improves clinical skills and promotes a positive attitude toward exercise among heath professionals working with active individuals with diabetes.
- Promotes networking, support, and sharing of experiences among physically active people with diabetes.
- Provides a forum for exchanging information and access to resources and role models.
- Increases knowledge and promotes positive attitudes about diabetes and exercise among coaches and physical education teachers.

With chapters in a dozen U.S. cites, DESA holds forums annually. These forums include regional, national, and international conferences that provide up-to-date information from medical professionals and an opportunity to exchange ideas with athletes with practical experience. In addition, quarterly newsletters enable networking support and further sharing of experiences. Membership costs $30.00 per year. For more information about DESA, contact the following:

Diabetes Exercise and Sports Association
1647 West Bethany Home Road #B
Phoenix, AZ 85015-2507
Tel: 602-433-2113
Fax: 602-433-9331
www.diabetes-exercise.org

National Coalition for Promoting Physical Activity

The National Coalition for Promoting Physical Activity (NCPPA) was formed "to unite the strengths of public, private, and industry efforts into a collaborative partnership to inspire and empower all Americans to lead physically active lifestyles to enhance their health and quality of life."

The framework for the Coalition's initial efforts has been built around the following areas: the development of one, consistent physical activity message to clarify for Americans the confusing array of messages that currently exist; the coordination of education efforts between the public and private sectors; and public policy as it relates to exercise. To that end, the NCPPA channels its collective energies into the following segmented activities:

- NCPPA State Coalitions: the State Coalitions are the key to achievement at the grassroots level, with State Coalitions being provided a range of tools, reports, alerts, and program options for effective action at the state and community level.
- Health Communications Campaign: annual physical activity and health promotional campaigns at the national, state, and local levels.
- Political Education and Advocacy: federal and state legislative, administrative, and regulatory agenda for physical activity and health developed and implemented by NCPPA.
- Healthy People 2010: relevant organizations are encouraged to increase their involvement with the activity and fitness aims of the national health objectives.

- Organizational Outreach: tools to help provide information on the Surgeon General's Report on Physical Activity and Health to other organizations.

The NCPPA as an Organization

The NCPPA has more than 150 member organizations and is led by an elected president and one executive board member representative from each of the following organizations:

American Alliance for Health, Physical Education, Recreation & Dance
American Cancer Society
American College of Sports Medicine
American Heart Association
Association for Worksite Health Promotion
International Health, Racquet & Sportsclub Association
National Association of Governor's Councils on Physical Fitness and Sports
National Athletic Trainers' Association
National Recreation and Park Association

Individuals who are members of organizations belonging to the NCPPA may volunteer to serve on committees and to participate in other activities of the Coalition. For more information, visit the NCPPA website at www.ncppa.org, or contact the NCPPA at 317-637-0349 or natcoal@ncppa.org.

Index

About the American Diabetes Association

The American Diabetes Association is the nation's leading voluntary health organization supporting diabetes research, information, and advocacy. Its mission is to prevent and cure diabetes and to improve the lives of all people affected by diabetes. The American Diabetes Association is the leading publisher of comprehensive diabetes information. Its huge library of practical and authoritative books for people with diabetes covers every aspect of self-care—cooking and nutrition, fitness, weight control, medications, complications, emotional issues, and general self-care.`

To order American Diabetes Association books: Call 1-800-232-6733. http://store.diabetes.org [Note: there is no need to use **www** when typing this particular Web address]

To join the American Diabetes Association: Call 1-800-806-7801. www.diabetes.org/membership

For more information about diabetes or ADA programs and services: Call 1-800-342-2383. E-mail: Customerservice@diabetes.org www.diabetes.org

To locate an ADA/NCQA Recognized Provider of quality diabetes care in your area: Call 1-703-549-1500 ext. 2202. www.diabetes.org/recognition/Physicians/ListAll.asp

To find an ADA Recognized Education Program in your area: Call 1-888-232-0822. www.diabetes.org/recognition/education.asp

To join the fight to increase funding for diabetes research, end discrimination, and improve insurance coverage: Call 1-800-342-2383. www.diabetes.org/advocacy

To find out how you can get involved with the programs in your community: Call 1-800-342-2383. See below for program Web addresses.

- *American Diabetes Month:* Educational activities aimed at those diagnosed with diabetes—month of November. www.diabetes.org/ADM
- *American Diabetes Alert:* Annual public awareness campaign to find the undiagnosed—held the fourth Tuesday in March. www.diabetes.org/alert
- *The Diabetes Assistance & Resources Program (DAR):* diabetes awareness program targeted to the Latino community. www.diabetes.org/DAR
- *African American Program:* diabetes awareness program targeted to the African American community. www.diabetes.org/africanamerican
- *Awakening the Spirit: Pathways to Diabetes Prevention & Control:* diabetes awareness program targeted to the Native American community. www.diabetes.org/awakening

To find out about an important research project regarding type 2 diabetes: www.diabetes.org/ada/research.asp

To obtain information on making a planned gift or charitable bequest: Call 1-888-700-7029. www.diabetes.org/ada/plan.asp

To make a donation or memorial contribution: Call 1-800-342-2383. www.diabetes.org/ada/cont.asp